Point-of-Care Testing

Second Edition

Point-of-Care Testing

Second Edition

Edited by
Christopher P. Price, PhD, FRCPath, FACB
Andrew St John, PhD, MAACB
Jocelyn M. Hicks, PhD, FRCPath

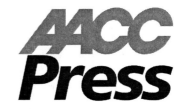

2101 L Street, NW, Suite 202
Washington, DC 20037-1558

2 3 4 5 6 7 8 9 0   PCP   06 05 04

Printed in the United States of America

Library of Congress Cataloging-in-Publication Data

Point-of-care testing / edited by Christopher P. Price, Andrew St John, Jocelyn M.
  Hicks.—2nd ed.
      p. ; cm.
  Includes bibliographical references and index.
  ISBN 1-59425-012-X (alk. paper)
  1. Point-of-care testing. 2. Evidence-based medicine. I. Price, Christopher P. II. St
John, Andrew. III. Hicks, Jocelyn M.
  [DNLM: 1. Point-of-Care Systems. 2. Delivery of Health Care—methods. W 84.7 P752 2004]
RC71.7P656 2004
616.07′5—dc22

                                                                                    2004051633

Contents

Part Five: Conclusions

Preface

In the preface to the first edition of this book, Morton Schwartz pointed out that "Point-of-Care Testing (POCT) introduced a revolutionary but not new concept." He went on to make the point that laboratorians have "for decades . . . gone to the patient, or had him or her come to a phlebotomy station, obtained a specimen, taken it to a central laboratory, performed the analysis, and reported the data to the individual who initially requested the test(s)." This is a fair reflection of the practice of laboratory medicine over much of the past two centuries. However, the discipline of laboratory medicine was born at the bedside, and the specialty only migrated to the laboratory as the tests became more complex, the workload became greater, and instrumentation became more sophisticated.

Such an evolution is not confined to laboratory medicine, and the practice of clinical medicine has also undergone considerable change, both in terms of the place in which much of the practice is undertaken and the specialization that has occurred. Indeed, it is a change that is seen throughout all walks of life, and is founded on a number of factors including advances in technology, increased knowledge, and changing human values. Every one of these traits applies to POCT.

Thus, technology has evolved to the level where it is now possible to measure any of the genomic, proteomic, and metabolomic markers of clinical interest, using techniques that meet the fundamental requirement of a POCT device—namely that the result is generated within a short time interval of the request being made. It might be argued that the speed of response is not quite quick enough to enable all POCT to be integrated seamlessly into the clinician–patient interaction—as, for example, in the case of the clinical thermometer, surely one of the most successful POCT devices. Miniaturization will ensure that the criteria of short assay time, as well as minimal sample requirement and mobility, will take POCT devices that one step further, overcoming some of the barriers to greater implementation of POCT.

Two key barriers related to concerns about the quality of POCT are gradually being eroded as the reproducibility of manufacture improves and procedures are put into place to ensure that the devices are used properly. The reproducible manufacture of devices relies on fabrication technology that is employed in other important industrial sectors where reliability is crucial, e.g., components in life support systems, cars, airplanes, and space vehicles. In parallel with this we have seen great steps made in the reagents that underpin the analytical methods used for recognizing and quantitating the analytes of interest. The second important development has been the bridging of the gap between the laboratory professional (the professional analyst) and the patient's caregiver, through the implementation of point-of-care coordinating committees. This development acknowledges the need to train and support staff, who do not generally have much technical training, in the basic skills of analytical science. In addition, it recognizes the wider issues surrounding the fact that many patients will be managed by a combination of POCT and laboratory-generated results. What will be the next stage in this particular evolutionary cycle?

However, technology is by no means the only driver in the development of POCT. There are acute clinical situations where the rapid availability of a result is important for the safe and effective treatment of a patient; these applications were at the vanguard of the early development of POCT. Now there are other reasons for considering the use of POCT, which can lead to improved benefits for the patient, as well as for the clinician and the health provider organization. These developments are very exciting, as they offer the potential to bring genuine improvements to patient care. However, they also bring with them considerable challenges, particularly to the healthcare professional, and to the provider and payer organizations. There is no doubt that the introduction of POCT brings with it the need for change, if the benefits are to be delivered. There will be changes to the laboratory staff and organization, in terms of the potential reduction in workload and support for the POCT operators, as well as implications for the individuals performing the tests. The greatest challenge, however, is probably for those receiving and acting upon the test result, and for the whole infrastructure of the changed clinical process that ensues. Practically, this amounts to changes in working practices and also in resource allocation (including reimbursement).

Technology has also brought with it improved communication, best exemplified by the Internet. This has probably had the greatest influence on the public's understanding of health and disease, and on human values and expectations. It is in these spheres of influence that we are likely to see some of the greatest, and perhaps unexpected, adoption of POCT. A test result can help to guide a clinician in the use of a particular treatment protocol as well as offering the same support to the patient. It therefore provides a natural vehicle for the transition of a long-term objective of health planners, that being to encourage the patient to take greater responsibility for his or her own care. This then brings in other cultural changes associated with patient empowerment and patient choice—and thence into health promotion. POCT is already beginning to play a role in these major cultural changes, and will continue to do so as speed and convenience become more of an important attribute for the purchaser—which may increasingly be the patient and the healthy person.

All of these issues are addressed in the second edition of this book. The book is enlightening on technology and supporting on regulation and management issues. The comprehensive chapters on clinical application of POCT are challenging because they illustrate the potential utility of this modality of testing in a wide range of settings, and the benefits that can be achieved. POCT has the potential to facilitate radical change in the way that healthcare is delivered. The reader should make that judgment from the evidence presented.

Christopher P. Price
Andrew St John
Jocelyn M. Hicks

Editors

Christopher P. Price, MA, PhD, MCB, FRSC, FRCPath, FACB
Vice President, Global Clinical Research
Diagnostics Division, Bayer HealthCare
Newbury
    and Visiting Professor in Clinical Biochemistry
University of Oxford
Oxford
United Kingdom
Tel: 44 1285 644105
Fax: 44 1285 644105
E-mail: chris.price.cp@bayer.co.uk

Andrew St John, PhD, MAACB
Consultant
ARC Consulting
Perth
Western Australia
Tel: 61 8 9271 1036
Fax: 61 8 9271 1036
E-mail: stjohn@starwon.com.au

Jocelyn M. B. Hicks, PhD, FRCPath
President
JMBH Associates, Health Care Management Consultants
    and Professor Emeritus, Pediatrics and Pathology
George Washington School of Medicine
    and Executive Director Emeritus
Children's Hospital
Washington, DC
United States of America
Tel: 1 202 363 5330
Fax: 1 202 263 5322
E-mail: jmbhassoc@aol.com

Other Contributors

Marvin M. Adner, MD
Chief of Medicine
Department of Medicine
Metrowest Medical Center
Framingham, Massachusetts
United States of America
E-mail: marvin.adner@tenethealth.com

Ian C. Barnes, BSc, MSc, PhD, FRCPath
Head of Pathology
Clinical Support Services
Pathology Clinical Management Team
Department of Clinical Biochemistry and Immunology
Leeds Teaching Hospitals NHS Trust
Leeds
　　and Pathology Adviser
Department of Health
London
United Kingdom

Michael J. Bennett, PhD, FRCPath, DABCC
Professor of Pathology
Department of Pathology and Laboratory Medicine
University of Pennsylvania
The Children's Hospital of Philadelphia
Philadelphia, Pennsylvania
United States of America
E-mail: bennettmi@email.chop.edu

Thomas P. Benson
Senior Research Scientist
Self Testing R & D
Bayer HealthCare LLC
Elkhart, Indiana
United States of America

James C. Boyd, MD
Associate Professor
Department of Pathology
University of Virginia Health System
Charlottesville, Virginia
United States of America
E-mail: jboyd@virginia.edu

David G. Bullock, BA, MSc, PhD, DipCB
Director, Wolfson EQA Laboratory
UK NEQAS
Queen Elizabeth Medical Center
Birmingham
United Kingdom
E-mail: d.g.bullock@bham.ac.uk

David Burnett, OBE, BSc, PhD, FRCPath
Consultant in Quality and Accreditation
Penarth
United Kingdom

Christopher D. Byrne, PhD, FRCP, FRCPath
Professor of Endocrinology & Metabolism
Southampton General Hospital
Southampton
United Kingdom

Maria R. Calaminici, MD, PhD, MRCPath
Consultant Histopathologist
Department of Histopathology
Bart and The London NHS Trust
London
United Kingdom

Scott E. Carpenter, MS, PhD
Staff Scientist
Applied Research
Bayer HealthCare LLC
Elkhart, Indiana
United States of America

Robert H. Christenson, PhD, DABCC, FACB
Professor of Pathology
Professor of Medical and Research Technology
University of Maryland School of Medicine
Director, Rapid Response and Clinical Chemistry
　　Laboratories
Laboratories of Pathology
University of Maryland Medical Center
Baltimore, Maryland
United States of America
E-mail: RCHRISTENSON@umm.edu

Paul O. Collinson, MD, FRCPath
Consultant Chemical Pathologist
Department of Chemical Pathology
St. Georges Hospital and Medical School
London
United Kingdom

Robert Cramb, BSc, MSc, MB, ChB, FRCPath
Consultant Chemical Pathologist
Department of Clinical Biochemistry
University Hospital Birmingham NHS Trust
Queen Elizabeth Hospital
Birmingham
United Kingdom
E-mail: rob.cramb@uhb.nhs.uk

Laurence M. Demers, PhD, DABCC, FACB
Distinguished Professor of Pathology and Medicine
Department of Pathology and Laboratory Medicine
The Pennsylvania State University, M. S. Hershey
    Medical Center
Hershey, Pennsylvania
United States of America
E-mail: lmd4@psu.edu

George J. Despotis, MD
Associate Professor
Department of Anesthesiology and Pathology and
    Immunology
Washington University School of Medicine
St. Louis, Missouri
United States of America

Charles Eby, MD
Associate Professor
Department of Pathology and Immunology
Division of Laboratory Medicine
Washington University School of Medicine
St. Louis, Missouri
United States of America

Sharon S. Ehrmeyer, PhD, MT(ASCP)
Professor, Pathology and Laboratory Medicine
University of Wisconsin Medical School
Madison, Wisconsin
United States of America

Reinhard Fend, BSc, MSc
Research Fellow
Cranfield BioMedical Centre
Institute of BioScience and Technology
Cranfield University at Silsoe
Bedfordshire
United Kingdom

Callum G. Fraser, BSc, PhD, FAACB
Clinical Leader
Department of Biochemical Medicine
Ninewells Hospital and Medical School
Dundee
Scotland
E-mail: callum.fraser@tuht.scot.nhs.uk

Danielle B. Freedman, MB, BS, FRCPath
Consultant Chemical Pathologist and Associate Medical
    Director
Department of Chemical Pathology
Luton and Dunstable Hospital NHS Trust
Bedfordshire
United Kingdom
E-mail: danielle.freedman@ldh-tr.anglox.nhs.uk

Franke N. Gill, MS, MT(ASCP)
Director of Ancillary Testing
Department of Pathology
Children's Medical Center of Dallas
Dallas, Texas
United States of America

Peter Gosling, PhD, FRCPath
Consultant Clinical Scientist
Department of Clinical Biochemistry
University Hospital Birmingham NHS Trust
Selly Oak Hospital
Birmingham
United Kingdom
E-mail: Peter.Gosling@uhb.nhs.uk

James W. Gray, MB ChB, MRCP(UK), FRCPath
Consultant Medical Microbiologist
Department of Microbiology
Birmingham Children's Hospital
Birmingham
United Kingdom
E-mail: jim.gray@bch.nhs.uk

Robert W. Hardy, PhD, DABCC, FACB
Section Head of Clinical Chemistry
Associate Professor
Department of Pathology
Division of Laboratory Medicine
University of Alabama at Birmingham
Birmingham, Alabama
United States of America
E-mail: hardy@path.uab.edu

Paul A. H. Holloway, BSc, PhD, BM, BCh, MRCPath
Consultant Chemical Pathologist
Department of Chemical Pathology
St. Mary's Hospital
    and Honorary Senior Lecturer in Metabolic Medicine
Imperial College
London
    and Consultant Chemical Pathologist in
        Intensive Care
    and Honorary Reader in Medicine
Nuffield Department of Medicine
University of Oxford
Oxford
United Kingdom

Glen L. Hortin, MD, PhD
Chief of Clinical Chemistry
Department of Laboratory Medicine
National Institutes of Health
Bethesda, Maryland
United States of America

Michael P. Houlne, PhD
Research Scientist
Self Testing R & D
Bayer HealthCare LLC
Elkhart, Indiana
United States of America

Albert Huisman, PhD
Clinical Biochemist
Department of Laboratory Medicine
University Medical Center Utrecht
Utrecht
The Netherlands

Richard G. Jones, MA, DM, MRCP, FRCPath
Senior Lecturer in Chemical Pathology
University of Leeds
Department of Clinical Biochemistry & Immunology
Leeds Teaching Hospitals Trust
Leeds
United Kingdom
E-mail: rick.jones@leedsth.nhs.uk

Joseph H. Keffer, MD, FACB, FASCP, FCAP
Clinical Professor
Department of Pathology
University of Texas Southwestern
Dallas, Texas
United States of America
E-mail: jhkeffer@earthlink.net

Roger E. H. Kirkbride, BPharm, MRPharmS, CdipAF, MBA
Strategic Project Manager
Healthcare Development
Boots the Chemists
Nottingham
United Kingdom
E-mail: roger.kirkbride@ntlworld.com

Andrew J. Krentz, MD, FRCP
Consultant Physician and Clinical Lead in Diabetes & Endocrinology
Southampton University Hospitals NHS Trust
Southampton
United Kingdom
E-mail: A.J.Krentz@soton.ac.uk

Larry J. Kricka, DPhil, FACB, CChem FRSC, FRCPath
Professor
Department of Pathology and Laboratory Medicine
University of Pennsylvania
    and Director
Department of General Chemistry
University of Pennsylvania Medical Center
Philadelphia, Pennsylvania
United States of America
E-mail: kricka@mail.med.upenn.edu

Edmund J. Lamb, PhD, FRCPath
Consultant Clinical Scientist
Department of Clinical Biochemistry
Kent and Canterbury Hospital
East Kent Hospitals NHS Trust
Canterbury
United Kingdom

Craig A. Lehmann, PhD, CC (NRCC), FACB
Dean/Professor
School of Health Technology and Management
Health Sciences Center
Stony Brook University
State University of New York
Stony Brook, New York
United States of America
E-mail: clehmann@notes.cc.sunysb.edu

Joanne E. Martin, MA, MB BS, PhD, MRCPath
Professor of Neuropathology
ICMS Pathology
Queen Mary, University of London
London
United Kingdom
E-mail: J.E.Martin@qmul.ac.uk

Richard P. Moriarty, MD, FCAP
Medical Director of Laboratories
Department of Pathology
Sentara Healthcare
Norfolk, Virginia
United States of America
E-mail: RPMORIAR@sentara.com

Krsty Nale, MD
Specialist Registrar in Histopathology
Department of Histopathology
Royal Lancaster Infirmary
Lancaster
United Kingdom

Rasaq Olufadi, MB BS, MMed
Specialist Registrar in Chemical Pathology
Southampton University Hospitals NHS Trust
Southampton
United Kingdom

Donald R. Parker, PhD, FACB, DABCC
Director, Clinical & Outcomes Research
Bayer HealthCare LLC
Elkhart, Indiana
United States of America

M. Joan Pearson, BA, BSc, MSc, PhD, CChem MRSC, MIHM
Clinical Scientist
Department of Clinical Biochemistry and Immunology
Leeds Teaching Hospitals NHS Trust
Leeds
United Kingdom
E-mail: Joan.Pearson@leedsth.nhs.uk

David L. Phillips
Director of Marketing
Abbott Point-of-Care
East Windsor, New Jersey
United States of America
E-mail: david.phillips@i-stat.com

John D. Piette, PhD
Research Career Scientist
    and Associate Professor of Internal Medicine
Veterans Affairs Health Services Research and
    Development Program
    and Michigan Diabetes Research and Training Center
University of Michigan
Ann Arbor, Michigan
United States of America
E-mail: jpiette@umich.edu

Michael J. Pugia, PhD
Director, New Product Development
Research & Development
Bayer HealthCare LLC
Elkhart, Indiana
United States of America
E-mail: michael.pugia@bayer.com

Mihailo V. Rebec, PhD
Staff Scientist
Self Testing R & D
Bayer HealthCare LLC
Elkhart, Indiana
United States of America

Majed A. Refaai, MD
Resident Physician
Department of Pathology and Immunology
Division of Laboratory Medicine
Washington University and Barnes-Jewish Hospital
St. Louis, Missouri
United States of America

Paul M. Ripley, PhD, CPhys, MIP
Research Scientist
Self Testing R & D
Bayer HealthCare LLC
Elkhart, Indiana
United States of America
E-mail: paul.ripley@bayer.com

Mitchell G. Scott, PhD, DABCC
Professor
Department of Pathology and Immunology
Division of Laboratory Medicine
Washington University School of Medicine
St. Louis, Missouri
United States of America
E-mail: mscott@pathbox.wustl.edu

Andrew H. Shennan, MD, MRCOG
Professor, Obstetrics and Maternal Medicine
Department of Women's Health, Maternal and Fetal
    Research Unit
Guy's King's and St. Thomas' School of Medicine
London
United Kingdom

Mark D. S. Shephard, BSc, MSc, MAACB
Director and Senior Research Fellow
Community Point-of-Care Services
Flinders University Rural Clinical School
Flinders University
South Australia
Australia
E-mail: Mark.Shephard@flinders.edu.au

Terry Shirey, PhD
Director of Scientific Affairs
Nova Biomedical Corporation
Waltham, Massachusetts
United States of America

Tanu Singhal, MRCOG
Specialist Registrar
Directorate of Women's, Perinatal, and Sexual Health
University Hospitals of Leicester NHS Trust
Leicester
United Kingdom

Kevin Spencer, BSc, MSc, DSc, CSci, CBiol, MIBiol, EurClinChem, CChem, FRSC, FRCPath
Honorary Senior Lecturer
Harris Birthright Research Centre for Fetal Medicine
King's College Hospital
University of London
    and Director of Biochemical Screening
Fetal Medicine Foundation
London
    and Consultant Biochemist
Endocrine Unit
Clinical Biochemistry Department
Harold Wood Hospital
Romford
United Kingdom
E-mail: KevinSpencer1@aol.com

Helen Spriggs
Patient
London
United Kingdom
E-mail: helen.spriggs@bayer.co.uk

Anne Sutcliffe, BSc, MB, ChB, FRCA
Consultant Anesthetist
Department of Anesthetics
University Hospital Birmingham NHS Trust
Birmingham
United Kingdom

Richard P. Taylor, PhD, FRCPath
Consultant Clinical Scientist
Department of Clinical Biochemistry
John Radcliffe Hospital
Oxford Radcliffe Hospitals NHS Trust
Oxford
United Kingdom
E-mail: richard.taylor@orh.nhs.uk

Wouter W. van Solinge, PhD
Professor of Laboratory Medicine
University Medical Center Utrecht
Utrecht
The Netherlands
E-mail: w.w.vansolinge@azu.nl

Ian D. Watson, MSc, PhD, FRCPath
Consultant Biochemist and Toxicologist
Department of Clinical Biochemistry
University Hospital, Aintree
Liverpool
United Kingdom
E-mail: IAN.WATSON@aht.nwest.nhs.uk

Jason J. S. Waugh, BSc (hons), MB BS, DA, MRCOG
Consultant/Senior Lecturer
Department of Obstetrics and Maternal Medicine
Directorate of Women's, Perinatal and Sexual Health
University Hospitals of Leicester NHS Trust
Leicester
United Kingdom
E-mail: jason.waugh@uhl-tr.nhs.uk

Gilbert E. Wieringa, MSc, MRCPath
Consultant Clinical Scientist
Department of Biochemistry
Christie Hospital NHS Trust
Manchester
United Kingdom
E-mail: Gilbert.Wieringa@christie-tr.nwest.nhs.uk

John F. Wood, DBMS, CSci, FIBMS
Operational Director
Department of Laboratory Medicine
Southampton University Hospitals (NHS) Trust
Southampton
United Kingdom
E-mail: John.Wood@suht.swest.nhs.uk

Anthony C. Woodman, BSc, MSc, PhD
Reader in Translational Medicine
Head, Cranfield BioMedical Centre
Institute of BioScience and Technology
Cranfield University at Silsoe
Bedfordshire
United Kingdom
E-mail: a.c.woodman@cranfield.ac.uk

Jeremy Wyatt, DM (Oxon), FRCP, FACMI, MB BS
Professor
Associate Director for Research and Development
National Institute for Clinical Excellence
London
United Kingdom

Sylvia Wyatt, MA
Future Healthcare Network Manager
NHS Confederation
London
United Kingdom
E-mail: Sylvia.Wyatt@nhsconfed.org

Lou Ann Wyer, MT(ASCP)
Clinical Specialist, POCT
Laboratory Services
Sentara Healthcare
Norfolk, Virginia
United States of America

Part **One**

Introduction

Chapter 1

Point-of-Care Testing: What, Why, When, and Where?

*Christopher P. Price, Andrew St John,
and Jocelyn M. Hicks*

Medicine is said to have its origins in magic and priestly activities; early rock engravings have been interpreted as showing a relationship between doctor and priest, with the former wearing a mask to frighten away demons (1). Hippocrates is regarded as the father of medicine. He stressed the role of the doctor at the patient's bedside (the doctor-patient relationship), the importance of observation, the need to establish hypotheses (recognizing that it might be necessary to change views on the cause of a particular set of symptoms), and the need to maintain the trust of the patient during this period (2). The transition to the study of body fluids has gone hand in hand with an increasing understanding of the pathophysiology of disease and of the treatment and eradication of disease.

THE ORIGIN OF DIAGNOSTIC TESTS

Diabetes mellitus was first recognized about 1500 B.C, when early healers noticed that ants were attracted to the urine of people with a mysterious emaciating disease (3). There are many subsequent references to observations of diabetes mellitus. Once the deductive process was born, together with the links between recognizing the disease, then an understanding of its pathology and subsequent treatment followed.

Some of the earliest references to diagnostic methods are found in the teaching of Ayurveda medicine, which provided a detailed description concerning the inspection of urine. A diagnostic method known as the "examination of the eight bases" included the examination of urine and feces. A prognostic marker was determined by dropping a bead of oil on the urine—the spreading of the oil being indicative of the patient's remaining life span (4). The foundation of observation and deduction was established both in terms of seeking to identify the origin of an illness and the effect of treatment. There was also a great deal of knowledge available to early healthcare practitioners, although personal experience and opinion played a greater part as communication was poor. The relationship between the doctor and the patient was established early in the history of medicine with the doctor seen as the expert in whom the patient could trust and be encouraged to trust. Individual responsibility for health is a more modern concept, perhaps because major diseases are often being seen as a consequence of man's own choice of lifestyle, rather than being the consequence of infectious diseases.

In the late 15th century, a book on the subject of urinoscopy was published. It provided a description of a physician who was called to inspect a full flask of urine in the presence of the patient (5). In the latter part of the 17th century, Willis described the sweet taste of urine in a publication, *Treatise of Urines* (6). Also, in the 17th century, the discipline of laboratory medicine was born, with a transition from testing for research purposes to making a diagnosis (2).

Many diagnostic tests became available in the 18th and 19th centuries It soon became obvious that testing could no longer take place at the bedside and thus, the first laboratory was born. The first laboratory was set up in a ward-side room, which is still a characteristic of many hospitals, particularly in association with intensive care units. However, this ward-based laboratory was still inadequate so the central hospital laboratory was proposed. In the late 19th century, Sir William Osler recognized laboratories "as essential to the proper equipment of the hospital as the intern. They are to the physician as the knife and the scalpel are to the surgeon." Also, Osler advocated for adequate laboratories under the leadership of a specialist pathologist in all large hospitals (7). However, the first diagnostic tests were performed at the bedside and point of care.

Today, laboratory test results play a key role in 60% to 70% of all diagnostic decisions (8). The revolution of the past two decades in cellular and molecular biology not only has enhanced our knowledge of disease but also has pointed the way to future opportunities in both diagnosis and treatment as well as eradication of disease. The genomics revolution is widely seen as fueling a proteomics revolution that will lead to a flood of new markers, many appearing in unison with new therapies. With the knowledge of the mechanism of action as well as, invariably, the molecular origin of the disease, we are beginning to see the appearance of new drugs that target particular tissues or cells. We know that there is significant interpersonal variation in response to drugs, and now we have the tools in many cases to measure that variability. As a consequence, the in vitro tests that previously were used to support a whole battery of observations and investigations are now beginning to take center stage in the investigation of the patient. This trend has been termed "personalized medicine" (9).

In parallel with the chemistry of diagnostic testing, there has been an equally large evolution in instrumentation, which began with the development of the colorimeter and the use of the test tube. In many respects instrumentation grew in parallel with the repertoire of tests and the workload. As the testing repertoire increased and the demands on the laboratory grew, it became clear that there were at least two streams of development—the large automated workhorse and the rapid stat analyzer. The extremes in instrumentation today are seen, on the one hand with the modern integrated platforms of analyzers as well as analyzers that are linked to specimen tube tracking, operating in large core laboratories, and on the other hand with the handheld glucose measuring system, and the miniaturized devices. The two address quite different needs—from the relatively slow turnaround, high-volume testing needs to the rapid response required in order to take action immediately. This evolution has not solely been due to advances in technology but has also been driven by changes to the way healthcare is delivered.

CHANGES IN HEALTHCARE DELIVERY

Clearly, the first references to healthcare are founded in the home and the workplace. The first idea of moving patients away from their home environment was probably rooted in the recognition of infectious diseases such as the early plagues. In the United Kingdom the last isolation hospital closed in the early 1960s, although some were kept in readiness against the possibility of an outbreak of smallpox until the early 1980s (10). The impact of an epidemic was seen recently with the outbreak of SARS and its impact on healthcare institutions. There has been a transition to a multiplicity of caregiving environments including the home (visited by the physician) and hospitals of varying sizes depending upon the size and needs of the local population or community. In the past two decades, there have been considerable changes in the way that healthcare is delivered, and although experience varies according to different countries and different styles of healthcare system (e.g., socialized and private healthcare systems), there is a consistent underlying pattern. Thus, there is a move toward:

- A more patient-centered approach to care
- A greater emphasis on primary care
- More rapid (efficient) triage of patients through the hospital system
- Greater use of one-stop clinics
- A reduction in dependence on the hospital as the focus of clinical care
- Consolidation of hospital facilities
- A reduced length of stay in hospital units (e.g., emergency room, admissions unit)
- Use of the pharmacy as an alternative community environment for healthcare provision

- Use of helplines (e.g., NHS Direct in the United Kingdom)
- Use of the Internet

The number of studies that focus on reducing the length of stay illustrate the trend toward reducing the emphasis on hospital care, both from an economic as well as a quality-of-care perspective. Statistics show that there is still a considerable variation in the average length of hospital stay in different countries. There have been specific initiatives to reduce the length of hospital stay, and the number of beds associated with hospital care in several countries including the United States, the United Kingdom, and Germany. However it would be dangerous to make too much of these statistics as reducing the dependence on hospital care does require a viable primary care sector. A key feature of an effective primary care sector will include access to rapid diagnostic testing. The trends are depicted in Figure 1-1.

CHANGES IN LABORATORY MEDICINE PROVISION

In parallel with changes in the way that clinical services have been delivered, there have been changes in the organization of laboratory services. This has been led by the United States and Australia with the development of core laboratories and laboratory service networks. This trend has now spread to Europe with changes being proposed in the United Kingdom (8), Germany, and Italy. This trend is depicted in Figure 1-1; consolidation of laboratory facilities creates the need for point-of-care testing (POCT), especially when seen in terms of the trends in patient care delivery.

PATIENTS AND THEIR EXPECTATIONS

The patient of the 21st century is a more informed individual as far as his/her health and well being are concerned. In

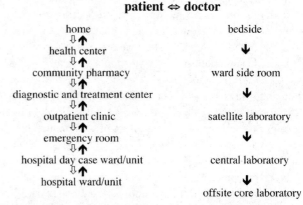

Figure 1-1 Trends in patient care. Diagram indicating the way in which care delivery has evolved ⇧ and is currently trending ← (*left-hand panel*), and a diagram of diagnostic testing, indicating the way in which much of the testing has been consolidated ← (*right-hand panel*). Current trends indicate the need for more point-of-care testing.

addition the patient is a more demanding customer for health-care services. The information age has resulted in the patient having greater access to information and as a consequence becoming a more knowledgeable patient. Greater affluence, travel, and choice have increased exposure to other healthcare environments, which has led to pressure for change in many countries. Healthcare has become an important feature of political agendas for the major political parties in many countries of the developed world.

Patients are increasingly aware, and being made aware, of the standards of healthcare available to them. There are support groups, which are sometimes seen as pressure groups, because they lobby for improved healthcare in their particular area of interest (e.g., osteoporosis, diabetes, prostate cancer). These groups are increasingly influencing the health agenda in many countries. There is also a wide range of disease registries that provide information on the performance of individual services (11, 12). In addition, a wide range of professional organizations publish guidelines on the Internet covering the diagnosis and management of diseases (13, 14).

With the Internet, patients now realize that they can purchase diagnostic tests directly; indeed, there are advertisements encouraging people to "know their number" (e.g., cholesterol values). The availability of diagnostic tests for home testing has long been used in the management of diabetes, and more recently in relation to the management of anticoagulation therapy. With statin therapy becoming available over-the-counter and widely used, more cholesterol testing is likely in the future. There has also been a trend toward cholesterol testing being seen as a test of wellness, because the patient is taking charge of their own health.

WHAT IS POINT-OF-CARE TESTING?

There have been many descriptive names given to the subject of this book, including bedside testing (15), near patient testing (16), physician's office testing (17), extra-laboratory testing (18), decentralized testing (19), and offsite, ancillary, and alternative site testing (20) as well as POCT. Handorf (21), in an attempt to rationalize terminology, attempted to differentiate alternative site testing from POCT. He identified alternative site testing as being undertaken within a hospital's jurisdiction but outside of the traditional hospital laboratory setting. POCT was equated with physicians' office laboratory testing as well as testing in mobile vehicles. Testing at the bedside and in vivo testing was considered to come within the definitions of both alternative site and POCT. However, the author recognized that with the "popularization of vertical integration strategies" some physicians' office laboratories may come under the domain of the hospital laboratory; the flaw of this delineation lies in the original recognition of two apparent testing paradigms, both appearing to be based on what might be termed management arrangements.

POCT can therefore be defined as the provision of a test when the result will be used to make a decision and to take appropriate action, which will lead to an improved health outcome.

APPROPRIATE SITES FOR POINT-OF-CARE TESTING

The two most common sites for POCT are probably the patient's routine living environment (e.g., home, leisure, and work place) where self-monitoring of blood glucose is widely performed and the intensive care unit where blood gas and electrolyte measurements are common. There has now been considerable expansion of the places where POCT is used (Table 1-1). Subsequent chapters of this book will present evidence with regard to the effectiveness and benefits associated with POCT in these environments.

WHY POINT-OF-CARE TESTING?

The utility of POCT lies in the value of the immediacy of response. The diagnostic performance of the tests is likely to have already been established using a central laboratory style of service, but the benefits and outcomes will only have been established in the point-of-care setting—if the unique benefit is to be proven. POCT brings the tools of laboratory medicine closer to both doctor and patient, and more broadly to the carer-patient relationship. In addition, it enables the patient to become more closely involved in his/her own disease management.

The initiation of the diagnostic process begins with the patient and the doctor having a question that requires an answer. It may be a question relating to the diagnosis of a disease, to the screening for disease, to the therapy, or to the outcome. The question may be directly related to the clinical situation and its resolution or outcome, or it may be indirect and more related to operational issues. Some examples of diagnostic questions are given in Table 1-2.

The second stage in the process is the initiation of the procedure for specimen collection, which in the past depended

Table 1-1 Sites at Which Point-of-Care Testing Is Performed

Home
Workplace
Leisure facility
Community pharmacy
Health center (general practitioner/physician's office)
Diagnostic and treatment center
Outpatient clinic (physician's office)
Ambulance/helicopter
Mobile hospital
Emergency room
Admissions unit
Operating room
Intensive care unit (adult, pediatric, and coronary care units)
Ward (unit)

Table 1-2 Some Clinical Questions Relevant to the Use of Point-of-Care Testing

Can urinalysis be used to rule out urinary tract infection in an asymptomatic at-risk woman?

Can chlamydial screening reduce the prevalence of complications of infection?

Does screening for urine protein give earlier detection of renal disease in at-risk populations?

Does frequent self-monitoring of blood glucose improve glycemic control?

Does self-monitoring of prothrombin time improve maintenance of a patient's INR?

Does hemoglobin A1c at the time of the clinic visit improve compliance with treatment protocol?

Does regular monitoring of serum cholesterol improve compliance with statin therapy?

Does a rapid cardiac marker service enable effective rule-out of myocardial infarction in patients with chest pain?

Does regular monitoring of blood gas and electrolytes reduce length of stay in intensive care units?

on the written instruction on a request form to the nurse and/or phlebotomist. But in more recent times, this process has been aided by various electronic-ordering processes. Collection of the specimen is then followed by transportation to the laboratory and registration in the laboratory information system (a daily logbook prior to the introduction of computers). There are many variations in this part of the process based on the geographical disposition of the patient facilities (e.g., units, wards, clinics) and the laboratory. In the laboratory, there are a series of procedures that encompass sample preparation prior to analysis and may include centrifugation and removal of the cellular components, as in the case of blood. The sample is then subjected to a range of analytical procedures culminating in the production of a valid analytical result. A valid result at this stage signifies that the analytical procedure has been completed within prescribed analytical standards, including quality control. In the case of a histopathological sample, quality control can only ensure that the sample has been processed in a suitable way to enable interpretation.

The interpretative phase is fundamentally a comparative exercise against a reference point associated with normality, taking account of any confounding issues such as biological variation and changes seen in the disease suspected or established, if the objective of the investigation is disease monitoring. Interpretation may also take into account any previous results. In the case of numerical results, this interpretative step may be partially completed automatically by the laboratory computer using an established algorithm (e.g., delta checks, use of cut-off values, and decision protocols). In the case of histopathological specimens, the comparison is based on pattern recognition and is more qualitative and subjective.

In all cases a report is prepared which may include commentary that indicates the likelihood of the outcome that the requesting clinician was questioning at the outset such as is the patient suffering from a particular condition, or is the treatment

effective, or is there a risk of a further event? This information is then transmitted back to the requesting doctor and the cycle is complete when the action is taken in relation to the question posed at the outset.

This diagnostic cycle is illustrated in Figure 1-2 and has been described at some length in order to: (a) highlight the number of steps that are involved, (b) indicate the supporting activities required to ensure that the process is conducted effectively, and (c) enable the reader to appreciate the potential benefits that might accrue in an operational sense from the use of POCT, while also recognizing the potential pitfalls. Many of these issues are dealt with in subsequent chapters of this book. In a report from one management consultant a few years ago, there were as many as 56 steps identified between a doctor requesting a test and receiving the result. In a recent analysis, the time taken from test request to receipt of a result from a central laboratory ranged from 3 h to 4 days (22)! Simple analysis of the processes involved in generating a test result often fails to recognize the activities that support this cycle of events. These activities include training of the staff involved (ensuring that staff are competent in the practice of each step) and targeting the relevant decision maker to receive the result (ensuring that there is sufficient knowledge for the result to be used effectively). Self-testing may be regarded as a unique situation in that a doctor is not directly involved; however, when self-testing is used as part of the management of a chronic disease (e.g., diabetes mellitus), the doctor will wish to ensure that the diabetic patient is properly trained and informed on the use of blood glucose monitoring, including the appropriate action to take with abnormal results. Previous studies have supported the need for proper education and training. Backing up the many anecdotal observations, Kirkpatrick and Holding (23) provided documentary evidence that a significant proportion of results transmitted electronically to an emergency room were never accessed. Raine (24) showed that 16% of diabetics in one study were found to be using an incorrect

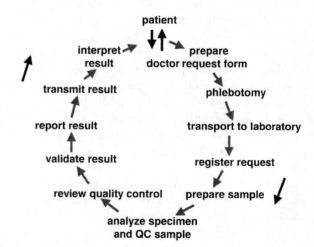

Figure 1-2 The diagnostic cycle. Representation of the activities associated with the delivery of a diagnostic investigation; from request to interpretation.

calibration code when asked to bring their glucose meters in for checking at the time of their routine clinic visit.

HEALTH OUTCOMES AND POINT-OF-CARE TESTING: BENEFITS AND VALUE

Clearly, the patient is at the center of any discussion on the benefits of POCT. The goal of any healthcare intervention has to be to bring maximum benefit, with minimal risk and at reasonable cost. Thus, while the focus of attention is on the patient there are benefits that can be realized by the doctor as well as other care givers, the provider organization, the purchaser, and society. These are typically considered clinical and economic benefits, although it can be helpful in the context of POCT to consider the latter in terms of both operational and economic benefits. Much of the early literature on POCT dealt with issues of technical performance and microeconomic analysis of cost per test, as exemplified in the health technology assessment of POCT in the primary care setting undertaken by Hobbs et al. (25).

The Clinical Outcomes

Developments in both diagnostic and intervention procedures as well as our understanding of diseases and their management are the fundamental and primary reasons for the increasing interest in POCT. The secondary financial pressures provide the momentum. These developments have led to the near eradication of some diseases and the earlier diagnosis and better management of other diseases. Other diseases have emerged as a consequence of the change in age profile of the population. In addition, social change has resulted in the appearance of previously unrecognized diseases as well as an increasing expectation on the part of the patient to be treated or even cured.

The provision of a stat result may avert a life threatening crisis and may also ensure that there is a more rapid and effective change in patient management (26). This is a description of ruling in a diagnosis and a particular decision pathway. There are several examples of these clinical scenarios and these will be explored in subsequent chapters of this book. Similarly an immediate test result may help to rule out a diagnosis and lead the clinician to consider another alternative (27, 28). Sometimes the most difficult scenario to explore in relation to POCT is the benefit that can accrue from the provision of a result, for example, in diabetes mellitus, to aid counseling in relation to therapeutic management. Studies now show that a hemoglobin A1c (HbA1c) result at the time of consultation has been more effective than a result communicated at a later date to the patient (29, 30). Similar evidence for better compliance exists for other tests and treatments. It may sometimes be difficult to demonstrate the benefit in terms of morbidity and mortality, although intuitively it is clearly more effective to guide a patient's management with hard evidence or proof, rather than the more vague exhortation to do better, particularly when there are no other symptoms that can be used to guide the patient. The use of POCT to support compliance with treatment protocols will be extremely important in the future because it touches on the concept of the patient taking more responsibility for his/her care—but obviously guided by the knowledge and evidence provided by the doctor and other healthcare professionals (27, 28).

The clinical outcome should also be seen in terms of the help it provides to the caregiver, both in terms of improving the quality of diagnostic information (enabling better decision-making) and providing additional tools for patient counseling. Consequently this achieves improved satisfaction for both the patient and the caregiver.

The Operational Outcomes

There are three major reasons for investigating changes in the way in which healthcare services are delivered: (a) improved clinical outcomes, (b) patient demand, and (c) the escalating costs of healthcare. Improved clinical outcomes take into account the appropriate availability of expertise in the context of the disposition of primary, secondary, and tertiary care, set against the risks associated with the different care settings. Access to specialist care in a hospital setting (e.g., trauma, major surgery) has to be balanced against the risks associated with hospital care as well as the economic considerations. The risks will include exposure to nosocomial infection and speed of access. The advent of less invasive procedures has helped to reduce these risks considerably, but has also enabled the rise of day case surgery and the inherent need for faster diagnostic support services. There is an increasing interest in devolving chronic disease management away from the hospital setting, bringing operational benefits to both the healthcare provider as well as to the patient. The consolidation of facilities in order to improve productivity is a feature of most primary, secondary, and tertiary care facilities, including laboratories. The focus on the costs of care has produced initiatives other than consolidation of services including rationing of services as well as benchmarking of costs and outcomes.

The Economic Outcomes

The overwhelming focus on the costs of care is reflected in the limited perspective or microeconomic approach. This approach is taken to the cost of diagnostic testing by many people involved in healthcare, including laboratory professionals. Thus, efforts are always being made to reduce the cost per test, rather than taking a more holistic or macroeconomic approach looking more broadly at the cost per patient episode. Invariably, POCT is seen as more expensive when viewed in the light of cost per test, and yet in many cases the benefits are seen not only in terms of improved outcomes but also in terms of reduced utilization of resources (eg., reduced length of hospital stay, use of blood products, better use of staff time) (27, 28, 31). Clearly, in order for a more holistic approach to gain acceptance, there has to be a recognized system for transfer of resources between cost centers. Despite the difficulty associated with such a major change in thinking, failure to recognize the need for change in the management of resources will mean the stifling of future development, particularly in the situation where diagnostic testing budgets are held down.

CHANGING THE PATTERN OF DELIVERY

Changes in the way healthcare is delivered are due to a variety of factors. These include an increasing technological approach to medicine balanced by an awareness of the need to focus on better communication with patients and the public, an increasing burden of disease associated with social change, and an aging population set within the constraints of increasing costs.

Thus, as suggested earlier, there is a greater focus on the primary care physician as the crucial interface with the patient. The physician serves as the health educator as well as the filter or gatekeeper for entry to the secondary and tertiary levels of care. The corollary of this observation is that the primary care physician may in future undertake more testing: (a) to exclude uncomplicated conditions, (b) to rule in those patients that require urgent specialist services, (c) to provide an initial workup of tests prior to the patient being seen by a specialist physician, and (d) as part of a strategy for management of chronic diseases. Similar reasons for testing may apply to the patient sent to the hospital either as an emergency or an elective referral.

If the secondary and tertiary services are consolidated into fewer centers, then the primary care physician may take on additional responsibilities including that of seeing patients in a small district or community hospital. POCT may then become part of the testing procedure at this type of facility or be used to cover evening and night shifts for intensive care facilities in smaller hospitals when central laboratory coverage is not available on a 24-h basis. The greater consolidation of specialist medical services brings with it the benefits of a greater critical mass of expertise. However, it also demands that these services are used effectively; one of the practical consequences of this is the rapid triage of patients and the necessity for rapid turnaround of results.

Thus, the changing pattern of delivery, with the two extremes of more clinical activity in primary care and consolidated tertiary care, suggests the possibility of more POCT. In addition, the consolidation of laboratory facilities—especially when a core laboratory is created—automatically creates the need for POCT. Indeed, there appears to be an increasing organizational conflict between the consolidation of laboratory facilities and the devolution of patient care. POCT can therefore be seen as a vehicle for facilitating organizational change, providing an exciting means of achieving some of the benefits expected from newer approaches to healthcare delivery.

A change in testing delivery invariably requires that other aspects of the process of care must also change if the real benefits are to be realized. This point has been alluded to in a number of studies and has been explicitly recognized in others. Thus, Rink et al. (32) in an early study of POCT in primary care found that general practitioners did not change their approach of practice, and saw little value in POCT. Kendall et al.

(33), while able to show greatly reduced times to produce a result, were unable to demonstrate a reduced length of stay in the emergency room. This in part may have been due to a lack of change in practice—specifically being available to receive the results when they became available. Murray et al. (34) performed a similar study, however, they did show a reduced length of stay. The authors attributed the reduced length of stay to the ability to discharge a proportion of the patients earlier when normal results were produced. These authors also pointed out that lengths of stay may not be reduced by POCT if test results are required from the laboratory in addition to POCT, in order to make a triage decision. Nichols et al. (35) made explicit reference to this issue in a study of POCT in the interventional radiology and invasive cardiology settings. These authors found that there was no change in the clinical practice in these settings upon implementation of POCT until the clinical protocol was revised. The importance of this was emphasized in an accompanying editorial (36).

CONCLUSIONS

The key objective of POCT is to produce a result more quickly. There are several reasons why speed may be important, covering both clinical and operational considerations. The sophistication of technology today is such that the reliability or technical performance of POCT devices can be assured. Thus, problems related to the technical quality of results are now more likely to be due to poor compliance with standard operating procedures, which is analogous to compliance with treatment protocols and should be addressed as part of the overall approach to maintaining good clinical practice. The testing phase is only one part of the diagnostic process. Users of any diagnostic service need proper support in training on the use of the service, interpretation of results, and development of the service. Thus, understanding the preanalytical and postanalytical phases are vital to the decision whether to adopt POCT. In addition, to integrate any modification of the testing phase with commensurate change in the clinical management practice protocol is vital. Any consideration of the economics of POCT should take into account the wider perspective on benefits rather than simply focus on the cost of the test. This book maintains the goals of the first edition, namely to assist the laboratorian and clinician in determining how to organize and deliver a high-quality POCT service and to determine whether this approach to testing will be clinically and operationally cost effective.

REFERENCES

1. Hinnells J, Porter R, eds. Religion, suffering and healing. London:Kegan Paul, 1998.
2. Porter R. The greatest benefit to mankind. A medical history of humanity from antiquity to the present. London: Harper Collins, 1997:831pp.
3. MacCracken J, Hoel D. From ants to analogues. Puzzles and promises in diabetes management. Postgrad Med 1997;101:138–40.

4. Bynum WF, Porter R, eds. Companion encyclopedia of the history of medicine. London: Routledge, 1993:297pp.

5. Copeman WSC. Doctors and disease in Tudor times. London: Dawson, 1960:116–21.

6. Foster WD. Genesis of a specialty. In: Pathology as a profession in Great Britain. London: Royal College of Pathologists, 1981: 1–18.

7. Cushing H. The life of Sir William Osler. Oxford, UK: Oxford University Press, 1926:367pp.

8. Department of Health Pathology Modernisation Team. Modernising pathology services. http://www.dh.gov.uk/assetRoot/04/07/31/12/04073112.pdf (accessed February 22, 2004).

9. Kalow W. Pharmacogenetics and personalised medicine. Fundam Clin Pharmacol 2002:16:337–42.

10. Rivett G. From cradle to grave; fifty years of the NHS. London: King's Fund Publishing, 1997:506pp.

11. Renal Registry. http://www.renalreg.com (accessed February 22, 2004).

12. European Network of Cancer Registries. http://www.encr.com.fr (accessed February 22, 2004).

13. National Kidney Foundation K/DOQI Clinical practice guidelines for chronic kidney disease; evaluation, classification and stratification. http://www.kidney.org/professional/doqi/kdoqi/p1_exec.htm (accessed February 22, 2004).

14. American Diabetes Association. Clinical practice recommendations. http://www.diabetes.org/for-health-professional-and-scientists/cpr/jsp (accessed February 22, 2004).

15. Oliver G. On bedside urine testing. London: HK Lewis, 1884:1–128.

16. Marks V, Alberti KGMM, eds. Clinical biochemistry nearer the patient. London: Churchill Livingstone, 1988.

17. Mass D. Consulting to physician office laboratories. In: Snyder JR, Wilkinson DS, eds. Management in laboratory medicine, 3rd ed. New York: Lippincott, 1998:443–50.

18. Price CP. Quality assurance of extra-laboratory analyses. In: Clinical biochemistry nearer the patient II. Eds Marks V, Alberti KGMM. London: Bailliere Tindall, 1987:166–78.

19. Ashby JP, ed. The patient and decentralized testing. Lancaster, UK: MTP Press, 1988:128pp.

20. Handorf CR. College of American Pathologists Conference XXVIII on alternate site testing: Introduction. Pathol Lab Med 1995;119:867–71.

21. Handorf CR. Background: Setting the stage for alternative-site laboratory testing. Clin Lab Med 1994;14:451–8.

22. Severson C. Decentralisation of patient services; cost analysis for testing point of care vs central lab. SMI Conference on Market Opportunities and Technology Trends in Point of Care Diagnostics, The Hatton, London, February 16–17, 2004.

23. Kilpatrick ES, Holding S. Use of computer terminals on wards to access emergency test results; a retrospective audit. BMJ 2001; 322:1101–3.

24. Raine CH. Self-monitored blood glucose: A common pitfall. Endo Pract 2003;9(11):137–9.

25. Hobbs FD, Delaney BC, Fitzmaurice DA, Wilson S, Hyde CJ, Thorpe GH, et al. A review of near patient testing in primary care. Health Technol Assess 1997;1:1–230.

26. Strickland RA, Hill TR, Zaluga GP. Rapid bedside analysis of arterial blood gases and electrolytes improve patient care during and after cardiac surgery. Anesthesiology 1988;69:A257.

27. Price CP. Point-of-care testing. BMJ 2001;322:1285–8.

28. Price CP. Point of care testing. Potential for tracking disease management outcomes. Dis Manage Health Outcomes 2002;10: 749–61.

29. Cagliero E, Levina E, Nathan D. Immediate feedback of HbA1c levels improves glycemic control in type 1 and insulin-treated type 2 diabetic patients. Diabetes Care 1999;22:1785–9.

30. Thaler LM, Ziemer DC, Gallina DL, Cook CB, Dunbar VG, Phillips LS, et al. Diabetes in urban african-americans. XVII. Availability of rapid HbA1c measurements enhances clinical decision-making. Diabetes Care 1999;22:1415–21.

31. Price CP. Medical and economic outcomes of point-of-care testing. Clin Chem Lab Med 2002;40:246–51.

32. Rink E, Hilton S, Szczepura A, Fletcher J, Sibbald B, Davies C, et al. Impact of introducing near patient testing for standard investigations in general practice. BMJ 1993;307:775–8.

33. Kendall J, Reeves B, Clancy M. Point of care testing: randomised, controlled trial of clinical outcome. BMJ 1998;316:1052–7.

34. Murray RP, Leroux M, Sabga E, Palatnick W, Ludwig L. Effect of point of care testing on length of stay in an adult emergency department. J Emer Med 1999;17:811–4.

35. Nichols JH, Kickler TS, Dyer KL, Humbertson SK, Cooper PC, Maughan WL, et al. Clinical outcomes of point-of-care testing in the interventional radiology and invasive cardiology setting. Clin Chem 2000;46:543–50.

36. Scott MG. Faster is better—it's rarely that simple! Clin Chem 2000;46:441–2.

Part Two

Technology

Chapter 2

Technology of Handheld Devices for Point-of-Care Testing

Michael J. Pugia and Christopher P. Price

The market of handheld devices for rapid analysis of diagnostic biomarkers has grown 20% annually from 1980 to 2000 (1). The application of devices has grown from solely measuring glucose into an increasing array of devices capable of measuring many more analytes. These devices are not only used by the patient but also by a wide range of healthcare professionals in many point-of-care testing (POCT) environments, including the patient's bedside, clinics, the home, and the physician office as well as the small, moderately complex, and Clinical Laboratory Improvement Amendments (CLIA)-waived laboratories.

There has been a significant change in the technology applied to POCT devices over the past two decades (2–7). Prior to 1985, the majority of applications were (*a*) blood glucose assays, (*b*) simple chemistries for urinalysis, and (*c*) pregnancy tests. Many of these early devices required several manual interventions prior to obtaining result, with the inherent risk of a multistep process. Later a range of devices were developed to measure (*i*) a wide range of metabolites (e.g., cholesterol, uric acid, and lactate), (*ii*) enzymes (e.g., aspartate and alanine aminotransferase, creatine kinase, and γ-glutamyl transferase), and (*iii*) haptens, peptides, and proteins by immunoassay. In addition, the number of steps that the operator is required to perform has been significantly reduced, and the reproducibility of manufacture has improved along with improvements in the stability of reagents and the calibration of the methods. This has led to improvements in the convenience and reliability for the patient.

The primary motives for these handheld devices are clinical need with either high frequency or time urgency for the clinical result as well as the need for convenience (8–11). In addition, there are economic reasons for the use of POCT. The market is dominated by blood glucose testing, which is a multibillion dollar business. However, pregnancy testing, urinalysis, screening for drugs-of abuse, cardiac markers, hepatitis testing, hemoglobin testing, blood gas/electrolyte, HIV, cholesterol, occult blood, infectious disease testing, coagulation testing, and fertility testing are also now significant contributors to this growing market (2–7).

The reasons for this growth are driven both by needs for immediate testing at or near the patient and by advances in technology. Advances in the designs and manufacture of detectors and analytical enablers have increased accuracy and precision (12–13). The handling of fluids has evolved from the use of simple absorbent matrices or layers to the use of chromatographic, capillary, and other systems that add more functionality to the device. Smaller and lower-cost devices can now serve as transducers of signals from the chemical reaction environment to the readout device. The development of electronic components, molding, machining, packaging, and software have allowed large-volume, low-cost manufacture of detectors and devices. These advances have brought new devices into the hands of lay users (14–15).

In the last few years, there has also been a change in the way in which healthcare is delivered with a lesser emphasis on referral of patients to the hospital and greater provision of services in the community at the primary care level. This is combined with a desire to triage the patient through the hospital system more efficiently, adopting a more patient-centered (friendly) approach. In addition, there has been an evolution in the awareness of the population with regard to the following: (*a*) health and well-being; (*b*) the presence, risk, or absence of disease, and (*c*) the desire to know more about certain diagnostic test results (e.g., their cholesterol value). Although this trend and growth in testing has realized improvements in healthcare for both the patient and the physician, little has been written about the factors that have and will continue to affect the design and development of handheld POCT devices.

DEVICE DESIGN CONCEPTS

Three Types of Handheld Device

To simplify the review of the large number of handheld devices on the market today, a classification of three major types will be used (Figure 2-1). It is not possible to review all systems individually, but representative examples rated best-in-class, first-in-class, or uniqueness will be used as examples to describe the principles of the system design. For those requiring a survey of all devices, several sources are available (7).

In Type 1, reagents are included in a porous matrix that is affixed to some kind of holder to facilitate easy handling. Sample is applied to the matrix and mixes with reagent to produce a signal that is interpreted by a reader or visually by the operator. The readers can vary in size. They are either portable and handheld or more static tabletop systems. In addition, systems can vary by the number of results produced in a fixed period of time.

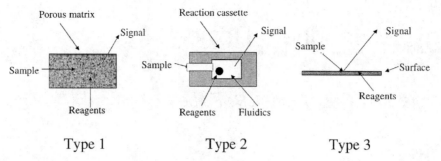

Figure 2-1 Three types of handheld devices: Type 1 (*left*), Type 2 (*center*), and Type 3 (*right*).

In Type 2, reagents are held in a reaction cassette. When the sample enters the cassette, it is mixed in one or more processes with reagents. In this configuration, the reaction signal is invariably interpreted with a reader.

In Type 3 (the least common type), reagents and specimen react on the surface of the device, then the signal is read on the surface or coupled to some form of transducer, which converts the signal to produce some form of electrical response. This type of system does not always need fluidic manipulations, but the reaction signal is invariably interpreted by a reader.

Overview of Technology

The advent of enabling technologies in the areas of detection methods (detector), recognition methods (recognition), fluid handling (fluidics), signal reading (transduction), and analytical processing (enabler) have allowed devices to meet the needs of the patient and the healthcare professional and to achieve commercial success.

The primary enabling technologies have been in the development of detection and recognition strategies; the early methods used colorimetric or fluorometric chemistries. These were then combined with recognition technologies such as enzymatic degradation, immunological recognition and latterly molecular recognition. The development of detection reactions continued with luminescence and electrochemistries, optical motion detection, and ion-selective materials. Today, simple devices exist that will detect extremely low levels of circulating proteins using handheld immunoassay systems (14). However, the availability of simplified detection and recognition technology also continues to limit the scope of POCT devices. Thus, handheld devices that perform complete blood counts are not available and devices to detect DNA and RNA (i.e., low copy numbers) are not commonly available.

Second, complex fluidic handling has been achieved by advances in papers, membranes, plastic molding, micromachining, surface treatment, moisture barriers, layered material, chromatography, capillary, and pressure systems. Today's successful devices have eliminated the need for many operations including: (*a*) wiping to remove sample at the end of the prescribed reaction period, (*b*) mixing reagents, (*c*) pipetting reagents, (*d*) addition of secondary reagents or washes, and (*e*) timing of reactions or washes.

The third major advance came with the ability to produce devices that read a range of signals at low cost, with accuracy and precision. This became possible with processors, displays, touch screens, photocells, and memory, and as electronic components and circuit boards advanced in design and fabrication. In addition, large-scale and reproducible reagent-manufacturing techniques such as dry reagent formulation, thin-film casting, screen and inkjet printing, coating and dosing techniques, surface treatment, cassette and channel molding, and fabrication have also been introduced. The innovative use of some raw materials to enhance reagent stability has allowed the low-cost manufacture of electrode sensors, dry reagents, and film-based devices.

Finally, data processing as an enabling technology perhaps represents the most fundamental advance but one that is often overlooked. For example, analytical calibration and quality-control methods are invisible to the lay user but these methods have facilitated performance improvements toward laboratory standards. This has resulted from large-scale reagent production, input and output devices, calibration algorithms, barcoded lot identification, quality-control systems in the machines, and bidirectional instrument communication (connectivity; see Chapter 20).

Detection Methods (Detector)

Detection methods can be broken into two components: recognition and signal generation. These components are generally biological or chemical, but they can also be polymeric and inorganic. Together, they form the essential components of the analytical device, capable of producing a signal related to concentration of the analyte to be detected.

Clinical analysis at the point of care has traditionally used optical signals, electrochemical signals, optical motion, and surface interrogation (12, 13, 16) (Table 2-1). As POCT device designs are miniaturized, the specimen volumes used are smaller; the ability to detect lower concentrations of analyte becomes even more challenging. This is particularly disappointing, because detection of many of the new proteomic markers will require sensitivity ranging from the femtomolar (10^{-15} mol/L) to the attomolar (10^{-18} mol/L) range (17). Today, the lower limits of protein detection only ranges from nanomolar

Table 2-1 Approaches Taken to Signal Generation in POCT Handheld Devices

Signal generation	Types
Optical detection	Absorbance, reflectance, transmission, fluorescence, luminescence, turbidimetry and nephelometry
Electrochemical signals	Amperometric, impedimetric, potentiometric
Optical motion	Light scattering, paramagnetic particles, interference pattern, image analysis
Surface interrogation	Optical interference, pattern recognition, surface enhancement, diffraction, ellipsometry, surface plasmon resonance

(10^{-9} mol/L) to picomolar (10^{-12} mol/L), within the time frames used in POCT devices (generally <10 min) (7).

With detection materials (e.g., reflectance, transmission, fluorescence, phosphorescence, luminescence, conductivity, resistance, magnetic field, evanescent wave, electrical field, and coulometry), size limitations dominate many physical and chemical properties (18–24). Detection is limited by the reporter molecule, the size of the detected molecule, and the distance between detection surfaces and detected molecule. Multiplexing signals into multiple determinations with the same or separate reagent areas (often called channels) have been used to increase sensitivity in, for example, particle-flow cytometry (25). Detection methods applied to micrometer-sized detectors and to nanometer-sized analytes have yet to provide sufficient sensitivity for POCT devices.

Optical detection is inclusive of all spectroscopic methods or reactions which can be grouped as direct, indicators, catalytic, particles, and scattering (16, 26). Direct measurement of the analyte's spectra over other components is only useful when the analyte is the primary component and accounts for a significant total mass of the sample (>0.1%). Examples of this are the oximetry parameters measured in blood by blood gas analyzers, such as carboxyhemoglobin, oxygenated hemoglobin, and methemoglobin, as well as optical hematcrit and oxygen measurements (27, 28). Indicators such as binding dyes allow detection at the micromolar level. Catalytic reactions can be used for the micromolar detection of substrates, and for enzymes through reactions with signal-forming substrates. Catalysis can also amplify detection down to nanomolar levels with use of oxidizers, reducers, and activators to regenerate reagents and enzymes (enzyme amplification methods). Particle labels are primarily used for detectable signals in immunoassay based on chromatograpy, flow-through, and cassette devices that are capable of detection down in to the picomolar range (29, 30). Light scattering can be used for the direct detection of aggregation of large molecules such as protein analytes and their complementary antibodies, but the limit of detection is in the micromolar range (31).

Electrochemical signal generation can be grouped into amperometric, impedimetric, and potentimetric detection methods. Most handheld glucose systems now rely on electrochemical reactions to generate signals for detection (6, 7, 32). Amperometric and potentiometric glucose methods are now perfected to the point of allowing the required precision and accuracy to be achieved at sample volumes as low as 0.3 to 4 μL and assay times from 5 to 30 s.

The electrochemical detector typically has two or three types of electrodes: a bioactive material called a working or common electrode, a nonbioactive reference electrode, and a counter electrode when there is an oxidation at the common electrode. The common electrode is responsive to a chemical reaction produced directly or indirectly by the analyte. The reference electrode measures potential; no reaction occurs at the reference electrode, and the counter electrode maintains charge balance if needed.

In the amperometric device, the current of the common electrode (vs. the reference electrode) is held at a constant value. Change in current due to a chemical reaction is measured by the potential observed at the reference electrode. In the potentiometric process, the change in current is measured across the working and reference electrode. When a sample or other solution connects the electrodes, a measurable signal relates to the concentration of the analyte being measured. Potentials can be turned on or off to allow multistep assays in which biochemical and chemical reactions occur prior to detection. Common electrodes can be simple metals, solid-state, or incorporated into the membrane with a recognition element. The signal can require specific conditions such as pH, oxidizing agents, potentials, reductants, and mediators.

Glucose-measuring systems provide excellent examples of the evolution in enzyme-based electrochemical detectors (6). Originally, common electrode detectors used glucose oxidases to generate H_2O_2 or consume O_2 (33), either by direct or indirect reactions. Glucose oxidase catalyzes the oxidation of glucose to gluconic acid by the transfer of electrons to flavin-adenine dinucleotide (FAD). In a second version, glucose is detected when the reduced FAD molecule is oxidized through an electrochemical mediator, ferrocene, which produces a signal (34). A number of alternative mediators have been described. Mediators allow electrodes to operate at potentials less subject to interference by uric acid, vitamin C, oxygen, paracetamol, and other specimen components.

The other device that has made the most use of electrochemical methods has been the blood gas and electrolyte system. Some of these systems have extended the application of electrochemistries beyond blood gases and electrolytes into hematocrit and enzyme-mediated chemistries, such as the completely handheld i-STAT® system (i-STAT Corporation, East Windsor, NJ, USA) (35–36).

Optical motion detection is a very important detection method in handheld devices for coagulation testing (37–39). This is partly because the first systems using optical motion detection were designed to mimic the reference mechanical method of the Lee-White clotting time (40–42). The Hemochron® 400 is an early example, manufactured in 1969 by International Technidyne Corporation (ITC, Edison, NJ, USA) (40). In general, the specimen is applied to a reagent solution containing a clotting activator that causes a blood specimen to clot. The time in which the clot forms is measured by the ability of a magnet or magnetic particle to move out of alignment with a magnet detector.

Optical motion detection technology was modified by the use of nanoparticles such as paramagnetic iron oxide particles in an oscillating magnetic field under controlled temperatures. The Rapidpoint Coag system developed by Pharmanetics (formerly Cardiovascular Diagnostics, Morrisville, NC, USA) is an example of the design first introduced as the Thrombolytic Assessment System (TAS) by Cardiovascular Diagnostics in 1985 (37–38). Another design is called speckle detection, which was technology developed by Biotrack in 1990 and marketed as the CoaguChek Plus™ (Roche Diagnostics, Mannheim, Germany) (43). Red blood cells move through a molded capillary and pass by a pair of photodetectors that create and measure the speckle or interference pattern. Clot formation decreases fluctuations in the pattern. Once a predetermined threshold is met, the instrument displays the clotting time.

The surface-interrogation signal is typically optical and conducted by measuring spectroscopic changes on the surface of an optical element. Recognition agents coat the optical element and the sample is directly applied to the surface. Optical changes are due to optical interference, pattern recognition or surface enhancement upon association of an analyte. For example, the optical element can be a diffraction grating with reflectance changes measured upon binding. Looking for changes in a given area allows diffraction pattern recognition as in an optical grating printed with antibody on a reflective surface (44). The surface-interrogation method has also been applied to the following: (*a*) optical fibers by measuring a fluorescent reaction product (45), (*b*) the polycarbonate surface of a conventional compact disc (CD) (46), (*c*) nanoparticle-based barcodes (21), (*d*) ellipsometry (47), and (*e*) light-wave guides using evanescent wave fluorescence (48, 49).

Recognition Methods (Recognition)

The recognition component takes advantage of the ability of a molecule or material to specifically recognize the target substance (16, 50–53). This component allows the detection signal to be specific to the analyte being detected. The greater the specificity of the recognition component to the analyte, the less interference observed.

Recognition can be grouped as indicators, catalytic reactions, and association host reactions (16, 50–53) (Table 2-2). Indicators are molecules that interact directly with the analyte to be detected in favor of other components of the specimen. Catalytic reactions involve molecules that interact directly with the analyte and catalyze a secondary reaction for detection; these could include degradation, activation, or inhibition. Association hosts are molecules or materials that bind or associate with analytes to be detected in favor of other components (e.g.,

Table 2-2 Approaches Taken to Analyte Recognition in POCT Handheld Devices

Recognition	Types
Indicators	Direct conjugation, ion pairing, hydrophobic binding
Catalytic reactions	Enzyme substrate, enzyme detection, catalysis reaction product, inhibitor or activation detection
Association host	Proteins, molecular imprints, selective membranes, antibodies, macromolecules, nucleic acids, lectins

as occurs with an antibody binding to its complementary antigen).

The urinalysis reagent strip, with multiple reagent pads affixed to a plastic handle, is a good example of the panel of indicators and catalytic reactions of recognition components. This panel measures glucose (catalytic), protein (indicator), ketone (indicator), pH (indicator), occult blood (catalytic), bilirubin (indicator), urobilinogen (indicator), nitrite (indicator), specific gravity (indicator), leukocytes (catalytic), microalbumin (indicator), and creatinine (catalytic) (16, 51). One reagent area can contain all of the chemicals needed to generate color response to the analyte, resulting from five or more timed and competing reactions, all containing a recognition component (16). This example has used several types of indicator recognition reactions such as direct conjugation to a molecular feature of the analyte, hydrophobic binding, ion-pairing conjugation, and the detection of electrolytes by pH indicators. The specificity of the recognition component can impact the performance of the assay by reducing interference. For example, the improvement in the affinity of indicator dyes to bind to albumin has allowed detection of microalbuminuria (54).

In catalytic recognition reactions, the analyte can be the catalyst or the reactant. Elastase from white blood cells can be recognized by serving as a catalyst for enzyme substrates. The reacted enzyme substrates provide a signal. Enzymes also act as natural recognition agents, as in the example of glucose detection by glucose oxidase. There are also molecules other than enzymes that can act as catalysts, such as in the example of the catalytic detection of creatinine by formation of an active complex with copper (55).

The reduction of interference in catalyst recognition reactions has long been a goal, such as reduced oxygen and hemoglobin dependencies to enable shorter read times and smaller sample volumes. For example, blood glucose measuring systems now use a variety of different enzymes, each with various strengths and weakness (6, 7). The recognition enzyme for glucose devices is now changing from glucose oxidase to glucose dehydrogenase, which does not require oxygen and is suitable for small samples to prevent interferences from hematocrit, altitude, environmental temperature or humidity, hypotension, hypoxia, and high triglyceride concentrations (32, 56).

Recognition through an association host has been one of the most flexible methods. Association host techniques can be grouped as proteins in coagulation tests, selective membranes in blood gas assays, macromolecules in electrolyte methods, antibodies in immunoassays, and nucleic acids in DNA/RNA testing (37, 52, 53, 57). Most of these association host techniques have been applied to handheld POCT devices, with the current exception of DNA/RNA. In the future, immunoassay is likely to continue to be the method that is most commonly exploited as the number of proteomic markers is expected to increase (17).

Recognition proteins that are used in coagulation testing also include clotting activators such as thromboplastin; these are added to the specimen as a recognition element to convert proteins in the blood-clotting cascade. Thromboplastin converts prothrombin to thrombin. The time to conversion to prothrombin is a measurement of the presence of Factors II, V, VII, and X. The testing menu has expanded from prothrombin time to partial thromboplastin time to enoxaparin, heparin, and protamine; it is now possible to measure the levels of a number of thrombolytic drugs and other clotting factors (37–43).

Selective membranes have been used as recognition techniques for blood gas analysis since 1953 (57). The handheld configurations include the i-STAT system and the Immediate Response Mobile Analysis (IRMA, Diametrics Medical, Roseville, MN, USA) blood analysis system (35, 36, 58). The common menu includes pH, oxygen and carbon dioxide (57–59). In the early blood gas systems, a pH-sensitive glass membrane produced an electrochemical potential as a function of the hydrogen ion concentration on the outer bulb surface. In the case of carbon dioxide, the gas selectively diffused across the membrane and carbon dioxide concentration was quantified as a change in pH of the electrolyte. For oxygen, molecules selectively diffused through the semipermeable membrane and reduction of oxygen was detected. In general, recognition elements are used to extract or exclude the passage of the analyte from the specimen across one or more barriers which constitute the membrane. Selective membranes can be fabricated from glass, polymers, and other materials; they can be films, liquids, or planar configurations. For both electrode and optical signal devices, the goal is to make the membrane permeable to analytes but not contaminants of the sample (60). The fundamental means to achieve this involve changes to the membrane composition and the ability of the recognition elements to bind to the analyte (61).

Menus have been built around analytes needed for the clinical assessment of oxygen uptake, oxygen transport, oxygen release, and tissue oxygenation and have been expanded to include sodium, potassium, calcium, chloride, and lactate (35, 36, 57–59). This expansion occurred with new recognition elements (e.g., ionophores) that were added to membranes, use of enzymes as an additional recognition element, and the combination of multiple selective membranes in layers. Enzymes added to the membrane allow for selectivity to metabolites such as urea, lactate, creatinine, and glucose (57). For example, in the detection of urea the primary analyte recognition can be accomplished with enzymatic cleavage to ammonium ion; then, secondary detection can be accomplished with an ammonium-selective membrane. First discovered in 1969, ionophores are macromolecular structures that are used as recognition elements for ions and are applied to membranes for selective detection of metals (62). Neutral molecules used as recognition elements for molecules such as creatinine are now being applied as they have been discovered, and molecules as small as water can be selectively passed through channels in structures (63, 64).

Application of immunological recognition of antigens with antibodies has been a key advance, and has allowed the POCT menu of tests to be greatly expanded to include assays for drugs, hormones, proteins, and pathogens. These support the diagnosis of a number of conditions such as ovulation, cardiac risk assessment, and the detection of infections, cancer, and other diseases (65, 66). There are various immunoassay methods that could be applied to handheld devices, such as microparticle capture immunoassay, latex agglutination inhibition, solid-phase immunochromatography, enzyme immunoassay, fluoroimmunoassay, luminescence immunoassay, rare earth metals–labeled immunoassay, and optical color label assay with labels such as colored latex particles and colloidal gold (26, 65–66). Electrochemical signal transducers based on amperometric, impedimetric, and potentiometric detection methods have similarly been proposed (50, 67, 68). Optical motion detection of immunoassay has been explored for assays such as thyroid stimulating hormone but as an immunoassay detection technology, they are limited by sensitivity (39).

Most handheld systems for immunoassay use similar basic technology with some variation. Solid-phase immunoassays are commonly based on the immunochromatography format (65, 69). In general, the immunochromatography reaction takes place in one or more layers, which constitutes several reagent and reaction zones. The main reaction takes place in the test or capture zone, typically a nitrocellulose membrane (69). In the layers prior to the capture zone, an analyte-specific antibody reacts with the analyte in the sample zone and is chromatographically transferred to the nitrocellulose membrane. The first antibody, typically bound to colored latex particles as a signal label, is initially impregnated in the sample zone (e.g., by printing); the sample contains the analyte, which binds to the labeled antibody. In the capture zone, a second antibody is immobilized (typically covalently coupled) in a band and captures particles when the analyte is present (effectively the analyte forms a sandwich of the two antibody reagents). The presence of analyte creates a test line in the test band area and a signal is produced (Figure 2-2). Excess labeled antibody can also continue to migrate along the solid phase and be captured by an immoblized antispecies antibody, creating a second signal line. This is used as an internal quality control check to indicate that the device has worked.

Immunochromatographic devices have been designed for urine, whole blood, plasma, saliva, and other specimens by changes to pretreatment and condition steps or materials prior to the capture zone. Pretreatment steps that require the operator

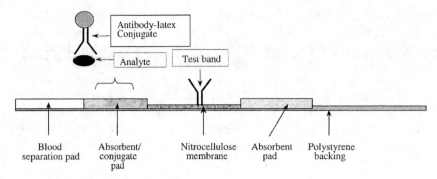

Figure 2-2 Immunochromatographic assay format with porous matrix.

to manipulate the specimen by mixing with other fluids or handling other parts in addition to the strip are less preferred. Optical signal generation is also preferred, because of a lack of interference, washing or treatment steps, and high sensitivity. An example of this sensitivity is the TropT® assay developed by Roche Diagnostics (Mannheim, Germany) for the cardiac biomarker Troponin T, which has a detection limit of 0.05 μg/L (16 pmol/L) in whole blood (70, 71).

In principle, the immunoassay format can be either heterogeneous, which requires a separation step, or homogeneous, without separation; these generally constitute noncompetitive and competitive formats respectively. For heterogeneous assays, solid phases can be used to separate bound antigen from free antigen and can include plastic wells, tubes, capillaries, membranes, latex particles, and magnetic particles. Capture antibodies are attached to the solid phases. Antibodies can also be attached or conjugated or labeled with signal reagents that directly or indirectly produce detectable responses. Strong affinity labels such as streptavidin and biotin are often used to enhance capture phases. An immunoassay can also use multiple and different antibodies in a variety of manners (e.g., by immobilization onto different areas of the solid phase; and the use of more than one label to create a multianalyte assay). Some devices available can perform multiple assays on one specimen. The Triage™ Panel for eight different drug classes or for four different cardiac markers (72, 73) are two examples (Biosite Diagnostics, San Diego, CA, USA). CARDIAC STATus™ from Spectral Diagnostics (Toronto, Ontario, CAN) can detect myoglobin, troponin I, and creatine kinase isoenzymes in one handheld device (30).

The homogeneous format is best suited for hapten detection. In addition, this format can be used for a large molecule, when the presence of very high levels of the analyte may lead to a hook effect and an erroneous result. An example of a homogeneous format is the DCA 2000 assay for hemoglobin A_{1C} (HbA$_{1C}$; Bayer Diagnostics, Tarrytown, NY, USA) which is primarily designed for diabetics to detect changes in glycated protein as a measure of glucose control (31).

Fluidic Technology (Fluidics)

Fluidics primarily minimize the steps in a POCT device and increase ease of use. Analytical procedures typically require

multiple steps such as sample and reagent metering, sample dilution, sample conditioning, and converting the analyte to prepare it for subsequent reactions (e.g., use of a reagent; removing interfering components; mixing reagents; lysing cells; capturing biological molecules; enabling enzymatic reactions; and enabling incubation for binding events, staining, or deposition) These steps may be carried out before, during, or after the metering of the sample from the primary specimen, or after metering but before carrying out reactions that provide a measure of the analyte.

Fluidic processes or designs can be categorized by the absorbent, flow-through, lateral flow, cassette, capillary, tubing, or centrifugal system that is used in the device (73–76) (Table 2-3). Fluidic designs can contain materials for analysis of one or more specimens, and multiple analytes may be detected per specimen (16, 30, 36). The fluidic elements are typically single-use and intended to be disposable after use. Consequently, to the extent possible they are made of inexpensive materials, while being compatible with the reagents and the samples that are to be analyzed. In most instances, the element is made of a combination of hydrophilic and hydrophobic substrates. These include a long list of polymers (e.g., polycarbonate, polystyrene, polyacrylate, polyurethene) as well as natural fibers, silicates, glass, waxes, and metal foils (77). Techniques have expanded not only the substrates that can be used but also to the number of packaging techniques that keep the ingredients stored in their most active form. This typically means keeping water vapor out, either by sealing or

Table 2-3   Key Elements of Fluidics Systems Employed in POCT Handheld Devices

Fluidics	Types
Format	Absorbent, flow-through, lateral flow, cassette, capillary, tubing, centrifugal system
Matrix	Papers, plastic, membranes and films
Flow propulsion	Adsorption, chromatographic, capillary action, centrifugal force, pumping, vacuum, electro-osmosis, heating, mechanical

desiccation, or keeping the ingredients from migrating within or out of the device. The formulation of dry reagents has been one of the fundamental developments that aided the evolution of stable POCT reagent and calibration systems.

Fluidic handling of specimens and reagents by clinical analyzers in the hospital laboratory allows greater flexibility than is possible in a handheld POCT device; the concentration and treatment steps would inconvenience the user. Fluidic handling can occur through flow propulsion, most simply by chromatographic or capillary actions, or alternatively by centrifugal force, pumping, vacuum, electro-osmosis, or by heating; although the last five actions are generally more costly. This allows liquids to be moved from one region of the device to another as required for the analysis being carried out.

Moving chemical and biological reagents (through absorbence and drying) into a matrix (e.g., paper) was one of the first fluidic technologies to drive the evolution of POCT devices (78, 79). Absorbent substrates or carriers can include polymers, glass, wetting agents, and other additives. Membranes and films can also serve as absorbent substrates. In general, the specimen or treated specimen enters the matrix through pores and is absorbed. This absorbance allows mixing and metering to occur. The earliest forms of dry reagent paper strips were Clinistix®, introduced in 1956 for urine (51), and Dextrostix® (both Miles-Ames, now Bayer Diagnostics), introduced in 1966 for blood glucose analysis. A series of blood chemistries were then developed, such as Ektachem® (Kodak, now Johnson and Johnson, Rochester, NY, USA), AccuMeter® (Accu-Tech, LLC, Vista, CA, USA), Vision® (Abbott Laboratories, Abbott Park, IL, USA), Reflotron® (Boehringer, now Roche Diagnostics, Mannheim, Germany), and the Seralyzer® instrument (Miles-Ames, now Bayer Diagnostics) (4, 78, 79). Examples of reactive agents now included in the matrix are dyes, enzyme substrates, antigens, nucleic acids, antibodies, ionophores, intercalators, enzymes, proteins, and peptides, along with a host of secondary chemicals used for polymers, activators, and surfactants.

Absorbant substrates can be used in a format to move fluid vertically along a strip or cassette base (Figure 2-1). This principle of lateral flow has been especially useful for chromatographic separation in immunoassay strips (65, 69) and has also been applied to chemistry by immobilization of an enzyme or reagent and by passage of sample through reagent pads such as the cholesterol esterase and oxidase in the AccuTech product (80). The fluidic flow is dependent on a series of factors, including pore size, surfactant, and selection of substrate materials (81–83). The substrates can also be included in a flow-through format that moves fluid through the center of a device as in the Vision product. An example of a flow-through separation is the removal of erythrocytes and white cells from a whole blood sample, allowing only plasma to move forward for testing (4).

Use of multiple matrices allows a chemical reagent to be placed into distinct areas provided for reaction steps such as filtration, timed chemical reactions, and removal of interference (84). The first matrix layer at the point of sample application must overlap or lie adjacent (abut) the next matrix layer, providing for transfer of the fluid through the area. Migration can be driven by a matrix pad that takes up the excess specimen. Stacking matrix layers, as in films such as Ektachem, allow multiple separating, spreading, and color-forming layers to enhance colors; this also enables the incorporation of incompatible reagents into the same device.

The majority of disposable devices now use a cassette format to hold reagents and to interface with or connect the specimen to the reagent and to the measurement system. The cassettes also serve as holders for multiple matrix layers to allow adequate pressure points. The Triage Immunocassette Panel for Drugs of Abuse enables 10-min testing for up to eight of the most commonly overdosed prescription and illicit drugs (Figure 2-3). Devices for both B-type natriuretic peptide and a panel of cardiac muscle damage markers use a similar cassette format to hold reagents (72, 85). The Pharmanetic's coagulation tests are based on optical motion principles, with magnetic particles in a dry reagent cassette.

Reagents are more often dried into the matrix sensors, but can be applied directly onto the fluidic cassette. Cassettes are typically molded plastic with some form of surface treatment to allow compatibility with reagents. The Bayer HbA1c DCA 2000, Cholestech GDX™, and LDX (Cholestech, Hayward, CA, USA) are immunoassay, chemistry, and enzymatic assay systems that use fluidic cassettes (31, 86) (Figure 2-4). The cassette is typically inserted into a reader and may be manipulated by movement, heat, or other conditions to aid fluidic movements. Metrika's NTX bone-resorption test (Metrika, Sunnyvale, CA, USA) is an example of a cassette that also

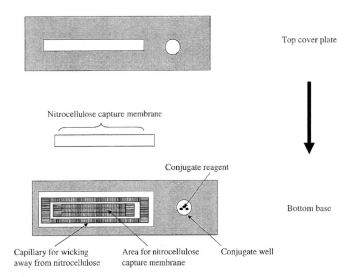

Figure 2-3 Immunofluidic cassette with external dilution solution: The Triage Panel for eight different drug classes (Biosite Diagnostics, San Diego, CA, USA) is represented as an example. The cassette also serves as a holder for nitrocellulose layers to allow adequate pressure points and has capillaries molded into the base to allow the solution to wick out of the capture phase and into the bottom base. The sample is mixed with a dry reagent in a well and the user then pipettes it onto the nitrocellulose along with a liquid to develop a color.

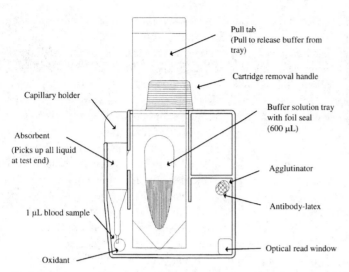

Figure 2-4 Immunofluidic cassette with internal dilution solution: The DCA 2000 hemoglobin A_{1c} reagent cartridge is represented as an example of a fully integrated fluidic cassette. The user adds the capillary holder for the specimen into the cartridge, then releases liquid reagent solution by pulling a tab. Liquid reagent, antibodies, and other reagents are dried onto the cartridge, and the specimen is mixed through a series of mechanical movements performed by the reader until the detection signal is generated.

contains electronic, optics, and display to facilitate production of the result (87). Finally, the cassette serves as the containment vessel for the specimen after use An example of a blood gas and electrolyte cassette is the i-STAT electrochemical-based reader, which uses a fluidic cassette (35, 36).

Capillaries have long been used as a disposable format in both optical and electrochemical sensors. A microcuvette can be a capillary cavity, which collects a fixed amount of specimen and contains reagents deposited on its inner walls. The blood sample is drawn into the cavity by capillary action and spontaneously mixed with the reagents. The B-Hemoglobin Test System (Hemocue, Angelholm, Sweden) is an example of a microcuvette for hemoglobin and glucose that is placed into the portable analyzer to give a value on a display screen in <1 min (27, 88).

Movement of liquids through capillaries is dependent on the nature of the fluid, the geometry of the capillary, and the surface energy of the materials used (69, 75–79). Movement of liquids through the capillaries is usually prevented by capillary stops. There are several ways in which the capillaries and sample wells can be formed, such as injection molding, laser ablation, diamond milling, embossing, printing, and layering. Layering, printing, and molding are often preferred in order to reduce the cost of the device. Capillary networks were first identified in designs applicable to POCT devices as fluidic formats in 1975 (89). Generally, a base portion of the device will create the desired geometry of sample well and capillaries. After reagent compounds have been placed in the wells, then a top portion will be attached over the base to complete the capillary.

Tubing for fluidics can be included in a cartridge with electrochemical or other sensors. This type of system typically has two parts, the fluidic cartridges and the analyzer. The cartridges can include a calibrant solution, sample handling system, waste chamber, and heating elements. For example, blood gas and electrolyte systems can package all of the solutions, valves, and tubing into one continuous-use cartridge (33–34, 57–59). Each cartridge can perform a set number of tests, packaged in a contained unit, and inserted directly into the analyzer. Each cartridge also includes the sensors and carrier information regarding the maintenance and calibration. The analyzer allows active pumping of the sample and reagent mixture back and forth through an aperture in the cartridges to allow timing control and direction.

Many devices have had several types of fluidics applied; for example, the use of dry reagents (37–40) and a cassette containing a molded capillary (43) in coagulation testing. The devices that are more quantitative have often used liquids as diluents, autocalibrants, and wash solutions. This is particularly true with analytes requiring measurement over a wide continuous range or without large separations between clinical decisions (positives and negatives). In many cases, POCT blood chemistry analyzers also require CLIA-waived status (highest degree of accuracy with essentially error-free use). Liquid reagent containing device systems can be factory calibrated as well and yet can automatically treat specimens with the liquids needed to reduce matrix effects and improve accuracy. An example of these POCT systems is the HbA_{1c} assay system on the DCA 2000+® Analyzer (Figure 2-4).

Recent trends toward microfluidics are creating miniaturized measurement devices such as micrototal analysis systems, biological microelectromechanical systems, or lab-on-a chip devices by a variety of companies for application outside of POCT (90–92). Through the use of micrometer-scale geometries, these systems have one or more channels of <1 mm and are produced by a variety of microfabrication techniques. These devices perform operations such as mixing, presenting arrays of reagents (e.g., capture antibodies, multiplexing, amplification, multichanneling, separation, reaction pumping, gating, and signal evaluation) (93–97). Multistep microfluidic designs are possible for complex clinical diagnostic assays and are being provided by several companies for potential application in POCT.

Signal Reading (Transduction)

A transducer must read the reagent signal, translate it into numerical output, and provide output to the user. The device transducer captures the signal, processes the signal to a digital result, and displays the output. The output can be printed, displayed, or sent to a networked device.

The signals that handheld POCT devices are most capable of reading are either electrochemical or optical (Table 2-4). Optical readers require a light source, a means of wavelength selection, a detector, and an optical system to deliver light to and from the sample to the detector. The optical system may be imaging when exact spatial resolution is required. However,

Table 2-4 Types of Transducers Employed in POCT Handheld Devices

Transducers	Types
Signal engine	Optical, electrochemical, magnetic
Component	Microprocessors, buttons, printer, case, table, power board
Electronic displays	LED, graphic display, LCD, touch screen
Connectivity	Serial ports, USB, Ethernet card, wireless

many systems have taken advantage of the advances in non-imaging optics. Depending on the angle of incidence and detection as well as the surface character of the media, reflectance measures light reflected off a surface that is either specular or diffuse. Transmission is a measure of incident light passing through a media. Reflectance and transmission can be linearly related to concentration by the use of a relation like the Kubelka-Munk equation or used as a percentage of a usable range. In all cases, the changes are measured at the absorbing wavelength, calibrated against white or transparent standards, and often corrected by nonabsorbing wavelengths. Electrochemical readers require only a means of reading a voltage or current.

Signals are amplified and processed by the main electronic circuit board, and translated into numerical output. Microprocessors have decreased in size and cost, and memory has increased in capacity as the technology has evolved (e.g., the number of transistors on a microprocessor doubles every 18 months). This has led to increased speed, decreased board size, and increased memory, allowing more calculations and outputs. Electronic displays have improved from difficult-to-read, passive light liquid-crystal displays (LCDs) to high-resolution, backlit, or light-emitting diode (LED) displays. Also, the ability of the user to enter data into the device has significantly improved from mechanically activated switches to touch screens. Connectivity has advanced from low-speed RS232 serial ports to high-speed universal serial bus (USB) and Internet interfaces. Specimen and patient information has progressed from key entry to magnetic-card or barcode entry. In addition, reagent or consumable lot calibration can be read off the disposable unit by many devices—although the obvious goal is achieving minimal lot-to-lot variation.

Glucose meters were the first instruments to be made at a sufficiently low cost and ease of use to allow general POCT, even home use. This first became possible with Miles Laboratories' Ames Reflectance Meter, introduced in 1966, when analyzers used reflectance photometry with dry reagent. In 1981, the meter progressed to the low-cost digital components (Glucometer®, Bayer Diagnostics, Elkart, IN, USA). Glucose devices of today have almost entirely replaced the optical-based instruments of 20 years ago that required considerable operator intervention (7).

Today's meters can provide more than just glucose concentration measurement by inclusion of additional features such as sampling, temperature control, reagent feed, and automatic controls. Also, meters have extended the range of analytes measured with transduction immunoassay reactions such as the reflectance refractometers (98, 99). Metrika's A1cNow Monitor uses miniaturized digital electronics, a mini-LCD, microoptics, and solid-state chemistries to provide a handheld single-use instrument for measurement by immunochromatography of HbA$_{1C}$ (Figure 2-5). They all transduce color into a result by using a collection cartridge that is placed into, or is part of, the instrument. Signal readers have continued to evolve to include more features such as greater accuracy, data documentation, and graphical user interfaces, thus, removing the subjectivity of traditional methods such as visual reading.

Analytical Processing (Enabler)

Devices provide threshold or quantitative results from the signal detected by the transducer. First, the signal is converted by an enabler system into a result that a patient and/or healthcare professional can understand. Next, the result is sent to a graphics display, a printer, or exported to an information network or system. Examples of enablers are operating systems, algorithms, data management, and method performance parameters (Table 2-5). Typically, enablers are written into software code, but they can also be included into chip sets.

Operating systems are typically low-cost and low-level programs that run on flash chips However, they are evolving to use standard software packages like those found in handheld computers or personal data assistants (PDAs; e.g., Windows CE and Palm OS) as the cost of these systems decrease. The

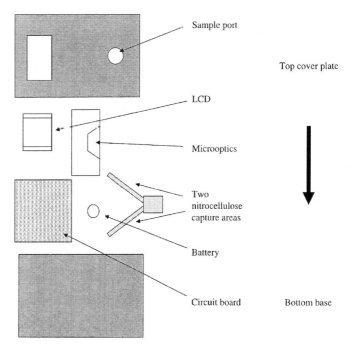

Figure 2-5 Immunofluidic cassette enclosed in reader: the Metrika Now Monitor hemoglobin A$_{1c}$ analyzer is represented as an example of a cassette containing electronics, optics, and display for the result. The specimen must be mixed with liquid reagent in a separate vial, incubated, and added to the specimen application port.

Table 2-5 Examples of the Enablers Used in POCT Handheld Devices

Enablers	Types
Operation systems	ALU, compiled C code, computer OS
Algorithms	Data processing, communication, signal-to-noise reduction, measurement calibration, data distribution
Data management	Held, directed, stored, recalled
Parameters	Lot correction, reference agreement, calibration, error trapping, calculation factor, error budget

operating system communicates with and controls the hardware and devices of the transducer by interaction with a series of operations, drivers, functions, and routines. Programming languages conduct numerical analyses using algorithms.

Algorithms are for data processing, communication, signal-to-noise reduction, measurement, calibration, and data distribution. Algorithms convert the data through a series of calculations into various levels and forms leading to the final result. Data must be managed throughout the process by being held, directed, stored and recalled. Parameters are factors, set-points, and other calibration information. The complexity of enablers has increased along with the demands on calibration, error trapping, and increased output- and input-device options. The number of parameter set-points has increased from tens to thousands over the past 20 years, because the complexity of device qualification has increased.

Setting parameters allow calibration by the manufacturer. They are based on agreement to a reference point while accounting for as many sources of errors as possible. The dynamic range of the detector is centered on the clinical decision threshold to allow optimal decision making. The parameters are entered at the time of manufacture and are sometimes adjusted to account for detector lot differences. Thereafter, the transducer automatically self-adjusts via the enabler during first-time power-up and during each assay. In the event the system is unable to make appropriate internal adjustments, an error message is displayed.

In practice, parameter setting is not as straightforward as just described (72, 100). Before judging how the device meets decision limits and reference ranges, the reference methods and solution must be selected, which are typically quantitative but not always. Standardization among older devices has reduced the complexity but does not always address underlying problems. Threshold decision limits can be applied to analytes with well-established clinical decision limits, based on large outcomes studies (e.g., albuminuria, human chorionic gonadotropin, drugs of abuse in urine) and have well-defined separations between positive and negative test results (54, 72, 99). Quantitative tests are more often applied to analytes that require measuring of the specific levels present over a continuous range of values (e.g., glucose, therapeutic drug monitoring,

HbA1c) or having smaller separations between decision levels (e.g., cholesterol risk assessment) (6, 31, 42, 86, 101).

Parameters attempt to correct for as many sources of analytical variation as possible. Typically device performance accounts for worst-case scenarios such as reagent performance aging, poor testing environments, potential misuse, and interference. Performance is proven in elaborate validation schemes. When detectors are stored and used properly, acceptable performance (up to the expiration date) is ensured. Lot-specific calibration number or coding numbers are factors used in the standard curve to increase accuracy and are derived from characterization of manufacturing lots. The use of calibration solutions reduces the ease of use, provides additional sources of analytical error (the process of doing calibration) and does not provide greater accuracy potential. Lot-specific calibration cannot offer as much user control of accuracy and requires far greater analysis, characterization, and process control by the manufacturer. Factory calibration uses tight process controls specified by the manufacturer for the device; each lot released undergoes a thorough analysis and characterization.

DESIGN APPROACHES USED FOR POCT HANDHELD DEVICES

Designing new devices requires approaches that must handle many constraints represented by the system performance requirements to allow the device to meet clinical requirements. Meeting these requirements demonstrates how technologies can be designed into the device to minimize operator errors, ensure quality, and meet the needs of patients. Detector, fluidic, transducer, and enabler technologies play key roles in defining the design approach. Together they are considered a system. The closer that a technology component is able to meet design constraints, the easier the design approach. Some typical solutions are discussed in this section.

Preventing Errors

Errors that are prevented can be grouped as sample, component, operator, and performance. Sample errors can be preanalytical or interference-related, whereas operator errors can be procedural or accidental. Component errors can be stability or failure-related, whereas performance errors can be accuracy or bias-related. Choice of the detection and fluidic technology is the first step to reduce or prevent these errors, and transducer and enablers can offer solutions in cases of limitations.

The collection, handling, and storing of specimens in clinical analysis creates a preanalytical dependency on how specimens should be handled. Criteria defined for laboratory analyses will generally apply to POCT devices. Choice of the detection methods can reduce sensitivity to accommodate sample storage; for example, an immunoassay might use an antibody that is not dependent on an unstable protein conformation to work (102). In general, all devices are manufactured to ensure stability for specimens stored over several hours at room temperature, days for refrigeration, and months for freezing.

Even for a detection method, unstable analytes can present problems A minimum response time can be required for a fresh sample. However, the fresh time can refer to hours in the case of an organism or seconds in the case of a fingerstick. Choice of fluidics can increase the fresh time window by acting as a collection, purification, and storage device. Examples include extraction solutions used to test for infectious diseases such as *Helicobacter pylori, Influenza A/B,* infectious mononucleosis, and group A β-hemolytic streptococci (103). In whole-blood testing, often a separation of plasma from cells eliminates irrelevant signals and instabilities from cellular material such as hemoglobin (104). One fluidic example is the use of a trapping layer placed directly over the signal-generating layer.

In general, every effort is made to ensure that a device will offer complete or sufficient resistance to interference, but it is not always possible to achieve this due to the detection method or fluidics used. Several methods are used to obtain a reasonable protection from common biological components, detergents, preservatives, matrix affects, and drugs. Interference can be destroyed by reactions in the detector, as in urinalysis and glucose-testing systems (16, 105). Fluidic designs prevent interference in the specimen from migrating to a signal-generating layer through a trap in a pretreatment layer. Treatment with a diluent is also a common solution to this problem (31, 72, 73). Although the potential for device interference is usually known and mentioned in the labeling, contamination of specimens with any additive may affect results and should be avoided.

Operator error can be procedural or accidental. Procedural errors increase if the device is technique-dependent. Two key ergonomic factors are the placement of specimen into the reactor matrix and of the reactor matrix in the transducer. The use of calibration numbers, calibration solutions, sample treatment steps, and multistep instructions are all factors in whether a device is prone to procedural errors. The device can be designed to minimize errors by using detection and fluidic technology that require the user to perform only one step; the other steps are incorporated into the device. Glucose systems provide evidence of this, which includes being able to obtain results directly from a fingerstick, to autocalibration of the device and elimination of precise volume measurement (106).

Accidental errors are often not obvious to the laboratory professional but occur with untrained lay users, many of whom are not familiar with electronics and lack understanding of analysis and clinical results. Error trapping and alarm reporting help to minimize impact, but built-in tolerances are often needed as repeat error messages reduce the usefulness of the device Tolerances reflect a built-in safety. For example, an immunochromatography cassette minimizes the effect on sample handling by allowing overfills and flagging errors for underfills (73).

Component errors due to instability or failure must be prevented in design. Stability of the detector and fluidics must be ensured over the shelf life of the device and the defined storage condition requirement. This can be accomplished either by minimizing any change in the consumables or by correcting

for the change. Instability errors are typically invisible to the lay user until the product reaches a critical environment or age. Many ingredients and materials are used to solve instability (78, 79).

Failure errors are prevented by simplicity in instructions and operation. Specimen application and placement of the disposable into the analyzer must be operator-independent. Read-times are typically set for convenience but not all detectors are read-time independent. Specimen application must prevent crossover, carryover between tests, and leaching of reagent out of the device. Prolonged exposure to the sample can leach chemical from the reagent, which can produce an aberrant result. Instrument contamination due to sample carryover and between-detector crossover can be avoided by designing an instrument that cleans completely and does not hold contamination introduced into the device.

Factory calibration procedures can reduce accuracy problems. At the time of manufacture, calibration solutions with known concentrations of each analyte are introduced to the sensors and the signals are then stored as set-points. When a patient sample is analyzed, the analyzer compares the signal obtained from the calibration solution to the signal from the patient's sample and calculates the analyte concentration. Reusable sensors can use live calibration prior to testing; disposable sensors use representatives out of a batch to characterize the lot. Most handheld devices must produce a numerical result with some degree of accuracy and minimal bias affecting the clinical decision limit. Bias is inherent to the detection method and specimen variation or matrix effects (e.g., hematocrit effects). Dilution steps eliminate matrix effects in all cases (31). The degree of accuracy as defined by the range around the average number can also vary with the fluidic and detection method. Thus, to increase accuracy a device can be prewarmed so testing can proceed at a set temperature.

Assurance of Quality

Quality defines the essential performance requirements, and compliance with the protocol assures standardization. This is accomplished by three methods: (a) control systems, (b) checks, and (c) compliance. These three methods ensure that requirements are met when the device reaches the market. Development approaches for new devices apply some form of these methods, depending on the design. Technology is used to overcome the constraints that may be recognized in a system, or in the sample. As an example, the results produced by the early blood glucose testing systems were influenced by the hematocrit of the sample—a problem that does not exist in the majority of the more modern devices.

Control systems are used for assurance of claims. Release limits are set for large-scale manufacturing lots, which are based on calibration settings in instruments. These settings allow claims and account for variations in the overall system Variations between lots, operators, days, and specimens as well as in stability are typically used. Release of meters and reagents is performed with factory-designated calibration reagents. In-lot calibration control system characteristics (defined by the manufacturing lot) are entered into the instrument by assignment numbers. The transducer identifies the test to be performed by reading the code (electronic signature or barcode) on each disposable unit. In total control systems, the process to make the detector and transducer is held tighter than the requirements, or lot variations are small in comparison to specimen variations.

Checks are examples of safety controls that are now included in the device. This ensures that the device has not failed in its the ability to store quality-control data, information relating to date and time of operation, and operator and specimen identification. To counteract the effects of color-blindness, differences in reading method, and interpretation of color, checks are part of the trend toward instrument reading of the reaction and away from subjective visual color-reading. Remote control checks of devices outside of the central clinical laboratory are a new trend. Other systems now lock out the user every 24 h unless a quality-control function is completed. Control samples, either real or electronically simulated, are used as checks in a given time period. Immunochromatography strips are a good example of an application of checks for false results in the detector (70). Negative-control lines are used to ensure the reagent is present, whereas a positive-control line confirms the reagent is reactive to analyte. Fluidics-control lines are used to verify correct flow through the device.

Compliance to standards allows greater quality of results and safety across manufacturers. Standards such as for safety, performance, medical decision limits, clinical and laboratory practice, and others are considered along with processes such as risk analysis, traceability and good development practices; together they ensure that a certain level of work was applied for approval. Standards for electrical discharge, dangerous reagents, sampling device or lancet, and environmentally friendly disposal of the analytical consumables are accounted for in device designs.

User Requirements

Convenience of use is a fundamental user requirement. One measure of convenience is the minimization of training or periodic retraining. Others include avoiding multiple steps for activation, seamless calibration, quality control, data entry, sample presentation, result reading, and data transfer to maintenance. Durability is another absolute requirement, and the fragility of the device is controlled by designs that account for display screen stability, drop test, reliability tests, and accelerated use-testing. High instrument cost or disposable expenses reduce the effectiveness of the design to compete with the laboratory-based service. Physical size and weight requirements are important, as working space for the device is always limited.

Requirements are dependent upon what technology can achieve, what the user generally accepts, what is best-in-class, or what is possible within a generation. Today, glucose meters are as small as the smallest PDA, whereas the majority of blood gas meters are still benchtop size. This discrepancy may be explained in part by the complexity of the blood gas

technology and the fact that they are generally reusable systems that are used to measure a relatively large number of specimens each day. In some clinical settings, a handheld device is ideal, whereas in others a benchtop system may be more useful (e.g., a multianalyte device in the emergency room or primary care physician's office). Another effort to meet user requirements is to keep the time to result to a minimum. In cases where there is a requirement for high sensitivity, accuracy must not be compromised at the expense of size and timing, particularly in critical care devices (57–59). Data entry, management, and transfer are increasingly important requirements that have become essential as technology has allowed standards of class to progress.

DEVICE EXAMPLES

Nine cases of devices are described to illustrate the principles and the importance of design concepts (Table 2-6). It is not the purpose of this chapter to describe all devices or to compare performance, but to use key systems to increase understanding of the design concepts in common use. General lists of products represented by the case example have been compiled in several reviews (7).

The examples are split among the three types of devices and span the variety of detector, fluidic, transducer, and enabler technologies used. Type 1 examples include glucose meters for strips or sensors, urinalysis strips, immunochromatography devices, and flow-through devices. Type 2 examples include microcuvette immunoassay, blood gas and electrolyte cassette, fluidic cassette, and coagulation cassette. Type 3 examples include immunoassay surface-responsive devices.

Often, design is as constrained by the selection of detector and fluidic technologies as it is by the requirements. Although transducer and enabler technologies offer solutions, in some cases an overall system will still face constraints. Flexibility of the systems can be evaluated when comparing the typical performance and the limitations they possess.

Performance Characteristics

There are several tools that have been developed to check the performance of devices within a particular class. Device types that have been on the market longer (>20 years) generally have greater compliance with the standardization procedures and tools than newer devices, which are often left to be assessed by the manufacturer, receive mixed reports on performance, or lack standards for performance checks.

Several good performance standards are available for glucose meters (107). The Clarke plot assesses and rates performance by risk areas. For example, meter errors that could lead to hypoglycemia are given more weight. Although it would be easier to just recommend a level of imprecision across the range for blood glucose (e.g., CV < 10%), there needs to be greater detail to support how this is determined and measured. For example, a device may meet the stated imprecision overall but fail at a critical decision point. This type of risk assessment is necessary for almost all devices.

Table 2-6 Detection and Fluidic Methods Used in Device Examples

Example	Signal detection method		Fluidic method		
	Signal generation	Recognition	Format	Matrix	Flow propulsion
Glucose meter	Electrochemical (amperometric, potentiometric) Optical detection (catalytic)	Catalytic reactions (enzyme substrate, catalysis reaction product)	Absorbent, flow-through, capillary	Paper, plastic, membranes, films	Adsorption, capillary action
Urine multiple strip	Optical detection (indicators, catalytic)	Indicators (direct conjugation, ion pairing, hydrophobic binding) Catalytic reactions (enzyme substrate, enzyme detection, catalysis reaction product, inhibitor detection)	Absorbent	Paper	Adsorption
Immuno-chromatography	Optical detection (catalytic, particles)	Association host (antibodies, selective membranes, macromolecule)	Lateral flow, cassette	Paper, membranes	Chromatography
Flow-through	Optical detection (catalytic and particles)	Association host (antibodies, selective membranes, macromolecules)	Flow-through, cassette	Paper, membranes	Adsorption
Microcuvette	Optical detection (direct, indicators, catalytic)	Indicators (direct conjugation) Catalytic reactions (catalysis reaction product)	Capillary, cassette	Plastic	Capillary action
Immunofluidic cassette	Optical detection (catalytic and particles)	Association host (antibodies, selective membranes, macromolecule)	Cassette	Plastic	Capillary action, centrifugal, pumping, vacuum, mechanical
Blood gas and electrolyte cassette	Electrochemical (amperometric, potentiometric)	Association host (selective membranes, macromolecules)	Cassette, capillary, tubing	Plastic, membranes, films	Pumping, vacuum, heating, mechanical
Coagulation cassette	Optical motion (nanoparticles, paramagnetic particles, interference pattern)	Catalytic reactions (enzyme substrate, enzyme detection, catalysis reaction product)	Lateral flow, cassette	Paper, plastic	Chromatography capillary action
Immuno–wave guide	Surface induction (surface enhancement, pattern recognition)	Association host (antibodies, macromolecules)	Cassette, fiber, surface	Plastic, inorganic	Pumping, pipetting

Almost all devices have performance characteristics that are given more weight to allow optimal performance to be achieved at critical decision points. Thus, urinalysis strips, drug-of-abuse testing devices, pregnancy tests, and devices for cholesterol, HbA_{1C}, cardiac panels, blood gas, and infectious disease markers all have defined decision levels and claim criteria. To understand the differences in performance within a class, it is necessary to understand the various approaches used to assess them. Imprecision is often suggested and disputed as the method (107). Threshold tests often use negative and positive agreement at a defined claim level and degree of uncertainty based on a medical decision limit (72). Performance in the hands of lay users compared to professional users is often part of the criteria used (108), since such differences clearly exist (109). In general, it is the design team and opinion leaders who develop standards for performance before choosing and designing a device.

Limitations of Devices

The design cases can be used to illustrate the limitations of certain technologies and the importance that these characteristics may have across the range of users. For example, a limitation might not exclude utility to a physician in a particular case, but it might present a problem to a patient (e.g., a child) This should be considered by the POCT administrator and steps should be taken to ensure that the operation of the device is properly explained to the patient. Issues can often be discussed more effectively in terms of the performance characteristic rather than according to the technologies. The three key performance factors are sample integrity, operator usage, and design.

Sample Integrity. Correct patient and sample identification, sample age, viscosity, cell lysis, timing of collection, and collection procedure are all factors that can limit the successful use of the device. Degradation or deterioration of the analyte will interfere with accurate detection unless prescribed sample storage conditions are followed. Interference from contaminating substances and naturally occurring biological constituents also occur (110). Interference can be addressed by either signal generation, recognition, and fluidic methods to remove interference or by instrument compensation using the transducer or enablers (111).

Operator Usage. Inexperienced users and procedural issues can limit the success of a device. Technique dependencies such as multiple steps needed to get a result, critical timings, and sample volumes can cause operator-to-operator variation (e.g., occurrence of bias). Stringent storage and operating conditions for consumables and systems also increase the risk of bias; for example, the need for prewarming of refrigerated ingredients can lead to errors, especially when an urgent result is required. Minimizing maintenance and training requirements by engineering out operator-dependent steps can help to decrease operator errors. Reducing the risk of cross contamination can be addressed by considering all of the components of a device that the specimen is able to touch (e.g., optical windows, electrical contact points, tables, drawers) Strategic placement or protection of critical areas away from the specimen can minimize these types of errors.

Considerations such as temperature, air conditioning, high humidity, poor lighting, altitude, and storage are usually accounted for at the design stage in order to increase the consumable shelf life, and to a lesser extent, to reduce operator error. However, there have still been instances in which device performance has been shown to decline when used outside the clinical laboratory environment (112–114). Certain devices are less prone to decline due to minimal requirements for training, minimal procedural steps, reduced specimen handling requirements, and convenient operation conditions (115).

Design. Design is critical to how limited a device will be and it can directly affect the variation in performance seen between devices, specimens, and operators. The analytical approach used, the number of operator steps involved, and the use of onboard calibration and quality control will all need to be considered in the light of the performance criteria set for the test, as well as knowledge of the environment in which the test is going to be used. Each class and design has best- or worst-case limits of performance as well as performance characteristics for sample integrity and operator usage. Thus, a different design might be considered for a device to be used in the home, versus the paramedical vehicle, the emergency room, the operating room, and the outpatient clinic or doctor's office.

Glucose-meter systems present an example where the device can be affected by sample integrity depending on the fluidics and signal generation technology used. Thus, the system performance can be affected by hematocrit, hemolysis, differences between plasma and blood, and oxygen tension depending on the design (104, 116). In the case of glucose devices, the catalytic reaction chosen defines the oxygen dependence. Oxygen-independent systems with minimal reaction times are characteristics of the best designs available today. Glucose systems can also have operator-dependent issues with regard to sample volume (107). Devices that are resistant to underfills, overfills, and time delays have less dependence on technique. The number of parts and pieces that a user has to handle also increases the chances for operator-induced errors. Thus, autocalibration, autosensor presentation, and disposable units are all features of best-of-class systems.

Although sample integrity can lead to erroneous results, it is possible to minimize these effects by specific changes to the fluidics. Thus, in the case of the urinalysis strip, the sample serves as solvent and dilution is not possible; therefore, specimen-to-specimen differences can be large and dependent on the indicators and catalytic reagents used for detection. Newer methods have taken into account the potential specimen interference, with a consequent reduction in errors (16, 54). The lack of sample processing (dilution or washing) limits these tests to the detection of analytes at defined threshold limits (e.g., $\geq$ or $\leq$). These types of semiquantitative or yes/no tests can be very predictive at the limits, but are not quantitative and often rely heavily on confirmation testing. Corrections can be done for sample issues; for example, creatinine can be measured to correct for the concentration of urine. This also reduces operator dependence by removing the need for timed urine collection (117). Instrumentation for strips further reduces operator-associated dependencies with visual subjectivity (98).

Fluidic designs such as lateral-flow or flow-through designs allow for separation of the analyte from other, potentially interfering, specimen components, with or without the need for additional fluid. This separation is the key method of reducing sample integrity effects, although it does mean that an interferent is present in the reaction mixture at a higher concentration than in the comparable laboratory method. More complex designs with greater fluidic handling, such as in the case of the HbA1c and cholesterol cassette assays that include additional washings or allow larger dilutions, can greatly decrease the dependency (31, 86). These types of devices are typically used when the analyte measurement requires a high level of precision and accuracy. Blood gas and electrolyte cassettes with tubing are an example of a case with high requirements to meet the performance standards of critical care medicine, and these requirements are met with good fluidic and gas handling.

The choice of detection method can also help to reduce sample integrity effects. For example, in immunoassay systems, the choice of antibody used in the device influences the risks associated with cross-reactivity and the potential for a hook effect (65). Even microcuvette systems, which lack additional fluids and are limited to analytes such as the direct detection of hemoglobin, can still be affected by the presence of a hemoglobin variant.

Design solutions are also required to take account of operator dependencies, such as errors in sample application, mixing, incubation periods, extractions, and the timing of detection endpoints. The choice of proper fluidic systems can eliminate, internalize, or reduce some of these operator dependencies. Thus, as stated earlier, devices that require greater care in storage and stability are more prone to operator-induced errors. Between-instrument variations are reduced by using reagents that are calibrated specifically for the meter and meet the manufacturer-defined thresholds.

FUTURE PROSPECTS

Handheld devices are expected to rapidly evolve with recent technological advances in microfabrication, ultrasensitive detection methods, electronics, solid-state chemistry, and molecular pathology. The dominant role of blood glucose, urinalysis, HbA_{1C}, infectious disease, drugs of abuse, cardiac markers, coagulation, and blood gases in testing will continue, but new analytes will be discovered as a consequence of the advances in genomics and proteomics. Cancer markers, rapid assessment of cardiac function, and more infectious disease agents are currently key growth areas. It is also envisaged that there will be more markers associated with inherited and lifestyle disease susceptibility and drug efficacy as well as tools to aid in diagnostic reasoning. In addition, device connectivity will become essential for POCT in all environments.

The needs of patients and healthcare professionals are driving the technological solutions toward a common platform that will fit easily into small operating spaces and be truly portable—being implanted in some cases (e.g., blood glucose monitoring in diabetes patients). Systems capable of serving the needs of several clinical environments and of offering broader capabilities will undoubtedly require further advances in technology for detection, fluidics, transducers, and enablers.

Miniaturization has already been applied in several devices with respect to electronics, optics, detectors, and fluidics. The functionality of these devices is expected to increase exponentially; for example, by the number of test results produced per device, the types of analyses available, and the number of analytes that can be measured. Chip-based technologies (used in genomics and proteomics, and other high-throughput screening applications) are currently at test densities of 10,000 and are able to detect as many new markers. Miniaturization also offers the possibility of meeting other requirements, such as microsampling, more sensitive and accurate detection methods, universal processes and platforms, reduced reagent and material requirements, and lower costs.

However, before products can reach the user, technology advancements are still needed in the areas of materials, surfaces, and fluidic-control methods (e.g., gating, triggering, venting, separation, metering, mixing, splitting; improvements in specimen application ports and applicators; microdetectors capable of higher sensitivity and greater accuracy). The recent advent of enabling microfluidic technology promises to give POCT devices this flexibility while still maintaining the simplicity for the end-user (see Chapter 6).

Although current user requirements are typically defined by what can be achieved, trends will emerge based on needs; for example, a need for devices that are smaller (cm range), accommodate more specimen types, work with lower sample volumes ($<\mu L$), perform across wide environmental changes (20–80% relative humidity, 15–30 °C), use less power (AA batteries), and are better able to store, transfer, and receive information (identify and store disease management changes). In addition, greater attention will be placed on correct patient identification, the disposable device, and the test result through the use of machine-readable identifiers (e.g., barcodes, magnetic strips, and biometric recognition systems). A great deal of work has already been accomplished in the area of glucose monitoring (118–119). The evolution of the glucose-measuring systems is an excellent testament to the progress that has been made in POCT device design and manufacture. Progress has also been achieved for nucleic acid chips (120) and protein chips (121). The trends experienced by these established systems are likely to affect the development of all devices and will eventually lead to devices for identification of even the smallest molecular difference at the point of care.

REFERENCES

1. Research and markets: point of care diagnostic testing world markets. London: M2 Communications, Trimark Publications, 2003.
2. Gilbert HC, Vender JS. The current status of point-of-care monitoring. Intl Anesth Clin 1996;32:243–61.
3. Dirks JL. Diagnostic blood analysis using point-of-care technology. AACN Clin Issues 1996;7:249–59.
4. Maclin E, Mahoney WC. Point-of-care testing technology. J Clin Lig Assay 1995;18:929–38.

5. Kost GJ, Hague C. The current and future status of critical care testing and patient monitoring. Am J Clin Pathol 1995;104:S2–17.

6. Gough DA, Armour JC, Baker DA. Advances and prospects in glucose assay technology. Diabetologia 1997;40:5102–7.

7. Nichols JH (editor) Point-of-care testing. Performance improvements and evidence-based outcomes. New York: Marcel Dekker, 2003.

8. Fleisher M. Point-of-care testing: Does it really improve patient care? Clin Biochem 1993;26:6–8.

9. Shirey TL. Critical care profiling for informed treatment of severely ill patients. Am J Clin Pathol 1996;104:S79–87.

10. Smith BL, Vender JS. Point-of-care testing. Resp Care Clin N Amer 1995;1:133–41.

11. Castro HJ, Oropello JM, Halpern N. Point-of-care testing in the intensive care unit: The intensive care physician's perspective. Am J Clin Pathol 1995;104:S95–9.

12. Turner AP. Biosensors. Curr Opin Biotech 1994;4:49–53.

13. Cooper JC, Hall EA. The nature of biosensor technology. J Biomed Eng 1988;10:210–9.

14. Despotis GJ, Joist JH, Goodnough LT. Monitoring of hemostasis in cardiac surgical patients: Impact of point-of-care testing on blood loss and transfusion outcomes. Clin Chem 1997;43:1684–96.

15. Males RG, Stephenson J, Harris P. Cardiac markers and point-of-care testing: a perfect fit. Crit Care Nurs Q 2001;24:54–61.

16. Pugia MJ. The technology behind diagnostic strips. Lab Med 2000;31:92–6.

17. Clark BF. Towards a total human protein map. Nature 1981;292:491–2.

18. Ostroff RM, Hopkins D, Haeberli AB, Baouchi W, Polisky B. Thin film biosensor for rapid visual detection of nucleic acid targets. Clin Chem 1999;45:1659–64.

19. Loscher F, Bohme S, Martin J, Seeger S. Counting of single protein molecules at interfaces and application of this technique in early-stage diagnosis. Anal Chem 1998;70:3202–5.

20. Kurner JM, Klimant I, Krause C, Preu H, Kunz W, Wolfbeis OS. Inert phosphorescent nanospheres as markers for optical assays. Bioconjugate Chem 2001;12:883–9.

21. Nam J-M, Thaxton CS, Mirkin CA. Nanoparticle-based bio–bar codes for the ultrasensitive detection of proteins. Science 2003;301:1884–6.

22. Grant KM, Hemmert JW, White HS. Magnetic field-controlled microfluidic transport. JACS 2002;124:462–7.

23. Cook TA, Slovacek RE, Love WF, Schulkind RL, Walczek IM. Multiple output referencing system for evanescent wave sensor. US Patent 5,738,992, April 14, 1998.

24. Huang Y, Ewalt KL, Tirado M, Haigis R, Forster A, Ackley D, et al. Electric manipulation of bioparticles and macromolecules on microfabricated electrodes. Anal Chem 2001;73:1549–59.

25. Herzenberg LA, Parks D, Sahaf B, Perez O, Roederer M, Herzenberg LA. The history and future of the fluorescence activated cell sorter and flow cytometry: A view from Stanford. Clin Chem 2002;48:1819–27.

26. Bangs LB. New developments in particle-based immunoassays: introduction. Pure Appl Chem 1996;68:1873–79.

27. Gehring H, Hornberger C, Dibbelt L, Rothsigkeit A, Gerlach K, Schumacher J, et al Accuracy of point-of-care-testing (POCT) for determining hemoglobin concentrations. Acta Anaesthesiol Scand 2002;46:980–6.

28. Lugara PM. Current approaches to non-invasive optical oximetry. Clin Hemorheol Microcirc 1999;21:307–10.

29. Hoeschen C, Gholdmann BU, Moeller RH, Hamm CW. Analytical performance and clinical application of a new rapid bedside assay for the detection of serum cardiac troponin I. Clin Chem 1998;44:1925–30.

30. Schouten Y, de Winter RJ, Gorgels JMC, Koster RW, Adams R, Sanders GT. Clinical evaluation of the CARDIAC STATus™, a rapid immuno-chromatrographic assay for simultaneous detection of elevated concentrations of CK-MB and myoglobin in whole blood. Clin Chem Lab Med 1998;35:469–73.

31. Guthrie R, Hellman R, Kilo C, Hiar CE, Crowley LE, Childs B, et al. A multisite physician's office laboratory evaluation of an immunological method for the measurement of HbA1c. Diabetes Care 1992;15:1494–98.

32. D'Costa EJ, Higgins IJ, Turner AP. Quinoprotein glucose dehydrogenase and its application in an amperometric glucose sensor. Biosensors 1986;2:71–87.

33. Clark LC, Lyons C. Electrode systems for continuous monitoring in cardiovascular surgery. Ann NY Acad Sci 1962;102:29–45A.

34. Cass AEG, Davis G, Francis CD, Hill HAO, Aston WJ, Higgins IJ, et al. Ferrocene-mediated enzyme electrode for amperometric determination of glucose. JACS 1984;56:667–71.

35. Erickson KA, Wilding P. Evaluation of a novel point-of-care system: the i-STAT® portable clinical analyzer. Clin Chem 1993;39:283–7.

36. Gault MH, Harding CE. Evaluation of the i-STAT® portable clinical analyzer in a hemo-dialysis unit. Clin Biochem 1996;29:117–24.

37. Oberhardt BJ. Thrombosis and homeostasis testing at the point of care. Am J Clin Pathol 1995;104:S72–8.

38. Oberhardt BJ, Dermott SC, Taylor M, Alkadi ZY, Abruzzini AF, Gresalfi NJ. Dry reagent technology for rapid, convenient measurement of blood coagulation and fibrinolysis. Clin Chem 1991;37:520–6.

39. Merenbloom HK, Oberhardt BJ. Homogeneous immunoassay of whole-blood samples. Clin Chem 1995;41:1385–90.

40. Blumenthal RS, Carter AJ, Resar JR, Coombs V, Gloth ST, Dalal J, et al. Comparison of bedside and hospital laboratory coagulation studies during and after coronary intervention. Cathet Cardiovasc Diagn 1995;35:9–17.

41. Lee RI, White PD. A clinical study of coagulation time of blood. Am J Med Sci 1913;145:495–503.

42. Pam CM, Jobes D, Van Riper D, Ogilby JD, Lin CY, Horrow J, et al. Modified microsample ACT test for heparin monitoring. J Extra-Corporeal Technol 1996;28:16–20.

43. Solomon H, Mullins R, Lyden P, Thompson P, Hudoff S. The diagnostic accuracy of bedside and laboratory coagulation procedures used to monitor the anticoagulation status of patients treated with heparin. Am J Clin Pathol 1998;109:371–8.

44. Kubitschko S, Spinke J, Bruckner T, Pohl S, Oranthe N. Sensitivity enhancement of optical immunosensors with nanoparticles. Anal Biochem 1997;253:111–22.

45. Vo-Dinh T, Tromberg BJ, Griffen GD, Ambrose KR, Sepaniak MJ, Gardenhire EM. Antibody-based fiberoptics biosensor for the carcinogen benzo(a)pyrene. Appl Spectrosc 1987;41:735–8.

46. La Clair JJ, Burkart MD. Molecular screening on a compact disc. Org Biomol Chem 2003;1:3244–9.

47. Ostroff RM, Maul D, Bogart GR, Yang S, Christian J, Hopkins D, et al. Fixed polarizer ellipsometry for simple and sensitive

detection of thin films generated by specific molecular interactions: Applications in immunoassays and DNA sequence detection. Clin Chem 1998;44:2031–5.

48. Silzel JW, Cercek B, Dodson C, Tsay T, Obremski RJ. Mass-sensing, multianalyte microarray immunoassay with imaging detection. Clin Chem 1998;44:2036–43.

49. Sutherland RM, Dahne C, Place JF, Ringrose AS. Optical detection of antibody-antigen reactions at a glass-liquid interface Clin Chem. 1984;30:1533–8.

50. Morgan CL, Newman DJ, Price CP. Immunosensors: technology and opportunities in laboratory medicine. Clin Chem 1996; 42:193–209.

51. Free A, Free H. Urinanalysis in clinical laboratory practice. Cleveland, OH: CRC Press, 1975:217–24.

52. Hage DS. Affinity chromatography: A review of clinical applications. Clin Chem 1999;45:593–615.

53. Kricka LK. Nucleic acid detection technologies—labels, strategies, and formats. Clin Chem 1999;45:453–8.

54. Pugia MJ, Lott JA, Profitt JA, Cast TK. High-sensitivity dye binding assay for albumin in urine. J Clin Lab Anal 1999;13: 180–7.

55. Pugia MJ, Lott JA, Bierbaum LD, Cast TK. Assay of creatinine using the peroxidase activity of copper-creatinine complexes. Clin Biochem 2000;33:63–73.

56. Banauch D, Brummer W, Ebeling W, Metz H, Rindfrey H, Lang H, et al. A glucose dehydrogenase for the determination of glucose concentrations in body fluids. Z Klin Chem Klin Biochem 1975;13:101–7.

57. Severinghaus JW. The invention and development of blood gas analysis apparatus. Anesthesiology 2002;97:253–6.

58. Hedlund KD, Oen S, LaFauce L, Sanford DM. Clinical experience with the diametrics IRMA (Immediate Response Mobile Analysis) blood analysis system. Perfusion 1997;12:27–30.

59. Kozlowski-Templin R. Blood gas analyzers. Respir Care Clin N Am 1995;1:35–46.

60. Johnson RD, Bachas LG. Ionophore-based ion-selective potentiometric and optical sensors. Anal Bioanal Chem 2003;376: 328–41.

61. Qin Y, Bakker E. Evaluation of the separate equilibrium processes that dictate the upper detection limit of neutral ionophore-based potentiometric sensors. Anal Chem 2002;74:3134–41.

62. F Vogtle, E Weber. Host quest complex chemistry. Macrocycles synthesis, structure and application. Berlin/Heidelberg/New York: Springer Verlag, 1985.

63. Magalhaes JM, Machado AA. Array of potentiometric sensors for the analysis of creatinine in urine samples. Analyst 2002; 127:1069–75.

64. Olsher U, Frolow F, Bartsch RA, Pugia MJ, Shoham G. Crown ether alcohols. I. Crystal and molecular structure of the complex between sym-hydroxydibenzo-14-crown-4 and water molecules including interesting water-methanol channels JACS 1989;111: 9217–21.

65. Price CP. The evolution of immunoassay as seen through the journal Clinical Chemistry. Clin Chem 1998;44:2071–4.

66. Purvis DR, Pollard-Knight D, Lowe CR. Direct immunosensors. In: Price CP, Newman DJ, eds. Principles and practice of immunoassay. London: Macmillan, 1997:511–43.

67. Rickert J, Gopel W, Beck W, Jung G, Heiduschka P. A "mixed" self-assembled monolayer for an impedimetric immunosensor. Biosens Bioelectron 1996;11:757–68.

68. Menon VP, Martin CR. Fabrication and evaluation of nanoelectrode ensembles. Anal Chem 1995;67:1920–8.

69. Qian S, Bau HH. A mathematical model of lateral flow bioreactions applied to sandwich assays. Anal Biochem 2003;322: 89–98.

70. Collinson PO, Gerhardt W, Katus HA, Muller-Bardoff M, Braun S, Schricke U, et al. Multicenter evaluation of an immunological rapid test for the detection of Troponin T in whole blood samples. Eur J Clin Chem Clin Biochem 1996;34:591–8.

71. Baum H, Bertsch T, Bohner J, von Pap KW, Hoff T, Wilke B, et al. Detection limit, cut-off and specificity of an improved rapid assay for cardiac troponin T. Clin Lab 2001;47:549–54.

72. Buechler KF, Moi S, Noar B, McGrath D, Villela J, Clancy M, et al. Simultaneous detection of seven drugs of abuse by the Triage™ Panel for Drugs of Abuse. Clin Chem 1992;38:1678–84.

73. Apple FS, Christenson RH, Valdes R, Wu AHB, Andriak AJ, Duh SH, et al. Simultaneous rapid measurement of whole blood myoglobin, creatine kinase MB, and cardiac troponin I by the Triage Cardiac Panel for detection of myocardial infarction. Clin Chem 1999;45:199–205.

74. Volles DF, McKenney JM, Miller WG, Ruffen D, Zhang D. Analytic and clinical performance of two compact cholesterol-testing devices. Pharmacotherapy 1998;18:184–92.

75. Bunce R, Thorpe G, Keen L. Disposable analytical devices permitting automatic, timed, sequential delivery of multiple reagents. Anal Chim Acta 1992;248:263–9.

76. Schembri C, Burd TL, Kopf-Sill AR, Shea LR, Braynin B. Centrifugation and capillarity integrated into a multiple analyte whole blood analyzer. J Auto Chem 1995;3:1799–104.

77. LaPorte R, ed. Hydrophilic polymer coatings for medical devices, structure/properties, development, manufacture and application. Lancaster, PA: Technomic Publishing, 1997.

78. Zipp A, Hornby WE. Solid phase chemistry: Its principles and application in clinical analyses. Talanta 1984;31:863–77.

79. Walter B. Dry reagent chemistries in clinical analysis. Anal Chem 1983;55:498A–514A.

80. Allen MP, DeLizza A, Ramel U, Jeong H, Singh P. A non-instrumented quantitative test system and its application for determining cholesterol concentration in whole blood. Clin Chem 1990;36:1591–7.

81. Batteiger B, Newhall V, Jones RB. The use of Tween 20 as a blocking agent in the immunological detection of proteins transferred to nitrocellulose membranes. J Immuno Meth 1982;55: 297–307.

82. Jones KD. Troubleshooting protein binding in nitrocellulose membranes, Part 1: principles. IVD Technology 1999;5:32–41.

83. Schneider Z. Aliphatic alcohols improve the adsorptive performance of cellulose nitrate membranes—application in chromatography and enzyme assays. Ann Biochem 1980;108:96–103.

84. Curme HG, Columbus RL, Dappen GM, Eder TW, Fellows WD, Figueras J, et al. Multi-layer film elements for clinical analysis: General concepts. Clin Chem 1978;24:1335–42.

85. Antman EM, Grudzien C, Sacks DB. Evaluation of a rapid bedside assay for detection of serum cardiac troponin T. JAMA 1995;273:1279–82.

86. Santee J. Accuracy and precision of the Cholestech LDX System in monitoring blood lipid levels. Am J Health Syst Pharm 2002;59:1774–9.

87. Blatt JM, Allen MP, Baddam S, Chase CL, Dasu BN, Dickens DM, et al. A miniaturized, self-contained, single-use, disposable

assay device for the quantitative determination of the bone resorption marker, NTx, in urine. Clin Chem 1998;44:2051–2.

88. Ashworth L, Gibb I, Alberti KGMM. HemoCue: Evaluation of a portable photometric system for determining glucose in whole blood. Clin Chem 1992;38:1479–82.

89. Burtis CA, Bostick WD, Johnson WF. Development of a multipurpose optical system for use with a centrifugal fast analyzer. Clin Chem 1975;21:1225–33.

90. Wang J. Survey and summary. From DNA biosensors to gene chips. Nucl Acid Res 2000;26:3011–6.

91. Figeys D, Pinto D. Lab-on-a-chip: A revolution in biological and medical sciences. Anal Chem 2000;71:330A–335A.

92. Chiem NH, Harrison DJ. Microchip systems for immunoassay: An integrated immunoreactor with electrophoretic separation for serum theophylline determination. Clin Chem 1998;44:591–8.

93. Johnson RD, Badr IHA, Barrett G, Lai S, Lu Y, Marc J, et al. Development of a fully analysis integrated system for ions based on ion-selective optodes and centrifugal microfluidics. Anal Chem 2001;73:3940–6.

94. LJ Kricka. Miniaturization of analytical systems. Clin Chem 1998;44:2008–14.

95. He B, Tan L, Regnier F. Microfabricated filters for microfluidic analytical systems. Anal Chem 1999;71:1464–8.

96. Kamholz AE, Weigl BH, Finlayson BA, Yager P. Quantitative analysis of molecular interaction in a microfluidic channel: the T-sensor. Anal Chem 1999;71:5340–7.

97. Cunningham DD. Fluidics and sample handling in clinical chemical analysis. Anal Chim Acta 2001;429:1–18.

98. Rumley A. Urine dipstick testing: Comparison of results obtained by visual reading and with the Bayer CLINITEK 50. Ann Clin Biochem 2000;37:220–1.

99. May K. Unipath clearblue one step™, clearplan one step™ and clearview™, In: Wild D, ed. The immunoassay handbook. London: The Macmillan Press. 1994:233–5.

100. Lott JA, Johnson WR, Luke KE. Evaluation of an automated urine chemistry reagent strip analyzer. J Clin Lab Anal 1995;9: 212–7.

101. Parsons MP, Newman DJ, Newall RG, Price CP. Validation of a point-of-care assay for the urinary albumin:creatinine ratio. Clin Chem 1999;45:414–7.

102. Spitznagel TM, Clark DS. Surface density and orientation effects on immobilized antibodies and fragments. Biotechnology 1993;11:825–9.

103. Campos J. Diagnosis of infectious disease with point of care assays. J Clin Lig Assay 2002;25:333–41.

104. Kilpatrick ES, Rumley AG, Myint H, Dominiczak MH, Small M. The effect of variations in hematocrit, mean cell volume, and red blood cell count on reagent strip tests for glucose. Ann Clin Biochem 1993;30:485–7.

105. Steinhausen RL, Price CP. Principles and practice of dry chemistry systems. In: Price CP, Alberti KGMM, eds. Recent advances in clinical biochemistry. Edinburgh, Scotland: Churchill Livingstone, 1985:273–96.

106. Powell M. A novel blood glucose testing system: first impressions of the Glucometer Esprit. Pract Diabetes Int 1998;15: 7–8.

107. Chen ET, Nichols JH, Duh SH, Hortin G. Performance evaluation of blood glucose monitoring devices. Diab Tech Ther 2003;5:749–68.

108. Weiss SL, Cembrowski GS, Mazze RS. Patient and physician analytical goals for self-monitoring blood glucose instruments. Am J Clin Pathol 1994;102:611–5.

109. Skeie S, Thue G, Nerhus K, Sandberg S. Instruments for self-monitoring of blood glucose: Comparisons of testing quality achieved by patients and a technician. Clin Chem 2002;48:994–1003.

110. Young DS. Effects of drugs on clinical laboratory tests, 4th ed. Washington, DC: AACC Press, 1995:1–643.

111. Kroll MH, Elin RJ. Interference with clinical laboratory analyses. Clin Chem 1994;40:1996–2005.

112. Sedor FA, Holleman CM, Heyden S, Schneider KA. Reflotron cholesterol measurement evaluated as a screening technique. Clin Chem 1988;34:3542–5.

113. Wong RJ, Mahoney JJ, Harvey JA, Van Kessel AL. StatPal II pH and blood gas analysis system evaluated. Clin Chem 1994; 40:124–9.

114. Gosselin RC, Owings JT, Larkin E, White RH, Hutchinson R, Branch J. Monitoring oral anticoagulant therapy with point-of-care devices. Clin Chem 1997;43:1785–6.

115. Stahl M, Branslund I, Iversen S. Filtenbord JA. Quality assessment of blood glucose testing in general practitioners' offices improves quality. Clin Chem 1997;43:1926–31.

116. Sylvester ECJ, Price CP, Burrin JM. Investigation of the potential for interference with whole blood glucose strips. Ann Clin Biochem 1994;31:94–6.

117. Newman DJ, Pugia MJ, Lott JA, Wallace JF, Hiar AM. Urinary protein and albumin excretion corrected by creatinine and specific gravity. Clin Chim Acta 2000;294:139–55.

118. Wilkins E, Atanasov P. Glucose monitoring: state of the art and future possibilities. Med Eng Phys 1996;18:273–88.

119. Yang Q, Atanasov P, Wilkins E. A needle-type sensor for monitoring glucose in whole blood. Biomed Instr Technol 1997;31:54–62.

120. Ibrahim MS, Lofts RS, Jahrling PB, Henchal EA, Weedn VW, Northrup MA, et al. Real-time microchip PCR for detecting single base differences in viral and human DNA. Anal Chem 1998;70:2013–7.

121. Wang J, Chatrathi MP. Microfabricated electrophoresis chip for bioassay of renal markers. Anal Chem 2003;75:525–9.

Chapter **3**

Benchtop Instruments for Point-of-Care Testing
Andrew St John

This chapter will examine the technology behind benchtop point-of-care testing (POCT) devices. There is no sharp demarcation in terms of physical size between these devices and the handheld type of instruments described in the previous chapter. A wide range of instruments will be discussed in this chapter. In general, benchtop devices are not used directly at the patient's bedside but are located in areas attached to critical care areas, certain general inpatient clinical areas (wards), outpatient clinics, and doctors' offices. Many of the systems employ technology that was developed for automated analyzers used in the central laboratory and have been adapted and miniaturized to a degree for use in a more confined environment. Some of the instruments in this category are quantitative versions of the qualitative strip devices previously described where the size of the instruments has increased through the incorporation of a reader device. The main features that describe the evolution of the benchtop analyzer are those that 'engineer in' all of the operator steps necessary to produce a result and, where possible, 'engineer out' the steps that might give rise to operator errors. This is achieved in part by reducing the complexity of the operator interface.

The commonest type of benchtop devices are blood gas or critical care testing analyzers, which have been in existence for many decades but have become steadily more sophisticated, primarily through the expansion of the test menu, so that some devices, in effect, provide a mini–point-of-care laboratory. In the past decade, whole-blood sensor technology has been extended to measure many other analytes, including proteins, hormones, enzymes, and blood cell and coagulation parameters. Benchtop devices also exist for measurement of many urine parameters.

This chapter will focus on devices that require no pretreatment of the sample prior to placement in the analyzer, and particular attention will be given to devices that have appeared in the time since publication of the first edition of this book (1).

GENERAL DESIGN PRINCIPLES OF BENCHTOP DEVICES

The same general goals behind the design of POCT devices that were described in the previous chapter, for handheld devices, are similarly applicable to benchtop devices. Most important, the fact that they are often used by personnel with a limited technical background or training means that the user interface is a critical feature that can inhibit the successful

application of that device. Information technology is also important not only for communication and control of components within the instrument but also for linking the device to external information systems.

The design requirements of simple stand-alone test strips will differ from those of large benchtop instruments where there will be a much higher degree of complexity. Whatever the size, all POCT devices should meet the following overall requirements:

- Be simple to use, i.e., require the minimum of steps to produce a result
- Use reagents that are robust in terms of storage and usage, including calibration
- Produce results concordant with the central laboratory and consistent with the clinical need
- Be safe in terms of storage, usage, and disposal

After the analytical technology, the operator or user interface is the most important design feature; it also provides a way for manufacturers to differentiate their products. Many benchtop instruments have liquid crystal display (LCD) screens as the primary interface now that these have become relatively inexpensive to manufacture (2). Other interfaces include key pads, barcode readers, and printers. The latter are now almost obligatory in terms of ensuring that a hard copy of the results is available. Patient safety and the need for positive patient, sample, and operator identification have led to many devices incorporating barcode readers. These are also included for identifying reagents and other consumables to the system, some of which will incorporate factory calibration as well as informing the instrument how to process a particular test. Finally, operator ID can also be achieved via a barcode reader, thus ensuring that there is traceability to the person who performed the test.

Sample access and delivery of the sample to the actual sensing component of the strip, cassette or cartridge are key processes and ideally may be the only interactions of the user with the device. Clearly, a well-defined interface should guide the user through the operation and tolerate or warn the operator of minor errors, such as delays in pressing the appropriate keys or buttons on a touch screen.

Control and communications systems are a major component of all benchtop POCT devices. Even the smallest device has a control subsystem that coordinates all the other systems and ensures that all the required processes for an analysis take place in the correct order. Operations to control include insertion or removal of the strip, cartridge or cassette; temperature control; sample injection or aspiration; sample metering; sample detection; mixing; incubation; timing of the detection process; and waste removal. Fluid movement can often be accomplished by mechanical means through pumps, centrifugation—commonly used in benchtop systems, and fluidic properties such as surface tension, which is often a critical element in the design of the simple strip tests, and in microfabricated systems (3). The fluidics of a typical blood gas analyzer are shown in Figure 3-1.

In benchtop systems, where size constraints are not so important, it is now possible with modern electronics to have sophisticated data processing, management, and storage capabilities. Data storage will include calibration-curve data and quality-control limits as well as patient results. In some systems data transfer and management takes place when the meter or reader is linked to a small benchtop device called a docking station. These and other devices include communication protocols that allow data to be transferred to other data management systems, a subject that will be discussed in more detail in Chapter 20.

CRITICAL CARE ANALYZERS

Blood gas instruments represent one of the earliest forms of POCT devices, having been in existence for nearly 50 years. While instruments that measure just hydrogen ion (pH) and blood gases are still produced, many laboratories and critical care units now purchase devices that measure many additional parameters and are more correctly called critical care analyzers. As well as measuring more analytes, several decades of development have seen major advances in design and ease of use. With appropriate training and management, these complex devices can be used safely by many non–laboratory trained personnel, in a wide variety of point-of-care locations.

Most blood gas and electrolyte instruments contain electrochemical sensors or electrodes that rely on potentiometric or amperometric measurement of the signal (4). The analytical principles of these electrodes are largely the same as those used in the first generation of instruments, but technological advances have enabled electrodes to be constructed in a number of different ways, and this has resulted in several distinct types of critical care analyzers (Table 3-1). These include the single-use, handheld, critical care analyzers, which were mentioned in the previous chapter. In addition, alternatives to electrochemical technology using optical measurement of critical care parameters have appeared in recent years and are now available as commercial devices (5, 6).

Conventional Benchtop Analyzers

The larger or so-called benchtop critical care analyzers use conventional electrodes that are much reduced in size compared to designs of 10–20 years ago (7). These miniature electrodes are hand built and complex in design but have the following user-friendly features:

- A flow-through design that reduces the sample volume needed for analysis and protects the ion-selective membrane
- A visible sample path
- Maintenance-free operation; i.e., no need to refill with electrolyte, or change the membranes
- A working lifetime of 6–12 months

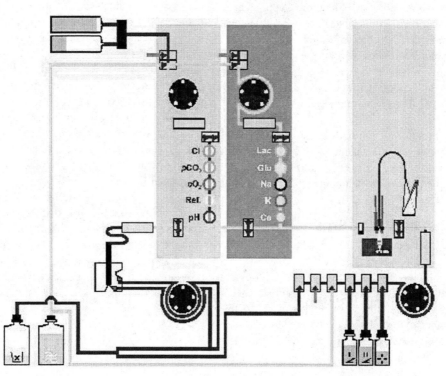

Figure 3-1 Flow diagram of a typical blood gas analyzer. Courtesy of Radiometer Copenhagen.

Table 3-1 Main Features of Conventional Benchtop, Cartridge-Based, and Single-Use or Handheld Critical Care Analyzers

Benchtop	Cartridge-based	Single-use or handheld
Electrochemical detection	Electrochemical detection	Electrochemical and optical detection
Multiple use	Multiple use	Single-use cassette or cartridge
Largest menu of tests on one sample	Menu expanding including integrated CO-oximetry	Full menu only obtained through the use of multiple cassettes
Not portable	Semiportable	Truly portable
Amount of maintenance is progressively reducing	Little maintenance	Least maintenance
May be the most cost-effective system for medium to large test volumes	May be cost-effective for medium to large test volumes	May be only be cost effective for small to medium volumes

- Easy and rapid user replacement of failed electrodes, with a minimum of downtime for the instrument.

The easy access to electrodes and modular nature of modern blood gas analyzers is illustrated by Figure 3-2, which shows an exploded view of the EasyLite critical care analyzer (Medica Corporation, Bedford, MA, USA). Of all the types of critical care analyzers, benchtop instruments generally have the largest possible menu of tests, and these include blood gases; electrolytes; metabolites such as glucose, lactate, urea and creatinine; CO-oximetry; and bilirubin. In such a multianalyte device the flow of blood, calibrants, wash, and quality-control (QC) solutions through the device will be controlled by an extensive arrangement of detectors, valves, pumps, and software. The device will include a range of analytical technologies apart from the typical microelectrodes previously described. These include thick-film technology (discussed later) for measurement of parameters such as glucose, lactate, and urea. These are biosensors using enzymes in reactions similar to those used in the central laboratory, but the challenge for

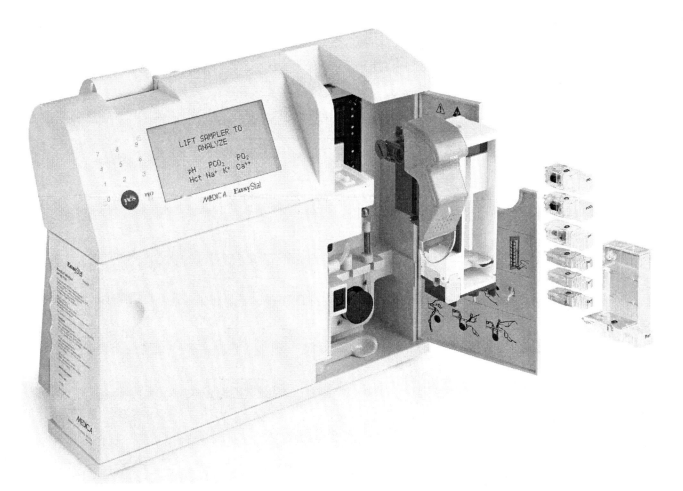

Figure 3-2 Exploded view of the EasyStat critical care analyzer. Courtesy of Medica Corporation.

manufacturers has been to devise reusable enzyme-based sensors that will function after repeated exposure to whole-blood samples.

In addition to being reusable, important design features of this type of sensor are how substances such as drugs are prevented from causing interference. Manufacturers use a variety of methods to overcome these problems, shown in Figure 3.3. Selective membranes can physically prevent the interferent molecule from reaching the sensor. By using a lower polarization voltage at the anode, it is possible to polarize and thereby measure the lactate or glucose concentration in the sample without also polarizing most of the interferent molecules. Some instruments also use a compensation electrode to overcome interference. The compensation or interference electrode is identical to the sensing electrode except that it contains no glucose or lactate oxidase. Thus it has no response to the glucose or lactate in the sample, but only responds to the interfering substances. The signal from the compensation electrode is deducted from the sensing electrode to yield that signal due to glucose or lactate alone (8).

Many benchtop critical care instruments can also determine hemoglobin and in some cases hematocrit levels. The latter is determined by conductivity, but the values obtained by this method in certain situations, such as when performing open-heart surgery, may not provide accurate results. Treatment of such patients should be based on hemoglobin results or on packed cell volume (PCV) hematocrit methods (9). The various hemoglobin species in blood, including oxy- and carboxyhemoglobin, are determined by CO-oximetry. CO-oximeters are an integral part of many benchtop analyzers and rely on multiwavelength spectrophotometry, where light absorption by hemolyzed blood is measured at up to 60 or more wavelengths

to determine the concentration of the five required hemoglobin species (10). In this way, determination of the fraction of oxyhemoglobin (Fo_2Hb) avoids the potential problems that can result from relying upon an estimated oxygen saturation produced by blood gas devices without a CO-oximeter. One manufacturer has recently extended multiwavelength spectrophotometry to measure bilirubin directly in whole blood, and more devices are likely to appear using this technology (11). These technological advances reflect the desire of clinicians to have the ability to measure parameters beyond the classical menu of gases and electrolytes, on relatively small specimens of whole blood. This is a considerable advantage, not only for neonatal and pediatric patients but also for adult patients where there is increasing concern about anemia resulting from excessive blood collections.

The ability to measure a much larger number of analytes has undoubtedly added to the complexity of the device, but all critical care analyzers now include many features that facilitate operation of the instrument (Table 3-2). Most critical care parameters are measured on specimens inserted directly from the collection syringe. Until recently, it was the usual practice to inject blood into devices. Now almost all instruments use sample aspiration as the form of specimen delivery, thus avoiding analytical problems from excessive injection pressure (12) as well as potential safety hazards such as blood spraying back onto the operator or into the instrument. The sample volume required for analysis has also decreased, in some instruments down to 35 μL for pH and blood gases, but the increasing menu of tests means that >100 μL may be required for a full panel of tests.

The main disadvantage associated with electrochemical sensors is that over time the electrodes drift from their baseline

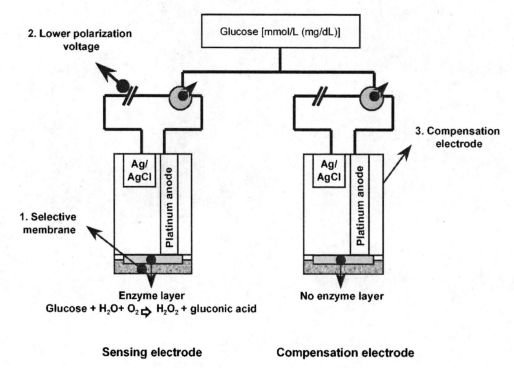

Figure 3-3   Various strategies to overcome interference in the amperometric measurement of glucose.

Table 3-2 Features of Critical Care Analyzers That Minimize Risk of Errors and Contribute to Ease of Use

Long-life, maintenance-free electrodes or disposable sensor packs
Touch screens as the user interface
Software that can demand user and patient identification
Built-in barcode scanners
Sample aspiration instead of injection
Reduced sample sizes
Clot detection within the analysis chamber
Sample detection to prevent short samples
Liquid calibration systems instead of gas bottles
Automated calibrations
Automated QC sampling
Sophisticated QC programs including interpretation of data
Connectivity to information systems allowing remote monitoring and control
Inbuilt videos for training purposes

and require recalibration. One of the most common causes of drift is the build up of protein layers on the electrode or in the sample path. This type of drift can be corrected with a one-point calibration that can be programmed to occur automatically, in many instruments every 30–60 min. Slower changes, as well as drift in the baseline, occur in the slope of the electrode response. This can be corrected using a two-point calibration, which may be required and programmed to occur every 4–8 h.

Until recently, high-quality gases of two different tensions of CO_2 and O_2 were required to calibrate blood gas analyzers. To overcome the expense and inconvenience of gas cylinders, several manufacturers use, either exclusively or in combination, liquid calibration systems, room air, and an internal O_2-zero solution. In the Roche Omni (Roche Diagnostics, Graz, Austria), the calibration solution is generated from two aqueous base solutions immediately before calibration is required, and conductance measurements are used to determine the composition of the final calibration mixture (13).

Ion-selective electrodes (ISEs) also require periodic calibration. Most ISEs exhibit what is called Nernstian behavior, which means that there is a semilogarithmic relationship between the detection signal and the activity (concentration) of the ion to be measured. In such cases, the ISE can be calibrated using a two-point procedure. However, some ISEs (e.g., lithium and magnesium), do not exhibit such linear behavior, and in these cases more than two calibration points may be needed. With the development of combination instruments measuring multiple parameters, considerable care has to be taken with formulating the calibration solutions so that they have ionic strength similar to that of the sample to be analyzed, since ionic strength is a major determinant of ion activity. This can only be achieved in urine by prediluting the sample in appropriate diluent.

Benchtop blood gas analyzers remain the best choice for medium to large workloads of critical care testing because of their wide menu and their status as generally the most cost-effective form of analysis.

Cartridge-Based Portable Analyzers

The design of this more recent type of critical care analyzer came about through advances in technology and the desire among users for easier-to-operate blood gas devices. The latter has become all-important, as more and more critical care testing is located outside of the central laboratory and at the point of care. Some 15 years ago, advances in microfabrication of printed circuit boards enabled the development of an array of electrochemical sensors on a plastic card. This was the basis of the Mallinckrodt multiuse cartridge blood gas analyzer, which is now the Gem Premier 3000 (Instrumentation Laboratory, Lexington, MA, USA) (14). The more recent development of thick-film–type sensors, mentioned previously, has led to the development of chemical and biosensor arrays with capabilities including measurement of glucose and lactate in the Gem Premier and other cartridge-based systems, such as the Rapidpoint 400 (Bayer Diagnostics, Medfield, MA, USA) and the Radiometer ABL 77 (Radiometer Copenhagen, Bronshoj, Denmark).

Thick-film manufacturing involves the application of specially formulated pastes and inks to specific areas on an inert support base, often using screen-printing techniques. The result is well-defined sensor zones with electrical conduction and electrical isolation zones. Cocktails containing the recognition agent, such as an enzyme or antibody in the case of biosensors, are then dispensed over the sensor zone using robotic techniques, after which the device is fired to a high temperature to remove interfering binding agents in the paste and to bond the various materials to the support layer (15). Thick-film sensors are usually about 10–25 μm in thickness, with the sensor spot approximately 1 mm in size.

This contrasts with thin-film sensors, which are fabricated using wafers of thin metal oxide films and which are of submicrometer thickness. To date, the single-use, handheld i-STAT analyzer is the only example of a thin-film–based critical care analyzer (16); its design was discussed in Chapter 2. Thick-film technology has a number of advantages compared to thin-film sensors. It is a very robust technology that is particularly compatible with enzymatic reagents that have a stable lifetime in a sensor of between 1–8 weeks. Their relatively low cost of production compared to thin-film sensors means that replacement of a sensor after several weeks of use is not an economic problem. The ability to put different multiparameter combinations on one cartridge, easily achieved interference compensation, and the potential to be further reduced in size are all advantageous features (8). One disadvantage of thick-film sensors, however, is that they generally require a period of time to equilibrate after being removed from the storage pack and placed in the instrument. With thin-film sensors, because the sensor layer is of micrometer dimensions, blood can permeate very quickly and the sensor cartridge can be used immediately after it is unwrapped from its packing.

However, this so-called wet-up time for thick-film sensors is becoming shorter with advances in design.

Sensor arrays can now be incorporated into a single cartridge or pack that contains all the reagents that are necessary for analysis of patient samples. The cartridge is placed in the body of a small benchtop analyzer that is significantly smaller than the previously described conventional benchtop analyzers, but it incorporates similar functionality and is therefore portable. Because the sensor/reagent packs have a limited life once placed into the instrument, they are produced in a number of different sizes that are sufficient for 75–700 analyses per pack, depending on the manufacturer. This confers a degree of flexibility that enables this type of device to be used cost-effectively for a variety of workloads. The cartridge design varies among manufacturers but some are now available that include calibrants, in addition to the sensors and reagents for patient and QC analysis.

The major advantage of these devices is their convenience—the only major task of the operator is to change the cartridge or cassette when it has performed the stated number of analyses. One device even includes a video that can assist users with such tasks (17). While the analytical performance of these types of devices has been published (17, 18, 19), there appear to be no reports in the literature evaluating their effect on operational aspects, such as potential staff savings or whether such devices are better in locations such as emergency rooms compared to larger and more labor-intensive critical care analyzers. This information would be useful in evaluating the business case for the purchase of such devices. Despite this, it is likely that more devices will appear in cartridge-based format in the future and incorporate the same comprehensive menu that is available on their larger counterparts.

Optical Blood Gas Analyzers

One of the major disadvantages of electrochemical measurements is that they require regular calibration due to electrode drift. Optical measurements overcome this problem because they can be calibrated at the time of manufacture (20). The sensor chemistry is placed on a rigid and optically transparent support termed a planar optode. In the Osmetech OPTI™ instrument (Osmetech, Roswell, GA, USA) six optodes for measurement of pH, P_{CO_2}, P_{O_2}, Na^+, K^+, and Ca^{2+} are incorporated into a single-use, flow-through measurement cassette that is placed into a small, portable, microprocessor-based instrument that measures optical fluorescence. In addition, the P_{O_2} sensor optode provides measurement of total hemoglobin (tHb) and calculated oxygen saturation (S_{O_2}) by reflectance. After blood is aspirated into the cassette, it lies immediately above each of the optodes and then diffuses through an optical isolation layer into the sensor layer. Here, interaction between the indicator and analyte either increases or decreases the fluorescence, depending on the analyte concentration.

Optodes are easy to manufacture because of their simple planar structure, which has no electrical connectors and no reference electrodes. They are prepared as compound sheets or foils that comprise the sensing layer sandwiched between the

upper optical isolation layer and a lower optically transmissive adhesive layer. Individual sensor or optode discs are punched out and inserted into the plastic, disposable cassette. A key part of the optode manufacturing process is that they are also calibrated during production, and the calibration curve is incorporated into a barcode. This accompanies the cassette and is entered into the instrument software when the cassette in placed in the instrument. The factory calibration is checked once with precision buffers and gas mixtures immediately before use.

All of the above features, together with the fact that no reagents, other than a single gas cylinder, are required with the OPTI measurement system represent advantages over electrochemical systems. The major disadvantage of optical systems is that relatively complex and expensive devices are required to measure the optical signals. The Radiometer NPT 7 (Radiometer Copenhagen, Bronshoj, Denmark) is another critical care analyzer that uses optical detection but has a multiple-use format through a cartridge design (Figure 3-4) (6). Despite their stated advantages, it remains to be seen whether optical systems will gain a significant share of the critical care testing market compared to electrochemical analyzers.

Quality Control and Management of Critical Care Analyzers

During the past decade, there have been significant advances in reducing the workload associated with ensuring the quality of critical care testing results. Instruments still require whole blood, and this demands that operators remain aware of all the various preanalytical requirements for critical care analytes. However, manufacturers have addressed some of these preanalytical issues, such as the move to sample aspiration mentioned previously. There are also systems to prevent clotted samples, formerly the bane of a blood gas machine operator's life, from entering key areas of the instrument. This is particularly important for cartridge-based instruments, where a clot has the potential to result in failure of a whole cartridge long before its normal expiration time, with all the attendant costs. While sample size has decreased over the years, the reality is that operators will continue to periodically test the capabilities of the instrument by presenting the minimum volume of sample. Thus, sophisticated sample detection and control systems are present in most instruments to ensure that sufficient sample enters the measurement or sensor areas. If this does not occur, error signals are generated to ensure that false results are not given and acted on.

Multiple-use benchtop and cartridge-based instruments continue to require calibration at regular intervals, and quality-control samples must be analyzed at intervals set by local quality and accreditation guidelines. Calibration procedures have been automated for many years, and this has been followed recently by automated procedures for QC analysis. There are a variety of designs, including mechanical sampling of material from glass vials or aspiration of material from reagent pouches. A key part of the design is to ensure, as far as is possible, that the auto-QC sample follows the same pathway

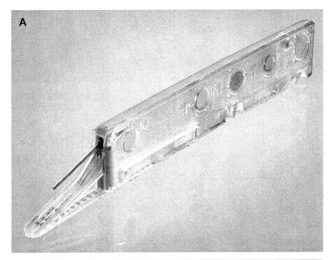

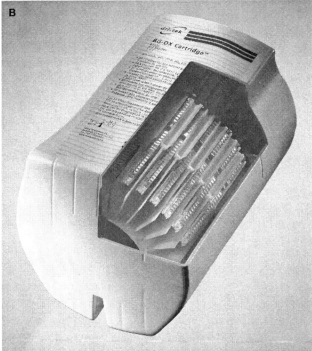

Figure 3-4 (*A*) Single-use cuvette for optical measurement of blood gases. (*B*) CO-oximetry cartridge with 30 single-use cuvettes for optical measurement of blood gases and CO-oximetry. Courtesy of Radiometer Copenhagen.

and process as that of a patient sample. All systems allow the operator to set the time intervals at which the material is sampled, and some are operated by software systems that monitor the results and will shut down the channel of the analyzer that is out of control, or even the whole instrument. An evaluation of one of these systems shows that their deployment has the potential to save significant resources, particularly in remotely located devices (21).

Many critical care devices now come with LCD screens or are linked to PCs or data managers on which can be displayed the internal QC data. Presentations of QC data commonly include Levy-Jennings charts, and some include so-called

Westgard rules (22). One manufacturer has recently released a more sophisticated software package that claims a much quicker error detection process than conventional batch quality-control procedures. It is likely that other manufacturers will adopt similar software features as processing power becomes ever less expensive and ways are sought to differentiate products other than by analyte alone.

Batch-based quality-control procedures generally used on benchtop instruments are clearly not applicable to single-use critical care devices such as the i-STAT, OPTI, or IRMA (ITC, Edison, NJ, USA) devices. Unit-use devices employ a variety of QC procedures, which include processes that take place at the time of manufacturing and are integral to that process (i.e., good manufacturing practices) (23). In addition, most unit devices are subjected to various electronic checks when they are placed in the measurement device and just prior to placement of the blood sample in the device. Such checks are not a substitute for periodic liquid QC testing, since they do not check all of the events that take place with a patient analysis. However, they remain a valuable QC procedure, and this now seems to be accepted by most laboratory scientists (24). Anecdotal reports suggest that a continuing source of misunderstanding is how often a batch of unit devices should be subjected to conventional liquid QC procedures. Manufacturers make recommendations, but a clearer understanding is required by the profession. The quality control of unit- or single-use devices is explained in more detail in Chapter 14.

The linking or interfacing of critical care testing instruments to information systems is not yet mandatory, but given the clinical importance of the data, it is not difficult to envisage that it might become so in the not too distant future. The interfacing of devices can be direct to laboratory or hospital information systems or, as is more common in countries such as the United States, to data managers. Connectivity is not only important for ensuring that patient results reach the patient's medical record but also because of the availability of software to remotely monitor and control critical care analyzers in locations remote from the central laboratory. These informatic aspects of critical care testing analyzers and the whole area of connectivity will be discussed in more detail in Chapter 20.

Chemistry and Immunochemistry Analyzers

The basic analytical principles of many benchtop POCT chemistry and immunochemistry analyzers are similar to those of their counterparts in the main laboratory. An obvious key difference is that in order to minimize the sample handling involved with POCT devices, it is necessary to include either analytical methods or sensors that can directly utilize whole blood or include steps that remove the red cells prior to analysis. The devices described next all use whole-blood samples, but in most cases serum or plasma can also be used.

The Reflotron® system (Roche Diagnostics, Mannheim, Germany) is one of the oldest POCT chemistry systems, having evolved from the earlier Reflomat® and Reflochek® models, and is still used in a variety of different locations throughout the world (25). In this device, multiple reagents are located adjacent to a plasma-separating layer in which a glass filter traps red blood cells, after which the plasma flows into a glass-fiber reservoir. Initiation of the reaction takes place when the strip is inserted into a photometer that presses the reagent layers into contact with the plasma in the reservoir. The relationship between the measured reflectance and the concentration of analyte is described by the Kubelka-Munk function:

$$C\alpha \frac{K}{S} = \frac{(1-R)^2}{2R}$$

where C is the analyte concentration, K is the absorption coefficient, S is the scattering coefficient, and R is the percentage of reflectance. The constants required to solve this function, together with other calibration information, are stored in a magnetic strip on the underside of each test strip. The system is relatively tolerant of sample volume ($\pm 10\%$), but extremes of hematocrit can cause aberrant results. The performance of the system for many of the common analytes has been documented in the literature (26).

Several analytical devices overcome the problem of interfering red cells by incorporating centrifugation within the instrument. One of these is the Piccolo® analyzer (Abaxis, Union City CA, USA) which incorporates a centrifuge not only to separate cells from plasma but also for the purposes of distribution and mixing of both sample and reagents (27). All the reactions take place in small disposable rotors that contain the required diluents and reagents for a particular and related group of tests. An analysis is initiated by placing a few drops of blood directly into the rotor sample port, after which the rotor is placed in the drawer of the analyzer; closing the drawer positions the rotor on top of a centrifuge spindle. A combination of capillarity and centrifugal force results in metering the correct amount of blood, separating the cells from the plasma, sampling the required amount of plasma, mixing the sample with the correct volume of diluent, distributing the mixture to the reaction cuvettes, and, finally, mixing the sample and diluent with the reagents. The spectrophotometer is a stroboscopic xenon lamp that monitors the reactions in the cuvettes at nine wavelengths and calculates the results from the absorbance data, which are available ~15 min after the sample is placed in the analyzer.

All of these steps proceed without operator intervention. In addition, various quality-control procedures are automatically included in many of the processes. Thus the Piccolo iQC program checks on the composition and delivery of all substances involved in the analytical reactions, validates the optics, quantifies interferents such as hemolysis or lipemia, and suppresses results where the interference limits have been exceeded. Of particular importance are checks on the rotors to ensure that the variation in performance among rotors is minimal. A comparison of the device to a conventional laboratory analyzer showed the results of the Piccolo to be acceptable (28).

The Abbott Vision™ (Abbott Diagnostics, Abbott Park, IL, USA) is another point-of-care chemistry device that relies on rotating cuvettes and centrifugation to separate plasma from whole blood (29). Sample requirements are not critical; all reagent cuvettes are barcoded, and results are produced in approximately 15 min. The instrument was one of the first to introduce the feature of long-term analytical stability so that calibrations are required only infrequently; this again minimizes the interaction of the operator with the device. Other devices that can perform general chemistry tests include the Careside® analyzer (Careside, Culver City, CA, USA), which is based on single-use test cartridges that include a plasma separation step, and the LDX™ system (Cholestech, Hayward CA, USA), which has cartridge-based tests for lipids, glucose, and alanine aminotransferase. Both devices are designed to minimize the tasks required of the operator once a blood sample has been placed in the cartridge or device. The relative simplicity of the Cholestech device is indicated by the fact that it is classified as a waived device under the Clinical Laboratory Improvement Amendments (CLIA) (30).

The clinical utility of performing cardiac marker tests at the point of care has led many manufacturers to devise instruments for this market. Many of these use lateral flow strips in conjunction with a reader device, and this technology has been discussed in the previous chapter. The Stratus CS® analyzer (Dade Behring, Deerfield, IL, USA) uses enhanced radial partition immunoassay to detect cardiac markers including troponin I (31). The device incorporates a centrifuge, which makes it one of the larger benchtop devices, but it also incorporates sampling direct from the blood collection tube, thus minimizing preanalytical errors. This feature, together with its better analytical sensitivity for troponin I compared to many other methods, makes it a popular POCT device.

Diabetes testing and monitoring is another clinical area where POCT can deliver patient benefits, and several small cassette or strip-based devices are available for measurement of HbA1C and urine albumin. The Bayer DCA™ (Bayer HealthCare, Tarrytown, NY, USA) is a small benchtop device that can measure both these key analytes as well as creatinine so that the albumin measurement can be corrected for urine concentration (32). The device is a cartridge-based system that uses a light-scattering immunoassay to measure glycated hemoglobin, together with a colorimetric assay for total hemoglobin. The cartridge is a relatively complex structure that contains antigen-coated latex particles, antibodies to HbA1C and lysing reagents that are mixed following addition of the whole-blood or urine sample. Measurement takes place when the cartridge is placed into a temperature-controlled reader. The analytical performance is sufficient for quantitative monitoring of diabetic control, and the device can also measure urinary albumin and creatinine (33, 34). The size of the device allows it to be used in diabetic clinics and doctors' offices.

In recent years, several benchtop immunoassay instruments have appeared that potentially have a larger menu of tests than can be performed on the smaller strip-based tests, yet are of a size that can be accommodated in clinics or doctors' practices. The Innotrac Aio!™ (Innotrac Diagnostics, Oy, Finland) is a fully automated random-access immunoanalyzer based on a universal all-in-one (AIO) reagent concept that uses time-resolved fluorescence for detection of parameters such as C-reactive protein, human chorionic gonadotropin (hCG), and cardiac markers (35). A range of sample types can be used, including whole blood. The assay is initiated by adding a defined amount of whole blood, serum, or plasma, plus buffer, to a cup in which all the necessary reagents, including a europium lanthanide chelate, are dry coated. The mixture is incubated for 15 min at 36 °C, washed and dried, and the europium signal is then measured; results are available 18 min after sample addition. Twelve analyte cups are packed into a so-called analyte pen that is barcoded with the factory calibration, and a new calibration is required only if there is a change in lot number. The assays are both sensitive and have a broad working range that limits the number of samples requiring dilution. Recent publications indicate that this technology can be extended to rapid homogeneous assays for urinary albumin and pregnancy-associated plasma protein A (PAPP-A), which will facilitate their measurement at the point of care (36, 37). This europium technology, with some modifications, will appear later this year in a similar benchtop instrument suitable for clinics, called the Delfia Express (Perkin Elmer, Turku, Finland).

Rapid point-of-care measurement of PAPP-A and other related parameters are also possible using the Kryptor,™ a benchtop immunoassay analyzer marketed by Brahms Diagnostics (Brahms Diagnostica GmbH, Berlin, Germany). The measuring principle is time-resolved amplified cryptate emission (TRACE) technology, which combines a europium cryptate donor with an acceptor protein molecule isolated from red algae (38). When these are combined in an immunocomplex with the analyte of interest and the complex is excited, the emission signal of the bound complex is amplified and has a relatively long half-life, while excitation of the unbound acceptor is followed by a much shorter emission. The technology has user-friendly features, such as barcoded cassettes containing all the reagents, including donor chelate and acceptor, while sample addition is automated with a sample carousel. The instrument is operated via a computer and can be operated in random-access, batch, or stat mode (39). An account of a clinical application is given in Chapter 33.

The Kryptor technology can also be used for measurement of procalcitonin, a precursor of calcitonin that is increased in concentration by various infections (40). A recent study using a high-sensitivity assay in patients with suspected lower respiratory tract infections showed that a rapid procalcitonin assay could be used to guide appropriate treatment (41).

COAGULATION MONITORS

There is a well-defined clinical need to monitor anticoagulant therapy in both acute and chronic medical settings, and the value of POCT devices has been demonstrated in several studies (42). The number of patients requiring long-term anticoagulant therapy is growing, and coagulation monitoring is one of the largest sectors of the POCT market after glucose

monitoring and pregnancy testing. Consequently, there are trends in coagulation instrumentation similar to those that have taken place in glucose meters. However, coagulation measurement poses greater challenges to manufacturers, and consequently coagulation devices do not yet display all of the features that are incorporated in the more sophisticated glucose meters.

One of the difficulties of coagulation measurement is that a test such as prothrombin time (PT) is in fact a functional test of a whole pathway. The pathway is dependent on several enzymes, all of which are present at far lower levels than those of glucose; furthermore, they are temperature dependent. These factors have required designs that have resulted in first- and second-generation coagulation meters generally being smaller than benchtop critical care analyzers but much larger than glucose meters. More recently, smaller, handheld devices have become available for home monitoring.

General features of a typical coagulation meter include a design that can utilize fingerstick samples in the case of home or clinic monitoring, with minimal demands on the user in terms of sample application. The reaction usually takes place in a cassette or test strip that is maintained at a temperature above 37 °C in order to maximize the reaction kinetics and minimize changes in outside temperature. Portable meters of the latest generation that are now generally used in hospital locations are much easier to use than earlier systems, although some still require relatively large specimen volumes of 100–400 μL.

In the case of PT, thromboplastin is a key reagent component, needed to initiate the external coagulation pathway, while for activated clotting time (ACT), kaolin or celite are important components of the reagent systems. Different sources of these reagents can lead to variations in the performance of the test system, a problem that in some cases is accentuated by the use of dried reagents in comparison to liquid systems (43). Another important initiator of coagulation is calcium, and this may or may not be added to the dried test mixture in the cassette or strip, depending on the test.

Manufacturers have used a variety of systems to detect the clotting event in coagulation meters. Automated coagulation instruments first appeared in the early 1970s and used magnets to detect the decrease in sample flow or movement that results from the clotting process. In the Hemochron system for ACT measurement (International Technodyne Corporation, Edison, NJ, USA), the magnet is located in the sample tube, together with appropriate reagents. After adding the patient sample, the tube is placed in the well of the instrument, thereby triggering a timer. A detector monitors a magnet in the tube that becomes misaligned due to the clotting process and eventually stops the timer. While this classic type of technology is still used in various devices, it has some disadvantages, such as the need for accurate and large sample volumes and the fact that with only one detector or sensor, some samples may produce clots that are too fragile to displace the magnet.

Newer generations of instruments have incorporated features that have overcome these problems. While using the same basic detection principle, the Actalyke XL, from Helena Point of Care (Helena Laboratories, Beaumont, TX, USA) uses a two-point electromechanical "soft-clot" process. Measurement of ACT relies upon two magnets or detectors, positioned at $0°$ and $90°$, and with such an arrangement it is possible for smaller and more fragile clots to trigger the detector (44).

More user-friendly features such as barcoded cuvettes containing reagents for a specific test and smaller sample volumes are incorporated in the Hemochron Jr. Signature. Besides requiring only a drop, or 15 μL, of whole blood, the sample is contained entirely within the cuvette, an important requirement for devices being used at the point of care. The detection principle is different from that in other Hemochron devices in that it relies on optical monitoring of the clotting process in a narrow channel. Following addition of the sample to the test cartridge, a precise quantity of sample is added to the reagents and the mixture passes into a test channel, where it is moved backward and forward through a narrow aperture. Two optical sensors or light-emitting diodes (LEDs) monitor the speed at which the sample moves between them; as the clot forms, the sample speed slows and when it reaches a predetermined level the instrument indicates the time. The same technology is used in the Gem® PCL Plus analyzer (Instrumentation Laboratory, Lexington, MA, USA), which can measure ACT, activated partial thromboplastin time (APTT), and PT. An evaluation of this device found that although the PT and APTT parameters showed a bias compared to those from a central laboratory, the PCL values were sufficiently reliable for clinical use (45).

Successive generations of coagulation monitors from Medtronic (Medtronic, Minneapolis, MN, USA) use a mechanical detection principle. The movement of a plunger-flag assembly in and out of the patient sample is monitored by optical sensors. After activation of the reagents by the patient sample, the clotting process is detected by the decreased drop rate of the plunger (46).

Several companies have used paramagnetic iron oxide particles as the clot detection principle, an approach originally developed by Cardiovascular Diagnostics. The particles are incorporated in the reaction chamber of a test cassette together with test-specific reagents for PT, APTT, or ACT. The iron particles move in a characteristic pattern in response to an oscillating magnetic field. Addition of a drop of blood to the cassette results in the formation of a clot that changes the movement of the particles, and this is detected by an infrared sensor; the time taken to reach this state is an indication of the clotting time (47).

The measurement principle of the Roche CoaguChek Pro/DM (Roche Diagnostics, Mannheim, Germany) relies on speckle detection technology to measure PT, APTT, and ACT. The patient sample is added to a cartridge that contains the reagents for a specific test. While the sample moves down the sample channel by capillary action, it mixes with the reagents and is oscillated. The instrument contains an infrared light source that directs a coherent light beam onto the oscillating sample. The movement of the red cells in the blood defracts the light to produce an interference or "speckle" pattern that is recorded by the photodetector. This speckle pattern changes when the capillary flow slows as the sample clots. The time taken for this to happen is a measure of the clotting time (48).

Newer detection technologies that can be classified broadly as electrochemical are used in the Hemosense and i-STAT instruments. The ACT cartridge of the i-STAT handheld analyzer contains celite and a substrate that has an amide linkage cleaved by thrombin in the patient sample. Clotting results in cleavage of a product that can be detected amperometrically as an indication of the ACT. A study of patients undergoing cardiac surgery and dialysis showed that i-STAT ACT results compared favorably to those from the Hemochron instrument and to overall heparin levels (49).

In the HemoSense InRatio™ coagulation meter for measurement of PT, (HemoSense, Milpitas, CA, USA), clotting is detected by impedance rather than current (50). Because this is a device likely to be used by patients, the device has various features designed to make QC automatic or that require minimal involvement of the patient. These include a test strip that has three channels, one for the patient test and two for different levels of internal QC; all three channels operate simultaneously when a patient sample is applied to the strip (Figure 3-5). Similar features of integrated onboard QC operate in other smaller meters or devices likely to be used by patients such as the ITC ProTime Microcoagulation System (ITC, Edison, NJ, USA). Several studies have shown that the ProTime device can be used satisfactorily by patients for self-testing purposes (51, 52). Many meters have QC lockout features that prevent operation of the device if the QC results are not within prescribed limits, as well as software to detect common errors such as expired reagents or incorrect specimen placement or volume.

Recent instruments now include either onboard data management facilities or software that easily allows them to be linked to laboratory or hospital information systems, so-called

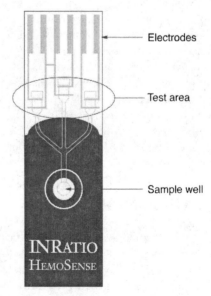

Figure 3-5 Hemosense test strip with three electrodes for patient and QC samples. Courtesy of HemoSense.

connectivity. Software features in devices used as part of the process to administer heparin or other anticoagulants include the ability to calculate doses through input of data such as the height and weight of the patient. Thus the Bayer Rapidpoint Accent device (Bayer Diagnostics, Tarrytown, NY, USA) has the ability to calculate the amount of protamine required to reverse heparin-induced anticoagulation following open heart surgery (53).

One of the major issues that still remain for point-of-care coagulation testing is comparison of POCT data to results from coagulation analyzers in the central laboratory. This is a particular problem for ACT, where a gold standard for comparison does not exist (44). Reports in the literature indicate that despite improvements and progress with standardization, lack of agreement can still be a major problem (54).

PLATELET FUNCTION ANALYZERS

Over the years, a number of techniques and devices have been designed to measure platelet function. The use and function of these devices overlaps to some extent with those described previously, and this reflects the fact that platelets are an integral part of both the coagulation and hemostasis processes. Several studies of open-heart surgery patients have shown the potential for point-of-care coagulation and platelet assays to reduce both bleeding and the use of transfused blood products in these patients (55). This section will focus on instruments specifically designed to measure platelet function, some of which have been designed to be used at the point of care (Table 3-3).

The thromboelastograph was originally developed in the 1940s but has enjoyed renewed interest in recent times as a bedside monitor of hemostasis in patients who have undergone cardiac or liver surgery. The TEG® thromboelastograph (Haemoscope, Niles, IL, USA) comprises a sample cup that oscillates back and forth constantly at a set speed through an arc of 4° 45′. Whole blood is placed into the cup, and a stationary pin attached to a torsion wire is immersed into the blood. When the first fibrin forms, it begins to bind the cup and pin, causing the pin to oscillate in phase with the clot. The acceleration of the movement of the pin is a function of the kinetics of clot development and is displayed on a chart recorder. Older thromboelastographs required considerable skill to use and maintain,

but the latest model from Haemoscope is an ergonomically designed, user-friendly benchtop device that is a combined hemostasis-coagulation analyzer. Software enables the operator to perform a completely automated platelet function assessment and functional fibrinogen assay. Application of the TEG has been shown to reduce the postoperative transfusion of blood products from 25% in a standard-test-guided group to 5.6% in the TEG-guided group (56).

The Sonoclot analyzer (Sienco, Wheat Ridge, CO, USA) measures changes in the viscoelastic properties of a blood clot. An ultrasonic probe is placed in a cuvette containing the blood sample and celite. As the sample clots, the viscous force creates an impedance to the vibrating probe, and the output signal is displayed as a graph (Sonoclot signature). The graph has various characteristic features that reflect the clotting process, including the time to peak, which is an indicator of platelet count and function (44). The performance of the analyzer has been reviewed by Forestier et al. (57), and it has been shown to be a useful investigation in patients undergoing cardiac surgery (58).

Platelet function can also be assessed from the ability of blood to clot when exposed to high shearing forces (59). A commercial instrument, the PFA-100 (Dade Behring, Deerfield, IL, USA) has been developed from this principle. It measures the closure time required for platelets to occlude an aperture in a membrane coated with different agonists. The closure time is dependent on the platelet activity. The instrument has not been specifically designed for point-of-care use, and there is only limited data on its usefulness for monitoring patients undergoing cardiac surgery (60). However, the PFA-100 has many user-friendly features including self-contained test cartridges and minimal sample manipulation, and it produces results in a few minutes.

A platelet-activated clotting test can be performed on the Hemochron Hemostasis Management System (Medtronic, Minneapolis, MN, USA) The kaolin-activated clotting time is measured in the presence or absence of increasing concentrations of platelet-activating factor (PAF). The final result is a clot ratio that is related to postoperative blood loss in certain patients undergoing cardiac surgery (61, 62). The test is conveniently packaged as a six-channel cartridge containing kaolin, heparin, and increasing levels of PAF.

Table 3-3 Benchtop Devices Used for Assessment of Platelet Function

Device	Measured parameter	Detection principle
TEG thromboelastograph (Haemoscope)	Clot physical properties	Electrical transduction of clot formation in a rotating cup
Sonoclot analyzer (Sienco)	Clot viscoelastic properties	Change in impedance of an ultrasonic, vibrating probe
PFA-100 (Dade Behring)	Closure time following activation with epinephrine or ADP	Change in pressure across aperture as platelets form a plug
Hemostasis Management System (Medtronic)	Effect on clotting process of platelet-activating factor	Optical measurement of the change in the rise and fall of a plunger

HEMOGLOBIN AND COMPLETE BLOOD COUNT MEASUREMENTS

A number of dedicated devices are available for point-of-care measurement of hemoglobin. The HemoCue device (HemoCue AB, Angelholm, Sweden) comprises a factory-calibrated small, portable analyzer and a single-use disposable cuvette. The latter has walls precoated with sodium deoxycholate to lyse erythrocytes, sodium nitrite to oxidize hemoglobin to hemiglobin, and sodium azide to form the final colored product, which is measured at 565 and 880 nm. The latter measurement is to correct for turbidity. Only 10 μL of the specimen is required, and the cuvette is self-filling. The accuracy and precision of the system has been proven in various studies (63, 64). Since its introduction, various other useful POCT features have been introduced to the system, including an internal, electronic self-test that is performed every time the analyzer is switched on, and data storage of up to 600 results. More recently the optics have been further improved to allow accurate measurement of hemoglobin levels down to 0.2 g/L (65).

The GDS Stat Site hemoglobin method (Stanbio Laboratory, Boeme, TX, USA) uses similar analytical principles, but measurement is by reflectance, using a single wavelength (66). The meter is calibrated using a lot-specific code card, the code from which is then stored in the meter's memory. The instrument optics are checked prior to placing a drop of blood on the reagent pad of the card, which is then inserted into the reflectance meter. The design of the meter does not allow blood to contaminate the meter itself. Only values between 60 and 210 g/L (6.0–21 g/dL) are reported; values outside of this range are reported as low or high.

The manufacturers of conventional laboratory hematology instruments have miniaturized their machines to produce models suitable for use in locations such as clinics or doctors' offices. These include the Beckman Coulter A^c.T diff2™ (Beckman Coulter, Brea, CA, USA), earlier models of which have been evaluated in point-of-care locations (67). The Sysmex KX-21N (Sysmex Corp., Kobe, Japan), which can perform a three-part differential, has an automated startup routine, and sampling only requires the pressing of a single button. While some of these devices have user-friendly features such as closed-tube sampling, they retain a degree of complexity and size that makes them less than ideal for bedside testing. In the future, we may see smaller and simpler complete blood count analyzers that use novel measurement technology with the capability to offer full white cell differentiation and which can be used easily at the point of care.

URINE TESTING

A large proportion of urine dipstick testing is performed at the point of care, and the majority of urine dipsticks are read visually. However, small desktop instruments are available to measure the color changes in the strips and are used increasingly in clinics and surgeries. All the manufacturers of urine strips make reflectance devices to measure their strips, such as the Bayer Clinitek® 50 (Bayer Diagnostics, Medfield, MA, USA) or the Roche Chemstrip® 101 (Roche Diagnostics, Mannheim, Germany). In both these devices, strips have to be manually placed in the device following placement of the sample on the strip, but the timing of incubation, measurement, calculation of results, and printout are all automatic. The major advantage of these devices is in avoiding the errors that occur from poor timing, as well as those from the visual reading of marginal color changes and operator-to-operator variability (68).

In the typical physician's office practice, where a variety of different tests may be performed, space to locate instrumentation may be at a premium. Thus the attractiveness and utility of automated urine strip readers is likely to be increased if the same instrumentation can be used to perform other tests. The Bayer Clinitek Status™ is an example of a device that combines reading of urine dipsticks with the qualitative measurement of urine hCG using a lateral flow immunoassay (69). The latter is also a test that can be subject to the vagaries of visual interpretation and would therefore benefit from automated reading. Besides combining tests, the Status offers a touch screen and automatic printout of results, both useful operator features in a busy practice or ward. Later-generation devices can also be easily linked to information systems via connectivity software, thus helping to ensure that results will appear in the patient record.

CONCLUSIONS

Advances in design and manufacturing are now capable of incorporating what is essentially a minilaboratory into a relatively small benchtop device. The most sophisticated critical care analyzers can now measure directly nearly 20 parameters, and an even larger number if you include derived indices. Not only has a degree of miniaturization been achieved but the designs include features that prevent many of the potential operator errors from occurring. Equally important, the analytical performance of these devices is as good as that seen for analysis in the central laboratory, as shown in Table 3-4, which compares the precision of sodium and potassium analytes in relation to external quality control data.

The same technological trends have taken place with devices dedicated to measurement of single or small panels of analytes, including coagulation parameters and diabetes-related analytes such as cholesterol. In the latter case, Table 3-4 shows that the precision of POCT cholesterol is not as good as that achieved by the central laboratory, as judged by quality control materials, but it may be sufficient for certain clinical purposes and is likely to improve with further technological innovation.

Other future developments are likely to include a similar evolution in capability for immunoassay instruments as has occurred for critical care analyzers and also for DNA measurements. There is probably already a need to perform PCR and other molecular techniques closer to the patient, such as for

Table 3-4   Quality of Analysis of Electrolytes and Cholesterol on Central Laboratory Equipment Compared to Point-of-Care Devices

Performance measured	Sodium		Potassium		Cholesterol	
	SD	CV %	SD	CV %	SD	CV %
Best central laboratories	0.6	0.4	0.02	0.5	0.025	0.6
50% of central laboratories	1.5	1.1	0.07	1.7	0.102	2.5
Best POCT sites	0.3	0.2	0.00	0.1	0.076	1.8
50% of POCT sites	1.0	0.7	0.06	1.6	0.183	4.4

Data courtesy of the Royal College of Pathologists of Australasia Quality Assurance Programs Ltd. Data quoted is average performance obtained from analysis of 12 linearly related samples over 24 weeks.

infectious disease detection or for pharmacogenomics testing. However, a suitable instrument to perform such tasks has yet to be developed.

At the moment, many common panels of tests have to be performed on different analyzers. Thus, despite the large menus of many sophisticated critical care analyzers, they do not incorporate the ability to measure coagulation parameters or cardiac makers on a single sample, cassette, or cartridge. Such a development may not be far away. In the case of chronic disease management, the ability to measure the common diabetes-related tests on a single instrument would also be very useful.

Finally, while the design of these devices now precludes many of the typical operating errors, no device yet made is foolproof. The latter is an elusive goal, but one that will continue to drive innovation and design in the development of benchtop POCT analyzers.

REFERENCES

1. Kallner A. Benchtop technology. In: Price CP, Hicks JM, eds. Point-of-care testing. Washington, DC: AACC Press, 1999:67–98.
2. McClelland I, Adamson K, Black ND. Information issues in telemedicine systems. J Telemed Telcare 1995;1:7–12.
3. Khandurina J, Guttman A. Bioanalysis in microfluidic devices. J Chromatogr A 2002;943:159–83.
4. Scott MG, Heusal JW, LeGrys VA, Siggaard-Andersen O. Electrolytes and blood gases. In: Eds Burtis CA, Ashwood ER, ed. Tietz textbook of clinical chemistry, 3rd ed. Philadelphia: WB Saunders, 1999:1056–92.
5. Schlebusch H, Paffenholz I, Zerbach R, Leinberger R. Analytical performance of a portable critical care analyser. Clin Chim Acta 2001;307:107–12.
6. Boalth N, Wandrup J, Larsson L, Frischauf PA, Lundsgaard FC, Andersen WL, et al. Blood gases and oximetry: calibration-free new dry-chemistry and optical technology for near-patient testing. Clin Chim Acta 2001;307:225–33.
7. Ritter C, Gharamani M, Krysl FJ, Lang S, Poltl C, Weis L. A new family of maintenance free sensors for blood gas analysis in micro volumes. In: D'Orzio P, ed. Preparing for critical care analyses in the 21st century. Proceedings of the 16th International Symposium. Washington, DC. AACC Press, 1996.
8. Schaffar BH, Kontschieder H, Ritter C, Berger H. Highly miniaturized and integrated biosensor for analysis of whole blood samples. Clin Chem 1999;45:1678–9.
9. Stott RA, Hortin GL, Wilhite TR, Miller SB, Smith CH, Landt M. Analytical artifacts in hematocrit measurements by whole-blood chemistry analysers Clin Chem 1995;41:306–11.
10. Brunelle JA, Degtiarov AM, Moran RF, Race LA. Simultaneous measurement of total hemoglobin and its derivatives in blood using CO-oximeters; Analytical principles; their application in selecting analytical wavelengths and reference methods; a comparison of the results and the choices made. Scand J Clin Lab Invest 1996;56(Suppl 224):47–69.
11. Rolinski B, Kuster H, Ugele B, Gruber R, Horn K. Total bilirubin measurement by photometry on a blood gas analyser: potential for use in neonatal testing at the point of care. Clin Chem 2001;47:1845–7.
12. Gosling P, Dickson G. Syringe injection pressure: a neglected factor in blood PO_2 determination. Ann Clin Biochem 1990;27:147–51.
13. Mollard J-F. Single phase calibration for blood gas and electrolyte analysis. In: D'Orazio P, ed., Preparing for critical care analyses in the 21st century. Proceedings of the 16th International Symposium. Washington, DC: AACC Press, 1996.
14. Jacobs E, Nowakowski M, Colman N. Performance of Gem Premier blood gas/electrolyte analyser evaluated. Clin Chem 1993;39:189–93.
15. D'Orazio P, Maley T, McCaffrey RR. Planar (bio)sensors for critical care diagnostics. Clin Chem 1997;43:1804–5.
16. Davis G. Microfabricated sensors and the commercial development of the i-STAT point-of-care system. In Ramsay G, ed. Commercial biosensors. New York: John Wiley & Sons, 1998; 47–76.
17. Magny E, Renard MF, Launay JM. Analytical evaluation of Rapidpoint 400 blood gas analyser. Ann Biol Clin (Paris) 2001; 59:622–8.
18. Lindemans J, Hoefkens P, van Kessel AL, Bonnay M, Kulpmann WR, van Suijlen JD. Portable blood gas and electrolyte analyser evaluated in a multiinstitutional study. Clin Chem 1999;45: 111–7.
19. Jacobs E, Ancy JJ, Smith M. Multi-site performance evaluation of pH, blood gas, electrolyte, glucose, and lactate determinations with the Gem Premier 3000 critical care analyzer. Point of Care 2002;1:135–44.
20. Lubbers DW. Optical sensors for clinical monitoring. Acta Anaesthesiol Scand 1995;35:37–54.
21. Hirst D, St John A. Keeping the spotlight on quality from a distance. Accred Qual Assur 2000;5:9–13.
22. Westgard JO, Stein B. Automated selection of statistical quality-control procedures to assure meeting clinical or analytical quality requirements. Clin Chem 1997;43:400–3.

23. Phillips DL. Quality systems for unit-use testing devices. Clin Chem 1997;43:893–6.

24. Westgard JO. Electronic quality control, the total testing process, and the total quality control system. Clin Chim Acta 2001;307: 45–8.

25. Steinhausen RL, Price CP. Principles and practices of dry chemistry systems. In: Price CP, Alberti KGMM, eds. Recent advances in clinical biochemistry. Edinburgh, Scotland: Churchill Livingstone, 1985;273–96.

26. CP Price, PU Koller. A multicentre study of the new Reflotron system for the measurement of urea, glucose, triacylglycerols, cholesterol, gamma-glutamyltransferase and haemoglobin. J Clin Chem Clin Biochem 1988;26:233–50.

27. Schembri CT, Ostoich V, Lingane PJ, Burd TL, Buhl SN. Portable simultaneous multiple analyte whole-blood analyser for point-of-care testing. Clin Chem 1992;38:1665–70.

28. Boncheva M, Pascaleva I, Dineva D. Performance of POCT-chemistry analyzer Picollo (Abaxis) in primary health care. Gen Med 2002;4:28–31.

29. Schultz SG, Holen JT, Donohue JP, Francoeur TA. Two-dimensional centrifugation for desktop clinical chemistry. Clin Chem 1985;31:1457–63.

30. Cobbaert C, Boerma GJ, Lindemans J. Evaluation of the Cholestech LDX desktop analyser for cholesterol, HDL-cholesterol and triglycerides in heparinised venous blood. Eur J Clin Chem & Clin Biochem 1994;32:391–4.

31. Heeschen C, Goldmann BU, Langenbrink L, Matschuck G, Hamm CW. Evaluation of a rapid whole blood ELISA for quantification of troponin I in patients with acute chest pain. Clin Chem 1999;45:1789–96.

32. Pope RM, Apps JM, Page MD, Allen K, Bodansky HJ. A novel device for the rapid in-clinic measurement of haemoglobin A1c. Diabet Med 1993;3:260–3.

33. Parsons MP, Newman DJ, Newall RG, Price CP. Validation of a point-of-care assay for the urinary albumin: creatinine ratio. Clin Chem 1999;45:414–7.

34. ECRI. Evaluation Glycohemoglobin Analyzers. Health Devices 2003;32:409–35.

35. Hedberg P, Valkama J, Puukka M. Analytical performance of time-resolved fluorometry-based Innotrac Aio! cardiac marker immunoassays. Scand J Clin Lab Invest 2003;63:55–64.

36. Qin QP, Christiansen M, Pettersson K. Point-of-care time-resolved immunofluorometric assay for human pregnancy-associated plasma protein A: use in first-trimester screening for Down syndrome. Clin Chem 2002;48:473–83.

37. Qin QP, Peltola O, Pettersson K. Time-resolved fluorescence resonance energy transfer assay for point-of-care testing of urinary albumin. Clin Chem 2003;49:1105–13.

38. Mathis G, Metzler J, Fussenegger D, Sutterlutti G, Feurstein M, Fritzsche H. Sonographic observation of pulmonary infarction and early infarctions by pulmonary embolism. Eur Heart J 1993; 14:804–8.

39. Spencer K, Spencer CE, Power M, Dawson C, Nicolaides KH. Screening for chromosomal abnormalities in the first trimester using ultrasound and maternal serum biochemistry in a one-stop clinic: a review of three years prospective experience. BJOG 2003;110:281–6.

40. Meisner M. Pathobiochemistry and clinical use of procalcitonin. Clin Chim Acta 2002;323:17–29.

41. Christ-Chain M, Jaccard-Stolz D, Bingisser R, Gencay MM, Huber PR, Tamm M, et al. Effect of procalcitonin-guided treatment on antibiotic use and outcome in lower respiratory tract infections: cluster-randomised, single-blinded intervention trial. Lancet 2004;363:600–7.

42. Laposata M. Point-of-care coagulation testing: stepping gently forward. Clin Chem 2001;47:801–2.

43. Zweig SE. Dry reagent prothrombin time and other hemostasis methods. In: Kost GJ, ed. Principles and practice of point-of-care testing. Philadelphia: Lippincott Williams & Wilkins, 2002;57–66.

44. Prisco D, Paniccia R. Point-of-care testing of hemostasis in cardiac surgery. Thromb J 2003;1:1–10.

45. Hirsch J, Wendt T, Kuhly P, Schaffartzik W. Point-of-care testing apparatus. Measurement of coagulation. Anaesthesia 2001;56: 760–3.

46. Oberhardt BJ. Thrombosis and homeostasis testing at the point of care. Am J Clin Pathol 1995;104(4 Suppl 1):S72–8.

47. Oberhardt BJ, Dermott SC, Taylor M, Alkadi ZY, Abruzzini AF, Gresalfi NJ. Dry reagent technology for rapid convenient measurement of blood coagulation and fibrinolysis. Clin Chem 1991; 37:520–6.

48. Solomon H, Mullins R, Lyden P, Thompson P, Hudoff S. The diagnostic accuracy of bedside and laboratory coagulation procedures used to monitor the anticoagulation status of patients treated with heparin. Am J Clin Pathol 1998;109:371–8.

49. Paniccia RF, Fedi S, Carbonetto F, Noferi D, Conti PF, Bandinelli B, et al. Evaluation of a new point-of-care celite-activated clotting time analyzer in different clinical settings. The i-STAT celite-activated clotting time test. Anesthesiology 2003;99:54–9.

50. Jina A. A novel point-of-care prothrombin time monitoring system Chest 2000;118(Suppl): 2835.

51. Oral Anticoagulation Monitoring Study Group. Point-of-care prothrombin time measurement for professional and patient self-testing use. A multicenter clinical experience. Am J Clin Pathol 2001;115:288–96.

52. Oral Anticoagulation Monitoring Study Group. Prothrombin measurement using a patient self-testing system. Am J Clin Pathol 2001;115:280–7.

53. Fitch JC, Geary KL, Mirto GP, Byrne DW, Hines RL. Heparin management test versus activated coagulation time during cardiovascular surgery: correlation with anti-Xa activity. J Cardiothorac Vasc Anesth 1999;13:53–7.

54. Tripodi A, Chantarangkul V, Mannucci P. Near-patient testing devices to monitor oral anticoagulant therapy. Br J Haematol 2001;113:847–52.

55. Despotis GJ, Joist JH, Goodnough LT. Monitoring of hemostasis in cardiac surgical patients: impact of point-of-care testing on blood loss and transfusion outcomes. Clin Chem 1997;43:1684–96.

56. Shore-Lesserson L, Manspeizer HE, DePerio M, Francis S, Vela-Cantos F, Ergin MA. Thromboelastography-guided transfusion algorithm reduces transfusions in complex cardiac surgery. Anesth Analg 1999;88:312–9.

57. Forestier F, Belisle S, Contant C, Harel F, Janvier G, Hardy JF. Reproducibility and interchangeability of the Thromboelastograph, Sonoclot and Hemochron activated coagulation time in cardiac surgery. Can J Anaesth 2001;48:902–10.

58. Miyashita T, Kuro M. Evaluation of platelet function by Sonoclot analysis compared with other hemostatic variables in cardiac surgery. Anesth Analg 1998;87:1228–33.

59. Kratzer MA, Born GV. Simulation of primary haemostasis in vitro. Haemostasis 1985;15:357–62.

60. Slaughter TF, Sreeram G, Sharma AD, El Moalem H, East CJ, Greenberg CS. Reversible shear-mediated platelet dysfunction during cardiac surgery as assessed by the PFA-100 platelet function analyzer. Blood Coagul Fibrinolysis 2001;12:85–93.

61. Despotis GJ, Levine V, Saleem R, Spitznagel E, Joist JH. Use of point-of-care test in identification of patients who can benefit from desmopressin during cardiac surgery: a randomized controlled trial. Lancet 1999;354:106–10.

62. Despotis GJ, Levine V, Filos KS, Santoro SA, Joist JH, Spitznagel E, Goodnough LT. Evaluation of a new point-of-care test that measures PAF-mediated acceleration of coagulation in cardiac surgical patients. Anesthesiology 1996;85:1311–23.

63. Von Schenck H, Falkensson M, Lundberg B. Evaluation of HemoCue, a new device for determining hemoglobin. Clin Chem 1986;32:562–9.

64. Agarwal R, Heinz T. Bedside hemoglobinometry in hemodialysis patients: Lessons from point-of-care testing. ASAIO J 2001;47:240–3.

65. Morris LD, Pont A, Lewis SM. Use of a new HemoCue system for measuring haemoglobin at low concentrations. Clin Lab Haematol 2001;23:91–6.

66. Wu I, Peterson JR, Mohammad AA, Okorodudu AO. Evaluation of Stat-Site MHgb reflectance meter using hemosite for POC hemoglobin measurement Clin Chem 2002;48:A199.

67. Despotis GJ, Alsoufiev A, Hogue CW, Zoys TN, Goodnough LT, Santora SA, et al. Comparison of CBC results from a new, on-site hemocytometer to a laboratory-based hemocytometer. Crit Care Med 1996;24:1163–7.

68. Pugia MJ, Lott JA, Clark LW, Parker DR, Wallace JF, Willis TW. Comparisons of urine dipsticks with quantitative methods for microalbuminuria. Eur J Clin Chem Clin Biochem 1997;35:693–700.

69. Brock GH, Krauth KE, Luke KE, Zimmerle CT, Ledden DJ. An objectively read lateral flow immunoassay for urine hCG. Clin Chem 2003;49:A151.

Chapter 4

Noninvasive Technology for Point-of-Care Testing

Mihailo V. Rebec, Michael P. Houlne, Thomas P. Benson, Scott E. Carpenter, Donald R. Parker, and Paul M. Ripley

FUNDAMENTAL ANALYTICAL PRINCIPLES

Within the broad range of strategies used for clinical diagnostics, considerable effort has been directed to developing techniques and instrumentation that can lessen the discomfort and decrease the postprocedural complications that patients may experience during examination and diagnosis. The main objective of these initial efforts was to develop noninvasive techniques that would reduce the need for exploratory surgery as a diagnostic tool with its attendant complications and costs. Ultimately these strategies would employ noninvasive systems that use various technologies to visualize internal body structures and tissues without the need for surgery (1, 2). This led to the development of the most recognizable noninvasive diagnostic tools to date, such as computed tomography, magnetic resonance imaging (MRI), and ultrasound imaging. The dramatic impact of these new technologies has created high expectations within the medical community and led to an increased emphasis on the development of other new noninvasive tools.

The next area to receive considerable attention has been the development of noninvasive technologies that can detect a specific type of analyte within the living human body, in order to assist with managing important physiological problems. The precise detection of an individual analyte or molecule is an enormous challenge that places stringent demands on current technology and understanding. Consequently, most of the initial efforts have concentrated on the detection of analytes that require frequent analysis and that necessitate a sampling process that can be both difficult and painful. One area in which significant effort has been invested is the real-time monitoring of blood gases. Advances in this area have resulted in the development and commercialization of pulse oximeters, which are used to measure the oxygen saturation of hemoglobin in the blood in the form of oximetry (3–5), and are commonly found in most hospitals. This noninvasive approach is widely used with ambulatory patients and during anesthesia-assisted surgery. A second accomplishment of noninvasive technology has been the development and commercialization of the Bili-Check® device (6), which is used to monitor the concentration of bilirubin in newborn infants and eliminates the need for painful heelsticks. A third analyte that has attracted enormous ongoing attention is glucose, more specifically, monitoring the concentration of glucose in individuals with diabetes.

Recently it has been recognized that glucose monitoring is increasingly important and is of international concern. The World Health Organization has reported that the number of people with diabetes has grown significantly during the past 20 years (7), and this figure is predicted to double from approximately 170 million in 2000 to more than 350 million by 2030 (8). Furthermore, clinical evidence has clearly indicated that improved metabolic control leads to a dramatic reduction in microvascular complications associated with diabetes (9–11). Glucose is already the most widely tested analyte within medical diagnostics, and thus represents the single largest market segment in the diagnostic area; in the United States direct medical costs associated with disorders of glucose metabolism were estimated at $92 billion for 2002 (12). In the same study the indirect costs associated with such issues as work days lost through ill health and minor complications were estimated at $43 billion. Consequently, much time and effort has been invested in the development of more rapid, reliable, and less painful glucose analysis methods for both patients and medical professionals. Currently, glucose control for diabetic individuals may require several daily fingersticks, which are carried out with disposable lancets and testing strips. Multiple fingersticks can lead to both pain and discomfort. Over time these consumables can become costly and difficult to manage. Thus, scores of companies and research centers have been devoting significant effort in both time and money to the development of a noninvasive test for glucose.

METHODOLOGIES FOR NONINVASIVE GLUCOSE MONITORING

Two unique approaches are used for accomplishing a noninvasive glucose measurement. The first method involves removing the glucose from the body and conducting the analysis externally. The second approach is to analyze glucose within its natural living environment. Several systems that fit into the first category measure glucose contained in the interstitial fluid (ISF). These systems use different techniques for bringing the ISF that contains glucose to the surface of the skin. An example of one of these techniques, developed by Cygnus® (Redwood City, CA, USA), is reverse iontophoresis, in which an electrical potential is applied to the skin, which in turn drives ions through the skin to the surface along with glucose (13). The glucose is then analyzed by means of a conventional biosensor approach. Another group, Sontra (Franklin, MA, USA), uses a different technique for acquiring ISF. They use ultrasonic waves to increase the permeability of skin by perforating the protective stratum corneum. This creates a liquid bridge that allows ISF, with its glucose content, to diffuse to the surface of the skin. As in other methods, the glucose is then analyzed using a conventional biosensor.

These approaches have a distinct advantage in that glucose can be analyzed directly using a proven glucose-specific, analytical technique. These unique strategies also offer some other major advantages in that glucose measurements made outside of the body do not encounter interference from bulk tissue. Furthermore, if the ISF sample is extracted into a well-defined volume, then the glucose concentration can easily be calculated. However, there are other issues with these methodologies that are related to the consistency of the glucose sampling process, in particular how closely the glucose obtained from ISF that is brought to the skin matches the plasma glucose concentration. The relationship between ISF and plasma glucose is a very active area of research, especially the quantification of the time delays that occur for changes in the plasma glucose to be reflected in the ISF glucose. These time delays can be long because they represent the cumulative time for several linked events to occur. These include the time for ISF-based glucose changes to match plasma glucose changes and the time required to transport the glucose to the skin surface, have the glucose enter the analytical device, and finally allow the device time to perform an accurate analysis. The total time required for all of these functions can reach 30 min and presents a significant problem for the widespread use of these techniques where more rapid glucose control is required. Finally, with all of these techniques it should be emphasized that the glucose sample only comes from the ISF and this could be different from the actual plasma glucose concentration.

Measurement of glucose without removal from the body can be accomplished in three distinctive ways. Direct methods attempt to measure the optical or spectral properties of the glucose molecule in order to determine the glucose concentration in the body fluids. This approach is very similar in execution to the principles applying to both the BiliCheck and pulse oximeters. Indirect methods do not measure glucose directly but instead measure a particular property of living tissue that responds to specific changes in plasma glucose concentration. The tissue properties studied as a possible means of indirect glucose detection include optical scattering, changes in the indices of refraction, ionic strength, tissue conductance, and also impedance. A positive aspect of the indirect approach is that the secondary impact of glucose concentration changes could provide a much more superior signal for detection than some of the direct schemes (14, 15).

However, one significant drawback of indirect measurements is that changes in other analytes can also lead to similar alterations in the same tissue property. Furthermore, this change could produce a much larger signal than that observed with glucose. This type of problem was demonstrated in a study that investigated the potential of optical glucose sensors (16). The optical sensors were designed to measure changes in the optical scattering of skin as an indirect measure of glucose concentration. However, optical scattering was also found to change with the level of skin hydration (water), temperature, and other physiological processes involved with regulating blood flow. Therefore, changes associated with other tissue analytes have the potential to confuse the process of linking indirect measurements, which are specifically related to glucose concentration changes. Lastly, a combination of direct and indirect methods can be used. In this case the actual glucose concentration is derived by measuring changes in specific human physiology, which are associated with alterations in blood glucose concentration. Physiological events that have been investigated as potential indicators of changes in glucose concentration include blood flow, e.g., vasodilation, body core temperature, and changes in vision. It should be noted, however, that these types of indicators would be very specific to an individual and may not be appropriate for all patients.

OPTICAL-BASED TECHNIQUES FOR GLUCOSE MONITORING

The direct measurement of glucose seems to be the most desirable approach. Essentially, because glucose changes are based on glucose-specific molecular information, this could minimize interference from other analytes and also help to reduce other factors introduced by patient variability. Most of these direct techniques use some form of optical spectroscopy that uses light of specific wavelengths to identify glucose in bulk tissue (16, 17). The majority of all published reports in the area of noninvasive glucose analysis specifically report utilizing light from the near-infrared (NIR) spectral region (18–23). This region is of great interest because it combines glucose specificity and skin penetration properties that are not found in any other spectral regions, and has greatest potential for the eventual development of a noninvasive system. In this wavelength region NIR light interacts with the molecular structure of matter in a unique manner, which can be made very specific to glucose as well as other molecules or analytes (24–32). Therefore, NIR spectroscopy can be exploited to allow one to specifically observe glucose in tissue and quantify changes in its concentration. In addition to molecular specificity, light in this wavelength range also has excellent tissue penetration, minimizing optical interference such as tissue fluorescence. The ability of near-infrared light to penetrate tissue to a depth of centimeters, compared to millimeters for visible light, allows for a greater volume of analyte to be investigated. This in turn improves the accuracy of measuring the minute changes in glucose concentration.

Several different optical techniques have been employed for noninvasive glucose analysis (20). However, the most common have used either absorbance or Raman spectroscopy. In absorbance spectroscopy, light of a known intensity and wavelength is directed into the target tissue. A fraction of the light is absorbed by glucose and this can then be mathematically related to the quantity of glucose in that tissue site. Two experimental designs of the absorbance scheme have been most commonly used for glucose detection. The first is a transmission design in which light enters a tissue sample and transmits directly through to the opposite side for detection (32). The second is a reflectance design in which light impinges on a tissue sample, penetrates a small distance below the surface, and reflects back for detection (33–36).

Raman spectroscopy is performed by aiming a laser beam (single wavelength) at a particular tissue site. The incident laser light transfers energy to the tissue, which in turn scatters light back at wavelengths characteristic of the chemical composition of the tissue. The application of Raman spectroscopy for noninvasive glucose analysis is difficult because the size of the Raman signal is extremely small when compared to other optical techniques, such as absorbance- or transmission-based schemes. However, the advantage of Raman spectroscopy lies in the fact that the signal is very specific to the chemical composition of the tissue site. Thus it is easier to differentiate target molecules such as glucose in a complex tissue matrix using Raman compared to absorbance techniques. Another attractive aspect of Raman spectroscopy is that the water absorption features, which can create undesirable interference in most parts of the NIR region, have minimal impact on spectral information generated by the Raman technique.

Another spectroscopic technique that has received attention is optical rotation, which is a property of chiral molecules such as glucose. A chiral molecule has a molecular structure that cannot be superimposed on its own mirror image. Consequently, chiral molecules have the ability to rotate the polarization of monochromatic plane-polarized light that is passed through them. The degree of optical rotation depends on several factors such as the concentration of the compound, the path length the light traverses, and the wavelength of light used. This method has been used by several investigators to measure glucose by taking advantage of the chirality of the molecule (37–42). Optical rotation is not a particularly selective technique. It would be impossible to determine the concentration of a specific, single optically active species in a complex mixture of many other optically active compounds. Thus, most investigations have been done in vitro using aqueous samples or cell culture media (37–39). As different chiral species may be present in bulk tissue, several other investigators have explored the aqueous humor of the eye as a potential noninvasive approach to determining glucose concentration with polarimetry (40–42). The aqueous humor offers a much simpler biological medium, with a chemical environment containing considerably fewer interfering analytes.

The pursuit of noninvasive glucose detection has also given rise to some novel methodologies. An example is Kro-moscopy, which has recently been advanced (43–46) as a technique designed to correlate glucose concentration with the infrared color of tissue. It has been claimed that the technique has a direct analogy with the concept of human color perception. Kromoscopy is similar to absorbance spectroscopy except that the absorbance measurement is made with four overlapping wavelength bands as opposed to several single-wavelength channels. This unique approach claims to offer a simplified technique to perform a complex task (43). However, it is currently unknown how this technique would perform with real tissue samples in which light scattering dominates.

Photoacoustic spectroscopy has also been advanced as a possible technique for noninvasive glucose analysis (47–51). In photoacoustic spectroscopy light of a wavelength that is specific to the target molecule is focused in a small region within the tissue sample. As the target analyte in the tissue absorbs the light, it begins to heat up and expand, which in turn creates a pressure wave. This pressure wave is manifest as sound and can thus be detected with the use of a sensitive microphone. If the sample is scanned through several wavelengths, a fingerprint for glucose can be generated based on which wavelengths of light are optimum for creating sound waves for this particular analyte. Mackenzie and coworkers (52) have demonstrated that photoacoustic spectroscopy can be used to track glucose in both diabetic and nondiabetic subjects over the range of 5.5 to 27.7 mmol/L (100 to 500 mg/dL). However, in the same study the authors acknowledged that the possibility of interference from other analytes such as proteins exists, which would be the subject of further research.

CHALLENGES ASSOCIATED WITH NONINVASIVE MONITORING— ISSUES WITH TISSUES

Tissue is an inherently difficult matrix to study, regardless of the optical technique used, because its chemical composition and structural characteristics vary with time for each person as well as from person to person. These fleeting changes in tissue can have a significant effect on the optical nature of tissue (53), further complicating glucose analysis. Consequently, many noninvasive methods for glucose detection are still in development and have evolved from simpler in vitro experiments aimed at understanding the optical nature of tissue (53–56). These experiments have employed matrices in varying complexity ranging from tissue phantoms or artificial models (56–58), aqueous samples (59–65), and whole blood (66–68) to in vitro skin (54). Regardless of the optical technique deployed, several criteria common to all methods must be met to achieve success, including the strength of the optical signal to be measured, how specific the signal is to glucose, and finally the degree to which the measured glucose signal accurately represents the actual glucose in the body. Another important factor is the efficiency with which the diagnostic light is both delivered to the target site and collected. One of the most dominating tissue characteristics intrinsic to all light–tissue interactions is the scattering of light by cells within the tissue. Optical scattering in tissues is attributable predominantly to the difference in refractive index that exists between cell membranes and their cytoplasm. Other examples of refractive index mismatch that lead to scattering include that between the cell nucleus and organelles and the fluids that surround the actual cells. Variations in light scattering are critically dependent on many physical parameters such as temperature, wavelength, and tissue composition (water, blood, lipid, cell concentration, cell size, cell structure, etc.). Light scattering properties differ from one individual to the next, and can vary dynamically during a measurement process, thus making both calibration and the tracking of glucose trends very difficult. An illustrative example of how optical scattering can affect light traversing through tissue is shown in Figure 4-1. In the absorption case, Figure 4-1a, light that survives the absorption process is collected at the detector. In the presence of scattering (Figure 4-1b), some of the light that survives the absorption process undergoes scattering and is redistributed away from the detector, thus acting as another form of attenuation. A second significant contributor to the overall optical properties of tissue, especially in the infrared region, is absorbance by water. The glucose infrared spectral features are both broad and weak, and are located on two significantly stronger spectral features that are associated with scattering and water absorbance. This can be seen in the spectra shown in Figure 4-2. A relatively small path length, 50 μm, was used to emphasize how the main glucose peak in the near-infrared region is overlapped by water. In Figure 4-3, an exploded view of the "optical window" from 1 to 2 μm is shown, further indicating the weak absorption features of glucose in this region. If the path length is extended out to 1 mm, water absorption dominates from 2.5 μm onwards, preventing any of the strong glucose peaks from being observed. In Figures 4-2 to 4-4, the spectrum of glucose in the form of a pellet is displayed on all of the plots for comparison. Consequently, this combination of scattering and water absorbance can result in the attenuation of the diagnostic light to less than 1% of the original signal after it passes through tissue.

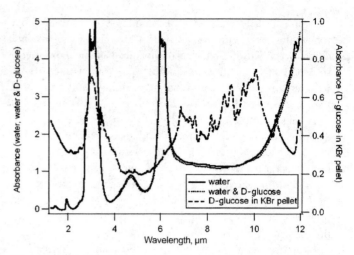

Figure 4-2 Absorption spectra of water and water containing 55.5 mmol/L (1000 mg/dL) of D-glucose. Both spectra were obtained using a path length of 50 μm. An absorption spectrum of pure D-glucose mounted in a KBr pellet is shown for comparison. The concentration of the pellet was 2 mmol/L (26 mg/dL); thickness was 2 mm.

IMPACT OF PHYSIOLOGICAL FACTORS ON NONINVASIVE DEVICES

As mentioned previously, indirect methods may have an advantage in that the signal they track tends to be greater in magnitude than those associated with the direct monitoring, thus making them easier to measure. Unfortunately, other plasma analytes can produce the same or even greater changes in signal. It is therefore imperative that the overlapping changes in analytes be decoupled in order to isolate glucose-related events. Early successes with these approaches have been slowed by this problem of decoupling (16). Methods that depend on a combination of direct and indirect methods rely on

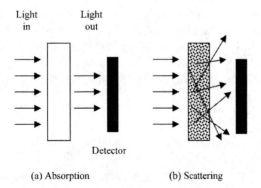

Figure 4-1 An illustrative example showing the difference between optical absorption (a) and scattering (b). In both cases the incident light is attenuated by the respective mechanism. However, in the case of optical scattering the light is redistributed by the target and not absorbed.

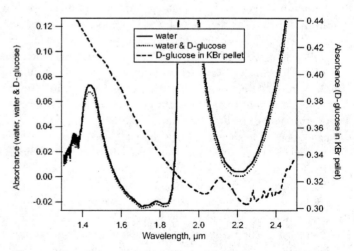

Figure 4-3 An exploded view of the spectra shown in Figure 4-1 over the optical window for human tissue between 1 and 2 μm. This part of the near-infrared spectrum includes areas referred to as the overtone and combination region. Note that water has low absorption in parts of this window, but glucose absorption is very weak.

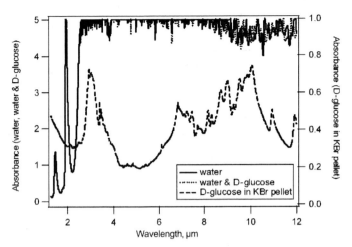

Figure 4-4 Absorption spectra obtained using the same concentration of D-glucose in water as in Figure 4-2. This time a path length of 1 mm was used in order to represent the amount of water typically sampled during a tissue-based optical measurement. Note how the strong water absorption completely dominates the main spectral peaks of D-glucose from 2.5 μm onward, and also obscures the optical window.

the physiological variations that result from changes in the blood glucose levels. Even though investigators can look for unique physiological signatures, such as the responsiveness of the human eye to varying patterns and frequencies at different glucose levels (69), a major challenge has been establishing how uniform these events are across the population. Furthermore, techniques that employ physiological events may be able to resolve large changes in concentration, such as between 8.3 and 13.9 mmol/L (150 to 250 mg/dL), but may not have the sensitivity to differentiate small differences, for example, 8.3 to 8.6 mmol/L (150 to 155 mg/dL).

Many groups have claimed success and some have announced that they will be launching a commercial noninvasive product in the near future. However, the technical hurdles associated with the development of a noninvasive monitoring system for glucose are understandably very high, and have prevented many ideas from being commercially realized. One of the most fundamental challenges is not technical but a direct physiological property of the body. In the blood of a healthy individual the normal concentration of glucose is about 5.6 mmol/L (100 mg/dL). The analyte typically represents 0.1% of the blood by mass. The relatively small mass of glucose plays a major role in determining the degree of accuracy required to track small changes in its concentration. For example, consider a noninvasive device that is attached to the finger as a target site. Any changes detected in the measured optical signal must be due to variations in the glucose concentration within the site. However, if the device were to move slightly or slip from the original location, a corresponding variation would occur in the optical signal. The variation could be caused by movement artifacts or by the fact that the signal is now sampling the same analyte in a different location. Both of these mechanisms have the potential to mask or confuse the original signal of interest,

resulting in unreliable tracking. Furthermore, the small optical signal emerging from the tissue site will easily be perturbed by tissue changes that can affect the most significant of tissue properties, optical scattering. These challenges can seem daunting, in particular when other issues such as the overall signal stability have yet to be considered, especially in the presence of an analyte whose concentration will also be dependent on other processes within the body. Consequently, a number of issues are related to noninvasive monitoring, which are independent of the analytical technique used, and can also have an effect on accuracy.

A glucose signal generated in the skin is the combination of information from two distinctively different locations—the intracellular and the extracellular space. Glucose in the extracellular space corresponds with glucose found in both the interstitial fluid and in the plasma located in the blood vessels. Intracellular glucose is found within the actual cells. Glucose originating in the intracellular space is very low compared to that found in the extracellular space. The question of how the concentration of glucose within the interstitial fluid relates to glucose in plasma has led to much debate within the clinical community. If we assume that most of the signal attributed to molecular glucose is found in the extracellular fluid, then we can deduce that 80% of this signal stems from glucose located specifically in the interstitial fluid. By comparison, if we were to break down the contributions of the total glucose signal that a noninvasive method obtains from the skin, less than 20% of the signal actually originates from plasma-based glucose. Therefore it is very apparent from these numbers that the relationship between ISF and plasma glucose is vital to the development of most noninvasive glucose systems. Furthermore, a clearer understanding of the contributions to the total glucose signal is needed as well as a clearly defined relationship between the interstitial and plasma glucose levels.

Another important consideration in the development of noninvasive glucose monitoring is the existence of glycated proteins within the skin. These create a static glucose background signal that will have to be distinguished from the dynamically changing glucose located in the ISF and plasma. Furthermore, tissue scattering properties, hydration levels, and glycation levels are different from one individual to the next. Consequently, these differences need to be accounted for and corrected in order for a noninvasive device to be used across a wide population base. In summary, the development of a noninvasive method for glucose monitoring represents a significant analytical challenge. Each technological approach represents parallel efforts involved in improving instrumentation to achieve better signal-to-noise ratios, refining the signal processing and developing more innovative calibration methods. Progress is being made in all of these key areas. Noninvasive techniques are being used for glucose that have reported >90% of predicted values to be in the A and B regions of the Clarke error grid (70, 71). However, performance standards for first- or second-generation noninvasive systems have yet to be defined, and these will ultimately affect when and where a noninvasive product reaches the public.

DESIGN CONCEPTS AND ILLUSTRATIVE EXAMPLES

The most familiar, widely recognized, and earliest noninvasive monitoring device used in the hospital was the infrared pulse oximeter. The development of the pulse oximeter dates as far back as 1874, when von Vieordt measured oxygen consumption by monitoring oxy- and deoxyhemoglobin bands spectroscopically (4, 5, 72–77). Aoygi is credited with developing the first commercial oximeter, which reached the market in 1974 (74). The miniaturization of electronics and sensors led to the development of a more practical device. By the mid-1980s, pulse oximetry had become a standard of care in the operating room (77), especially for monitoring blood oxygen saturation during anesthesia-assisted surgery. Even though noninvasive pulse oximetry does not provide an absolute measure of blood gases, as would be the case of laboratory testing, its ability to convey real-time, frequently updated information in an easily interpreted manner has contributed enormously to its acceptance in the clinical setting. Today, new applications of pulse oximetry continue to be developed (78).

By contrast, the most common noninvasive device to be found in the home would be the infrared ear thermometer. Invented by Phillips in 1986, the device measures the infrared radiation emitted from the eardrum. It has been successfully developed into a common home appliance, with several different variants readily available over the counter. Another hospital-based noninvasive device is the BiliCheck (79, 80), developed by SpectRx® (Norcross, GA, USA), which uses light reflected off the forehead to measure bilirubin levels in infants. Jaundice can affect up to 65% of all newborns and is the most common cause of hospital readmission during the first week of life. The measurement with the BiliCheck replaces a more time-consuming laboratory analysis of blood drawn from the heel of an infant, which is both painful and could lead to possible site infection with repeated measurements. This has helped to reduce the need for numerous painful heelsticks to obtain blood samples for bilirubin content analysis, thus increasing patient consent and compliance. The device received FDA approval in 1999, although it had been marketed in Europe for up to 1 year earlier. Hill-Rom AirShields® (Hatboro. PA, USA) also make a noninvasive bilirubinometer (80) as part of their line of infant care products.

The noninvasive measurement of glucose has tantalized researchers for some time as the search for an alternative to painful fingersticks for the growing population of diabetics has taken on greater importance. In the mid-1990s Futrex™ (Gaithersburg, MD, USA) promoted its DreamBeam™ analyzer, which measured glucose noninvasively with infrared light, as the first direct measurement device to be announced by a company. The device was never commercialized, amid protracted legal problems. BICO (Pittsburgh, PA, USA), formerly Biocontrol Technology, developed the Diasensor® 1000, which claimed to measure glucose from light reflected off the forearm. The FDA delayed making a final recommendation for approval in 1996 pending the presentation of additional data by the company. No such approval has been granted to date. BICO did receive Conformité Européene (CE) approval to market the device in Europe in 1998, although it is unclear how many such devices have been sold. Like Futrex, the company was involved in several legal difficulties. A new device, the Diasensor 2000, continues to be marketed in Europe today. Raman spectroscopy has recently been commercialized by LighTouch™ Medical. However, an actual device is not yet on the market (81).

The unfulfilled promises of the early devices of the 1990s appear to be partially realized with the development of the Glucowatch G2® Biographer (82–85) by Cygnus® (Redwood City, CA, USA). This second-generation device, which received FDA approval in 2002, is a follow-up on the initial Biographer approved in 1999. As its name would imply, the device is worn like a watch and applies an extremely low electric current to pull glucose from the interstitial fluid below the skin surface. The Biographer contains a single-use Autosensor® that collects and measures the glucose in the extracted sample. The Biographer is not intended as a replacement for fingerstick testing, but as an adjunctive device to track trends in glucose patterns that would otherwise be difficult to track with existing technology. A major benefit of the continuous monitoring provided by the device is the detection of hypoglycemic events. Cygnus acknowledges several limitations of the device, but further improvements in the technology are likely. Although Pendragon® Medical (Zurich, Switzerland) received CE certification in 2003 to market their Pendra® glucose monitor in Europe, such devices are not expected to be available in the United States until 2004. Like the Biographer, the device is intended for use in conjunction with conventional invasive monitoring methods, such as fingersticks, to track glucose trends. The watch-like device measures glucose by monitoring its effect on a physiological property such as tissue impedance.

Although the list of devices having received FDA approval or CE certification is short, there is no shortage of interest or effort in developing a noninvasive glucose monitor. A glimpse of what those devices may look like is provided by the myriad of patents and publications in the area. The range of technologies employed and practical embodiments is very diverse. The use of near-infrared reflectance in combination with sophisticated chemometric data analysis to measure glucose noninvasively has received the greatest amount of attention and development in the past 10 years. Sensys Medical® (Chandler, AZ, USA) has used a multidisciplinary approach to address the innumerable technical issues to develop the Sensys GTS®, which measures near infrared reflectance off the forearm. Although the device is not yet commercialized, the company claims a first-generation version provided accurate glucose readings 94% of the time in a multicenter trial (86). InLight Solutions® (Albuquerque, NM, USA) has developed a similar technology platform, but has sought to extend it to other applications such as blood alcohol and arterial blood gas measurement. SpectRx (Norcross, GA, USA) has started clinical studies of its continuous glucose monitoring system, which measures glucose in the ISF. The interstitial fluid, collected through a series of micropores that are created by a laser beam in the stratum corneum, reacts with a patch that serves as a glucose sensor. The simplicity of conducting a measurement off the eye, as in the manner done in an optometrist's office, has enticed several researchers to pursue the application of different technologies. The measurement of light reflectance off the retina as a means to monitor glucose has been proposed. The quantification of the change in optical rotation of the aqueous humor (40–42) due to glucose has also been suggested. Reflectance measurements in the mid-infrared region (35, 87) analogous to those in the near-infrared have been conducted. The measurement of thermal emission from various bodily structures has been suggested. One proposed embodiment is similar to the ear thermometer in that it measures the infrared emission from the tympanic membrane. Other forms of spectroscopy such as Raman, photoacoustic, and optical coherence topography also have their advocates.

Ultimately the successful design of a noninvasive device to measure glucose or any other analyte will require a multidisciplinary scientific and engineering approach to overcome the many challenges that have combined to make such a device elusive to date.

EVALUATING THE CAPABILITIES AND LIMITATIONS OF NONINVASIVE DEVICES

The analytical principles outlined in the first section have given an insight into the complex issues attendant with noninvasive blood glucose monitoring. The difficulties encountered in this field are made all the more tangible by the very limited scope of the commercial realization outlined in the previous section. The few successes in the noninvasive area have mainly been limited to pulse oximetry and bilirubin monitors, with glucose being all the more elusive. The extent of research and discovery in this area has been only partially discussed. Another important aspect of developing noninvasive technology is the evaluation and exploration of a device's strengths and weaknesses.

Experimental Considerations for Noninvasive Devices

In the process of assessing the performance of noninvasive devices and related technologies, it is not uncommon for researchers to begin with in vitro testing. This represents a stable and controllable environment in which the investigator can address the basic performance characteristics and handling of a device or technique. However, regardless of the level of complexity built into an in vitro test, there will still be considerable limitations when compared to in vivo testing, primarily because in vitro tests represent a static simulation of a device's ability to detect glucose in vivo. Unfortunately, in vivo tests are made on a dynamic system that possesses many different parameters over which the investigator has either limited or no control. Although in vitro testing does serve a useful purpose for proof of concept, caution must be exercised when evaluating the potential of a device based only on in vitro test results that have been extrapolated to in vivo performance.

Once in vivo testing of a noninvasive device is initiated, it is important to appreciate that measurements are greatly influenced by various aspects of sampling, i.e., the site to be targeted. This is quite crucial for devices that are based on internal measurements and utilize some form of spectroscopy. For these devices, highly desirable features for the chosen site would include the following:

- Good vascularization for high glucose signal; low fat/lipid content in order to reduce optical scattering
- Minimum interference from other body fluids such as sweat, oils, and saliva
- Little surface hair or dry skin that could introduce an artifact
- A site that is easy to prepare prior to use
- An accessible site that is convenient for regular testing

There are many articles in the literature that address the benefits and disadvantages of various sampling sites with their anatomical differences for a range of measurement techniques (35, 88–91). As mentioned previously, measurements made on a living organism can create a situation in which the composition of the sampling volume can change during and between readings. The ideal noninvasive device must ignore changes in tissue composition that may be detected along with glucose signal, but that are unrelated to the actual glucose level. For example, it is well known that the hydration level of human skin rapidly changes in response to many factors, such as environment and temperature (92–97). These changes in dermal composition can modify the "biomatrix" that contains the glucose, which is most undesirable. These environmental factors can introduce an apparent modification of the glucose concentration that is not linked to metabolism. Another important experimental consideration that is often overlooked is the way in which a device makes contact with or attaches to the skin. A clear illustration of this effect was reported in a recent article in which near-infrared imaging (optical tomography) was used to measure dynamic changes in optical properties of breast tissue as a function of pressure (98). The actual imaging of the breast tissue involves compressing the breast between glass plates or encircling the sample with an array of fiber bundles. The investigators demonstrated that a mild application of pressure changed the optical absorption and scattering of the tissue. Hence, the measurement technique itself, by its inherent design, is modifying the target it is supposed to measure. Jiang et al. recommend that, in this case, because the sampling process induces pressure, thereby causing changes in tissue composition and optical properties, these effects be considered in the design of medical instrumentation (98). Similarly, changes in tissue composition are also detrimental for detecting glucose or other analytes using noninvasive spectroscopic devices. Additional information about light scattering and absorption in biological media can be found in a collection of articles edited by Tuchin (99).

Device Testing Methods Unique to Glucose

Another important aspect of device testing that is very unique to glucose is the use of an oral glucose tolerance test (OGTT). In this test a known quantity of glucose is administered to a patient after fasting. The patient's glucose level is then monitored for a given length of time. In patients with normal insulin production, the blood glucose level should rise over the first hour to 8.9 to 10.0 mmol/L (160 to 180 mg/dL) and then fall back to normal levels between 5.6 and 6.7 mmol/L (100 to 120 mg/dL). In patients with diabetes, the high blood glucose level may be more than 11.1 mmol/L (200 mg/dL) and will take much longer to drop because of either impaired or nonexistent insulin production. During the test, frequent readings are taken with a noninvasive device, and these are then correlated with glucose readings obtained by a conventional method such as a fingerstick or an intravenous line used in conjunction with a benchtop analyzer. Important considerations for this type of test include the number of samples and the time interval between samples collected during the study. The data from the noninvasive device are then compared to the reference blood glucose values. The OGTT is an accepted medical procedure and represents the simplest and most low-cost method for noninvasive device testing. Another variation on this type of testing involves eating a carbohydrate-rich meal instead of drinking a high-glucose beverage. However, there is one critical concern with the OGTT and related forms of testing. Glucose levels change in a systematic way during an OGTT, which can cause a chance correlation between the analytical data from the noninvasive device and the measured glucose values (57). The noninvasive device may not be measuring glucose at all but another analyte that varies in a similar manner during the test, thus creating a phantom correlation.

An alternative to the OGTT method is to perform in vivo glucose clamping studies. This involves the controlled intravenous delivery of a specified concentration and volume of glucose using a variable rate pump (100). Using this approach, it is possible to select and hold a patient at several different glucose levels while specifying the precise times at which these levels are introduced. The clamping of the glucose level allows the decoupling of random interference from other analytes and removes chance correlations with glucose. Furthermore, by accurately monitoring the timing of events in a clamping study, lag times between plasma glucose and ISF can be accounted for. The flexibility of the clamping technique is particularly relevant for noninvasive devices that rely upon skin contact. Although in vivo glucose-clamping studies provide superior information for assessing the performance of a noninvasive device, they are more costly and must be supervised by a physician. Also, clamping studies are more inconvenient for the individuals tested, who must be attached to an intravenous line for several hours and will experience a range of glucose levels. As expected, clinical trails involving invasive procedures such as clamping also increase the risk of adverse complications, so liability issues must also be considered.

Data Analysis and Calibration Issues

In addition to the experimental protocol, the method of data analysis is critical in determining the capabilities and limitations of noninvasive devices. Optimal collection and analysis of data are integrally linked to the nature of the analytical signal generated by the device. For this discussion, devices that generate a single number or value will be termed *univariate*, an example being the standard fingerstick-based blood glucose meter. Devices that generate a vector or a sequence of related numbers will be termed *multivariate*, an appropriate example here being an optical spectrum generated by a device employing some type of spectroscopy. Standard statistical methods, such as regression analysis, are usually used to relate a set of single values generated by a univariate device to a corresponding set of blood glucose levels. These pairwise data are commonly referred to as a *calibration set*, or training set. The derived mathematical relationship, termed the *calibration model*, can then be used to predict blood glucose levels for new values, or observations, collected with the device. To evaluate device performance properly, the actual blood glucose level for each device observation must be known. Following accepted practices, the prediction set should not contain data that were used in the calibration set.

Most multivariate noninvasive devices are based on some form of spectroscopy and generate a sequence of numbers called a spectrum during each measurement, or observation. To form a calibration set, each spectrum must have a corresponding blood glucose value. At this point, data preprocessing (signal filtering) methods are sometimes applied to the original data, but this should be done with care so that important information is not lost. Multivariate data analysis methods, such as principal components regression (PCR) and partial least squares (PLS), are often used to analyze spectral data. The mathematical algorithms for these procedures are described in a number of sources (101–106). In general terms, these procedures identify linear combinations of variables within the signal, termed factors, which describe a large portion of the total variability in the data. These procedures offer several advantages, including the ability to decrease data complexity, reduce noise, and visualize complex internal relationships. Although there are a number of software packages for analyzing data by PCR or PLS, there are some official guidelines for their use. For example, ASTM Standard E 1655–00 (107) recommends that the total number of observations in the data set should be approximately four to five times the number of factors used in the PCR or PLS model. Otherwise, there is a chance of incorrectly modeling the data, thereby producing models that look good in calibration but perform poorly in prediction.

As most noninvasive glucose techniques generate multivariate data, an appropriate form of multivariate calibration must be used. In generating a multivariate calibration model the quality and stability of the model should be assessed. Most multivariate software packages generate a number of metrics that simplify the evaluation. In a similar manner, metrics such as correlation coefficient, *F*-test, and *t*-test can be used to gauge the statistical significance of univariate calibration models.

However, it is critical to judge the validity of univariate and multivariate models using an *independent* prediction set that does not contain data that were used to derive the calibration model. This is the only true test of in vivo performance. Good performance would be expected if: (*a*) the device is measuring a property directly related to glucose; (*b*) the calibration procedure has been performed correctly using an appropriate and representative data set; and (*c*) the prediction set contains observations that are very similar to the calibration set. Problems usually result when any of these assumptions is not correct or a data set has been corrupted by poor design. This third assumption is perhaps the most critical because ultimately there is a direct relationship to the feasibility of universal calibration. For any noninvasive glucose-monitoring device, it is desirable to have a calibration model that is transferable between different users.

In the broadest sense, a universal calibration model should accurately predict glucose, regardless of the user's race, gender, age, and so forth. Although an admirable goal, reliable glucose prediction for a given individual is often a demanding challenge in its own right. As mentioned earlier in the discussion on experimental considerations, skin and tissue changes are dynamic processes. The hydration level of skin can change quite dramatically depending on the stimuli it receives. For example, hydration levels can be altered easily by activities such as swimming, exercising, and showering. Another concern is possible changes in the device–sample interface caused by perspiration. If changes in the biomatrix or interface alter the device reading, and if these effects are not represented within the calibration set, then the predicted glucose values may not be reliable. The robustness of the calibration set and the specificity of a device for glucose (or its immunity to biomatrix changes) are critical factors in achieving a universal calibration. Device stability, in terms of signal drift and measurement repeatability, is also a prerequisite for attaining the goal of universal calibration. At present, true universal calibration still remains a vital foundation stone that must be put into place before noninvasive glucose monitoring can be realized.

Performance Characteristics and POCT Systems

An understanding of several factors is critical to the use of in vitro diagnostic (IVD) testing systems in a POCT environment. These include the medical criteria for making diagnostic or therapeutic decisions, system analytical performance (trueness, repeatability, and reproducibility), patient and physician information needs, and IVD convenience and ease of use. Regulatory, licensure, and quality assurance requirements for POCT environments also significantly influence selection and use of IVD testing systems. With the high level of current interest in the availability of noninvasive systems for the measurement of clinically useful analytes, particularly blood glucose, significant challenges still exist with respect to the ability to accurately detect and measure medically significant materials in the complex matrix of the human skin.

With the successful advent of noninvasive methods, key issues for laboratory staff will include the analytical accuracy of the measurement (trueness) and the ability of the system to satisfy well-established medical decision criteria. A continuing series of publications have focused on approaches to establishing these criteria (allowable error or measurement variation). Tonks (108), based on the analytical experience of 170 clinical laboratories, established an empirical formula for the definition of allowable limits of error:

$$\% \text{ Allowable error} = \frac{0.25(\text{assay reference range})}{\text{mean of the reference range}} \times 100$$

$$= \frac{0.25(95 - 65)}{80} = 9.4\%$$

As an example, a reference range of 3.6 to 5.3 mmol/L (65 to 95 mg/dL) would predict an empirically determined clinically allowable error of approximately 9.4% (CV < 4.7%) for blood glucose measurements.

Clarke et al. (70, 71) devised a system for assessing the accuracy of blood glucose monitoring systems, called error grid analysis (EGA). With this method, deviations of blood glucose monitoring system results from laboratory glucose results were grouped into five clinical outcomes categories based on the effect the inaccuracy of monitoring system results would have on glycemia management decisions. Based on treatment criteria, blood glucose monitoring system results within 20% of the laboratory result (EGA zone A) were thought to be clinically acceptable, leading to an appropriate clinical response. In 2000, an updated version of the blood glucose error grid was proposed by Parkes et al. (109), based on the consensus of 100 clinical experts as to the impact of glucose monitoring system inaccuracy on diabetes management. Rather than the discrete zones of comparative glucose results provided by the original error grid, the new error grid provided for five parallel or contiguous zones. In the Parkes error grid, the zone of clinically acceptable results was consistent with that recommended by Clarke (±20% of "true" glucose).

The development of performance criteria for laboratory testing results based on intra- and interindividual biological variability has been reviewed (110–112). The authors confirmed that measurements of clinical useful analytes are limited by the ability of a method to effectively detect clinically significant changes in levels in individuals (intraindividual biological variability; CV_{Bw}) or groups of patients (interindividual biological variability; CV_{Bb}). Consensus is that assay *total imprecision* should be less than one-half of the average within-subject biological variation (CV < ½CV_{Bw}) and that *method bias* should be less than one-quarter of the group biologic variation (CV < ¼CV_{Group}). With the specific example of glucose, one of the most commonly discussed analytes for noninvasive testing, the following are the published biological variation values: CV_{Bw} = 6.1%, CV_{Bb} = 7.8%, and CV_{Group} = 9.9%. Use of these CV values would indicate that expected performance for a glucose measurement system would be an imprecision of <3.1% and a bias of <2.5%, suggesting that glucose results obtained by a noninvasive system should be within ±10% of the target glucose value.

Two documents defining performance expectations for clinical systems, recently published by standards and clinical groups, include a standard defining expectations for blood glucose monitoring systems (113) and a medical association guidance on the performance expected for a number of clinical analytes (114). For the example of blood glucose, the standard indicates that 95% of results should be within ±20% of the target value, and the guidance (114) requires that results be within ±15% of the target blood glucose value. It is important to note that in determining the target value ("true glucose"), the reference analytical system must be traceable to a reference method and reference material of the highest metrologic order (115).

Considering the published sources (108–113), the widely published experience of clinicians and laboratorians over the past 10 years, and the physiological and technological challenges faced in the development of noninvasive methodologies; the following performance expectations are thought to be reasonable for blood glucose measurements in the near future (Table 4-1).

Although there is a stated need for increased accuracy in blood glucose assessment (whether determined using capillary blood, continuous, or noninvasive measurements), current technologies have not as yet delivered the desired level of accuracy. The 1993 ADA consensus conference (116) attendees published a recommendation for a blood glucose monitoring "total error (analytical plus user) of less than 10% at glucose concentrations ranging from 1.7 to 22.2 mmol/L (30 to 400 mg/dL)." In a more user-focused assessment, Skeie et al. (117) interviewed 201 diabetic individuals to determine the users' opinions of the differences in blood glucose measurements that would result in therapeutic responses on the user's part. Considering both hypoglycemic and hyperglycemic events, a summary of the glycemia management decisions of these 201 individuals suggested that an imprecision (CV) of ≤5% and bias of ≤5% (estimated error ≈ ±15%) was needed to effectively satisfy their clinical needs. Boyd and Bruns (118), using a Monte Carlo statistical simulation technique to assess the impact of measurement error on insulin use decisions, estimated that providing the correct insulin dosage 95% of the time requires measurement imprecision (CV) of ≤2% and bias of <1% (estimated error ≈ ±5–7%). Assessment of current blood glucose monitoring technologies (119, 120) has indicated that these monitoring devices are significantly chal-

lenged in meeting a total error [analytical plus user (10)] of <±20%.

FUTURE PROSPECTS

The previous accomplishments of noninvasive technology such as pulse-oximeters and bilirubin devices have set the standard for noninvasive devices. They provide considerable additional information that is of immediate benefit to both the health care professional and ultimately the patient. Furthermore, the impact of these devices is made all the more significant considering that they are relatively inexpensive to deploy and maintain. By comparison, noninvasive glucose monitoring seems to be struggling with many technical hurdles—a situation that often lends itself to the phrase the "quest for the Holy Grail." Indeed, not only does this reflect the elusive nature of a true noninvasive solution, but also highlights the disillusion created by broken promises and hollow statements of "in the next five years," from inventors and companies alike. However, it must be emphasized that the disparity with the previous success stories is due to glucose being part of a much larger and more complex picture, which truly belongs to the disease of diabetes. For example, a noninvasive bilirubin device is used to diagnose if a patient has jaundice. The task is very specific and well defined. By stark contrast, a noninvasive glucose device must accurately monitor the concentration of glucose in an exact and reliable manner on a regular basis. The situation becomes even more demanding when the device must perform this function within a complex tissue environment, which itself can be impacted by the chronic effects associated with the very disease of diabetes. Therefore, it is hardly surprising that a simple solution to this difficult and demanding problem has eluded the scientific and clinical communities for so long.

Against this background the authors have endeavored to give the reader an insight into some of the main challenges that exist in this field, and more importantly those that still need to be addressed. An attempt has been made to convey both the range and the complexity of some of the most difficult problems that are indeed specifically related to noninvasive monitoring. These have included appropriate analytical techniques, overcoming the protective biological barrier, issues related to instrument calibration, the degree of accuracy that is required or is acceptable, and finally that the technology is specific to the analyte of interest. All of these issues must be resolved for a noninvasive glucose monitoring device to succeed and gain both acceptance and trust with patient and clinician alike.

Before the matter of possible future devices is discussed, the status of current blood glucose meters should not go unmentioned, considering their important and continuing role in the management of diabetes. These meters have evolved tremendously over the last 20 years, from large, heavy reflectance-based meters to small, portable state-of-the-art devices that are widely accepted and used by individuals within the diabetes community. Even though these meters rely on a drop of blood obtained by a fingerstick to measure glucose, their ability to detect this vital analyte in an accurate and reproducible manner is a very elegant solution to an often overlooked,

Table 4-1 Performance Expectations in the Near Future

Time frame	Time window	Performance
Near term	Next 2 to 4 years	±20% of target
Midterm	Next 5 to 10 years	±15% of target
Long term	>10 years out	±10% of target

complex problem. Until a noninvasive solution is found these invasive devices will be the mainstay for the majority of people who require frequent, reliable, and accurate blood glucose monitoring.

With a view to the future, there is gathering evidence of a gradual phasing in of the first generation of noninvasive devices that are based on some of the concepts discussed in the introduction. Already there are products, such as the Cygnus Glucowatch, that have paved the way toward the concept of trending glucose over a period of time. The Pendra system produced by Pendragon (Zurich, Switzerland) is another continuous trending device. There is a growing inclination toward developing continuous devices that can monitor the glucose concentration within a subject, and thus act as an adjunct to pump users. This type of system would be a step closer to the concept of the artificial pancreas, in which the patient would have a self-regulating system that would both monitor glucose concentrations within the body and administer the appropriate bolus of insulin as required.

Regardless of which technology or type of system is proposed as a possible solution, it is very sobering to remember that progress in the medical community is both cautious and conservative. This is intentional, as the introduction of new ideas and products has the potential to affect people's lives not only for the better, but also for the worst. Therefore, as new concepts and products gain approval among the regulatory bodies and acceptance within the diabetic community, it may become clearer as to what the future may hold for noninvasive glucose monitoring.

REFERENCES

1. Winkelman JW, Tanasijevic MJ. Non-invasive testing in the clinical laboratory. Clin Lab Med 2002;22:547–58.
2. Coté GL, Lec RM, Pishko MV. Emerging biomedical sensing technologies and their applications. IEEE Sensors J 2003;3:255.
3. Fantini S, Franceschini-Fantini MA, Mair JS, Walker SA, Barbieri B, Gratton E. Frequency-domain multichannel optical detector for non-invasive tissue spectroscopy and oximetry. Opt Engin 1995;34:32–42.
4. Mendelson Y. Pulse oximetry: theory and applications for non-invasive monitoring. Clin Chem 1992;38:1601–7.
5. Jöbsis FF. Non-invasive, infrared monitoring of cerebral and myocardial oxygen sufficiency and circulatory parameters. Science 1977;198:1264–7.
6. Bhutani VK, Gourley GR, Adler S, Kreamer B, Dalin C, Johnson LH. Non-invasive measurement of total serum bilirubin in a multiracial predischarge population to assess the risk of severe hyperbilirubinemia. Pediatrics 2000;106:E17.
7. International Diabetes Federation (IDF). http://www.idf.org/e-atlas/home (accessed November 2003).
8. World Health Organization (WHO). http://www.who.int/ncd/dia (accessed November 2003).
9. Silverstein JH, Rosenbloom AL. New developments in type 1 (insulin-dependent) diabetes. Clin Pediatr 2000;39:257–66.
10. Nathan DM. Lifetime benefits and costs of intensive therapy as practiced in the Diabetes Control and Complications Trial. JAMA 1996;276:1409–15.
11. Shamoon H, Duffy H, Fleischer N, Engel S, Saenger P, Strelzyn M, et al. The effect of intensive treatment of diabetes on the development and progression of long-term complications in insulin-dependent diabetes mellitus. N Engl J Med 1993;329:977–86.
12. Centers for Disease Control and Prevention (CDC). http://www.cdc.gov/diabetes (accessed December 2003).
13. Rao G, Glikfeld P, Guy RH. Reverse iontophoresis: development of a non-invasive approach for glucose monitoring. Pharm Res 1993;10:1751–55.
14. Kalia YN, Merino V, Guy RH. Transdermal drug delivery. Dermatol Clin 1998;16:289–99.
15. Esenaliev RO. Application of light and ultrasound for medical diagnostics and treatment [Review]. In: Tuchin VV, ed. Proceedings of SPIE 2002;4707:158–64.
16. Heinemann L, Schmelzeisen-Redeker G. Non-invasive continuous glucose monitoring in type I diabetic patients with optical glucose sensors. Diabetologia 1998;41:848–54.
17. Heise HM. Non-invasive monitoring of metabolites using near infrared spectroscopy: state of the art. Horm Metab Res 1996;28:527–34.
18. Coté GL. Non-invasive and minimally-invasive optical monitoring technologies In: Bier DM, Finley D, eds. J Nutr 2001;[Suppl]:1596S–604S.
19. Khalil OS. Spectroscopic and clinical aspects of non-invasive glucose measurements. Clin Chem 1999;45:165–77.
20. Waynant RW, Chenault VM. Overview of non-invasive fluid glucose measurement using optical techniques to maintain glucose control in diabetes mellitus. LEOS 1998;12:3–6.
21. Klonoff DC. Non-invasive blood glucose monitoring. Diabetes Care 1997;20:433–7.
22. Arnold MA. Non-invasive glucose monitoring. Biotechnology 1996;7:46–9.
23. Lin J, Brown CW. Spectroscopic measurement of NaCl and seawater salinity in the near-IR region of 680–1230 nm. Appl Spectrosc 1993;47:239–41.
24. Lin J, Brown CW. Universal approach for determination of physical and chemical properties of water by near-IR spectroscopy. Appl Spectrosc 1993;47:1720–7.
25. Lin J, Brown CW. Near-IR spectroscopic determination of NaCl in aqueous solution. Appl Spectrosc 1992;46:1809–15.
26. Cael JJ, Koenig JL, Blackwell J. Infrared and raman spectroscopy of carbohydrates. Carbohydr Res 1974;32:79–91.
27. Vasko PD, Blackwell J, Koenig JL. Infrared and raman spectroscopy of carbohydrates Part II: Normal coordinate analysis of α-D-glucose. Carbohydr Res 1972;23:407–16.
28. Vasko PD, Blackwell J, Koenig JL. Infrared and raman spectroscopy of carbohydrates Part I: Identification of O-H and C-H-related vibrational modes for D-glucose, maltose, cellobiose, and dextran by deuterium-substitution methods. Carbohydr Res 1971;19:297–310.
29. Phelan MK, Barlow CH, Kelly JJ, Jinguji TM, Callis JB. Measurement of caustic and caustic brine solutions by spectroscopic detection of the hydroxide ion in the near-infrared region, 700–1150 nm. Anal Chem 1969;61:1419–24.
30. Bayly JG, Kartha VB, Stevens WH. The absorption spectra of liquid phase H_2O, HDO and D_2O from 0.7 μm to 10 μm. In: Infrared physics, vol. 3. Oxford: Pergamon Press, 1963:211–22.
31. Wheeler OH. Near Infrared spectra of organic compounds. Chem Rev 1959;59:629–66.

32. Fischbacher C, Jagemann KU, Danzer K, Müller, Papenkordt L, Schüler J. Enhancing calibration models for non-invasive near-infrared spectroscopical blood glucose determination. Fres J Anal Chem 1997;359:78–82.

33. Müller UA, Mertes B, FischBacher C, Jageman KU, Danzer K. Non-invasive blood glucose monitoring by means of near infrared spectroscopy: methods for improving the reliability of the calibration models. Int J Artific Organs 1997;20:285–90.

34. Heise HM, Marbach R, Koschinsky T, Gries FA. Non-invasive blood glucose sensors based on near-infrared spectroscopy. Artif Organs 1994;18:439–47.

35. Marback R, Koschinsky, Gries FA, Heise HM. Non-invasive blood glucose assay by near-infrared diffuse reflectance spectroscopy of the human inner lip. Appl Spectrosc 1993;47:875–81.

36. Robinson RM, Eaton PR, Haaland DM, Koepp GW, Thomas EV, Stallard BR, Robinson PL. Non-invasive glucose monitoring in diabetic patients: a preliminary evaluation. Clin Chem 1992;38:1618–22.

37. Coté GL, Cameron BD. Non-invasive polarimetric measurement of glucose in cell culture media. J Biomed Opt 1997;2:275–81.

38. Bell AF, Barron LD, Hecht L. Vibrational raman optical activity study of D-glucose. Carbohydr Res 1994;257:11–24.

39. Coté GL, Fox MD, Northop RB. Non-invasive optical polarimetric glucose sensing using a true phase measurement technique. IEEE Trans Biomed Eng 1992;39:752–6.

40. Gough DA. The composition and optical rotary dispersion of bovine aqueous humor. Diabetes Care 1982;5:266–70.

41. Rabinovitch B, March WF, Adams RL. Non-invasive glucose monitoring of the aqueous humor of the eye: Part I. Measurement of very small optical rotations. Diabetes Care 1982;5:254–8.

42. March WF, Rabinovitch B, Adams RL. Non-invasive glucose monitoring of the aqueous humor of the eye: Part II. Animal studies and the scleral lens. Diabetes Care 1982;5:259–65.

43. Misner MW, Block MJ. Non-invasive measurement by kromoscopic analysis. Spectroscopy 2000;15:51–5.

44. Sodickson LA. Improvements in multivariate analysis via kromoscopic measurement. Spectroscopy 1997;12:13–9, 22–4.

45. Misner MW, Block MJ. The raw data of kromoscopic analysis. Spectroscopy 1997;12:20–1.

46. Sodickson LA, Block MJ. Kromoscopic analysis: a possible alternative to spectroscopic analysis for non-invasive measurement of analytes in vivo. Clin Chem 1994;40:1838–44.

47. MacKenzie HA, Ashton HS, Shen YC, Lindberg J, Rae P, Quan KM, Spiers S. Blood glucose measurements by photoacoustics. In: Sevick-Muraca EM, Izatt JA, Ediger MN eds. OSA TOPS 1998;22:156–9.

48. Spanner G, Niessner R. Non-invasive determination of blood constituents using an array of modulated laser diodes and a photoacoustic sensor head. Fres J Anal Chem 1996;355:327–8.

49. Spanner G, Niessner R. A photoacoustic laser sensor for the non-invasive determination of blood contents. Anal Methods Instr 1993;1:208–12.

50. Quan KM, Christison GB, MacKenzie HA, Hodgson P. Glucose determination by a pulsed photoacoustic technique: an experimental study using a gelatin-based tissue phantom. Phys Med Biol 1993;38:1911–22.

51. Christison GB, MacKenzie HA. Laser photoacoustic determination of physiological glucose concentrations in human whole blood. Med Biol Eng Comput 1993;31:284–90.

52. MacKenzie HA, Ashton HS, Spiers S, Shen Y, Freeborn SS, Hannigan J, et al. Advances in photoacoustic non-invasive glucose testing. Clin Chem 1999;45:1587–95.

53. Chance B, Liu H, Kitai T, Zhang Y. Effects of solutes on optical properties of biological materials: models, cells, and tissues. Anal Biochem 1995;227:351–62.

54. Bruulsema JT, Hayward JE, Farrell TJ, Patterson MS, Heinemann L, Berger M, et al. correlation between blood glucose concentration in diabetics and non-invasively measured tissue optical scattering coefficient. Opt Lett 1997;22:190–2.

55. Maier JS, Walker SA, Fantini S, Franceschini MA, Gratton E. Possible correlation between blood glucose concentration and the reduced scattering coefficient of tissues in the near infrared. Opt Lett 1994;19:2062–4.

56. Burmeister JJ, Chung H, Arnold MA. Phantoms for non-invasive blood glucose sensing with near infrared transmission spectroscopy. Photochem Photobiol 1998;67:50–5.

57. Arnold MA, Burmeister JJ, Small GA. Phantom glucose calibration models from simulated non-invasive human near-infrared spectra. Anal Chem 1998;70:1773–81.

58. Kohl M, Cope M, Essenpreis M, Böcker. Influence of glucose concentration on light scattering in tissue-simulating phantoms. Opt Lett 1994;19:2170–2.

59. Dou X, Yamaguchi Y, Yamamoto H, Uenoyama H, Ozaki Y. Biological applications of anti-stokes raman spectroscopy: quantitative analysis of glucose in plasma and serum by a highly sensitive multichannel raman spectrometer. Appl Spectrosc 1996;50:1301–6.

60. Wicksted JP, Roel EJ, Motamedi M, March WF. Raman spectroscopy studies of metabolic concentrations in aqueous solutions and aqueous humor specimens. Appl Spectrosc 1995;49:987–93.

61. Wang SY, Hasty CE, Watson PA, Wicksted JP, Stith RD, March WF. Analysis of metabolites in aqueous solutions by using laser raman spectroscopy. Appl Opt 1993;32:925–9.

62. Pan S, Chung H, Arnold MA, Small GW. Near-infrared spectroscopic measurement of physiological glucose levels in variable matrices of protein and triglycerides. Anal Chem 1996;68:1124–35.

63. Spanner G, Niebner R. New concept for the non-invasive determination of physiological glucose concentrations using modulated laser diodes. Fres J Anal Chem 1996;354:306–10.

64. Hazen KH, Arnold MA, Small GW. Temperature-insensitive near-infrared spectroscopic measurement of glucose in aqueous solutions. Appl Spectrosc 1994;48:477–83.

65. Marquardt LS, Arnold MA, Small GW. Near-infrared spectroscopic measurement of glucose in a protein matrix. Anal Chem 1993;65:3271–8.

66. Berger AJ, Itzkan I, Feld MS. Feasibility of measuring blood glucose concentration by near-infrared raman spectroscopy. Spectrochim Acta A 1997;53:287–92.

67. Haaland DM, Robinson MR, Koepp GW, Thomas EV, Eaton RP. Reagentless near-infrared determination of glucose in whole blood using multivariate calibration. Appl Spectrosc 1992;46:1575–8.

68. Heise HM, Marbach R, Janatsch G, Kruse-Jones JD. Multivariate determination of glucose in whole blood by attenuated total reflection infrared spectroscopy. Anal Chem 1989;61:2009–15.

69. Castano J, Wang Y-Z, Chuang D. Blood glucose dependence of visual flicker threshold. Diabetes Technol Ther 2000;2:31–43.

70. Cox DJ, Clarke WL, Gonder-Frederick L, Pohl S, Hoover C, Snyder A, et al. Accuracy of perceiving blood glucose in IDDM. Diabetes Care 1985;8:529–36.

71. Clarke WL, Cox D, Gonder-Frederick LA, Carter W, Pohl SL. Evaluating clinical accuracy of systems for self-monitoring of blood glucose. Diabetes Care 1987;10:622–8.

72. Merrick EB, Hayes TJ. Continuous, non-invasive measurements of arterial blood oxygen levels. Hewlett-Packard J 1976;8:2–9.

73. Yoshiya I, Shimada Y, Tanaka K. Spectrophotometric monitoring of arterial oxygen saturation in the fingertip. Med Biol Engin Comput 1980;18:27–32.

74. Aoyagi T, Kishi M, Yamaguchi K, Watanabe S. Improvement of the earpiece oximeter. In: Abstracts of the 13th Annual Meeting of the Japanese Society of Medical Electronics and Biological Engineering. 1974:90–1.

75. Severinghaus JW, Astrup PB. History of blood gas analysis. VI: Oximetry. J Clin Monit 1986;2:270–88.

76. Severinghaus JW, Honda Y. History of blood gas analysis. VII: Pulse oximetry. J Clin Monit 1987;3:135–8.

77. Severinghaus JW, Honda Y. Blood gas analysis and critical care medicine. Am J Respir Crit Care Med 1998;4:S114–S122.

78. Mithall A. Pulse oximetry detects autonomic neuropathy in diabetes. J Diabet Complicat 1997;11:35–9.

79. Rubaltelli FF, Gourley GR, Loskamp N, Modi N, Roth-Kleiner M, Sender A, Vert P. Transcutaneous bilirubin measurement: a multicenter evaluation of a new device. Pediatrics 2001;107:1264–71.

80. Wong CM, van Dijk PJE, Laing IA. A comparison of transcutaneous bilirubinometers: SpectRx Bilicheck versus Minolta Air Shields. Arch Dis Child [Fetal and Neonatal ed.] 2002;87:F137–F140.

81. Light Touch Medical. http://www.lightouchmedical.com (accessed December 2003).

82. Tamada JA, Bohanon NJV, Potts RO. Measurement of blood glucose in diabetic subjects using non-invasive transdermal extraction. Nat Med 1995;1:1198–201.

83. Tierney MJ, Jayalakshmi Y, Parris NA, Reidy MP, Uhegbu C, Vijayakumar P. Design of a biosensor for continual, transdermal glucose monitoring. Clin Chem 1999;45:1681–3.

84. Garg SK, Potts RO, Ackerman NR, Fermi SJ, Tamanda JA, Chase HP. Correlation of fingerstick blood glucose measurements with GlucoWatch Biographer glucose results in young subjects with type 1 diabetes. Diabetes Care 1999;22:1708–14.

85. Tierney MJ, Tamanda JA, Potts RO, Jovanovic L, Garg S, and the Cygnus Research Team. Clinical valuation of the Gluco Watch Biographer: A continual, non-invasive glucose monitor for patients with diabetes. Biosens Bioelectron 2001;16:621–9.

86. Monfre S. European Association for the Study of Diabetes (EASD) 37th Annual Conference, Glasgow, Scotland, 2001.

87. Heise HM, Marbach TH, Koschinsky TH, Gries FA. Multicomponent assay for blood substrates in human plasma by mid-infrared spectroscopy and its evaluation for clinical analysis. Appl Spectrosc 1994;48:85–95.

88. Burmeister JJ, Arnold MA. Evaluation of measurement sites for non-invasive blood glucose sensing with near-infrared transmission spectroscopy. Clin Chem 1999;45:1621–7.

89. Burmeister JJ, Arnold MA, Small GW. Non-invasive blood glucose measurements by near-infrared transmission spectroscopy across human tongues. Diabetes Technol Ther 2000;2:5–15.

90. Cameron BD, Gorde HW, Satheesan B, Coté GL. The use of polarized laser light through the eye for non-invasive glucose monitoring. Diabetes Technol Ther 1999;1:135–43.

91. Steffes PG. Laser-based measurement of glucose in the ocular aqueous humor: an efficacious portal for determination of serum glucose levels. Diabetes Technol Ther 1999;1:129–33.

92. Grimnes S, Martinsen ØG. Bioimpedance and bioelectricity basics, chap. 4. San Diego: Academic Press, 2000.

93. Reilly JP. Applied bioelectricity: from electrical stimulation to electropathology, chap. 2. New York: Springer-Verlag, 1998.

94. Aberg P, Geladi P, Nicander I, Ollmar S. Variation of skin properties within human forearms demonstrated by non-invasive detection and multi-way analysis. Skin Res Technol 2002;8:194–201.

95. Nicander I, Ollmar S. Electrical impedance measurements at different skin sites related to seasonal variations. Skin Res Technol 2000;6:81–6.

96. Nicander I, Norlen L, Brockstedt U, Lundh-Rozell B, Forslind B, Ollmar S. Electrical impedance and other physical parameters as related to lipid content of human stratum corneum. Skin Res Technol 1998;4:213–21.

97. Xiao P, Imhof RE. Optothermal measurement of water distribution within the stratum corneum. In: Elsner P, Barel AO, Berardesca E, Gabard B, Serup J, eds. Skin bioengineering: techniques and applications in dermatology and cosmetology. Basel, Switzerland: Karger, 1998.

98. Jiang S, Pogue BW, Paulsen KD. In vivo near-infrared spectral detection of pressure-induced changes in breast tissue. Opt Lett 2003;28:1212–4.

99. Tuchin VV, ed. Handbook of optical biomedical diagnostics, chap. 1. Bellingham, WA: SPIE Press, 2002.

100. Clemens AH, Hough DL. Diagnostic method and apparatus for clamping blood glucose concentration. U.S. Patent 4526568, 1985.

101. Næs T, Isaksson T, Fearn T, Davies T. A user-friendly guide to multivariate calibration and classification, chap. 5, 6. Chichester, UK: NIR Publications, 2002.

102. Martens H., Næs T. Multivariate calibration. Chichester, UK: John Wiley & Sons, 1989.

103. Massart DL, Vandeginste BGM, Deming SN, Mishotte Y, Kaufman L. Chemometrics: a textbook, chap. 20, 21. Amsterdam: Elsevier, 1988.

104. Beebe KR, Pell RJ, Seasholtz MB. Chemometrics: a practical guide, chap. 5. New York: John Wiley & Sons, 1998.

105. Haaland DM, Thomas EV. Partial least squares methods for spectral analyses: 1. Relation to other quantitative calibration methods and the extraction of qualitative information. Anal Chem 1988;60:1193–208.

106. Thomas EV. A primer on multivariate calibration. Anal Chem 1994;66:795A–804A.

107. Standard practices for infrared multivariate quantitative analysis. ASTM Standard E 1655–00; 2000. http://www.astm.org (accessed December 2003).

108. Tonks DB. A study of the accuracy and precision of clinical chemistry determinations in 170 Canadian laboratories. Clin Chem 1963;9:217–33.

109. Parkes JL, Slatin SL, Pardo S, Ginsberg BH. A new consensus error grid to evaluate the clinical significance of inaccurcies in the measurement of blood glucose. Diabetes Care 2000;23:1143–8.

110. Fraser CG, Petersen PH. Desirable standards for laboratory tests if they are to fulfill medical needs. Clin Chem 1993;39:1447–55.

111. Fraser CG, Petersen PH, Ricos C, Haeckel R. Proposed quality specifications for the imprecision and inaccuracy of analytical systems for clinical chemistry. Eur J Clin Chem Clin Biochem 1992;30:311–7.

112. Sebastian-Gambaro MA, Liron-Hernandez FJ, Fuentes-Arderiu X. Intra- and inter-individual variability data bank. Eur J Clin Chem Clin Biochem 1997;35:845–52.

113. ISO 15197: 2003(E). In vitro diagnostic test systems—requirements for blood-glucose monitoring systems for self-testing in managing diabetes mellitus. Geneva, Switzerland: International Organization for Standardization, 2003.

114. Guidelines of the Federal Medical Council for the quality assurance of quantitative medical laboratory tests. Deutschen Ärzteblatt 2002;99:A1187.

115. ISO 17511:2002(E). In vitro diagnostic test systems—measurement of quantities in samples of biologic origin—metrological traceability of values assigned to calibrators and control materials. Geneva, Switzerland: International Organization for Standardization, 2002.

116. American Diabetes Association. Self-monitoring of blood glucose. Diabetes Care 1994;17:81–6.

117. Skeie S, Thue G, Sandberg S. Patient-derived quality specifications for instruments used in self-monitoring of blood glucose. Clin Chem 2001;47:67–73.

118. Boyd JC, Bruns DE. Quality specifications for glucose meters: assessment by simulation modeling of errors in insulin dose. Clin Chem 2001;47:209–14.

119. Bohme P, Floriot M, Sirveaux MA, Durain D, Ziegler O, Drouin P, Guerci B. Evolution of analytical performance in portable glucose meters in the last decade. Diabetes Care 2003;26:1170–5.

120. Chen ET, Nichols JH, Duh SH, Hortin G. Performance evaluation of blood glucose monitoring devices. Diabetes Technol Ther 2003;5:749–68.

Chapter **5**

Electronic-Nose Technology: Potential Applications in Point-of-Care Clinical Diagnosis and Management

Anthony C. Woodman and Reinhard Fend

Effective clinical care requires decision making based on multiple data inputs, e.g., gross symptoms, previous history, and biochemical tests. Rather surprisingly, such a broad approach has, in the main, not been the *modus operandi* for the development of point-of-care testing (POCT), which generally relies on a one target–one result approach. Developments in genomics have highlighted the concept of *array technologies* and the potential power of understanding disease signatures. Yet, as with many aspects of medicine, history provides numerous examples of where similar approaches have been deployed with great affect by past civilizations. One of the most graphic, yet still highly relevant, examples is the use of smell or, more correctly, olfactory diagnosis in medicine. Today, these same principals are being applied in machine olfaction or "electronic noses"; this chapter will review how "sniffing out" disease has considerable potential for revolutionizing point-of-care diagnostics.

The origins of odors as diagnostic indicators go back to around 400 B.C. and the father of medicine—Hippocrates (1). Descriptions at that time of the pouring of human sputum onto hot coal to thermally generate a smell could very well be considered a primitive pyrolysis of long-chain fatty acids, with release of volatile hydrocarbons or possibly lipid peroxidation from bacterial or infected tissue products. Similarly, traditional Chinese medicine also extolled the virtues of olfactory diagnosis (2). While early medical practitioners had not discovered bacterial pathogenicity, they clearly recognized that a disease–host interaction could change the odor of body excretions such as sweat, urine, vaginal fluid, and sputum (2). Diagnosis using the human sense of smell remained one of the most reliable methods in bedside medicine until the industrial and technological revolutions began in the 18th century. A collection of recorded diseases and infections liberating specific odors is presented in Table 5-1.

ANALYSIS OF VOLATILE BIOMARKERS: FROM HUMAN TO MACHINE OLFACTION

The human nose has 10^7 olfactory cells carrying G-receptor binding proteins that amplify and process odor signals through 5×10^4 glomeruli nodes (olfactory receptor) before being

further processed by 10^5 mitral cells (olfactory bulb) as the signal is sent to the central nervous system (3) (Figure 5-1). The human nose is a remarkable organ, and indeed is still considered the primary tool employed in industry to characterize the odor of a variety of consumer products. However, reliance on human olfaction to fully exploit odor analysis in clinical medicine is impractical.

During the 1950s and early 1960s, gas chromatography (GC) and GC-linked with mass spectrometry (GC-MS) provided the instrumentation with which to separate and identify volatile biomarkers [see (4) for a review of GC/GC-MS application in medical diagnostics]. While the introduction of GC-MS enabled the comprehensive study of possible disease markers, it has never emerged as a fully evaluated routine instrument for clinical diagnosis. Factors such as high capital costs and laborious and time-consuming methods requiring significant expertise and the sheer complexity of volatiles detected using GC-MS have all conspired to limit the application of this technology (5, 6). However, the wealth of knowledge generated by GC-MS has significantly enriched the understanding of the way the human body responds to disease and in particular the potential role of volatile organic compounds (VOC) as diagnostic markers. Consequently there has been a drive to develop instruments for routine clinical application without the drawbacks of GC-MS.

The term *electronic nose* was introduced by Julian Gardner in 1988 (7) and is the informal name encompassing an instrument comprised of chemical sensors combined with a pattern recognition system, so enabling discrimination between, or recognition of, both simple or complex odors or volatiles (8) (Figures 5-1 and 5-2). However, the origins of the technology go back more than 40 years.

In 1961, a mechanical olfactory instrument was described by Moncreiff (9), followed soon after by several attempts to mimic human olfaction through the study of redox reactions of odorants at an electrode (10), odorant conductivity (11), and odorant species contact potential (12). While these early devices might well now be viewed as primitive, they demonstrated that chemical reactions between volatile markers and various sensors could be amplified and be sensitive enough to enable qualitative differences to be measured at relatively low

Table 5-1 Diseases and Their Recorded Liberated Odors

Odor	Site/source	Disease
Baked brown bread	Skin	Typhoid
Stale beer	Skin	Tuberculosis lymphadenitis
Butcher's shop	Skin	Yellow fever
Grape	Skin/sweat	*Pseudomonas* infection
Rotten apples	Skin/sweat	Anerobic infection
Overripe Camembert	Skin	Bacterial proteolysis
Ammoniacal	Urine	Bladder infection
Amine-like	Vaginal discharge	Bacterial vaginosis
Rancid	Stool	Shigellosis
Full	Stool	*Rotavirus* gastroenteritis
Freshly plucked feathers	Sweat	Rubella
Sweet	Sweat	Diptheria
Full	Sputum	Bacterial infection
Putrid	Breath	Lung abscess, anerobic infection, necrotizing pneumonia
Full-offensive	Skin	Squamous cell carcinoma
Acetone-like	Breath	Diabetes mellitus
Musty/horsy	Infant skin	Phenylketonuria
Foul	Infant stool	Cystic fibrosis
Sweaty feet	Skin/sweat	Isovaleric acidemia
Burnt sugar	Urine	Maple syrup urine disease
Sweet/fruity or boiled cabbage	Infant breath	Hypermethionemia
Fishy	Skin/urine	Trimethylaminuria

Adapted from (4).

concentrations. This set the foundations for the work of Persaud and Dodd, who two decades later, in 1982, published the first report of an intelligent model of an artificial nose (13).

The aim of this "intelligent" artificial nose was simple—to try to detect different volatile compounds by simulating the different stages of the human olfactory system. To replicate this, the nose addressed the following aspects: the sampling and filtering of odors; the use of biochemical sensors with which volatiles could react and generate a signal that could be detected and amplified; the treatment of the sensor signal responses, including neural network analysis to evaluate key useful and relevant components of the data—with the end result *volatile odor recognition*. An appreciation as to how significant this breakthrough was can be gained by viewing the

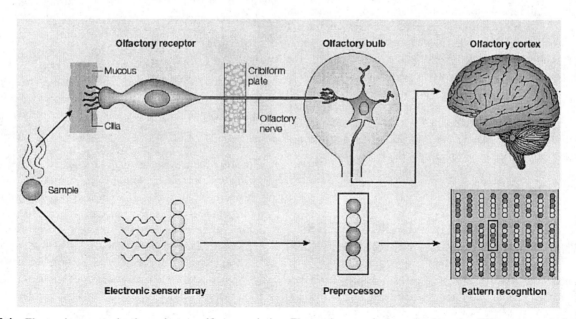

Figure 5-1 Electronic-nose technology: human olfactory mimics. Electronic-nose devices simulate the different stages of the human olfactory system, resulting in volatile odor recognition and discrimination between diseases and conditions (from 15).

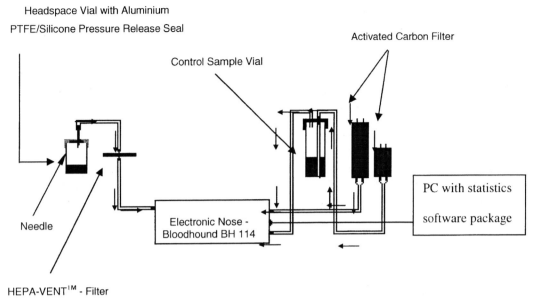

Figure 5-2 Overview of idealized electronic-nose configuration. The setup consists of the electronic-nose sensor array, a sample, and a control vial as well as two activated carbon filters and a HEPA-VENT filter. The carbon filters ensure an odorless airflow over the sensor surface and control and sample head space, whereas the HEPA-VENT filter prevents the fouling of the sensor surface. The electronic nose is connected to a PC running the control software and an appropriate data-analysis package.

number and breadth of patents filed that relate to the development of appropriate sensor arrays for: quality assurance and safety in the food and drinks industry (14); microbiological detection (15); and, of most relevance here, medical applications (reviewed in 4, 14, 16–18).

Mirroring the expansion in potential applications for the technology, the first commercial electronic noses were launched in the early 1990s (8). Among the first systems were devices from AlphaMOS in 1993, Neotronics and Aromascan in 1994, and Bloodhound Sensors and HKR Sensorsysteme in 1995 (8).

This chapter will primarily review the application of commercially produced systems in medicine, including commercially produced prototypes, and discuss when, where, how, and why electronic-nose (e-nose) technology has significant potential to affect POCT for a diverse range of diseases and conditions.

FUNDAMENTALS OF ELECTRONIC-NOSE TECHNOLOGY

While an in-depth description of analytical science, electronics and statistics is not really appropriate here, an insight into the key components helps illustrate both the potential and the pitfalls in applying electronic-nose technology.

As already indicated (Figure 5-1) the fundamental principle of the electronic nose is to mimic the human olfactory system. The human olfactory receptor cells are replaced by a nonspecific chemical sensor array, while the olfactory bulb is

replaced by *in silico* processing. Consequently the usefulness of electronic noses depends upon two key components—the sample must be presented in the correct format to optimize the interaction with the sensor array *and* the pattern recognition system must enable large data sets to be analyzed rapidly to provide appropriate and useful information.

Artificial Olfactory Receptor Cells—Nonspecific Chemical Sensor Arrays

Most electronic noses currently available contain between 6 and 32 sensors, although prototypes with up to 72 sensors are under development (AlphaMOS personal communication). All sensors share a common basic principle: the interaction between volatiles and sensor surface leads to a change in conductivity, resistance, or electrical frequency in the sensor, which generates a measurable time-dependent electrical signal (19, 20).

Metal Oxide Sensors

These sensors consist of an electrically heated ceramic pellet, onto which a thin porous film of SnO_2 doped with metal ions has been deposited (21). The doped SnO_2 film behaves as an n-type semiconductor, and the chemisorption of oxygen at the sensor surface results in the removal of electrons from the conducting band. Gases from the sample interact with the absorbed oxygen and thereby affect the conductivity of the SnO_2 film (21, 22).

Running at elevated temperatures (typically at 300–400 °C) these sensors achieve a fast response time and avoid interferences from water, which is important when using water-rich clinical samples. The response characteristics can be tailored to ensure optimal performance under a range of conditions by varying the operating temperatures and the doping agent (19, 22). Therefore, when combining short recovery time, resistance to humidity, and aging effects and little drift over time with an electrical output signal that is proportional to the odor concentration (23), metal oxide sensors offer considerable potential for application in clinical diagnostics. This said, these sensors are typified by demonstrating high power consumption (possibly limiting the point-of-care or nonspecialist facility application) and poor selectivity (23), which in turn places pressure on the downstream processing requirements and associated costs.

Conducting Polymers

The use of conducting polymers (CP) as sensors dates back to 1979, when Diaz and coworkers first electro-polymerized a thin film of polypyrrole (22). The sensors are fabricated by electropolymerizing thin polymer films across a narrow electrode gap (22, 24). The reversible absorption of molecules onto the film induces a temporary change in the electrical conductivity of the film by altering the amount of active charge carriers in the polymer structure (22, 24, 25). Conducting polymers in electronic noses are typically based on either poly(pyrolle) or poly(aniline) (22, 24). In both cases, it is easy to obtain a thin polymer film, and therefore reproducible sensors can be produced (7). The real advantage of conducting-polymer sensors is that the molecular-interaction capabilities of the polymer can be selectively modified by incorporating different counter-ions during polymerization or by attaching functional groups to the polymer backbone (22). Clearly this offers significant potential to increase the selectivity of the electronic nose in applications where chemicals of interest have been well-characterized, e.g., breath analysis for ketosis. Along with the high selectivity comes low power consumption (cf. metal oxides), although these are to some extent tempered by the shortcomings of long response times, inherent time and temperature drift, sensitivity to water and the high cost of sensor fabrication (22, 23). Despite this problem, we have used electronic noses containing conducting polymers extensively in our own research to great effect (see 4, 26–30, and in this chapter).

Piezoelectric-Based Sensors

The use of piezoelectric crystals as transducers for chemical analysis was first suggested by Sauerbrey in 1959 and demonstrated by King in 1964 (22). The two most commonly used piezoelectric based sensors in electronic noses are the surface acoustic wave (SAW) sensor and the bulk acoustic wave (BAW) sensor (7).

Surface Acoustic Wave (SAW) Sensor. SAW devices consist of interdigitated electrodes fabricated onto a piezoelectric substrate (e.g., quartz) onto which a thin film coating of a selective material is deposited (21, 22). An applied radio frequency produces an acoustic wave on the sensor surface (surface oscillation). The adsorption of odor molecules onto the thin film coating leads to an increase in the mass and elasticity module of the coating. This change in mass and elasticity perturbs the wave, leading to a frequency shift (21, 22). To compensate for pressure and temperature effects, the sample sensor is usually connected to a reference SAW device and the frequency difference is detected (7).

Bulk Acoustic Wave (BAW) Sensor. BAW devices consist of a piezoelectric resonator with one or both surfaces covered by a membrane such as acetyl cellulose or lecithin (31, 32). The BAW structure is connected to a suitable amplifier to form an oscillator. The resonant frequency of the oscillator is determined by the physical and geometrical properties of the device (32). Any changes in the physical properties of the membrane due to absorption of molecules affect the resonant frequency of the BAW device (31, 32), with the frequency shift being detected (22).

Data Analysis and Processing

Generally, volatile odor pattern data are received in the form of normalized data sets based upon the divergence, area and adsorption or desorption components of the individual sensor response (33). This generates a significant amount of data and requires effective data management (15). The techniques employed include simple supervised techniques such as discriminant function analysis (DFA), which can parametrically classify an unknown or random sample from a population. The commonest technique and the one we employ ourselves for initial data analysis is principle component analysis (PCA), which enables the visualization of large multivariate data sets and describes the relationships between samples identified.

However, for real-time sensing applicable in the clinical setting, more advanced data handling is required, with artificial neural networks (ANN), consisting of a series of algorithms capable of handling nonlinear sensor systems, being the method of choice. Through the collection of background "training data" and by using so-called back-propagation approaches, issues such as sensor drift and nonlinear data sets can be taken into account, thereby allowing accurate prediction of the classification of future real samples. Simplistically, using previous experience, the model is able to decide whether a new unseen sample has a similar profile to that seen previously. The greater the previous experience, the greater the probability of accurate prediction.

ELECTRONIC NOSE AND MEDICAL APPLICATIONS

The breadth of application for electronic-nose technology is massive. It includes monitoring the quality of food packaging (34) and dairy products (35); classification of vegetable oils (36), wines (37), and perfumes (38); together with the monitoring of sewage treatment (39) and sausage fermentation (40). Yet it is diagnostic medicine with its history of using smell that offers the greatest potential for mass application of the electronic nose, and never more so than in the arena of POCT.

Reviewing the literature concerning electronic-nose technology and medicine is baffling. Publications range from science of the highest caliber but with so many theoretical issues that any immediate routine application seems very unlikely, to such vigorous claims that the reader is left wondering why the author has not been awarded the Nobel Prize for medicine; the reality is of course somewhere in between. It is fair to say that to date no routine clinical diagnostic application for the electronic nose has been implemented, although several areas are very close to demonstrating this. However, the most striking observation is that the power of electronic-nose technology lies in the broad signature profiles generated. This is not a technology where every causative gene, protein or infectious agent needs to have been characterized in depth; like the diseases being analyzed, electronic-nose data describes all causative and consequential events.

When attempting to navigate through this technology in medicine, it soon becomes apparent that there is one clear delineator, namely, application of electronic nose in infectious diseases or noninfectious diseases. Using these two very broad subject headings, we will attempt to highlight both current and future applications of electronic-nose technology both in medicine in general and at the point of care.

Infectious Diseases

The analysis of infectious diseases represents by far the largest clinical research area for electronic-nose technology attracting both academic and commercial interest (see 15 for general review of this area). As a result, it is safe to speculate that this area will be the first to deliver a routine medical application for the technology.

What is the reason for such widespread interest? The answer is simple. Using conventional culture methods, diagnosis of infection can take 24–48 hours for bacterial infections (identification of *Mycobacterium tuberculosis* can require 4 weeks) and often around 7 days for fungal diseases. For appropriate early treatment including screening for therapeutic sensitivity, it is essential to obtain relevant rapid results in easily interpretable formats. Ideally such analysis should be amenable to use at the point of care and be the first step in rapid, responsive and appropriate anti-infectious therapy, reducing the incidence of unchecked infection and/or poorly targeted antibiotics.

Whether such analysis is following some degree of traditional culture (in vitro) or directly in/at the patient (in situ) has no bearing on how the sensor responses are generated: via the interaction of primary or secondary volatile bacterial metabolites either alone or in combination, where in most cases exactly which compounds are responsible is unknown or indeed irrelevant.

Diagnosis and Management of Sepsis in Wound Healing. The point-of-care analysis of the odors over the head spaces of 24 low-adherent contact dressings collected from 21 patients with leg ulcers was in fact one of first clinical

applications of electronic-nose technology (41). Using 20 conducting polymer sensors, a two-dimensional odor map demonstrated clear differences between ulcers of differing bacterial etiology. Ulcers infected with β-hemolytic streptococci formed a distinctive cluster away from the other three categories (mixed infection, *Staphylococcus aureus,* and control), which could not be resolved from each other. Despite this, the unambiguous separation of at least one bacterial species provided proof that host–pathogen interactions are identifiable by an electronic nose (4).

Today the analysis of wound healing remains at the forefront of clinical electronic-nose application. A recent European Union–funded project WUNSENS has integrated image capture technology with the electronic-nose technology of Alpha-MOS to develop a portable integrated wound assessment system for use at the point of care (IST-2001–52058).

Diagnosis and Management of Urogenital Infections. One of the areas where appropriate and effective therapy is most dependent upon early diagnosis is that of urogenital infections. Urinary tract infections (UTI) are a significant cause of morbidity, with three million cases each year in the US alone (27, 42). Estimates suggest that 20% of females between the ages of 20 and 65 years suffer at least one episode per year, which in turn increase the risk of contracting complicated or chronic urological disorders such as pyelonephritis, urethritis, and prostatitis (43, 44). Approximately 80% of uncomplicated UTI are caused by *Escherichia coli* and the remaining 20% by enteric pathogens such as *Enterocci, Klebsiella, Proteus,* and fungal opportunistic pathogens such as *Candida albicans* (27, 45, 46). Current diagnostics and antibiotic sensitivity tests require 24–48 hours to identify pathological species in a midstream specimen containing at least 10^5 CFU/mL.

A similar story is true for bacterial vaginosis; In the US alone there are an estimated 10 million doctor visits per for vaginal infections per year. Bacterial vaginosis (BV) is one of the most common causes of vaginal infection with high prevalence in women of childbearing age. Vaginal infection during pregnancy has been linked to preterm delivery (47) and spontaneous abortion in the third trimester and upper genital tract infections including histologic chorioamnionitis (48).

With a requirement for simple, accurate and, ideally, point-of-care analysis, the application of electronic-nose technology in managing urogenital infection has received considerable academic and commercial interest. The premise that analysis of volatiles generated from urine is clinically relevant stems from several gas-chromatographic studies during the 1970s (27). While these early studies lacked advanced computation to resolve data, they did demonstrate discrimination between *E. coli* and *Proteus spp.* (49).

Almost 25 years later, electronic-nose technology replicated these studies both in "spiked" urine samples where discrimination between *E. coli* and *P. mirabilis* was obtained after just four hours in culture (18) and clinical specimens (27, 50). Pavlou et al., using an array of 14 conducting polymer sensors (Bloodhound BH114) discriminated between *E. coli,*

Proteus spp., Staphylococcus spp., and no infection in a total of 70 patients with a combined positive predictive outcome of 99%, following 4.5-h liquid culture incubation (27). Aathithan et al. used an Osmetech microbial analyzer [Osmetech, Manchester, UK (51)], to diagnose bacteriuria. Analyzing 534 clinical urine specimens, the sensitivity and specificity of this device were 83.5% and 87.6%, respectively compared to traditional culture, when the cutoff was defined as 10^5 CFU/mL. While this data again shows the potential for electronic-nose technology, it is the Osmetech microbial analyzer (OMA) that warrants further discussion. Osmetech has received 510(k) approval from the FDA for the use of its microbial analyzer as a UTI sensor device. Offering both a centralized laboratory-based instrument and a smaller point-of-care option, Osmetech's view is that the device should enable negative samples to be screened out within minutes, enabling the number of cultured samples to be greatly reduced, resulting in cost savings.

The OMA is also marketed for the diagnosis of bacterial vaginosis. A case study on bacterial vaginosis in the United Kingdom has shown that conducting-polymer-based sensor arrays similar to that in the microbial analyzer could be used to successfully diagnose 89% of test subjects as being positive or negative for both bacterial and yeast infections (15, 52). Following the evaluation of over 1000 patients, the Osmetech device was given 510(k) approval by the FDA in January 2003, citing that the instrument had a sensitivity and specificity of 81.5% and 76.1% as compared to the current "gold standard" of the Amsel criteria, but with significant improvements in speed and expertise required (53).

The potential for electronic-nose technology in the detection, diagnosis, and management of urogenital infectious appears to be clear. The greatest challenge will be in establishing which is the most suitable environment for the technology to be deployed: centralized facility, clinic, GP surgery or, and possibly most interesting, community pharmacies. To a great extent where will depend on how and by whom the technology is commercialized.

Diagnosis and Management of Tuberculosis and Respiratory Disease. Tuberculosis represents one of the greatest global health challenges, with over one-third of the world's population being infected, leading to over 30 million deaths per year. Diagnostic tests such as microbiological culture, which require up to 4 weeks to obtain a definitive answer, and Ziehl-Neelson staining are time-consuming, while recently developed molecular tests, although extremely accurate, are prohibitively expensive for such a global problem. For the past 5 years our research at Cranfield University in collaboration with the Royal Tropical Institute in Amsterdam has focused upon the possibility of applying electronic-nose technology to diagnose tuberculosis (TB). Using a Bloodhound BH114 system consisting of 14 conducting polymers and primary cluster analysis (PCA) for data processing, we have investigated the feasibility of analyzing infected sputum samples either following a short period of "traditional" culture (3–4 days) or directly

following limited (2–4 h) incubation at 37 °C with and without an enzymatic cocktail (54, 55). We have been able to discriminate between different species of *Mycobacteria* (*M. tuberculosis, M. avium, M. scrofulaceum*) as well as other lung pathogens (*Pseudomonas aeruginosa*) compared to blank medium with an accuracy of 99% (Figure 5-3). This analysis worked equally well in culture as on sputum samples. The detection limit for *M. tuberculosis* was determined in culture and sputum and found to be as low as 10^4 CFU/mL, which is comparable to the gold standard of the Ziehl-Neelson stain. As part of an ongoing study funded by the World Health Organization (WHO), we are evaluating the Bloodhound electronic nose with 250 blind sputum samples obtained from the WHO sputum bank.

Gardner and coworkers have applied an Alpha-Mos Fox 2000 to identify bacteria that cause infections of the ears, nose and throat. These diseases are often associated with microorganisms such as *S. aureus, Legionalla pneumphilia*, and *E. coli*. Currently the diagnosis is based on taking a swab specimen of the infected area with subsequent culturing, assaying, and staining for classification. The entire procedure can take many days, causing a delay in treatment. In contrast, the electronic nose is not only able to detect the type of bacteria but also the growth phase in a relatively short period of time ($\approx$ hours). Gardner and his group analyzed 180 unknown samples using a neural network. A total of 100% of the *S. aureus* and 92% of the *E. coli* were correctly identified in the growth phase. These are remarkable findings, since all *Staphylococcus* samples collected during the initial lag phase were correctly predicted and this after an incubation period of only 10 min (14).

While we have highlighted a few of the infectious diseases where electronic-nose technology has received considerable attention, it is by no means an exhaustive review, but is an insight into which infectious areas may well see point-of-care applications. The limit to electronic-nose application in managing infectious disease appears to have no bounds. From the point-of-care diagnosis of eye infections (56) to detection of *Helicobacter pylori* in gastroesophageal isolates (26) and general clinical microbiology (see 15 for recent review), new potential applications are being explored.

Noninfectious Diseases

The application of electronic-nose technology for the investigation of noninfectious disease has not as yet received such detailed evaluation. The main specimens for these studies are blood, breath, and sweat. These body fluids are very complex, which, combined with complex disease pathology, makes noninfectious analysis much more difficult but not impossible.

Application of Electronic-Nose Technology in Renal Medicine. One noninfectious area that has received significant interest is renal medicine. The motivation for this most probably lies in the fact that well-characterized markers of renal disease are available. The first of these is microscopic hematuria. Di Natale and coworkers applied an electronic nose based on eight quartz microbalance sensors to analyze urine

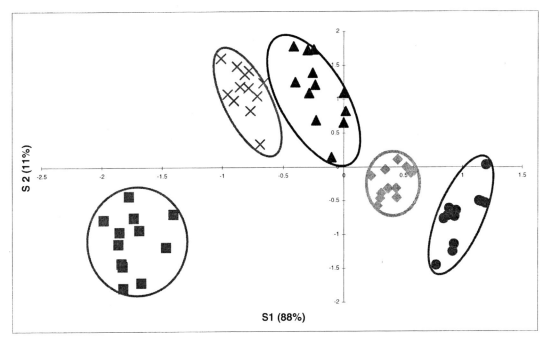

Figure 5-3 Identification of *Mycobacterium* and *Pseudomonas spp.* in human sputum using a 14 conducting-polymer sensor array and discriminate functional analysis (DFA). The DFA plot shows separate clusters of *M. avium* (×), *M. tuberculosis* (▲), *P. aeruginosa* (●), mixed infections (*P. aeruginosa* and *M. tuberculosis* = 1:1) (◆) and control sputum (■). The concentration of bacteria in the samples was 1×10^7 CFU/mL.

samples. Not only were they able to discriminate between urine containing blood compared to normal healthy urine, they were also able to correlate the sensor response to the amount of blood present in urine (57). However, this correlation was of a qualitative nature and no further attempts were made to find a quantitative correlation.

Patients suffering from kidney failure generally have a characteristic breath odor mainly caused by dimethylamine (DMA) and trimethylamine (TMA). Lin et al., using these two marker substances to investigate the potential of an electronic nose (six piezoelectric quartz crystals) as a diagnostic tool for uremia based on breath analysis, successfully distinguished between healthy individuals and chronic renal failure patients (58). There was, however, an overlap between patients suffering from renal insufficiency and hemodialysis patients. Nevertheless, the breath of kidney patients smelled significantly different from the breath of the healthy controls, indicating the potential of an electronic nose as an early, noninvasive diagnosis system for uremia.

An ever increasing number of patients have to undergo regular renal dialysis to compensate for acute or chronic renal failure. The estimated annual rate of patients starting renal replacement therapy (RRT) in England and Wales is 89 per million population, indicating that approximately 5350 patients started RRT in 2000, hemodialysis (HD) being the predominant form of RRT (59). The frequency and length of dialysis is generally determined empirically, with little or no online analysis available to ensure optimal dosage. Currently the dialysis dosage (accuracy) is estimated from the surrogate marker substance urea by calculating either the urea reduction rate (URR) or the normalized dialysis dose (kt/V). The behavior of urea during dialysis differs dramatically from the behavior of larger molecules such as α_2-macroglobulin (60, 61). However, these large molecules are the main causes of the long-term side effects of hemodialysis such as amyloidosis. In contrast, the electronic nose has the potential to assess the purity of blood by measuring several compounds simultaneously including alcohols, aldehydes, phenolic compounds, and ketones, and thus might lead to a more accurate description of dialysis. Our own studies using conducting-polymer sensors and PCA have indicated that it is possible to discriminate predialysis blood from postdialysis blood based on the volatile signature generated from blood (Figure 5-4), and this correlates well with biochemical data (30). Currently the analysis is undertaken off-line; however, future investigations are aimed at developing a device with which real-time online analysis can be undertaken, allowing tailoring of dialysis for every patient, every session.

Other Noninfectious Applications. Two further interesting applications for electronic-nose technology are in the noninvasive diagnosis and management of diabetes (62, 63) and in the diagnosis of lung cancer (64).

Ping et al. used electronic-nose technology to directly analyze expired breath from 18 patients with Type I diabetes and 14 healthy volunteers before and after eating, and demonstrated that such noninvasive monitoring could be a reliable method for monitoring diabetics (62). Mohamed et al. used an

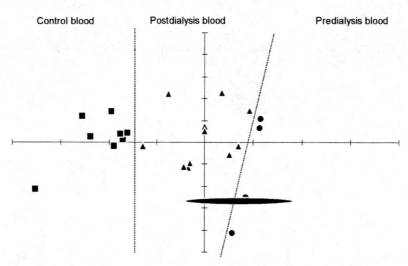

Figure 5-4 Shift in volatile signature detected in prehemodialysis blood compared to posthemodialysis blood using a 14 conducting-polymer array and primary cluster analysis (PCA). Control blood (■), Postdialysis blood (▲) and Predialysis blood (●) after 45-min incubation at 37 °C. Post- and Predialysis blood with the same number belong to the same patient.

electronic-nose and artificial neural network analysis to demonstrate that Type II diabetes could be detected via urine analysis with a 92% success rate (63).

Di Natale et al. have extended previous GC-MS studies (65) and demonstrated the utility of electronic-nose technology in detecting lung cancer (64). All patients with lung cancer and 94% of patients free from the disease were correctly classified following the analysis of alkenes and aromatic compounds in expired breath. While the sample size (42 patients) was relatively small, this study demonstrated just how broad is the potential application of electronic-nose technology in clinical practice.

FUTURE PROSPECTS

The development of robust instrumentation, particularly small handheld devices, coupled with remote data acquisition and central processing powered by hybrid intelligence systems could see electronic-nose technology commonplace in point-of-care diagnostics in 5–10 years.

As with all technologies, the electronic-nose technology has advantages and disadvantages (see Table 5-2), but the advantages far outweigh the disadvantages. Recent developments (materials, fabrication techniques) in sensor technology and in chemometric tools (data analysis) are steps toward more reliable and robust systems.

The promising studies reviewed herein indicate that there is a real potential for electronic noses at the point of medical delivery, where they could be used as a rapid screen for specific diseases or disorders. However, it is the combination of the POCT environment with the opportunity to gather data remotely and use advanced information-technology approaches, satellite communication and web-based knowledge systems to transfer them back to centralized facilities either for processing or disease management that add another dimension to this technology.

This would open up the potential for using such systems for epidemiological studies and, more importantly, aid in the diagnosis and management of disease locally, nationally or, indeed, globally. From tuberculosis and HIV to SARS and

Table 5-2 The Advantages and Disadvantages of Applying Electronic-Nose Technology

Advantages	Disadvantages
Quick response time (min)	Sensor drift
Simultaneous analysis of several compounds (fingerprint)	Not always reproducible
Combination of different sensor types possible (hybrid systems)	Susceptible to certain compounds (e.g., NH_3)
Simple sample preparation	Large amount of data accumulated → difficult to interpret
High throughput	Shelf life of sensors → data transferability
Low [$2 (£1)/test] running costs	Capital costs (up to £40,000)
Automation possible, real time	
Simple/robust system	
Operator independent	
High sensitivity (ppm range)	

cancer, both the individuals affected as well as the international bodies, such as the WHO, would be given the information with which to act almost immediately.

REFERENCES

1. Adams F. Hippocratic writings: Aphorisms IV, V. In: Stevenson DC, ed. The internet classic archive. New York: Web Atomics, 1994.
2. Porter R. The early years. In: Porter R, ed. The greatest benefit to mankind: a medical history of humanity from antiquity to the present. London: HarperCollins, 1997:147–62.
3. Kauer JS. Contributions of topography and parallel processing to odour coding in the vertebrate olfactory pathway. Trends Neurosci 1991;14:79–85.
4. Pavlou AK, Turner APF. Sniffing out the truth: clinical diagnosis using the electronic nose. Clin Chem Lab Med 2000;38:99–112.
5. Manolis A. The diagnostic potential of breath analysis. Clin Chem 1983;29:5–15.
6. Phillips M. Method for the collection and assay of volatile organic compounds in breath. Anal Biochem 1997;247:272–8.
7. Gardner JW, Bartlett PN. Electronic noses: principles and applications Oxford: Oxford University Press, 1999:1–243.
8. Gibson T, Prosser O, Hilbert J. Electronic noses: an inspired idea? Chemistry and Industry 2000;April 17:287–9.
9. Moncreiff RW. An instrument for measuring and classifying odours. J Appl Physiol 1961;16:742–3.
10. Wilkens WF, Hatman AD. An electronic analogue for the olfactory process. Ann NY Acad Sci 1964;116:608.
11. Buck TM, Allen FG, Dalton M. Detection of chemical species by surface effects on metals and semiconductors. In: Bregman T, Dravnieks A, eds. Surface effects in detection. New York: Spartan Books, 1965:156–66.
12. Dravnieks A, Trotter PJ. Polar vapour detection based on thermal modulation of contact potentials. J Sci Instrum 1965;42:64–6.
13. Persaud K, Dodd GH. Analysis of discrimination mechanisms of the mammalian olfactory system using a model nose. Nature 1982;299:353–5.
14. Gardner JW, Shin HW, Hines EL. An electronic nose system to diagnose illness Sensors and Actuators B 2000;70:19–24.
15. Turner APFT, Magan NM. Electronic noses and disease diagnostics. Nat Rev Microbiol 2004;2:1–7.
16. Mantini A, Di Natale C, Macagnano A, Paolesse R, Finazzi-Agro A, D'Amico A. Biomedical application of an electronic nose. Crit Rev Biomed Eng 2000;28:481–5.
17. Thaler ER, Bruney FC, Kennedy DW, Hanson CW. Use of electronic nose to distinguish cerebrospinal fluid from serum. Arch Otolaryngol Head Neck Surg 2000;126:71–4.
18. Saini S, Barr H, Bessant C. Sniffing out disease using the artificial nose. Biologist 2001;48:229–33.
19. Gardner JW, Bartlett PN. A brief history of electronic noses. Sensors and Actuators B 1994;18/19:211–20.
20. Pearce TC. Computational parallels between the biological olfactory pathway and its analogue "the electronic nose." 2 sensor based machine olfaction. Biosystems 1997;41:69–90.
21. Persuad KC, Travers PJ. Array of broad specificity film for sensing volatile chemicals. In: Kress-Rogers E, ed. Handbook of biosensors and electronic noses in medicine, food and the environment. New York: CRC Press, 1997;563–92.
22. Dickinson TA, White J, Kauer JS, Walt DR. Current trends in artificial-nose technology. Trends Biotechnol 1998;16:250–8.
23. Harper WJ. The strengths and weaknesses of the electronic-nose. In Cadwallader H, Rouseff RL, eds. Headspace analysis of food and flavors: theory and practice. New York: Kluwer Academic/Plenum Publishers, 2001:59–71.
24. Bartlett PN, Ling-Chung SK. Conducting polymer gas sensors part III: Results for four different polymers and five different vapours. Sensors and Actuators B 1989;20:287–92.
25. Shumer HV, Gardner JW. Odour discrimination with an electronic nose. Sensors and Actuators B 1992;8:1–11.
26. Pavlou AK, Magan N, Sharp D, Brown J, Barr H, Turner APF. An intelligent rapid odour recognition model in discrimination of *Helicobacter pylori* and other gastroesophageal isolates *in vitro*. Biosens Bioelectron 2000;15:333–42.
27. Pavlou AK, Magan N, McNulty C, Meedham-Jones J, Sharp D, Brown J, et al. Use of an electronic-nose system for diagnoses of urinary tract infections. Biosens Bioelectron 2002;17:893–9.
28. Fend R. Towards interactive dialysis: electronic nose analysis of volatile compounds generated and removed during dialysis [MPhil/PhD transfer thesis]. Cranfield University, 2002.
29. Fend R, Bessant C, Williams AJ, Woodman AC. Monitoring haemodialysis using electronic nose and chemometrics. Biosens Bioelectron 2004;19:1581–90.
30. Fend R, Geddes R, Lesellier S, Vodermeier H-M, Corner LAL, Gormley E, et al. The use of an electronic-nose to detect *Mycobacterium bovis* infection in badgers and cattle. Submitted J Clin Microbiol 2004.
31. Bartlett PN, Elliott JM, Gardner JW. Application of and developments in machine olfaction. Ann Chim 1997;87:33–44.
32. D'Amico A, Di Natale C, Verona E. Acoustic devices. In: Kress-Rogers E, ed. Handbook of biosensors and electronic noses—medicine, food and environment. New York: CRC Press, 1997;197–223.
33. Pearce TC, Schiffman SS, Nagle HT, Gardner JW, eds. Handbook of machine olfaction: electronic nose technology. London: Wiley, 2002:1–500.
34. Forgren G, Frisell H, Ericsson B. Taint and odour related quality monitoring of two food packaging board products using gas chromatography, gas sensors and sensing analysis. Nord Pulp Paper Res J 1999;14:5–16.
35. Schaller E, Bosset IO, Escher F. Practical experience with electronic nose systems for monitoring the quality of dairy products. Chimia 1999;53:98–102.
36. Martin YG, Pavon JLP, Cordero BM, Pinto CG. Classification of vegetable oils by linear discriminant analysis of electronic nose data. Anal Chim Acta 1999;384:83–94.
37. Baldacci S, Matsuno T, Toko K, Stella R, De Rossi D. Discrimination of wine using taste and smell sensors. Sens Mater 1998;10:185–200.
38. Carrasco A, Saby C, Bernadet P. Discrimination of Yves Saint Laurent perfumes by an electronic nose. Flav Fragn 1998;13:335–48.
39. Stuetz RM, Fennes RA, Engin G. assessment of odours from sewage treatment works by an electronic nose, H_2 S analysis and olfactometry. Water Res 1999;33:453–61.
40. Eklov T, Johansson G, Winquist F, Lundstrom I. Monitoring sausage fermentation using an electronic nose. J Sci Food Agric 1998;76:525–32.
41. Parry AD, Oppenheim B. Leg ulcer detection identifies beta-haemolytic streptococcal infection. J Wound Care 1995;4:404–6.

42. Schaechter M, Medoff G, Eisenstein BI (Eds) Mechanisms of microbial disease, 2nd ed. Baltimore: Williams and Wilkins, 2002:1–733.

43. Orenstein R, Wong ES. Urinary tract infections in adults. Am Fam Physician 1999;59:1225–34.

44. Lipsky BA. Prostatitis and urinary tract infection in men: what's new; what's true? Am J Med 1999;106:327–34.

45. Krcmery S, Dubrava M, Kcrmery V Jr. Fungal urinary infections in patients at risk. Int J Antimicro Agents 1983;11:289–91.

46. Honkinen O, Lehtonen OP, Ruuskanen O, Huovinen P, Mertsola J. Cohort study of bacterial species causing urinary tract infection and urinary tract abnormalities in children. BMJ 1999;318:770–1.

47. McGregor JA, French JI. Bacterial vaginosis in pregnancy. Obstet Gynecol Surv 2000;55:S1–19.

48. Hillier SL, Martius J, Krohn M, Kiviat N, Holmes KK, Eschenbach DA. A case-control study of chorioamnionic infection and histologic chorioamnionitis in prematurity. N Engl J Med 1988; 319:972–8.

49. Haywood NJ, Jeavons TH. Assessment of technique for rapid detection of *E. coli* and *Proteus sp* in urine by headspace gas liquid chromatography. J Clin Microbiol 1977;6:202–8.

50. Aathithan S, Plant JC, Chaudry AN, French GL. Diagnosis of bacteriuria by detection of volatile organic compounds in urine using an automated headspace analyser with multiple conducting polymer sensors. J Clin Microbiol 2001;39:2590–3.

51. Osmetech plc. http://www.osmetech.com/products/laboratory.html.

52. Persuad KC, Pisanelli AM, Evans P. In: Handbook of machine olfaction: electronic nose technology. London: Wiley, 2002:445–60.

53. Hay P, Tummon A, Ogunfile M, Adebiyi A, Adefowora A. Evaluation of a novel diagnostic test for bacterial vaginosis: "the electronic nose" Int J Std AIDS 2003;14:114–8.

54. Pavlou AK, Magan N, Meecham-Jones J, Brown J, Klatser P, Turner APF. Detection of *Mycobacterium tuberculosis* in vitro and in situ using an electronic nose in combination with a neural network system. Biosens Bioelectron 2004 [in press—available online at Elsevier Science Direct].

55. Fend R, Kolk A, Klatser P, Woodman AC. Early detection of *M. tuberculosis* infections in humans using electronic nose technology. 2004 [Submitted Nat Biotechnol].

56. Dutta R, Hines EL, Gardner JW, Bollot P. Bacteria classification using Cyranose 320 electronic nose. Bio Med Eng Online 2002; 1:1–7.

57. Di Natale C, Mantini A, Macagnano A, Antuzzi D, Paolasse R, D'Amico A. Electronic nose analysis of urine samples containing blood. Physiol Meas 1999;20:377–84.

58. Lin YJ, Guo H, Chang Y. Application of the electronic nose for uremia diagnosis. Sensors and Actuators B 2001;76:177–80.

59. Ansell D, Feest T. UK renal registry report, Bristol, UK, 2001.

60. Vanholder R, DeSmet R, Lesaffer G. Dissociation between dialysis adequacy and Kt/V. Sem Dial 2002;15:3–7.

61. Lowrie EG. The normalized treatment ration (Kt/V) is not the best dialysis dose parameter. Blood Purif 2000;18:286–94.

62. Ping W, Yi T, Haibao X, Farong S. A novel method for diabetes diagnosis based on electronic nose. Biosens Bioelectron 1997;12: 1031–6.

63. Mohamed EI, Linder R, Perriello G, Di Daniele N, Popple SJ, De Loren A. Predicting type 2 diabetes using an electronic nose-based artificial neural network analysis. Diabetes Nutr Metab 2002;15:215–21.

64. Di Natale C, Macagnano A, Martinelli E, Paolesse R, D'Arcangelo, Roscioni C et al. Lung cancer identification by the analysis of breath by means of an array of non-selective gas sensors. Biosens Bioelectron 2003;18:1209–18.

65. Philips M, Gleeson K, Hughes JMB, Greenberg J, Cataneo RN, Baker L, et al. Volatile organic compounds in breath as markers of lung cancer: a cross-sectional study. Lancet 1999;353: 1930–3.

Chapter **6**

Miniaturization Technology

Larry J. Kricka

Miniaturization is an ongoing goal for the designers and manufacturers of many devices and appliances, including those used for clinical analysis. The quest to make devices ever smaller has been enabled by the microelectronic chips essential to the operation of most, if not all, modern instruments and machines (1). Early work in microtechnology was spearheaded by engineers who saw the potential of combining the fabrication techniques developed in the microelectronics industry with the mechanical properties of silicon. They constructed micromachined devices ranging in complexity from a cantilever beam to an electric motor using micrometer-sized (10^{-6} m) silicon components (2, 3). Some of these microelectromechanical systems (MEMS) progressed to commercial products, such as the micromachined sensors for measuring blood pressure, monitoring fuel flow in engines, and triggering air bags in automobiles (4).

Now the techniques developed in the microelectronics industry, the high-speed printing industry, and MEMS research are being applied to medical diagnostic devices and have provided the foundation for microchip technology (e.g., microfluidic chips, biochips, bioelectronic chips), and microarray technology (protein, peptide, oligosaccharide, oligonucleotide, and cDNA chips) (5–8). These technologies provide a viable route to simplified assays (e.g., lab-on-a-chip devices), high-throughput simultaneous multianalyte testing (2-D and 3-D microarrays), and more sophisticated and easier-to-use portable analytical devices that have prospects for use at the point of care (9). If the current rate of development in miniaturization is maintained, then an intriguing prospect is the development of a handheld personal laboratory with an extensive menu of chemistry, hematology, coagulation, and even genetic tests.

This chapter reviews the current status of microtechnology and outlines its prospects in point-of-care applications. General information on miniaturization can be found on the following websites: http://www.gene-chips.com, http//:www.lab-on-a-chip.com, and www.functionalgenomics.org.uk. A future consideration is the effect of miniaturization at the nanoscale (nanotechnology) on point-of-care testing. The reader is directed to some recent literature for more information on nanotechnology and its potential applications (10–12).

RATIONALE FOR MICROMINIATURIZATION AND MICROMINIATURE DEVICES

Table 6-1 lists the advantages and disadvantages of miniaturization as it applies to clinical diagnostic devices. The principal advantage is the potential to integrate all of the steps in an analytical procedure onto a small chip-sized device (typically 1 × 1 cm). Such a device would only require that the user apply the sample and start the operation of the device. It would then take over and perform all of the analytical steps, beginning with sample preparation; subsequent analysis, data capture, and data processing; and finally, delivery of the analytical result via a display screen or a wireless link. However, this compelling advantage must be viewed in the context of some significant obstacles to miniaturization. These range from the inhibitory properties of materials used to construct microchips (e.g., inhibition of analytical reactions) to inherent insensitivity of detection for reactions reduced to submicroliter volumes (13–15). However, successes achieved with the current range of early-stage devices provide the basis for continued optimism for microminiaturization and the development of a broad range of microminiature analyzers that may be useful for point-of-care applications.

MICROCHIP FABRICATION TECHNIQUES AND MATERIALS

The current range of microfabrication techniques and materials used to produce microchips is listed in Table 6-2 (16–18). Photolithography is the most common technique for creating microscale features such as channels or chambers in silicon or glass microchips. For this process, the feature size of structures fabricated in or on a surface is determined by the choice of radiation source.

Conventional photolithography (405- or 436-nm light) is limited to features of approximately 1 μm, but with shorter wavelength light, such as deep UV (230–260 nm), a minimum feature size of 0.3 μm can be achieved. The even lower wavelength, x-ray, and e-beam sources can generate features as small as 0.1 μm. Molding and embossing techniques are applicable for the manufacture of plastic microchips, and ink-jet printing or spotting techniques derived from the printing industry are used extensively to create large two-dimensional

Table 6-1   Advantages and Disadvantages of Microtechnology

Feature	Advantage	Disadvantage
System integration	Microscale fabrication makes possible system integration (e.g., sample addition, processing, analysis, and read-out integrated in a single device).	Few examples of fully integrated devices have been produced, so the full extent of likely obstacles to implementation are not fully characterized.
Manufacture	Existing microelectronics; industry manufacturing processes or high-speed printing methods already geared to high-volume production can be adapted for the manufacture of microchips. High device density contributes to ease of mass production.	Few devices have progressed to full commercial manufacture, so exact manufacturing costs can only be extrapolated from data for related devices (e.g., integrated circuit chips).
Design iterations	Simultaneous fabrication of many different designs; speeds up design cycles and facilitates more design iterations.	—
Operation costs	Sample and test reagent consumption is greatly reduced due to the small internal volume of a microchip (submicroliter volumes), thus decreasing the reagent component of the overall cost per test.	—
Portability	Miniaturization facilitates the fabrication of compact, lightweight, handheld analyzers that are suitable for use in nonlaboratory settings, such as point-of-care testing.	The small size of microchip devices may pose human interface issues, i.e., the interface between the macro world of the human operator and the microworld of the microchip.
Speed of operation	Faster response times are possible using microscale devices.	—
Complex high-volume analysis	Massively parallel simultaneous testing of samples is possible with miniaturized arrays of different reagents on planar surfaces.	Quality control of all-in-one devices may be problematic. For example, regional failure of the analytical process on one part of a microarray may compromise the acceptability of data from other parts of the microarray.
Sample size	Low sample volume required.	In the case of heterogeneous biological specimens, a reduction in sample size may lead to nonrepresentative sampling and erroneous results. A reduction in sample size reduces the amount of analyte present and requires increasingly sensitive detection methods.
Disposal	Small size and low capacity of devices minimize the volume of waste fluids. It is also possible to entomb the entire reaction mixture and any unused reagents or sample in the microchip for safe disposal.	—
Safety	Small sample size reduces exposure of operators to potentially hazardous samples.	—
Reliability	Integration of operator-dependent steps increases reliability. Built-in redundancy provides an analytical safeguard (e.g., multiple test sites for simultaneous multiplicate assays).	—
Operational stability	Encapsulated microdevices provide extended operation over a wider range of environmental conditions of humidity and temperature	—
Range of fabrication materials	Tailor mechanical, electrical, or surface properties of a construction material to a particular application.	The surface chemistry of a construction material can have an adverse effect on reactions and processes performed in a microchip.
Assay speed	Diffusion distances are reduced in microvolume devices, and this contributes to increased rates of reaction.	—

Table 6-2   Construction Materials and Fabrication Methods for Microchips

Materials

Alumina, aluminium, ceramics, copper, diamond, fluorocarbon polymers, gallium arsenide, glass, gold, indium phosphide, polyester, polyethylene, polycarbonate, polyimide, polymethylmethacrylate, quartz, rubidium molybdenum oxide, silicon, silicon carbide

Microfabrication techniques

Anisotropic etching, electron-beam etching, electrodischarge drilling, focused ion-beam etching, isotropic etching, laser ablation, laser drilling, LIGA process [Lithographie, Galvanoformung, Abformung (deep x-ray lithography, electroforming, and plastic molding)], mechanical drilling, reactive ion etching, stereolithography

Assembly techniques

Adhesive bonding, anodic bonding, eutectic bonding, heat staking, mechanical clamping, solvent softening, thermal bonding

---

arrays of microsized spots of reagents on solid surfaces, e.g., the surface of a microscope slide.

Assembly is a key step in microchip fabrication. Bonding together the different parts that comprise a microchip is challenging (19). Delicate surface features must not be damaged during bonding of component parts, and the final assembly must not leak. For silicon and glass components, anodic bonding provides a liquid-tight bond. However, this process is performed at high temperatures, which restricts pre-loading the chip components with labile biological reagents. Plastic components can be bonded under milder conditions, and this provides a route to assembling microchips that are pre-loaded with reagents.

MICROCHIP DESIGN CONCEPTS

Microchips can be classified into three general types: microfluidic chips, bioelectronic chips, and microarray chips. I have used this classification because, currently, there is no internationally accepted nomenclature for the new generation of microsized analytical devices, and they are variously referred to as a chip, microchip, lab-on-a-chip, miniaturized total chemical analysis system (μ-TAS), biochip, gene chip, genome chip, proteome chip, or planar chip.

Many different microcomponents, such as microelectronics, electric motors, pumps, valves, refrigeration units, heaters, lasers, optical devices, and detectors have been fabricated, and in principle any of these components could be used in conjunction with any of the three basic types of microchips in the construction of highly sophisticated analytical microchips. In addition, there is ample surface area on most microchips for placement of the microelectronics that would be needed to operate the device.

Microfluidic Chips

A microfluidic chip contains interconnected microchambers, microchannels, filters, and other structures designed for manipulating liquid samples. The internal volume of a microfluidic chip depends on the geometry and cross-section of the particular structures in the chip, but volumes are usually in the nanoliter-to-microliter range. A capillary electrophoresis chip that simply consists of an arrangement of microchannels and reservoirs is a representative example of a microfluidic chip (Figure 6-1A) (20–22).

Bioelectronic Chips

A bioelectronic chip incorporates microelectronic components, e.g., electrodes that are designed to manipulate components of the biological sample introduced into the chip. It is embedded

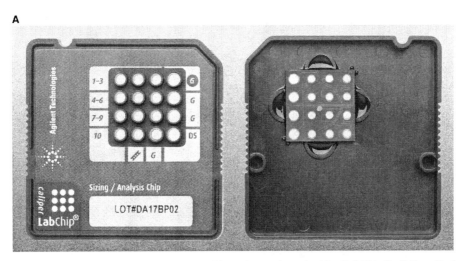

Figure 6-1   Microfluidic chips. (*A*) Top and underside of a capillary electrophoresis chip (LabChip®, Caliper Technologies Corporation).

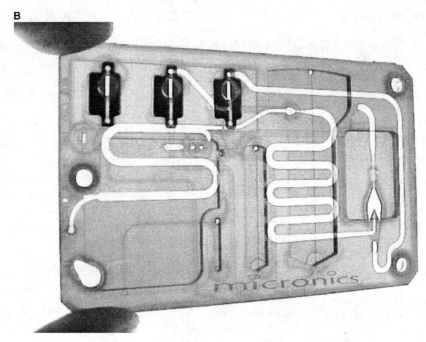

Figure 6-1 (*Continued*) Microfluidic chips. (*B*) Micronics Microcytometer™ lab card (images courtesy of Micronics, Inc., Redmond, WA).

on an electronic board, and this provides the connections to the electrical components within the chip, and links to a controller and output device (e.g., a display screen). Arrays of micrometer-sized electrodes located within a bioelectronic chip are effective for isolation of specific cells or microbes and for controlling DNA hybridization reactions within microchips (Figure 6-2A) (23, 24).

Microarray Chips

A microarray chip is an array of reagents (oligonucleotides, cDNA, peptides, proteins, tissue sections) synthesized in situ, spotted or assembled onto the surface of a small chip of silicon or a microscope slide, or immobilized on the surface of the

electrodes in a microelectrode array (25–29). These devices are also known as gene chips, genome chips, protein chips, proteome chips, or tissue microarrays depending on the identity of the arrayed sample or reagent (Figure 6-3). Microarrays are now used extensively in gene expression monitoring and drug discovery. Spot sizes are typically 100 μm or less, and arrays with hundreds of spots per square centimeter are in routine use. Very high densities of arrayed substances can be achieved using the in situ synthesis method for array fabrication (e.g., >1 million oligonucleotides/mm^2) (30). The scale of analysis possible with microarrays produces massive amounts of data and has necessitated a strong emphasis on bioinformatics techniques. Microarrays and the ancillary equipment for making,

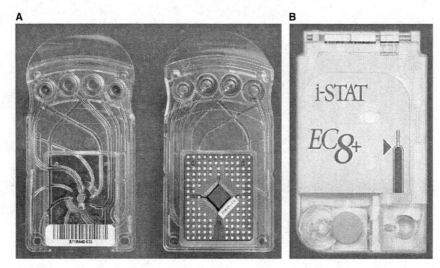

Figure 6-2 Bioelectronic chips. (*A*) Top and underside of a NanoChip™ (Nanogen, Inc., San Diego, CA); (*B*) i-STAT cartridge.

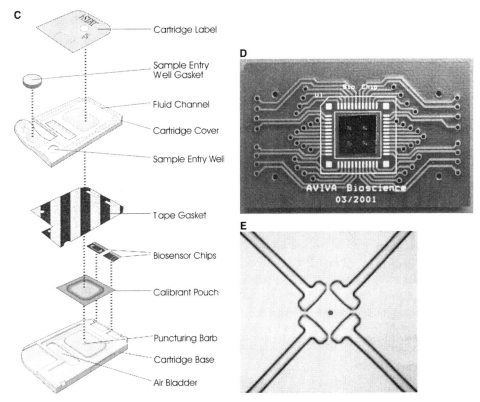

Figure 6-2 (*Continued*) Bioelectronic chips. (*C*) Exploded view of an i-STAT cartridge (images courtesy of i-STAT Corporation); (*D*) "patch-clamp" ion-channel analysis chip on its connection board; and (*E*) close up of electrodes for manipulating cells in the micromachined central well of the chip (images courtesy of AVIVA Biosystems Corporation, San Diego, CA).

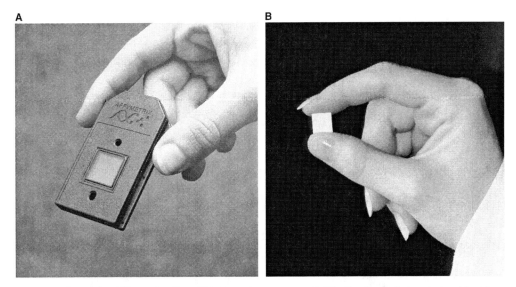

Figure 6-3 Microarray chips. (*A*) Affymetrix GeneChip® probe array; and (*B*) Randox® Laboratories biochip protein microarray. Reproduced with permission from Affymetrix Inc., Santa Clara, CA (Figure 6-3A) and Randox Laboratories Ltd., Crumlin, UK (Figure 6-3B).

processing, and reading microarrays are widely available, and the microarray is the most extensively used type of microchip.

In practice, many microchips combine design elements of microfluidic chips, bioelectronic chips, and microarray chips and can be considered hybrid microchips. An example of a hybrid microchip is the i-STAT cartridge for use in the i-STAT analyzer (www.i-stat.com) (31). The cartridge combines microfluidics, microelectrode-based sensors, an onboard calibrant solution, and an interface to a handheld analyzer that controls the operation of the cartridge and data handling (Figure 6-2, B and C). Another example of an hybrid miniaturized device is the Now™ Monitor (www.metrika.com) (Figure 6-4). This pager-sized single-use device combines a liquid-crystal display, microoptics, dry reagents, microelectronics, and a battery. It is designed to analyze hemoglobin A1c or lipids in blood, or microalbumin in urine (32). Although this device does not contain a planar microchip, it does integrate a broad range of miniaturized components and is a premier example of what is possible in the design and implementation of miniature components in a disposable integrated analyzer.

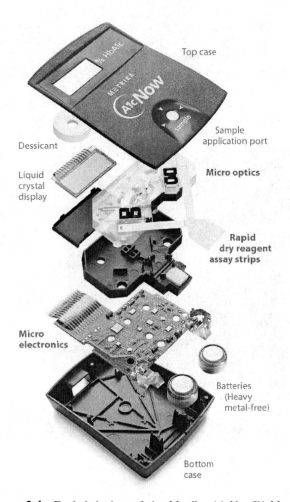

Figure 6-4 Exploded view of the Metrika A1cNow™ Monitor (image courtesy of Metrika, Inc., Sunnyvale, CA).

APPLICATIONS FOR MICROCHIP DEVICES

Currently, there are few examples of microchip devices in use at the point of care. The potential exists for many of the current range of microchip analyzers to be implemented in this manner, but regulations, consumer demand, and financial factors either currently prevent, or fail to drive this technology toward point-of-care applications.

Many of the conventional analytical separation techniques have been miniaturized to a microchip format, including capillary electrophoresis (CE) (33, 34), liquid chromatography (LC), (35) immunoassay (25–29), polymerase chain reaction (PCR) amplification reactions (36), mass spectrometry (37), and flow cytometry (38). In many instances the opportunity for system integration to produce total chemical analysis systems (TAS) on a microminiature scale (μ-TAS) has been a key motivating factor in the development of these devices (39). This type of device would provide total integration with all components of the analyzer (electronic control circuits, sample processing, analytical structures, reagents, communications) on a single chip-like device. It would put into the hands of the general public an analyzer with a menu of highly sophisticated tests that could be performed by anyone, anywhere, at any time. The full ramifications of this degree of enablement have yet to be evaluated. The following sections review the scope of the clinical applications of microchips that have potential for point-of-care applications.

Immunoassays

Many immunoassays have already been adapted to the point of care using dipstick and cassette devices (40, 41). These are mostly qualitative urine tests, and microchips offer a way of extending this to quantitative testing for multiple analytes in a range of fluids, including whole blood. Immunoassays have been implemented on each of the three major types of microchips, and representative examples are listed in Table 6-3 (42–56).

Microfluidic Chips. Microfluidic chip–based heterogeneous competitive and sandwich immunoassays and homogeneous (nonseparation) competitive immunoassays have been developed. In the heterogeneous type of immunoassays, reagents are immobilized either on beads loaded into a microfluidic structure [e.g., polystyrene (57), fluorescent latex (58), or magnetic beads (59)], or on internal surfaces within a microfluidic structure (60). Various cell filtration schemes have been developed in microchips, and these provide a route to preparing serum or plasma from whole blood or even isolating a specific cell subset for testing (61). Both qualitative immunoassays based on visual inspection of agglutination with the aid of a microscope and quantitative immunoassays in which bound and free fractions are separated by on-chip capillary electrophoresis have been devised.

Simple visual observation has been used to assess agglutination of red cells in an ABO typing immunoassay within 5-

Table 6-3 Microchip-Based Immunoassays

Analyte	Microfluidic chip	Bioelectronic chip	Microarray
Specific proteins	α-Fetoprotein [Song et al. (42)] Carcinoembryonic antigen [Sato et al. (43)] C-reactive protein [Pamme et al. (44)]	Cytokines [Huang et al. (51)]	Prostate specific antigen (PSA) (52)
Antibodies	Anti-HIV antibody [Karlsson et al. (45)]	—	IgE (55)
Hormones	Cortisol [Koutny et al. (46)] Thyroxine [Schmalzing et al. (47)]	—	Thyroid stimulating hormone [Ekins et al. (56)]
Drugs	Phenytoin [Hatch et al. (48)] Theophylline [Chiem et al. (49), von Heeren et al. (50)]	—	—
Microbes	—	*Bacillus globigii* [Huang et al. (52)] *Escherichia coli* [Huang et al. (52), Yang et al. (53)]	—
Toxins	—	Fluorescein-labeled cholera toxin B [Ewalt et al. (54)]	—

× 5-mm × 40-μm-deep silicon microchambers in a microfluidic chip, and in immunoassays for IgG using 4.55-μm-diameter fluorescent beads (58), and α-fetoprotein using 1.66-μm-diameter fluorescent latex beads (42). This AFP assay was rapid (~1 min) and detected concentrations of α-fetoprotein down to 10 pg/mL.

Capillary electrophoresis (CE) (46, 47, 49, 50) has emerged as a very popular means for rapid separation (<30 s) and quantitation of bound and free fractions in immunoassays in microfluidic chips. When combined with laser-induced fluorescence (LIF) detection, this technique is fast and sensitive and ideally suited for analysis of the nanoliter–picoliter volumes of reaction mixture in a chip. Another advantage is that it is easily integrated with microfluidic structures (e.g., mixing and reaction chambers) and with the electroosmotic type of pumping used to move fluid within an immunoassay chip.

There are now numerous examples of microchip fluoroimmunoassays that use capillary electrophoresis for both the separation and quantitation steps in a competitive immunoassay using liquid reagents (antibody and labeled antigen) (49, 62–64). Typically, these assays are performed in a microfluidic chip structure that includes a mixing channel that leads to an orthogonal capillary electrophoresis channel arrangement. The flow rate and length of the mixing channel determine the assay incubation time. A small portion of the reaction mixture is then delivered into the separation channel where the mixture is separated into bound and free species and quantitated by LIF. Fluorophore labels used as labels in this type of immunoassay include Cy-5 (62), and fluorescein (49). The analytical throughput of this type of system can be improved using a 6-channel microfluidic system. This has six independent mixing, reaction, and separation manifolds integrated onto one microfluidic wafer. Each of the manifolds is operated simultaneously and measured using a scanning fluorescence detection system (63). The current commercial equipment for microchip-based CE is benchtop in size (see http://www.chem.agilent.com), but further advances in miniaturization should effect an additional size reduction to the handheld size required for point-of-care immunoassay applications.

Bioelectronic Chip. A bioelectronic chip that contains an array of microelectrodes provides a format for multiplexed testing by virtue of its array design, and the electrodes facilitate an electric field-driven assay (53, 65). An array of capture antibodies is constructed by successive electronic biasing of the electrodes at each location so that biotinylated capture antibodies are attracted into an avidin-containing layer above the electrode. The biotinylated capture antibody then binds to the avidin and is immobilized at the electrode surface. This process is repeated for successive immobilization of capture antibodies at specific electrodes. The electric field is then used to direct the analyte, e.g., fluorescein-labeled staphylococcal enterotoxin B, to the appropriate electrode. Scanning the array for fluorescence reveals the presence of the different antigens in the test sample.

Microarray Chip. A major advantage of a microarray assay format is in simultaneous testing for a large panel of analytes. As yet, it is unclear what large panels of tests are appropriate or needed at the point-of-care, but allergen panels for detecting allergen-specific IgE antibodies and tests for different infectious agents or cytokines seem likely candidates.

Early microarray-based immunoassays used a high-sensitivity ambient analyte assay design, and an array of 100-μm-diameter (2) microspots of Texas Red–labeled capture antibody deposited on a substrate (e.g., polystyrene) and a fluorescein-labeled conjugate (25). Subsequently, the renewed interest in proteomics has led to many different types of protein microarrays (26–29). A protein microarray is usually produced by spotting different proteins onto defined locations on the surface of a solid substrate (e.g., glass microscope slide). In a sandwich-type assay, the array is then exposed to a sample, and after washing, detects captured proteins by reacting with a labeled detection antibody (66). Fluorescent (67, 68), chemiluminescent (51), and colorimetric endpoints (69) have been developed, and the latter in particular offers the possibility of direct inspection of an array in a point-of-care scenario. Microarray-based immunoassay products are in the commercialization phase, most notably the Evidence® analyzer (see http://www.randox.com) (Figure 6-3B). This is intended for the central laboratory, but it should help lay the foundation for microarray-based testing in a routine environment that could eventually lead to point-of-care applications.

Genetic Tests

Microchips currently provide the only viable technology for moving genetic testing to the point-of-care. Such a move is not likely in the near future, but nevertheless, the technology to enable point-of-care genetic testing now exists (Table 6-4) (70–87).

Microfluidic Chips. A key component of many genetic tests is the polymerase chain reaction. This reaction has been adapted to a microchip format in a both a time-domain and a space-domain format (36). In the time-domain format, the reaction mixture is kept stationary and the temperature of the microchip chamber is cycled between the different temperatures required for PCR, whereas in the space-domain format the reaction mixture is moved between different fixed temperature zones on the microchip. PCR microchips have been fabricated from various materials including silicon, glass, ceramics, and various polymers (e.g., polytetrafluoroethylene (PTFE), polydimethylsiloxane (PDMS), polyimide). The high thermal conductivity and low thermal expansion coefficient of silicon make it an excellent fabrication material for microvessels designed for performing the rapid and repeated heating and cooling cycles required by the polymerase chain reaction. However, plastics and the fabrication methods available for plastics offer greater flexibility and ease of integration as exemplified by the recent plastic microfluidic chips that have built-in microarrays (85).

A diverse range of targets has been amplified in a microchip using PCR or one of its variants, such as the reverse transcriptase (RT-PCR) or degenerate oligonucleotide primed polymerase chain reaction (DOP-PCR) (88). The amplicons synthesized in the reaction can be detected in reaction mixture removed from the microchip (89, 90) or, more relevant to point-of-care applications, by direct analysis methods. Microchips with transparent covers allow direct real-time optical readout of a PCR reaction in the microchip. This can be accomplished using a TaqMan® assay (91, 92) or by monitoring the increase in fluorescence intensity due to intercalation of a dye, such as ethidium bromide, into double-stranded amplicons (93).

Bioelectronic Chips. Microarrays formed on electrodes inside bioelectronic chips offer scope for manipulation of hybridization reactions and speeding up the hybridization reaction. Rapid analysis is an important consideration for point-of-care testing, and to be most useful, a test at the point-of-care must be completed as quickly as possible. Existing commercial bioelectronic chips (see www.nanogen.com) and emerging bioelectronic chips (see www.motorola.com/lifesciences/) are indicative of the potential of this analytical technique. A specific advantage is the versatility of this type of chip in both protein and nucleic acid analysis and in sample preparation, as illustrated by its successful use in cell isolation and cell sorting (94, 95).

Microarray Chips. Microarray chips have had a profound impact on the biological sciences and are now extensively used for massively parallel hybridization tests and comparative gene expression studies. This type of analysis is ideally suited to the testing for genetic diseases with many disease-causing mutations, such as in cystic fibrosis.

Simultaneous testing for all of these mutations could be accomplished in a single assay on an array device at the point-of-care and facilitate immediate medical decisions based on the results obtained. Currently, identifying which array test would be most suited or is urgently needed at the point-of-care is difficult. A case could be made for an array that screened for a large number of infectious disease agents, but it is harder to justify the array-based gene expression tests in view of the current state of our knowledge. Also, the sample preparation steps needed for a microarray test pose a significant barrier to point-of-care implementation. Finally, meeting the requirements of the regulations that govern diagnostic testing may not be a facile task as indicated by the recent controversy over a commercial microarray product (96).

Table 6-4   Representative Examples of Microchip-Based Genetic Tests

Microfluidic chips
  Duchenne muscular dystrophy diagnosis [Ferrance et al. (70)]
  Fragile X allele analysis [Sung et al. (71)]
  Microsatellite analysis (familial hypercholesterolemia) [Cantafora et al. (72)]
  Mitochondrial DNA analysis (diabetes) [Guttman et al. (73)]
Bioelectronic chips
  Papillomavirus detection [Vernon et al. (74)]
  Short tandem repeats analysis [Radtkey et al. (75)]
  SNP genotyping (β-2-adrenergic receptor) [Yoshida et al. (76)]
Microarray chips
  Assessing prostate cancer therapy [Luo et al. (77)]
  Campylobacter detection [Volokhov et al. (78)]
  Cancer diagnosis [Simon et al. (79)]
  Cardiovascular disease risk prediction [Cheek et al. (80)]
  CYP2D6 genotyping [Chou et al. (81)]
  Gene expression profiles (systemic lupus erythematosus) [Han et al. (82)]
  Gene expression profiling in cancer [Pusztai et al. (83)]
  Glioma progression assessment [van den Boom et al. (84)]
  K-ras mutation detection [Wang et al. (85)]
  Neuropsychiatric disorder characterization [Lehrmann et al. (86)]
  Single nucleotide polymorphism analysis (Factor V Leiden) [Schrijver et al. (87)]

Integrated Chips. Effective implementation of genetic tests will most likely require a PCR step, based on the current genetic testing technology. This will require integration of the pre-PCR and post-PCR steps on a chip if the overall genetic test is to be performed conveniently at the point of care. Considerable progress has been made toward this goal, and various pre-PCR and post-PCR reaction steps have been integrated into a single microchip device (97). These include pre-PCR sample preparation, such as white blood cell isolation using filters within a PCR chamber (98), and cell lysis (99, 100). Post-PCR processes integrated on a microchip include quantitation of amplicons by capillary or capillary gel electrophoresis, hybridization on oligonucleotide or cDNA microarrays (101–103), and enzymatic fragmentation of amplicons (104). The culmination of this research direction will be a handheld PCR analyzer capable of performing a wide range of genetic tests.

Cell Analysis

Shrinking the dimensions of an analyzer closer to the dimensions of a cell has been beneficial and has facilitated rapid and efficient cell isolation and analysis devices. As yet the opportunities for point-of-care cell analysis are limited. In theory, all of the current cell analyses performed on a flow cytometer or blood cell counter could be implemented on a microchip and moved to the point of care, and several different designs of miniaturized cytometers have been fabricated (38) (Figure 6-1B).

Microfluidic Chips. Red cell deformability can be measured using a micromachined silicon microhemorheometer (105). An imaging system monitors the flow and deformation of red cells in a series of eight 5- $\times$ 5- $\times$ 100-μm channels through a silicon dioxide window. Cell separation using microchip devices has proved to be very effective. Micromachined filters within microfluidic chips separate red and white blood cells and also filter other particulate mixtures (e.g., suspensions of latex microbeads) (106). The filters can be designed for a particular size separation and hence target the isolation of a specific cell type.

Micromachined silicon-glass microfluidic chips provide a route to point-of-care sperm testing and semen analysis (107, 108). It would be advantageous if some of the tests used to assess and investigate the infertile couple could be performed in a doctor's office. This would allow the physician to quickly determine an appropriate course of action during an office visit. Silicon microchannels capped with Pyrex glass are effective for the qualitative and quantitative assessment of sperm motility. A semen sample ($\sim$2 μL) is applied to the microchip through a hole in the Pyrex glass cover into an open chamber at one end of a 100-μm-wide, 40-μm-deep, fluid-filled tortuous microchannel constructed with a series of right-angle turns. Sperm enter the channel and swim along the tortuous channel. The distribution of sperm along the channel provides a measure of the motility and forward progression of sperm in the semen sample. Poorly motile sperm only migrate a short distance along the channel, whereas in a sample containing large numbers of highly motile sperm, many of the sperm swim rapidly to the far end of the channel. The time required for sperm to reach the end of the microchannel is monitored visually using a microscope, and this correlates with the conventional motility score. Other tests can also be adapted to the microchip format including sperm–cervical mucus penetration tests, and immunoassays for sperm antibodies.

Bioelectronic Chips. Several different bioelectronic chips have proved effective for cell isolation using dielectrophoresis (94, 95). AVIVA Biosciences has developed a bioelectronic chip–based method for patch-clamp analysis of cells and also for isolating rare cells from blood samples (Figure 6-2, D and E). Applications include isolating fetal red cells for prenatal testing for fetal genetic defects as an alternative to invasive procedures such as amniocentesis, and isolating cancer cells for development of cancer vaccines and dendritic cell therapy (see www.avivabio.com).

The microphysiometer is an example of a bioelectronic chip that allows the minute changes in pH that occur as a consequence of alterations in cellular metabolism to be measured (109). This device consists of an array of 125-pL wells in a flow chamber in contact with the pH-sensitive silicon surface of a light-addressable potentiometric sensor (LAPS) chip. Cells are trapped in the wells and exposed to a test substance and its effect on the cells trapped in the silicon wells assessed by monitoring changes in pH. The device is effective in a variety of applications including assessing cellular response to therapeutic agents (e.g., azidothymidine) (110).

Chemical Analyzers

The i-STAT analyzer, introduced in the 1980s, still represents the most advanced microchip-based chemical analyzer. This handheld instrument uses a single-use disposable cartridge containing microfabricated thin-film electrode sensors to test for a range of substances in whole blood (e.g., electrolytes, blood gases) (Figure 6-2, B and C). The cartridge contains a microfluidic system and a calibrant solution sealed in a pouch. Whole blood is applied to the sample well and the cartridge inserted into the handheld analyzer that controls the entire operation of the cartridge. The results of the analyses are displayed on a screen a few minutes after insertion of the cartridge into the analyzer. Numerous other miniature sensors have been fabricated and in some cases incorporated into miniature analyzers, e.g., a blood pH analyzer based on an ion-selective electrode field effect transistor (ISFET) within a silicon-glass structure (111) and a potassium-sensitive ISFET in a miniature analyzer (112).

Miniaturization has had an impact on many conventional analytical techniques. This raises the possibility of the development of miniature versions of the common analyzers and hence their deployment at the point-of-care. One of earliest examples was the miniaturization of the gas chromatograph in the 1970s (113). This instrument was fabricated on a 5-cm-diameter silicon wafer and comprised a 1.5-m-long spiral column (200 μm wide $\times$ 40 μm deep coated with OV-101 silicone oil) capped with a Pyrex glass cover plate. A 4-nL diaphragm valve was used for sample injection, and separated components were detected using a thermal conductivity detector clamped onto the wafer (113). Since that time many other instruments have been miniaturized, including the liquid chromatograph (15-cm-long spiral column (6 μm wide, 2 μm deep, total volume 1.8 nL) on a 5- $\times$ 5- $\times$ 0.4-mm silicon chip capped with Pyrex glass (114), and numerous electrophoresis devices (e.g., capillary electrophoresis chips) (20).

FUTURE PROSPECTS

The full impact of microtechnology on clinical testing has yet to be realized, but the foundations have been laid for future implementation. The various types of microchips are emerging as viable alternatives to conventional macroscale analytical systems, and in some applications providing analytical capabilities not possible using the macroscale systems. Commercialization of microchips for analytical applications has been slow, but the success of the capillary electrophoresis chips provides an example of the benefits of miniaturization of complex analytical techniques. The i-STAT analyzer is still the leading example of a microchip device for point-of-care testing.

The ever-broadening scope of analyses now possible using microchips will provide the basis for a greatly expanded point-of-care testing menu. Implementation of this menu of tests will be determined by regulations governing what tests and test methods can be used for point-of-care testing and by the cost–benefit ratio of their implementation. More problematic are the ethical issues that will emerge if highly sophisticated analyzers are developed as personal laboratories that can perform the current range of central laboratory tests. The prospect for genome snooping or proteome snooping will necessarily lead to careful evaluation of the development, sale, and deployment of these devices.

REFERENCES

1. Reid TR. The chip: how two Americans invented the microchip and launched a revolution. New York: Random House, 2001.
2. Petersen KE. Silicon as a mechanical material. Proc IEEE 1982; 70:420–56.
3. Stix G. Micron machinations. Sci Am 1992;267:106–17.
4. Bryzek J, Petersen K, McCulley W. Micromachines on the march. IEEE Spectrum 1994;31:20–31.
5. Kricka LJ. Hitchhiker's guide to analytical microchips. Washington, DC: AACC Press, 2002.
6. Cheng J, Kricka LJ, eds. Biochip technology. Philadelphia: Harwood Academic Publishers, 2001.
7. Schena M. DNA microarrays. A practical approach. Oxford: Oxford University Press, 1999.
8. Schena M. Microarray biochip technology. Natick: Eaton Publishing, 2000.
9. Tudos AJ, Besselink GAJ, Schasfoort RBM. Trends in miniaturized total analysis systems for point-of-care testing in clinical chemistry. Lab Chip 2001;1:83–95.
10. Kaehler T. Nanotechnology: basic concepts and definitions. Clin Chem 1994;40:1797–9.
11. Jain KK. Nanodiagnostics: application of nanotechnology in molecular diagnostics. Expert Rev Mol Diagn 2003;3:153–61.
12. Kricka LJ, Fortina P. Nanotechnology and applications: an all-language literature survey including books and patents. Clin Chem 2002;48:662–5.
13. Wilding P, Shoffner M, Kricka LJ. PCR in a silicon microstructure. Clin Chem 1994;40:1815–8.
14. Giordano BC, Ferrance J, Swedberg S, Huhmer AF, Landers JP. Polymerase chain reaction in polymeric microchips: DNA amplification in less than 240 seconds. Anal Biochem 2001;292:124–32.
15. Kricka LJ, Wilding P. Micromechanics and nanotechnology. In: Kost GJ, ed. Clinical automation, robotics, and optimization. New York: Wiley, 1996;45–77.
16. Shoji S, Esashi M. Microfabrication and microsensors. Appl Biochem Biotechnol 1993;41:21–34.
17. Becker H, Gartner C. Polymer microfabrication methods for microfluidic analytical applications. Electrophoresis 2000;21:12–26.
18. Ning Y, Fitzpatrick G. Microfabrication processes for silicon glass chips. In: Cheng J, Kricka LJ, eds. Biochip technology. Philadelphia: Harwood Academic Publishers, 2001;17–38.
19. Ko WH, Suminto JT, Yeh GJ. Bonding techniques for microsensors. In: Fung CD, Cheung PW, Ko WH, Fleming DG, eds. Micromachining and micropackaging of transducers. New York: Elsevier Science, 1985;41–61.
20. Manz A, Harrison DJ, Verpoorte EMJ, Fettinger JC, Paulus A, Lüdi H, et al. Planar chips technology for miniaturization and integration of separation techniques into monitoring systems: Capillary electrophoresis on a chip. J Chromatog 1992;593:253–8.
21. Harrison DJ, Manz A, Fan Z, Lüdi H, Widmer HM. Capillary Electrophoresis and sample injection systems integrated on a planar glass chip. Anal Chem 1992;64:1926–32.
22. Kricka LJ, Fortina P. Microchips: an all-language literature survey including books and patents. Clin Chem 2002;48:1620–2.
23. Heller MJ, Guttman A, eds. Integrated microfabricated biodevices. New York: Marcel Dekker, 2001.
24. Xing W-L, Cheng J, eds. Biochips. New York: Springer-Verlag, 2003.
25. Ekins R, Chu FW. Microarrays: their origins and applications. Trends Biotechnol 1999;17:217–8.
26. Zhu H, Snyder M. Protein arrays and microarrays. Curr Opin Chem Biol 2001;5:40–5.
27. Albala JS. Array-based proteomics: the latest chip challenge. Expert Rev Mol Diagn 2001;1:145–52.
28. Cahill DJ. Protein and antibody arrays and their medical applications. J Immunol Methods 2001;250:81–91.
29. MacBeath G. Proteomics comes to the surface. Nat Biotechnol 2001;19:828–9.
30. Lipshutz RJ, Fodor SP, Gingeras TR, Lockhart DJ. High density synthetic oligonucleotide arrays. Nat Genet 1999; 21(1 Suppl):20–4.
31. Erickson KA, Wilding P. Evaluation of a novel point-of-care system, the i-STAT portable clinical analyzer. Clin Chem 1993; 39:283–7.
32. Stivers CR, Baddam SR, Clark AL, Ammirati EB, Irvin BR, Blatt JM. A miniaturized self-contained single-use disposable quantitative test for hemoglobin A1c in blood at the point of care. Diabetes Technol Ther 2000;2:517–26.
33. Verpoorte E. Microfluidic chips for clinical and forensic analysis. Electrophoresis 2002;23:677–712.
34. Jin LJ, Ferrance J, Landers JP. Miniaturized electrophoresis: an evolving role in laboratory medicine. Biotechniques 2001;31: 1332–5, 1338–40, 1342, passim.

35. O'Neill AP, O'Brien P, Alderman J, Hoffman D, McEnery M, Murrihy J, et al. On-chip definition of picolitre sample injection plugs for miniaturised liquid chromatography. J Chromatogr A 2001;924:259–63.

36. Kricka LJ, Wilding P. Microchip PCR. Anal Bioanal Chem 2003;377:820–5.

37. De Mello AJ. Chip-MS: Coupling the large with the small. Lab Chip 2001;1:7N–12N.

38. Gawad S, Schild L, Renaud PH. Micromachined impedance spectroscopy flow cytometer for cell analysis and particle sizing. Lab Chip 2001;1:77–82.

39. Manz A, Graber N, Widmer HM. Miniaturized total analysis systems: a novel concept for chemical sensors. Sens Actuators 1990;B1:244–8.

40. Kricka LJ, Wilding P. Microfabricated immmunoassay devices, In: Price CP, Newman DJ, eds. Principles and practice of immunoassay, 2nd ed. New York: Stockton Press, 1997:605–24.

41. Kricka LJ. Prospects for microchips in immunoassays and immunoassay tests at the point-of-care. J Clin Ligand Assay 2002; 4:317–24.

42. Song MI, Iwata K, Yamada M, Yokoyama K, Takeuchi T, Tamiya E, et al. Multisample analysis using an array of micro-reactors for an alternating-current field-enhanced latex immunoassay. Anal Chem 1994;66:778–81.

43. Sato K, Tokeshi M, Kimura H, Kitamori T. Determination of carcinoembryonic antigen in human sera by integrated bead immunoassay in a microchip for cancer diagnosis. Anal Chem 2001;73:1213–8.

44. Pamme N, Koyama R, Manz A. Counting and sizing of particles and particle agglomerates in a microfluidic device using laser light scattering: application to a particle-enhanced immunoassay. Lab Chip 2003;3:187–92.

45. Karlsson R, Michaelsson A, Mattsson L. Kinetic analysis of monoclonal antibody-antigen interactions with a new biosensor based analytical system. J Immunol Methods 1991;145:229–40.

46. Koutny LB, Schmalzing D, Taylor TA, Fuchs M. Microchip electrophoretic immunoassay for serum cortisol. Anal Chem 1996;68:18–22.

47. Schmalzing D, Koutny LB, Taylor TA, Nashabeh W, Fuchs M. Immunoassay for thyroxine (T4) in serum using capillary electrophoresis and micromachined devices. J Chromatogr B 1997; 697:175–80.

48. Hatch A, Kamholz AE, Hawkins KR, Munson MS, Schilling EA, Weigl BH, et al. A rapid diffusion immunoassay in a T-sensor. Nat Biotechnol 2001;19:461–5.

49. Chiem N, Harrison DJ. Microchip-based capillary electrophoresis for immunoassays: Analysis of monoclonal antibodies and theophylline. Anal Chem 1997;69:373–8.

50. von Heeren F, Verpoorte E, Manz A, Thormann W. Micellar electrokinetic chromatography separations and analyses of biological samples on a cyclic planar microstructure. Anal Chem 1996;68:2044–53.

51. Huang RP, Huang R, Fan Y, Lin Y. Simultaneous detection of multiple cytokines from conditioned media and patient's sera by an antibody-based protein array system. Anal Biochem 2001; 294:55–62.

52. Huang Y, Ewalt KL, Tirado M, Haigis R, Forster A, Ackley D, et al. Electronic manipulation of bioparticles and macromolecules on microfabricated electrodes. Anal Chem 2001;73:1549–59.

53. Yang JM, Bell J, Huang Y, Tirado M, Thomas D, Forster AH, et al. An integrated, stacked microlaboratory for biological agent detection with DNA and immunoassays. Biosens Bioelectron 2002;17:605–18.

54. Ewalt KL, Haigis RW, Rooney R, Ackley D, Krihak M. Detection of biological toxins on an active electronic microchip. Anal Biochem 2001;289:162–72.

55. Fall BI, Eberlein-Konig B, Behrendt H, Niessner R, Ring J, Weller MG. Microarrays for the screening of allergen-specific IgE in human serum. Anal Chem 2003;75:556–62.

56. Ekins R, Chu F. Multianalyte testing. Clin Chem 1993;39:369–70.

57. Sato K, Tokeshi M, Kimura H, Kitamori T. Integration of immunoassay system into a microchip. Jpn J Electrophoresis 2000;44:73–7.

58. Wilding P, Kricka LJ, Zemel JN. Methods and apparatus for the detection of an analyte utilizing mesoscale flow systems. US Patent 5 637 469. 1997.

59. Jin-Woo C, Oh KW, Thomas JH, Heineman WR, Halsall HB, Nevin JH, et al. An integrated microfluidic biochemical detection system with magnetic bead-based sampling and analysis capabilities. Tech Dig MEMS 2001;447–50.

60. Yakovleva J, Davidsson R, Lobanova A, Bengtsson M Eremin S, Laurell T, et al. Microfluidic enzyme immunoassay using silicon microchip with immobilized antibodies and chemiluminescence detection. Anal Chem 2002;74:2994–3004.

61. Wilding P, Kricka LJ, Cheng J, Hvichia G, Shoffner MA, Fortina P. Integrated cell isolation and polymerase chain reaction analysis using silicon microfilter chambers. Anal Biochem 1998;257:95–100.

62. Guifeng J, Attiya S, Ocvirk G, Lee WE, Harrison DJ. Red diode laser induced fluorescence detection with a confocal microscope on a microchip for capillary electrophoresis. Biosens Bioelectron 2000;14:10–1.

63. Cheng SB, Skinner CD, Taylor J, Attiya S, Lee WE, Picelli G, et al. Development of a multichannel microfluidic analysis system employing affinity capillary electrophoresis for immunoassay. Anal Chem 2001;73:1472–9.

64. Mere L, Bennett T, Coassin P, England P, Hamman B, Rink T, et al. Miniaturized FRET assays and microfluidics: key components for ultra-high-throughput screening. Drug Discov Today 1999;4:363–9.

65. Ewalt KL, Haigis RW, Rooney R, Ackley D, Krihak M. Detection of biological toxins on an active electronic microchip. Anal Biochem 2001;289:162–72.

66. Templin MF, Stoll D, Schrenk M, Traub PC, Vohringer CF, Joos TO. Protein microarray technology. Trends Biotechnol 2002;20:160–6.

67. Urbanowska T, Mangialaio S, Hartmann C, Legay F. Development of protein microarray technology to monitor biomarkers of rheumatoid arthritis disease. Cell Biol Toxicol 2003;19:189–202.

68. Wiese R. Analysis of several fluorescent detector molecules for protein microarray use. Luminescence 2003;18:25–30.

69. Peck K, Sher Y-P. Application of enzyme colorimetry for cDNA microarray detection. In: Cheng J, Kricka LJ, eds. Biochip technology. Philadelphia: Harwood Academic Publishers, 2001; 325–40.

70. Ferrance J, Snow K, Landers JP. Evaluation of microchip electrophoresis as a molecular diagnostic method for Duchenne muscular dystrophy. Clin Chem 2002;48:380–3.

71. Sung WC, Lee GB, Tzeng CC, Chen SH. Plastic microchip electrophoresis for genetic screening: the analysis of polymerase chain reactions products of fragile X (CGG)n alleles. Electrophoresis 2001;22:1188–93.

72. Cantafora A, Blotta I, Bruzzese N, Calandra S, Bertolini S. Rapid sizing of microsatellite alleles by gel electrophoresis on microfabricated channels: application to the D19S394 tetranucleotide repeat for cosegregation study of familial hypercholesterolemia. Electrophoresis 2001;22:4012–5.

73. Guttman A, Gao HG, Haas R. Rapid analysis of mitochondrial DNA heteroplasmy in diabetes by gel-microchip electrophoresis. Clin Chem 2001;47:1469–72.

74. Vernon SD, Farkas DH, Unger ER, Chan V, Miller DL, Chen YP, et al. Bioelectronic DNA detection of human papillomaviruses using eSensor trade mark: a model system for detection of multiple pathogens. BMC Infect Dis 2003;3:12.

75. Radtkey R, Feng L, Muralhidar M, Duhon M, Canter D, DiPierro D, et al. Rapid, high fidelity analysis of simple sequence repeats on an electronically active DNA microchip. Nucleic Acids Res 2000;28:E17.

76. Yoshida N, Nishimaki Y, Sugiyama M, Abe T, Tatsumi T, Tanoue A, et al. SNP genotyping in the beta(2)-adrenergic receptor by electronic microchip assay, DHPLC, and direct sequencing. J Hum Genet 2002;47:500–3.

77. Luo J, Dunn TA, Ewing CM, Walsh PC, Isaacs WB. Decreased gene expression of steroid 5 alpha-reductase 2 in human prostate cancer: Implications for finasteride therapy of prostate carcinoma. Prostate 2003;57:134–9.

78. Volokhov D, Chizhikov V, Chumakov K, Rasooly A. Microarray-based identification of thermophilic *Campylobacter jejuni*, *C. coli*, *C. lari*, and *C. upsaliensis*. J Clin Microbiol 2003;41: 4071–80.

79. Simon R, Mirlacher M, Sauter G. Tissue microarrays in cancer diagnosis. Expert Rev Mol Diagn 2003;3:421–30.

80. Cheek DJ, Cesan A. Genetic predictors of cardiovascular disease: the use of chip technology. J Cardiovasc Nurs 2003;18: 50–6.

81. Chou WH, Yan FX, Robbins-Weilert DK, Ryder TB, Liu WW, Perbost C, et al. Comparison of two CYP2D6 genotyping methods and assessment of genotype-phenotype relationships. Clin Chem 2003;49:542–51.

82. Han GM, Chen SL, Shen N, Ye S, Bao CD, Gu YY. Analysis of gene expression profiles in human systemic lupus erythematosus using oligonucleotide microarray. Genes Immun 2003;4:177–86.

83. Pusztai L, Ayers M, Stec J, Clark E, Hess K, Stivers D, et al. Gene expression profiles obtained from fine-needle aspirations of breast cancer reliably identify routine prognostic markers and reveal large-scale molecular differences between estrogen-negative and estrogen-positive tumors. Clin Cancer Res 2003;9: 2406–15.

84. van den Boom J, Wolter M, Kuick R, Misek DE, Youkilis AS, Wechsler DS, et al. Characterization of gene expression profiles associated with glioma progression using oligonucleotide-based microarray analysis and real-time reverse transcription-polymerase chain reaction. Am J Pathol 2003;163:1033–43.

85. Wang Y, Vaidya B, Farquar HD, Stryjewski W, Hammer RP, McCarley RL, et al. Microarrays assembled in microfluidic chips fabricated from poly(methyl methacrylate) for the detection of low-abundant DNA mutations. Anal Chem 2003;75: 1130–40.

86. Lehrmann E, Hyde TM, Vawter MP, Becker KG, Kleinman JE, Freed WJ. The use of microarrays to characterize neuropsychiatric disorders: postmortem studies of substance abuse and schizophrenia. Curr Mol Med 2003;3:437–46.

87. Schrijver I, Lay MJ, Zehnder JL. Diagnostic single nucleotide polymorphism analysis of factor V Leiden and prothrombin 20210G > A. A comparison of the Nanogen Electronic Microarray with restriction enzyme digestion and the Roche LightCycler. Am J Clin Pathol 2003;119:490–6.

88. Fortina P, Cheng J, Kricka LJ, Waters LC, Jacobson SC, Wilding P, et al. DOP-PCR amplification of whole genomic DNA and microchip-based capillary electrophoresis. Methods Mol Biol 2001;163:211–9.

89. Waters LC, Jacobson SC, Kroutchinina N, Khandurina J, Foote RS, Ramsey MJ. Multiple sample PCR amplification and electrophoretic analysis on a microchip. Anal Chem 1998;70: 5172–6.

90. Ross PL, Davis PA, Belgrader P. Analysis of DNA fragments from conventional and microfabricated PCR devices using delayed extraction MALDI-TOF mass spectrometry. Anal Chem 1998;70:2067–73.

91. Taylor TB, Winn-Deen ES, Picozza E, Woudenberg TM, Albin M. Optimization of the performance of the polymerase chain reaction in silicon-based microstructures. Nucleic Acids Res 1997;25:3164–8.

92. Belgrader P, Benett W, Hadley D, Long G, Mariella R Jr., Milanovich F, et al. Rapid pathogen detection using a microchip PCR array instrument. Clin Chem 1998;44:2191–4.

93. Northrup MA, Benett B, Hadley D, Landre P, Lehew S, Richards J, et al. Miniature analytical instrument for nucleic acids based on micromachined silicon reaction chambers. Anal Chem 1998;70:918–22.

94. Cheng J, Sheldon EL, Wu L, Heller MJ, O'Connell JP. Isolation of cultured cervical carcinoma cells mixed with peripheral blood cells on a bioelectronic chip. Anal Chem 1998;70:2321–6.

95. Cheng J, Sheldon EL, Wu L, Uribe A, Gerrue LO, Carrino J, et al. Preparation and hybridization analysis of DNA/RNA from E. coli on microfabricated bioelectronic chips. Nat Biotechnol 1998;16:541–6.

96. Kling J. Roche's microarray tests US FDA's diagnostic policy. Nat Biotechnol 2003;21:959–60.

97. Burke DT, Burns MA, Mastrangelo C. Microfabrication technologies for integrated nucleic acid analysis. Genome Res 1997; 7:189–97.

98. Lee TMH, Hsing IM, Lao AI, Carles MC. A miniaturized DNA amplifier: its application in traditional Chinese medicine. Anal Chem 2000;72:4242–7.

99. Waters LC, Jacobson SC, Kroutchinina N, Khandurina J, Foote RS, Ramsey MJ. Microchip device for cell lysis, multiplex PCR amplification, and electrophoretic sizing. Anal Chem 1998;70: 158–62.

100. Lagally ET, Simpson PC, Mathies RA. Monolithic integrated microfluidic DNA amplification and capillary electrophoresis analysis system. Sens Actuators 2000;B 63:132–46.

101. Trau D, Lee TMH, Lao AIK, Lenigk R, Hsing I-M, Ip NY, et al. Genotyping on a complementary metal oxide semiconductor silicon polymerase chain reaction chip with integrated DNA microarray. Anal Chem 2002;74:3168–73.

102. Wooley AT, Hadley D, Landre P, deMello AJ, Mathies RA, Northrup MA. Functional integration of PCR amplification and capillary electrophoresis in a microfabricated DNA analysis device. Anal Chem 1996;68:4081–6.

103. Khandurina J, McKnight TE, Jacobsen SC, Waters LC, Foote RS, Ramsey MJ. Integrated system for rapid PCR-based DNA

analysis in microfluidic devices. Anal Chem 2000;72:2995–3000.

104. Anderson RC, Su X, Bogdan GJ, Fenton J. A miniature integrated device for automated multistep genetic assays. Nucleic Acids Res 2000;28:E60.

105. Tracy MC, Kaye PH, Shepherd JN. Microfabricated microhaemorheometer. IEEE International Conference on Solid-State Sensors and Actuators (Transducers'91). New York: IEEE, 199:82–4.

106. Wilding P, Pfahler J, Bau HH, Zemel JN, Kricka LJ. Manipulation and flow of biological fluids in straight channels micromachined in silicon. Clin Chem 1994;40:43–7.

107. Kricka LJ, Nozaki O, Heyner S, Garside WT, Wilding P. Applications of a microfabricated device for evaluating sperm function. Clin Chem 1993;39:1944–7.

108. Kricka LJ, Ji X, Nozaki O, Heyner S, Garside WT, Wilding P. Sperm testing with microfabricated glass-capped silicon microchannels. Clin Chem 1994;40:1823–4.

109. Owicki JC, Bousse LJ, Hafeman DG, Kirk GL, Olson JD, Wada HG, et al. The light-addressable potentiometric sensor. Annu Rev Biophys Biomol Struct 1994;23:87–113.

110. McConnell HM, Owicki JC, Parce JW, Miller DL, Baxter GT, Wada HG, et al. The cytosensor microphysiometer: biological applications of silicon technology. Science 1992;257:1906–12.

111. Shoji S, Esashi M, Masuo T. Prototype miniature blood gas analyzer fabricated on a silicon wafer. Sens Actuators 1988;14:101–7.

112. van der Schoot BH, van den Vlekkert HH, van den Berg A, Grisel A, de Rooij NF. A flow injection analysis system with a glass-bonded ISFETs for the simultaneous detection of calcium and potassium and pH. Sens Actuators B 1991;4:239–41.

113. Terry SC, Jerman JH, Angell JB. A gas chromatograph air analyzer fabricated on a silicon wafer. IEEE Trans Electron Devices 1979;ED-26:1880–6.

114. Manz A, Miyahara Y, Miura J, Watanabe Y, Miyagi H, Sato K. Design of an open-tubular column liquid chromatograph using silicon chip technology. Sens Actuators 1990;B1:249–55.

Chapter **7**

Approaches to Delivering a Laboratory Medicine Service: Distributed Laboratory Services

M. Joan Pearson and Ian C. Barnes

Worldwide, healthcare services differ in the way they operate, how they are funded, and in the professional structures that deliver laboratory medicine services. Developments are likely to be driven in part by organizational pressures. An example of this would be billing for services in the United States, so that US hospitals were mostly ahead of hospitals in the United Kingdom in implementing connectivity of point-of-care testing devices and patient data interface with laboratory information systems. Similarly, the extent to which patients wish to be involved in decisions about their treatment varies. However, healthcare services have much in common. The pressures of limited resources, shrinking workforces, requirements for different skill mixes, increasing regulation, and emphasis on quality and risk management are problems throughout much of the world. In addition, most countries now have more vocal patients who demand more involvement in their care and services that are convenient for them rather than for the healthcare providers.

At the same time, innovation continues, in information technology and analytical technology in particular, making new ways of delivering healthcare possible. Rising pressures on laboratory medicine (increased test requesting together with squeezes on costs) are particularly difficult to manage because traditionally most of their work has been out of sight to patients, managers, and policymakers, so their role has often been undervalued and underfunded. Political initiatives and reorganization of health services to meet pressures such as demographic changes and rising costs may place a further strain on the delivery of services.

CURRENT APPROACHES TO THE DELIVERY OF LABORATORY MEDICINE SERVICES

If one considers the way in which laboratory services have developed over the past six decades, we can see the early testing at the patient's bedside migrating to the ward side room and then to a discrete laboratory environment. As a consequence, the testing has gradually become distant from the patient, and the point at which the test result is used in clinical decision making. This evolution of laboratory services has probably peaked with the advent of the large offsite laboratories seen in the United States, and to a degree in Australia, handling more than 10,000 specimens a day. If one looks at all of the options for delivering a laboratory testing service, a number of modalities can be identified.

Central laboratories may be sited in hospitals or offsite, serving several local sites. Their demise has often been forecast, but workloads show few signs of declining. When based on hospital sites, the central laboratory usually provides the acute day and night services, often combining clinical biochemistry and hematology in core laboratories. Rising workloads and staffing costs, plus difficulties with recruitment and retention of staff, are managed in a number of ways. In more recent years, the strategy has been to move toward consolidation of laboratory services, improving efficiency and quality, with increased equipment, automation, and method standardization. Automated testing, robotic specimen handling, pneumatic tube delivery of specimens, electronic test requesting and ordering, and laboratory information management systems that interface with electronic patient records (EPRs) and hospital information systems are now routinely in place. Esoteric or specialized testing, which may be of low volume and require specialized equipment and staff with special expertise, may be provided in a central laboratory that serves several cities, a region, or even several regions.

Satellite laboratories, as the term implies, are small laboratories removed from, but related to, the central laboratory, and situated some distance away. They provide a more restricted range of tests than the central laboratory, at a smaller volume, and may cross specialties, providing, e.g., core chemistry, hematology, and microbiology tests. They may be situated in clinical areas on the same hospital site, e.g., in critical care areas such as emergency rooms (ERs), accident and emergency rooms (A&Es), intensive care units (ICUs) (1), and operating rooms (ORs), or in smaller peripheral hospitals, or, increasingly, in primary or community care. Management of patients with diabetes or on anticoagulant therapy may be provided in this way.

STAT laboratory is a term that is often used interchangeably with *satellite laboratory*, although short turnaround time (STAT) laboratories would generally provide a more restricted range of tests and serve critical care areas, rather than more general clinical areas. STAT laboratories are established specifically to provide short turnaround time testing for clinical situations that require results to be provided quickly. Examples are blood gas measurements for ventilated patients in ICUs or cardiac markers to diagnose or stratify patients with suspected myocardial infarction presenting to the ER.

Point-of-care testing (POCT) is variously defined, but is generally taken to be testing conducted away from the laboratory and near to the patient, often by personnel other than qualified laboratory staff. It may be conducted in small laboratories or side rooms off wards or clinics, or literally by the bedside or in the physician's office. POCT can be conducted in a huge variety of settings in addition to hospitals and primary care, including emergency vehicles, armed forces units in battle, pharmacies and other retail outlets, workplaces, and, increasingly, in patients' own homes. There may be some input by laboratory staff in nonhospital settings, e.g., in user training or managing quality-control or quality assessment systems, but this is not common. POCT systems often provide single tests on whole blood (i.e., no sample preparation) or urine, and have limited capacity in terms of sample throughput, although some semiautomated systems, e.g., in urinalysis, are becoming available. Connectivity of POCT test devices with main laboratory information technology (IT) systems, while usually possible, is often a problem for reasons of funding, organizational resistance, or professional practice. Increasingly, small analytical systems providing a limited range of tests, or handheld devices providing an array of tests, are being developed and marketed.

Definitions of the latter three modalities vary, depending on the health system, and should not be seen as restrictive—indeed, the various ways of providing analytical results on patient specimens should perhaps be seen as a spectrum and interchangeable in their nature. Satellite laboratories are usually staffed by laboratory scientists and technologists, who may rotate with their colleagues from the central laboratory. STAT laboratories may be staffed by laboratory personnel or may be available to nonlaboratory staff to use for POCT. POCT in some institutions is delivered from peripheral laboratories by laboratory personnel, whereas in others, POCT is regarded as any testing conducted outside a traditional laboratory environment by staff who are not trained scientists or technologists—generally nurses or junior doctors.

Data from testing that are distributed in this way can of course be integrated on the same laboratory information system (LIS) as well as most tests done at the point of care, as systems are becoming compliant with the National Committee for Clinical Laboratory Standards (NCCLS) connectivity standard POCT-1A (2). Efficient integration of POCT and STAT data with laboratory data and making the information available in the clinical area is a growing need, but many institutions still have a long way to go. Many POCT patient data are still paper based, with all the associated risks of transcription errors and mislaid paper. The Enterprise Analysis Corporation (3), in its 1999 US Hospitals POCT survey, stated that at that time fewer than 20% of patient results were recorded electronically in hospitals, and there may be little improvement on this figure in many areas. The ideal system of testing options available to suit local clinical needs and electronic data flow is illustrated in Figure 7-1.

DRIVERS OF CHANGE IN LABORATORY MEDICINE SERVICES

Strategies for delivering pathology services vary across the world and are influenced by such factors as reimbursement mechanisms and the extent of private sector involvement. However, the key drivers affecting pathology are similar across

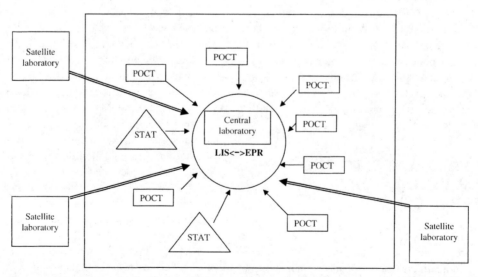

Figure 7-1   A representation of test information flow in a hospital environment: STAT, short turnaround testing (small laboratories in critical care areas); LIS, laboratory information system; EPR, electronic patient record. *Single arrows* indicate test result electronic information flow to the LIS from STAT laboratories and POCT in the same institution. *Double arrows* indicate test result electronic information flow to the LIS from satellite laboratories in peripheral hospitals. In this model, most testing is conducted in the central laboratory, with some STAT testing and POCT within the hospital and some satellite laboratories in peripheral hospitals. All information is transmitted electronically to the LIS, which interfaces with the EPR, where results are available to requesting staff in clinical areas.

continents, namely increasing demand, declining workforce, financial constraints, rising patient expectations, and rapid technological advances. Hospital patients suffer more acute problems and manifest more severe disease, while more cases are now treated by day surgery. The more chronic conditions, which once would have required hospital admission, are now being treated in primary care sites, and many patients with chronic illnesses are being treated and managed at home. Converging strategies appear to be developing across continents despite radical differences in healthcare systems, and are based on network formation bringing together pathology providers covering a wider healthcare community. Such programs are underway in Canada (British Columbia and Ontario), and there are numerous examples of networks in the United States, administered either by the independent sector or not-for-profit organizations. In England, the Department of Health has published "Modernising Pathology Services" (4), which sets out a strategy for improving the quality and efficiency of Pathology services in the National Health Service (NHS), with increased investment, and within the context of a more comprehensive healthcare delivery reorganization (5). Services will be redesigned and integrated into wider service developments and the workforce will be reviewed together with the skill mix required to deliver improved services by service redesign and flexible staffing. Strategic planning and service delivery, based on networks between NHS hospitals in several cities within a locality, is a model now used in other clinical areas in delivering service in critical care, coronary heart disease, and cancer (6). In particular, and most important, an outcomes approach is advocated for diagnostics, with closer collaboration with the diagnostics industry and building services around the needs of patients.

Another driver of change is increasing regulation: in the United States, the 1988 Clinical Laboratory Improvement Amendments (CLIA '88) legislation applies to all such testing, while in the United Kingdom, enrollment into accreditation schemes became compulsory in early 2004. The inclusion of POCT in laboratory accreditation in the United Kingdom is not yet as rigorous as the US system, although there are requirements for pathology supervision of POCT, user training, and quality systems. In the countries of the European Union, the In Vitro Medical Diagnostics Devices (IVDD) Directive (7) has established a regulatory framework, in conjunction with Conformité Européene (CE) marking of devices, for all laboratory testing, analyzers, and processes, including POCT. The purpose of the directive is to create a single market for medical devices within the European Union by harmonizing the regulations governing medical device manufacturers, and it aims to improve the level of protection of patients, users, and third parties and ensure that devices perform as intended.

The phrase "distributed laboratory services" implies that these services remain under the overall management of the existing laboratory system. However, in some respects, *devolution* of laboratory services may also develop outside of the historical environment of delivery, such as retail or commercial outlets and community diagnostic services, whether publicly or privately funded, where the ultimate responsibility for the results will not necessarily rest with the central laboratory. How the existing regulatory structures manage this change will differ from country to country. It is important that there is clarity on this when services are developed, that policymakers are aware of the risks in inadequately controlled POCT, and that lines of responsibility and accountability for the quality of testing and the competence of operators are clearly defined.

LOGISTIC CHALLENGES IN DELIVERY USING DISTRIBUTED LABORATORY SERVICES

While STAT and satellite laboratories may provide the shorter turnaround time required by clinicians and patients for the limited range of tests they provide, there are disadvantages. For those patients whose management requires additional tests that are available only in core laboratories, specimens often need to be transported long distances. The need to use both laboratory and POCT in order to make a clinical decision obviously negates the benefit that could be achieved from the latter.

Ideal arrangements as illustrated in Figure 7-1 are limited by the clinical, financial, and staffing pressures discussed earlier. Mergers and reorganizations may be forced on institutions situated in old buildings in large cities, with little or no scope for purpose-designed new buildings, and there are often differences in working practices, compounding staff recruitment and retention pressures that must be reconciled in managing the change. Transport of specimens within large hospital sites may be via pneumatic tube or by porters, with delays fairly common, but transport over the larger distances necessary in reconfigured services, when sites may be separated by several miles of busy urban roads, is expensive to operate and has significant problems—the inevitable time delays may compromise sample stability and quality and loss of samples is always a concern. The costs and delays must be balanced against the gains from savings on centralized and standardized equipment and lower staffing needs.

Compatible patient ID and IT systems are essential when services are consolidated and redistributed. In the United Kingdom, every person has a unique NHS number, and some hospitals are already using this as patient ID for test requests, rather than institution-specific "unit numbers," with universal use on the integrated care record service (ICRS) an NHS objective. Meanwhile, multiple files for one patient on the LIS are a common problem, compounded by inadequate information supplied by clinicians requesting or ordering tests, although electronic ordering can improve information quality. Greater emphasis on service quality and patient safety worldwide has raised awareness of the importance of accurate identification of patients, and the use of barcodes on patient wristbands when ordering and performing tests is now widespread.

Table 7-1 and Figure 7-2 illustrate an example of the actual organization of the laboratory services of three university teaching hospitals, working in partnership and providing acute services in two cities in northern England. Laboratory

Table 7-1   Basic Demographics of Hospital and Laboratory Services in a Major English City Partnership

Hospital	Approximate beds	Laboratory services	POCT
City A (pop. 720,000)			
Main sites			
1	1300	Central laboratory: most acute testing for inpatients, outpatients, community in city; limited STAT testing; some specialized supraregional services	25 blood gas analyzers (ICUs, neonatal units, delivery suites, ERs), 380 glucose meters, 20 urinalysis meters, 2 HbA1c analyzers
2	1100		
Peripheral sites			
1	240	No laboratory services	One blood gas analyzer (acute admissions), glucose meters
2	210	Satellite laboratories: limited services in biochemistry, hematology	One blood gas analyzer, glucose meters, some urinalysis meters
3	90		
4	80		
City B (pop 460,000)			
Main site	950	Central laboratory: most acute testing for inpatients, outpatients, community in city	Four blood gas analyzers, glucose meters, community HbA1c analyzers
Peripheral site	300	No laboratory services	One blood gas analyzer and glucose meters
Offsite laboratory		Serves both cities: some specialized nonacute pathology testing	

services at City A Main Site 1 and City B had merged, and an offsite laboratory was established between the two just prior to political changes in the NHS, which then resulted in the merger of the two acute care hospitals in City A, along with the peripheral hospitals associated with each. Progressive rationalization of services and centralization of low-volume testing has proceeded along with City A's acute clinical services reconfiguration, and this has involved equipment and method standardization and major restructuring of IT systems and transport arrangements between cities and intracity sites. The maximum distance between these sites is 12 miles (City B to both main sites in City A); other distances are 2 to 10 miles. The general principles of this process exist elsewhere in the United Kingdom, Europe, and the United States, and consolidation and rationalization of laboratory services are now widespread. During the past decade there has also been a reduction in the number of hospitals in the United States, a trend still seen, but to a lesser extent, in the United Kingdom.

Figure 7-3 illustrates the concept of a network of laboratories in a more rural environment, where the hospitals provide acute care services but are not teaching hospitals. In this situation the distances have a major effect on the ability to move specimens between sites, as well as on the movement of people, both patients and staff. Thus, although there is the opportunity for standardization of procedures, equipment, and methodology, there is less opportunity for consolidation of workstations, and consequently there is a greater level of duplication of testing sites throughout the network. Despite this, there is still plenty of scope for complementing the need for a common repertoire of tests on all sites with centralization

of more specialized tests on one site, possibly linked with a specialist clinical unit, e.g., a hemodialysis unit or oncology center.

The models differ in other respects besides the distances between the sites. Both provide services to primary care, but the second model covers a much wider area than the first. About 20% of the workload of the first is from primary care, but the second model has a much higher proportion of work for primary care and the community, and covers a much larger area. These considerations may affect future decision making involving the implementation of POCT.

CLINICAL REQUIREMENTS FOR TESTING SERVICES

The key clinical requirements for testing services will be those needed to deliver high-quality patient care. Universally, governments are developing policies and strategies for healthcare delivery that are focused on patient-centered care and a quality agenda. Key issues are access to services, patient choice, convenience and cost, and clinical effectiveness. In England, national clinical protocols have been introduced for a number of chronic diseases that specify standards of care and access targets and include diagnostic testing requirements. These National Service Frameworks include cancer (8), coronary heart disease (9), and diabetes (10). There is also a drive to decongest acute care hospitals and provide more healthcare in the primary sector. "Reforming Emergency Care" (11) proposed to reduce visits to ERs by providing access to treatment in local

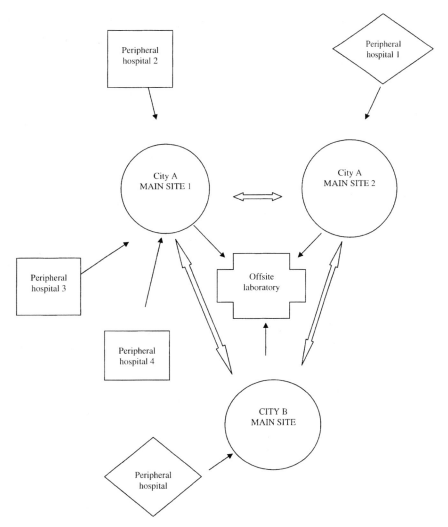

Figure 7-2 Map of the disposition of two laboratory medicine services in two adjacent English cities. Distances: Maximum distance (City A and City B main sites) = 12 miles. *Circles* indicate main city center hospital sites, with central laboratories providing acute core tests for the hospital, limited STAT tests, and specialized testing for the other sites (plus some supraregional services), with POCT in clinical areas. *Cross shape* indicates offsite laboratory providing nonurgent and specialized pathology testing. *Squares* indicate peripheral hospitals with satellite laboratories, staffed by laboratory staff, providing urea, creatinine, electrolyte, and some hematology readings, plus POCT in some clinical areas. *Diamonds* indicate peripheral hospitals with no laboratory service, only POCT (glucose, blood gases) in some clinical areas. *Double-headed arrows* indicate flows of specimens for noncore testing. *Single arrows* indicate flow of specimens for most testing other than POCT.

care centers. "Keeping the NHS Local: A New Direction of Travel" (12) provides a framework for treating more nonacute patients in primary care. These clinical requirements will require a balance of consolidated and distributed laboratory services, including POCT.

Wide Test Menu, Timeliness, and Maximum Quality

Clinicians generally want as many tests to be available as possible, to support the clinical service they provide. This may be in primary, secondary, or tertiary care settings, with esoteric testing required to support specialized clinical provision. Results that they can trust is a given, but laboratory professionals are better aware than clinicians and managers of how much

expertise and vigilance is needed to provide high-volume, high-quality and timely results, made available in a location and format that is clinically useful.

Short Turnaround Time

This is a major clinical pressure on laboratory services, although only a subset of results needs to be provided fast to ensure good clinical outcomes. Laboratory turnaround time (TAT) is generally assumed, sometimes incorrectly, to be a significant rate-limiting step in clinical processes. Reduced TAT is the main reason for clinicians wishing to implement POCT or to have satellite or STAT laboratories established, despite evidence that reduced TAT does not always improve outcomes [see, e.g., Kendall et al. (13)]. Pre- and postanalytical

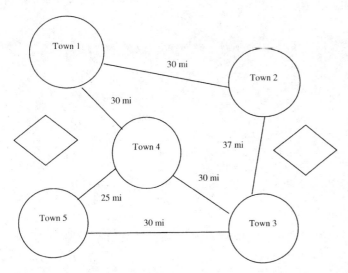

Figure 7-3 The disposition of a network of laboratories in a rural UK setting, indicating the distances between the hospitals served. *Circles* indicate a hospital with a laboratory. *Diamonds* indicate a hospital without a laboratory. *Lines* indicate distances between laboratory sites. mi = miles.

factors may increase the total TAT significantly, so examining the whole process (e.g., by process mapping) may allow changes to be made that meet the clinical TAT requirements.

The development of the electronic patient record (EPR) means that it will be essential to integrate the data from testing in satellite and STAT laboratories, and POCT, into the LIS and EPR. In making these observations about current practice, it is recognized that the style of care envisaged for the future, particularly from the perspective of the patient-centered approach, will demand a more rapid service—not just for diagnostics, but for other facets of care as well.

Response to and Support of Clinical Advances

Clinicians require diagnostic services to support clinical advances. These may be new treatment options requiring additional patient monitoring using new or existing tests, or day treatments, where reduced TAT may be particularly desirable. The likely changes in where and how clinical services are delivered (see Future Provision of Diagnostic Services section) will need to be understood and preferably anticipated.

Ease of use in POCT systems is a major factor in choice for clinicians, although there is rarely a good awareness of the importance of controlling pre- and postanalytical variables in minimizing errors (14). Interfacing of all diagnostic systems, including POCT equipment, with the EPR is increasingly desirable or obligatory in hospital testing, and systems for transferring data from home testing systems, for example, are available although not yet widely used in many countries. Portability is another requirement, depending on where the POCT system is to be used (e.g., ambulances or helicopters).

Reliability, Comparability, and Reproducibility of Results

Clinical attitudes to POCT services are mixed; there is some evidence that they trust POCT less than the central laboratory services (15) and this may make itself obvious by double testing (duplicate samples are sent to the laboratory to check POCT results), which does not help concerns about the costs of POCT, or the rising workload of central laboratories. Clinicians understandably want not only reliable results, but also POCT equipment and systems that do not break down frequently and that give results that are comparable with those from the laboratory for the same analyte. The fact that POCT systems often use different analytical methodologies from the laboratory test is often not understood, and differences in results may produce confusion and dissatisfaction among clinical users.

Clinical staff often have a poor awareness of the risks of POCT, in particular the necessity of using analytical quality control and quality assessment, and the risks inherent in poorly trained operators. The development of POCT systems that are simple to use and that may require very little preanalytical preparation will minimize these risks. Nevertheless, as services are devolved further and POCT in primary care and the community is increasingly integrated with patient treatment records, it is essential that lines of responsibility for the quality of results are clear. Laboratory staff, and in particular POC coordinators and managers, will need to develop skills in public relations and in communicating with and educating community clinicians, patients, and other users.

LIMITATIONS OF DELIVERY OPTIONS

Staff and Running Costs

Difficulties of recruitment and retention of laboratory personnel make POCT an attractive option for managers and planners, in addition to its other benefits. There are high fixed costs in establishing, staffing, and running satellite laboratories because of the low volume of testing done. However, the effect of POCT on clinical staff time of those who perform POCT must not be forgotten, as well as the need for laboratory supervision and management. The proposed network model of pathology provision in England has not yet been implemented, but experience with other NHS networks—in critical care, cancer and cardiac services—has provided some pointers to success. In managed networks, the manager is not connected to any of the existing individual providers (NHS Trust hospitals) but facilitates cooperation and joint planning leading to appropriate standardization of equipment and methodology and rationalization of services. Each member hospital retains its own financial autonomy, so success depends on good communication and a shared vision.

Costs and Benefits

There is a tension between the costs and benefits of POCT. On a purely cost-per-test basis, POCT is almost always more expensive than central laboratory testing. However, it has many advantages in addition to reduced TAT, and also the flexibility to provide diagnostic services near to patients wherever they are—in critical care, in primary care settings, in their own homes, or even when they are out shopping. This is probably where patients, judging the value of the service to them rather than the cost, will have a major effect on delivery, particularly in those countries where patient pressure has real effects on healthcare delivery; e.g., in the United Kingdom, patient choice in the NHS is a Department of Health priority (16). A major problem in many countries is in the way services are funded, and "silo budgeting" is widely seen as a barrier to the implementation of changes that bring benefits to parts of the organization, perhaps by reducing costs or increasing capacity and patient flows, while the changes are a cost to a different part of the organization that sees none of the benefits. Implementation of POCT is often blocked in this way, being seen purely as a cost to the user department rather than an overall benefit to the whole system (which may be a hospital or wider local health provision considered together). The remedy is to have system-wide planning of services, and to change the model of resource allocation, so that costs in one area are balanced by benefits in another.

The clinical and economic outcomes for proposed tests in the clinical context must be examined, taking a whole-system approach, and a joint judgment made. An outcomes-based approach to planning and implementing developments in testing services, however they are delivered, has not often been used, although the pressures of limited funding and staff recruitment and retention difficulties are increasingly forcing this approach to be considered. However, the complexities of healthcare funding often mean that assessing the economic outcomes and the benefits of POCT, despite its higher cost per test, cannot reliably be done in a generalized manner, and each institution must consider this in its own particular circumstances (17). Looking critically at economic outcomes is not easy, as it is necessary to study the effects of implementation of a new service separately from other variables that are almost inevitably present at the same time. Lee-Lewandrowski et al. (18) reported that they were unable to show the cost-effectiveness or otherwise of the POCT system they implemented in an ER STAT laboratory because their cost accounting system could not account for all the variables present. They stated, "In this situation, the decision to implement POCT in complex medical services remains largely intuitive."

Regulatory Framework

POCT in the United States is subject to regulation under CLIA '88 (19), and there are inspection bodies, e.g., the Joint Commission on Accreditation of Healthcare Organizations (JCAHO) (20), that ensure that institutions' conduct of POCT meets appropriate standards. The United Kingdom has no explicit legal framework for the regulation of POCT, but there is national guidance by the Medical and Healthcare Regulatory Agency (21) and others, which Clinical Pathology Accreditation uses when inspecting UK pathology departments for ac-

creditation of laboratory medicine services (compulsory from early 2004). In addition, the EU IVDD also regulates the way that CE-marked devices are used. There is therefore a considerable amount of guidance and regulation based on the concern that quality of POCT may be low if it is not conducted by trained operators, as systems may not be managed effectively, and analytical quality control and quality assessment may not be performed. The problems are likely to lie in making increasingly devolved users aware of the importance of following guidance.

Ethical Considerations

This is dealt with elsewhere in this book, but those providing or supporting POCT will increasingly need to be aware of the ethical implications of some POCT, e.g., drugs-of-abuse screening in workplaces and in the home, and questions of who should have access to patient results.

FUTURE PROVISION OF DIAGNOSTIC SERVICES

Laboratory medicine faces a number of challenges in delivering high-quality diagnostic services in the future.

New Scientific and Technical Developments

Developments in technology are providing new ways for delivering pathology services. On the one hand, large automated analyzers enable consolidation of a broad menu of high-throughput tests into central laboratories. These increasingly challenge the boundaries between traditional pathology disciplines and offer the possibility of multidisciplinary functional laboratories. New technologies, such as tandem mass spectrometry, provide the opportunity for improved analytical performance and reduced costs for specialist tests and some screening services, and will supersede more traditional techniques such as immunoassay. Developments in nanotechnology will provide portable systems capable of taking testing to the patient and challenging traditional laboratory locations and providers. Each of these innovations will impact on the type of staff required to deliver the testing in terms of training and competency.

Laboratory medicine has always worked closely with the diagnostics industry, which now takes on the role of method development, originally the role of the laboratory scientist. The risks and costs to industry of developing and implementing innovative technology are high, as opposed to incremental development of existing technology. Nevertheless, new technology will continue to become available, making more tests available at the point of care, e.g., genetics systems for pharmacogenomics, with equipment that is very simple to use, having inbuilt analytical quality control, miniaturization, and wireless communications for data transfer. Preanalytical error (14), particularly in sample preparation, will continue to be a concern in many systems, however, and data security and data quality will need careful management.

The likely growth in the use of new methods for continuous noninvasive monitoring of blood gases and electrolytes during surgery may in some clinical situations largely replace systems that currently use laboratory staff time for testing or equipment maintenance.

Changing Clinical Practice

As we have discussed previously, healthcare delivery is undergoing rapid and often radical change. Demand is outstripping resources and the aging population will put ever-increasing pressures on healthcare systems. The traditional models of referral for diagnosis and treatment to secondary and tertiary care facilities are being challenged. The focus is now on rapid, efficient, and cost-effective healthcare, with an expectation of more patient care being delivered in the primary care setting. Reducing the number of events in a patient care pathway and reducing bedstay is a key objective. In England, national access targets have been introduced that monitor waiting times for patients, and the diagnosis, treatment, and monitoring of chronic disease progression is being increasingly transferred to primary care. Clinical practice is changing to meet these demands, particularly with the introduction of one-stop clinics and treatment centers situated in the local community. There is an increasing reliance on diagnostic testing to support clinical management of patients. It is essential that diagnostic services are able to support the changes in patient flows and treatment regimens.

Information Technology

Telemedicine and virtual consultations are likely to increase in response to the pressures described earlier and to meet patient demand. This will have to be backed by diagnostic testing near the patient and results available to the consulting clinician together with other results in the patient's EPR. Patient privacy and confidentiality will continue to be central to the operation of efficient IT systems. The implications for the quality and integrity of patient records of increasing POCT outside the traditional hospital environment should not be underestimated.

The United Kingdom is implementing a national integrated care record service (ICRS) that will combine patient medical data, including pathology tests, into one record, accessible around the NHS by authorized staff caring for the patient. The increasing adoption of the patient's unique NHS number rather than a large number of institution-specific unit numbers will help this system to be a truly nationally accessible one. ICRS, together with the patient choice agenda and the drive to provision of more local services, will support devolution of diagnostic testing. The development of expert systems and decision support in conjunction with POCT to provide guidance on treatment or management to healthcare professionals or patients themselves, particularly in chronic disease management, will increasingly be an option.

Standards and Regulation

Most countries have some national regulation of laboratory services and inspection and accreditation arrangements to ensure compliance and user confidence in the quality of the service (see Chapter 16). NCCLS (2) develops and publishes standards for healthcare testing, including POCT and IT, which are used internationally, and the International Organization for Standardization (22) publishes standards for wider use. Work is proceeding internationally on harmonization of standards where possible. National accreditation bodies will need to acknowledge the likely increasing devolution of laboratory services and develop effective ways of ensuring that their testing and data management standards are of high quality.

However, the possible proliferation of many testing systems with different analytical methods, all providing input into a patient's record, could bring confusion about variation in results, so local standardization of methods and suppliers is desirable. Laboratory professionals will have an important responsibility in advising on implementation of testing in distributed or devolved sites so that standardization of methodology is implemented where possible and the extent of comparability of results from different systems is understood. Standardization of POCT equipment, IT connectivity of POCT systems, and interface with the LIS and EPR (in hospitals) and EPR and ICRS in other sites will be essential and will require coordinated local planning and implementation.

Safety and Risk Management

The risks associated with laboratory testing are generally understood by trained laboratory staff, but less so by users of POCT whether they are medical or nursing staff or patients themselves. The diagnostics industry has responded well to such concerns, incorporating implicit quality control checks in many of their products, advocating user training in their literature and device instructions, and often including external quality assessment (EQA schemes, proficiency testing) in purchase contracts with institutions. Advances in IT and data handling have also helped to ensure quality of results. Moves toward harmonization of international standards, device evaluations by national bodies such as the Medical and Healthcare Regulatory Agency in the United Kingdom, or multinational, such as the IVDD Directive issued by the European Union, help to establish standards not only for the manufacture and functioning of devices, but also their use and management.

Increasing litigation may result from the wider use of POCT devices in the community, and this should be borne in mind by staff in pathology who provide advice on system choice, purchase, management, and training to users, particularly those in developing delivery settings. This will extend many current roles of POCT managers and coordinators and should be seen as a very important obligation, with clear lines of responsibility agreed.

Staffing

Pathology services are facing increasing problems of retaining and recruiting appropriately trained staff in all areas (medical, scientific, technical, and support staff). An aging workforce and changing population demographics, coupled with increased competition from outside the healthcare sector, are making it difficult to maintain current staff levels with existing staffing structures and working practices. The introduction of new technology, particularly the larger automated systems for high-throughput analyses, are increasing capacity and leading to more efficient working in laboratories, but demand, not just in terms of volume, but also complexity and increased quality requirements is outstripping capacity. Increasing the workforce is only part of the process, and there is a need to review old and inefficient ways of working. Service redesign should take into account a review of workforce requirements and identify where skill mix changes and new ways of working can be introduced to support efficiency and effectiveness. This may include greater cross-disciplinary and multiprofessional collaboration.

The introduction of new technology and the balance between highly automated core laboratories, specialist testing sections, and distributed sites (POCT, satellite, or minilabs), and the potential devolution into the community of substantial amounts of routine testing, will create opportunities for changing roles of existing staff and the employment of other staff with different sets of skills and competencies to undertake new or extended roles. The increasing use of POCT will enable laboratory staff to become more integrated into direct patient care and management, either by providing direct analytical support or by providing quality assurance for nonlaboratory staff involvement. These will include junior doctors, nurses, pharmacists, and other allied health professionals. The role of the laboratory would include training, education, quality control, selection of equipment, maintenance, and troubleshooting. Essential to the efficiency and effectiveness of POCT will be advice from laboratory personnel on appropriate testing and interpretation of data.

In England, the government is implementing a series of coordinated human resource initiatives that will fundamentally alter the way in which nonmedical laboratory staff are employed. New pay structures and ways of working will be introduced [Agenda for Change (23)] that will be based on defined occupational standards and competency assessment for all grades of staff. This will be coupled with a new career progression framework that will enable more flexible working, guaranteed continuous professional development, and the opportunity to evolve new job roles. Overseeing this will be a regulatory framework that will require all staff to be registered on the basis of demonstrating competence against a set of proficiency standards [Health Professions Council (24)]. The standards expected of laboratory based staff should be extended to those using POCT systems.

Patient Choice and Public Perception

Patients worldwide are becoming more demanding about the quality of their care and expect choice of how and where they are treated. The recent consultation in the United Kingdom on patient choice and the subsequent publication of guidance (16) will affect the delivery of laboratory services in the United

Kingdom. Patients want health services to be provided locally, which must include testing services for screening, diagnosis, and monitoring treatment. This may mean small laboratories staffed by rotating staff from a hospital laboratory or locally employed staff who are trained to provide a limited range of tests on POCT equipment, which will be interfaced with electronic health records. Patients also want access to their health data and this may include test results, which is already the case in some countries.

Mintel (25), in a September 2003 report on over-the-counter (OTC) diagnostics in the United Kingdom, noted that "an increasing number of people are opting for self-diagnosis and turning their backs on doctors." In 2002, almost £55 million was spent on self-diagnostic products, including blood glucose monitors and pregnancy tests. The market had grown by 32% since 1998. Mintel expects this amount to rise to well over £60 million by 2007. People are becoming more willing to self-diagnose, suggesting that encouraging them to become better informed about their health and to seek other sources of reliable advice, such as from a pharmacist, is leading to greater self-reliance, as is the incidence of both chronic and acute conditions for which self-diagnosis and testing may be appropriate. The greater acceptance of the role of preventative medicine, the rising number of conditions appropriate for self-monitoring, and people's attitudes toward looking after their health suggest that these products will continue to be in high demand. Mintel's report on OTC diagnostics in the United States (March 2004) indicated that total sales of self-testing kits (for blood pressure, blood glucose, ovulation, and pregnancy) reached $842.9 million in 2003. Sales growth is expected to continue given the rising incidence of diabetes and hypertension and changing demographics in the United States. The aging of the baby boomers—whose numbers will reach 79.6 million in 2010—will result in much higher rates of diabetes and hypertension, both of which are conditions associated with aging, as well as obesity.

Diagnostic kits for the "worried well" are also widely available in pharmacies and other retail outlets, particularly for glucose monitoring, pregnancy testing, cholesterol, and fertility management (ovulation detection). Some pharmacies offer a diagnostic service to customers on a commercial basis. Other testing that is provided in some countries in primary care or the wider community, often by POCT, and is likely to be introduced elsewhere includes coagulation, cardiac markers including B-type natriuretic peptide, screening for drugs of abuse and infectious diseases, and tumor markers. As POCT systems and IT communications improve, however, it is likely that such services offered by community pharmacists will be integrated with other medical services in primary care such as diagnostic and treatment centers and the work of community physicians [general practitioners (GPs)], who, in the United Kingdom, for example, will be providing more medical care and taking over from secondary care some management of chronic diseases and medical procedures. The more locally available diagnostic services to support this could be provided by pharmacists, who may share chronic disease management and drug therapy with the GP.

POCT is the fastest growing segment of the diagnostics market in hospitals also; for example, an annual growth rate of about 8% up to 2007 is expected by Research and Markets (26) The Enterprise Analysis Corporation's survey of US hospital POCT in 2001 (3) suggested that in the following 5 years, one in four tests would be performed at the point of care and that POCT may represent 40% of pathology tests in future. The POCT market in 2001 was estimated at $4.9 billion and was expected to double within the following 5 to 10 years.

CONCLUSIONS

Optimal operation of distributed and devolved laboratory services, including POCT, will come about only through cooperation between the central laboratory and clinical departments (27). Existing laboratory personnel, not only POCT managers and coordinators, will need to develop leadership and influencing skills and increasingly work in teams with providers of healthcare services to ensure that distributed laboratory service and POCT are developed and delivered to the highest quality, are appropriate to clinical need, and operate within available resources.

REFERENCES

1. Naidoo R, Cox DJA. Intensive care laboratory. In: Tinker J, Browne DRG, Sibbald WJ, eds. Critical care, standards, audit and ethics. London: Edward Arnold, 1996:123–32.
2. National Committee on Clinical Laboratory Standards. http://www.nccls.org (accessed May 5, 2004).
3. Enterprise Analysis Corporation. http://www.eacorp.com (accessed May 5, 2004).
4. Modernising pathology services. London: Department of Health, February 2004.
5. The NHS Plan: a plan for investment, a plan for reform. London: Department of Health, July 2000.
6. NHS Modernisation Agency Innovation and Knowledge Group. http://www.modern.nhs.uk/scripts/default.asp?site_id=24 (accessed May 5, 2004).
7. Directive 98/79/EC to the European Parliaments and of the Council 1998-10-27 on in vitro diagnostic medical devices. Official J of the European Communities 1998;331:1–37.
8. The NHS cancer plan: a plan for investment, a plan for reform. London: Department of Health, September 2000.
9. Coronary heart disease—national service framework for coronary heart disease: modern standards and service models. London: Department of Health, March 2000
10. National service framework for diabetes standards. London: Department of Health, December 2000.
11. Reforming emergency care: first steps to a new approach. Department of Health, London, October 2001. http://www.dh.gov.uk/PolicyAndGuidance/OrganisationPolicy/EmergencyCare/fs/en (accessed May 6, 2004).
12. Keeping the NHS local: a new direction of travel. London: Department of Health, February 2003.
13. Kendall J, Reeves B, Clancy M. Point-of-care testing: randomised controlled trial of clinical outcome. Br Med J 1998;316:1052–7.
14. Plebani M Carraro P. Mistakes in a STAT laboratory: types and frequency. Clin Chem 1997;43:1348–51.
15. Gray TA Freedman DB Burnett D Szczepura A Price CP. Evidence based practice: clinicians' use and attitudes to near patient testing in hospitals. J Clin Pathol 1996;49:903–8.
16. Building on the best: choice, responsiveness and equity in the NHS. London: Department of Health, December 2003.
17. Foster K, Despotis G, Scott MG. Point of care testing: cost issues and impact on hospital operations. Clin Lab Med 2001;21:269–84.
18. Lee-Lewandrowski E, Corboy D, Lewandrowski K, Sinclair J, McDermot S, Benzer T. Implementation of a point-of-care satellite laboratory in the emergency department of an academic medical center. Arch Pathol Lab Med 2003;127:456–60.
19. CDC Division of Laboratory Systems (DLS). Clinical Laboratory Improvement Amendments (CLIA). http://www.phppo.cdc.gov/clia/default.asp (accessed May 5, 2004).
20. Joint Commission on Accreditation of Healthcare Organizations. http://www.jcaho.org
21. Device bulletin: management and use of IVD point of care test devices. London: MDA DB2002(03), March 2002.
22. International Organization for Standardization. http://www.iso.org (accessed May 5, 2004).
23. Department of Health. Agenda for change. http://www.dh.gov.uk/PolicyAndGuidance/HumanResourcesAndTraining/ModernisingPay/AgendaForChange/fs/en (accessedMay 5, 2004).
24. Health Professions Council. http://www.hpc-uk.org/ (accessed May 5, 2004).
25. Mintel International Group Ltd. http://www.mintel.com (accessed May 5, 2004).
26. Research and Markets. http://www.researchandmarkets.com (accessed May 5, 2004).
27. Halpern NA. Point of care testing: implementation is all: communication is key. J Crit Ill 2002;17:240–4.

Chapter 8

Analytical Performance Requirements for Point-of-Care Testing

Callum G. Fraser

Point-of-care testing (POCT) provides numerical test results rapidly. Minimizing the turnaround time that exists between the clinical decision to request a test and the availability of its result is one of the main reasons POCT was introduced. However, turnaround time is only one of the many performance characteristics of the analytical methodology used to generate the test result. Turnaround time is termed a practicability characteristic. There are also reliability performance characteristics, and the most important of these are imprecision and bias. Imprecision and bias have many ramifications for the clinical interpretation of numerical test results. These will be discussed in this chapter. Moreover, because imprecision and bias do have major influences on the interpretation of test results, it is vital to be able to define analytical performance requirements for POCT objectively in numerical format. The advantages and disadvantages of strategies to achieve these requirements will also be discussed.

EFFECT OF PERFORMANCE ON CLINICAL INTERPRETATION

Imprecision

Definition of Imprecision. *Imprecision* is the correct term for a quantitative estimate of random analytical variation. Imprecision is defined as the closeness of agreement between independent results of measurements obtained under stipulated conditions. Imprecision can be expressed quantitatively as a statistic such as standard deviation (SD) or coefficient of variation [CV; CV = relative SD = (SD/mean) · 100]. Imprecision can never be zero, although it can be reduced by careful selection of methodology and by adherence to strict standard operating procedures. Therefore, if internal quality control is regularly performed (e.g., replicate results on control sample material and calculation of SD and CV) in conjunction with POCT, then all users of this methodology should have knowledge of the imprecision of the analysis The importance of imprecision in clinical decision making has been reviewed in detail previously (1).

Sources of Test Result Variation. The test result reported by the laboratory as a single number actually represents a range of numbers that has a definable interval; the best measure of the interval is dispersion. The dispersion is made up of two major components. The first is imprecision, which is

random analytical variation. A second source of random test-result variation, and often the more important, is inherent biological variation. In the simplest and most widely used model of biological variation, each analyte in an individual varies around his or her individual homeostatic setting point. This variation can also be expressed quantitatively as a statistic such as SD or CV. Both the production and use of quantitative data on the components of biological variation have been fully described (2). The biological variation of many analytes has been well documented (3) and the data are available on the Internet (4). Because both imprecision and within-subject biological variation are random in nature, calculation of the total variation is possible. However, addition cannot be done by simply adding the SD or CV. Mathematical manipulations must use variance, which is SD^2. CV^2 is an allowable parameter for calculations, provided that the means of the components are the same. If the imprecision is termed CV_a and the within-subject biological variation is termed CV_b, then the total random variation [CV_t] can be calculated as $[CV_a^2 + CV_b^2]^{1/2}$. The total variation is the square root of the sum of the squares of the component variations, $CV_t = [CV_a^2 + CV_b^2]^{1/2}$. To calculate the dispersion, CV_t is multiplied by a covering factor, usually known as the Z-score, which is equal to the number of standard deviations appropriate for the selected probability. Generally, $P < 0.05$ is considered significant and the appropriate Z-score is 1.96. The dispersion that encompasses 95% of values is therefore $\pm 1.96 [CV_a^2 + CV_b^2]^{1/2}$. Sometimes, highly significant probablility is used, $P < 0.01$, and the appropriate Z-score is 2.58.

Imprecision and the Dispersion of a Single Test Result. Because of the potential effect on clinical decisions, those who interpret the single-number test result produced in POCT should be aware of the likely dispersion of the number, that is, the numerical interval in which a test result is likely to fall. A serum cholesterol concentration reported as 5.00 mmol/L (193 mg/dL) represents a range of numbers. For example, if the imprecision is 3.0% (within-subject biological variation of cholesterol is constant and is well documented to be 6.0%) (3), then the dispersion is $\pm 1.96 [CV_a^2 + CV_b^2]^{1/2} = \pm 1.96 [3.0^2 + 6.0^2]^{1/2} = \pm 13.1\%$. The 95% dispersion of the result of 5.00 mmol/L (193 mg/dL) is equivalent to a serum cholesterol interval of 4.34 to 5.66 mmol/L (168–219 mg/dL). This has significant ramifications for interpreting test results against fixed numerical criteria. An individual with a true homeostatic setting point of 4.60 mmol/L (178 mg/dL) might have the serum cholesterol value reported as 5.15 mmol/L (199 mg/dL), which is above the fixed limit of 5.00 mmol/L (193 mg/dL) considered by many to be ideal. In addition, an individual with a true cholesterol value of 5.45 mmol/L (210 mg/dL) might have the result reported as 4.80 mmol/L (185 mg/dL), which is less than the fixed limit that might stimulate some clinical action. Imprecision is important in this context, and the effect of imprecision on dispersion for cholesterol can be easily calculated. For CV_a of 2.0, 4.0, 6.0, 8.0, and 10.0%, the 95% dispersion is ± 12.4, 14.1, 16.6, 19.6, and 22.9%, respectively. Higher imprecision leads to widening of the dispersion, and in consequence, to poorer clinical decision making. POCT analytical methods very often have poorer imprecision than standard laboratory methods (5).

Imprecision and the Dispersion of the Reference Interval. Clinical interpretation is often undertaken against conventional population-based reference intervals (often erroneously termed normal or reference ranges). Users of POCT rarely develop their own specific reference intervals according to published guidelines (6), because this requires significant resources and expertise, although it is certainly appreciated that reference intervals can be influenced by analytical methodology. The components of the dispersion of a reference interval are within-subject and between-subject biological variation and, of course, imprecision. Higher levels of imprecision will lead to widening of the reference interval. A reference interval generated in the laboratory with a low-imprecision method will not be directly transferable to a POCT method with a higher level of imprecision. The true reference interval for the POCT method will cover a wider range. Use of the laboratory reference interval to interpret POCT test results will lead to more than the expected 5% of the population being classified as unusual, which might lead to an unnecessary clinical investigation and additional costs for both the individual and the healthcare system.

Imprecision and Number of Samples to Collect. Sometimes tests are done in replicate to generate a more reliable estimate of the true value for the individual. The number of samples needed for clinical decision making can be calculated objectively using the formula $n = (Z \cdot [CV_a^2 + CV_b^2]^{1/2} / D)^2$, where n is the number of samples needed to be within D% of the true homeostatic setting point with a Z-score appropriate for the probability (e.g., 1.96 for 95%), CV_a is the level of imprecision, and CV_b is the within-subject biological variation. As stated, the formula assumes analysis in singleton. Imprecision will have an effect on the number of samples. With cholesterol values as an example, if $CV_a = 3.0$%, then two samples would be needed to get an estimate within 10% for a probability of 95%. However, if $CV_a = 10.0$%, then five samples would be needed to achieve the same closeness for the same probability (i.e., 10% for a probability of 95%).

Imprecision and Monitoring Individuals over Time. One of the supposed advantages of POCT is that patients can be monitored more closely with frequent analyses. Monitoring involves comparison of serial test results obtained on an individual over time. Changes in numerical test results can be due to the patient's condition deteriorating or improving, but the variation must exceed the inherent preanalytical variation, within-subject biological variation, and imprecision. Thus, if preanalytical sources of variation are minimized by proper preparation of the individual prior to sampling, sample collection, and handling techniques (2), then the difference in the numerical test results must be greater than the inherent variation due to within-subject biological variation and imprecision. This difference is defined as the reference change value (RCV). The value is calculated as $RCV = 2^{1/2} \cdot Z \cdot [CV_a^2 + CV_b^2]^{1/2}$. The required change in cholesterol values (95% confidence) increases with deteriorating imprecision, because within-subject biological variation is constant. If CV_a was 2.0, 4.0, 6.0, 8.0, and 10.0%, then the RCV (the minimum change in serial values required to be significant) would be 17.5, 20.0, 23.5, 27.7, and 32.3%, respectively. In the evaluation of serial test results performed in clinical monitoring, imprecision has a direct effect on medical decision making.

BIAS

Definition of Bias

Bias is the correct term for a quantitative estimate of systematic analytical variation. Bias is defined as the difference between the results of the actual measurement and the true value. Allowable bias is usually described as a deviation in percentage terms and is often mathematically denoted as |B| (i.e., modulus of B or ±B). Through careful selection of analytical methodology with proper standardization and calibration procedures, bias can be zero. The comparative bias of POCT methodology may be investigated by comparison with a laboratory method of known bias, or better, through analysis of results attained in external quality assessment schemes (EQAS) or proficiency testing (PT) programs. The effects of bias on clinical test-result interpretation have been previously described in detail (7).

Bias and Reference Intervals/Fixed Limits

As noted previously, interpretation of test results generally makes use of population-based reference intervals. A reference interval generated in the laboratory using a method with either no bias or a known bias will not be directly transferable to a POCT method with a different bias. The true reference interval for the POCT method will be different. Use of the laboratory reference interval for POCT test-result interpretation will lead to a different group of the population being classified as unusual, which could result in further unnecessary investigation. Any analytical bias leads to greater than the expected 5% of the population being classified as outside the reference limits (2). This consideration also applies to clinical situations that use fixed limits to assist interpretation. For example, a serum cholesterol of >5.00 mmol/L (>193 mg/dL) is higher than the ideal, according to evidence-based clinical guidelines. If a POCT method had positive bias, then individuals with an ideal cholesterol of <5.00 mmol/L (<193 mg/dL) could be classified as having a concentration of >5.00 mmol/L (>193 mg/dL) and would be recalled for further tests, advised to change diet, or given drugs requiring lifelong monitoring. Any one of these would lead to increased personal and health service costs. In contrast, if the POCT had negative bias, then individuals with an unusual concentration could be missed, which could lead to early disease, again with personal and health service costs. POCT methods for glucose would have similar scenarios (i.e., POCT methods with positive bias leading to individuals being erroneously labeled as diabetic, or negative bias leading to a missed diagnosis), with serious consequences in both of these situations.

Bias and Clinical Characteristics

The clinical characteristics of sensitivity and specificity are affected by bias, because these involve fixed limits that have been set to give the desired clinical outcomes. Positive bias will lead to an increased number of individuals being labeled as diseased, because the number of true positives (i.e., individuals with the disease and an unusual test result) will increase with the number of false positives (i.e., individuals without the disease but with an unusual test result). Thus, the clinical sensitivity of the test will be higher and the specificity will be lower. Negative bias will lead to an increased number of individuals being labeled as healthy, because the number of true negatives (i.e., individuals without the disease and a usual test result) will increase with the number of false negatives (i.e., individuals with the disease but with a usual test result). Thus, the clinical specificity will be higher and the sensitivity of the test will be lower.

ANALYTICAL PERFORMANCE REQUIREMENTS

Analytical Performance and Interpretation of Test Results

Imprecision and bias, the important reliability characteristics of any analytical method, have important ramifications for test-result interpretation. Imprecision affects the dispersion of a single test result, the dispersion of the reference interval, the number of samples needed to estimate the homeostatic setting point of an individual, and the RCV. Bias affects the location of the reference interval, produces more outliers than the expected 5%, and affects clinical sensitivity and specificity. The challenge is to define in numerical terms, the analytical performance required to ensure that these effects are minimized and that clinical decision making is not compromised. Such analytical performance requirements have often been called analytical goals, but a better term is analytical quality specifications.

The Need for Analytical Quality Specifications

Quality specifications are required as necessary prerequisites for many facets of POCT (5). These specifications include

preparing procurement documents (generally including analytical performance requirements) for new POCT systems, assessing published work on the performance characteristics of POCT systems to assist objective selection, and evaluating procurement documents prepared by alternate suppliers (see Chapter 12). Moreover, quality specifications for acceptability (i.e., whether the performance achieved is acceptable) must be set before any data are generated in the POCT validation. Finally, quality specifications are vital to modern quality-planning models, to decide appropriate internal quality-control rules for the POCT, and to guarantee attainment of the specified analytical quality (8).

Setting Quality Specifications

Many publications are available to assist with the generation of quality specifications (2). However, some of these models are obsolete, and newer models continue to be published (9). In consequence, difficulties arise in deciding how to set numerical quality specifications for imprecision and bias. To investigate whether global agreement could be reached on strategies to set quality specifications in laboratory medicine, a consensus conference was held under the auspices of the International Union of Pure and Applied Chemistry, International Federation of Clinical Chemistry and Laboratory Medicine, and World Health Organization. An evidence-based model was published shortly before the conference (10), and in addition, a hierarchy of strategies to set quality specifications was published (11). The hierarchy of approaches is shown in Table 8-1.

Table 8-1 Hierarchy of Strategies to Set Quality Specifications

Level 1.	Assessment of the effect of analytical performance on specific clinical decision-making in specific clinical situations
Level 2.	Assessment of the effect of analytical performance on general clinical decision making
2A.	General quality specifications based on biological variation
2B.	General quality specifications based on medical opinions
Level 3.	Professional recommendations
3A.	Guidelines from national or international expert groups
3B.	Guidelines from expert individuals or institutional groups
Level 4.	Quality specifications laid down by regulation or by external quality assessment scheme (EQAS) organizers
4A.	Quality specifications laid down by regulation
4B.	Quality specifications laid down by EQAS organizers
Level 5.	Published data on the state of the art
5A.	Published data from EQAS and proficiency testing (PT) schemes
5B.	Publications on individual methodology

Level 1: Assessment of the Effect of Analytical Performance on Specific Clinical Decision Making in Specific Clinical Situations. At the top of the hierarchy is the ideal strategy for setting quality specifications. Ideally, test by test, the specifications will be derived by examining the effect of changing analytical quality on decision making per the specific clinical situation. The most commonly used methodology for this level of analysis has been discussed earlier in this chapter. As noted in the example of the cholesterol assay, if a POCT method had positive bias, individuals with ideal cholesterol concentrations could be classified as having an elevated concentration, with significant consequences (i.e., patient recalled for further tests, advised to change diet, and/or prescribed medication) In contrast, if the POCT method had negative bias, then an unusual cholesterol concentration could be missed, with a consequent lack of treatment and early disease for the patient. Both positive and negative bias lead to increased personal and health service cost. If a clinically acceptable misclassification rate can be defined, then it could be translated mathematically into a quality specification, in particular, for bias. Similar scenarios can be envisioned for glucose, glycated hemoglobin, microalbumin, and many other tests performed in POCT modalities (7). In this strategy, the crucial factor that allows clear definition of desirable analytical performance is deciding the acceptable clinical outcome. This, of course, is very difficult. In addition, few tests are used in single, well-defined clinical situations; another dilemma encountered in this strategy A recent study on quality specifications for glucose meters provides an excellent example of another approach to setting quality specifications with the use of mathematical modeling (12). The specifications were generated by an assessment of errors in insulin dose (i.e., delivery of the intended insulin dosage 95% of the time). This could be achieved when the bias and imprecision of the glucose meters was specified at <1% or <2% (depending on mean glucose concentrations and the rules for insulin dosing); as will be discussed later, these quality specifications are far more stringent than other strategies would give.

Level 2: Assessment of the Effect of Analytical Performance on General Clinical Decision Making. The second strategy for the development of quality specifications is based on general ways in which clinicians use test results.

The general approach (Level 2A) is to derive quality specifications from data on the components of biological variation, namely, within-subject (CV_i) and between-subject (CV_g) variation. In monitoring, RCV should be kept to a minimum, which will maximize the significance of any test result changes. As shown earlier, imprecision is important in this regard. Noise due to imprecision should be low enough to ensure that the biological signal is not confounded. For imprecision, the desirable general quality specification is that this should be less than half the mean within-subject biological variation; that is, $CV_a < 0.5CV_i$ (13). If this is achieved, then only a small amount of noise (~10%) is added to the signal. This approach has been widely accepted.

Population-based reference values are often used for the interpretation of laboratory test results. Because patients often have tests done in various locations and POCT is used as well as the central laboratory, the ideal is that all analytical methods providing test results for a single patient group should use reference values that do not have different levels of bias, for the reasons outlined earlier. To attain this ideal, bias should be less than one-quarter of the group biological variation (14), that is, $|B| < 0.25 [CV_i^2 + CV_g^2]^{1/2}$.

These well-established strategies have advantages in that data on components of biological variation are easy to obtain (3, 4), and the data seem independent of locale, methodology, and population. Moreover, quality specifications for imprecision, bias, and total allowable error (TE), calculated as TE = $|B| + 1.65CV_a$ (based on biological variation), are documented in these listings of data.

Second, general quality specifications (Level 2B) have been calculated from the responses of clinicians to a series of short theoretical case studies or vignettes on the general interpretation of test results. Essentially, the clinician defines change, and because the within-subject biological variation is known and the probability is usually assumed to be $P < 0.05$, use of a simple rearrangement of the aforementioned RCV formula allows CV_a to be calculated. Unfortunately, the majority of studies to date have significant deficiencies (15). In contrast, Thue et al. (16) and Skeie et al. (17) have used this approach to define quality specifications for hemoglobin and glucose meters, respectively. Their experimental work could be used as excellent models for further studies in this interesting, but rarely well done strategy.

Level 3: Professional Recommendations. Numerical quality specifications, particularly for imprecision, and less often for bias or total allowable error, have been proposed in many guidelines prepared by either national or international expert groups (Level 3A) or expert individuals or single institution groups (Level 3B). Of particular relevance to POCT are recommendations for self-monitoring of blood glucose and other associated analytes. Recently, the National Academy of Clinical Biochemistry (NACB) and the American Diabetes Association (ADA) have collaborated in providing a superb comprehensive set of guidelines and recommendations for the diagnosis and management of diabetes mellitus, many of which involve POCT (18). An interesting aspect of these guidelines is that the expert committee drafts were reviewed by an external panel of experts, then posted on the Internet to allow comments to be made by interested parties. Later, the material was presented at a major scientific meeting, the recommendations further modified, and finally, the guidelines underwent an internal review before publication. This approach minimizes the problems with generating quality specifications to date (e.g., guidelines are often empirical, conflicting quality specifications drawn up by different experts). This inclusive approach seems to be gaining favor, and the NACB, in particular, provides a model for others to emulate (19).

Level 4: Quality Specifications Laid Down by Regulation or by EQAS Organizers. Quality specifications have been laid down by regulation (Level 4A) in a number of countries. The best example is the U.S. Clinical Laboratory Improvement Amendments (CLIA) of 1988 (20), which document total allowable error for a number of commonly assayed analytes. Although widely used in quality management and planning models, these quality specifications are limited to the state of the art that was achievable at the time this legislation was prepared. Quality specifications are often laid down by EQAS organizers (Level 4B) to assist laboratorians in deciding whether their analyses meet acceptable performance standards. Although often based on expert opinion, these standards can be problematic, because they also tend to be subjective and are affected by the state of the art.

Level 5: Published Data on the State of the Art. Quality specifications could be derived from published data on the test performance achieved by laboratories in EQAS and PT (Level 5A). However, day-to-day analytical performance may not be accurately reflected by these estimates of the state of the art. Moreover, and most importantly, analytical performance in EQAS and PT reflects what can be achieved rather than what is desirable for good clinical decision making. Publications on individual methodology (Level 5B) usually give data on imprecision and comparative bias as well as information on other reliability and practicability performance characteristics. Since this type of work is usually done in an expert interested laboratory, the performance documented may well be the best possible rather than what could be attained by others in day-to-day practice. This is particularly relevant to POCT since many evaluations are performed only in laboratories with well-trained staff and are not undertaken by the staff members charged with both immediate patient care and the performance of the POCT procedure.

CHOOSING QUALITY SPECIFICATIONS— A CASE STUDY

The self-monitoring of blood glucose, which is probably the most widely used POCT, exemplifies well the real problems encountered in selecting quality specifications The NACB/ADA guidelines (18) document this dilemma in detail, and the material in this publication provides the basis for an excellent case study.

As mentioned in the guidelines, multiple quality specifications have been proposed for the performance of glucose meters. For potential users, adopting POCT technology is complicated by the conflicting specifications. Moreover, even if POCT users consulted the literature, the rationale for the competing proposals is not always clear.

Originally, the ADA recommended total error (user plus analytical) of <10% at glucose concentrations of 1.7 to 22.2 mmol/L (30–400 mg/dL), 100% of the time. In addition, values should differ by <15% from those obtained by a laboratory reference method (21). A recently revised specification from ADA proposed an analytical error of <5% (22). The

CLIA approach from the 1988 legislation says meters should be within 10% of target values or ±0.3 mmol/L (±6 mg/dL), whichever is larger (20). The National Committee for Clinical Laboratory Standards (NCCLS) recommendations vary with glucose concentration (i.e, ±20% of laboratory-generated glucose at >5.5 mmol/L (>100 mg/dL) and ± 0.83 mmol/L (±15 mg/dL) at ≤5.5 mmol/L (≤100 mg/dL) (23). These are undergoing revisions. Possible new NCCLS guidelines propose that for concentrations > 4.2 mmol/L (>75 mg/dL) the discrepancy between meter and the central laboratory results should be <20%, and for glucose concentrations ≤4.2 mmol/L (≤75 mg/dL) the discrepancy should not exceed 0.83 mmol/L (15 mg/dL). Using an approach similar to the use of vignettes, Skeie et al. (17), on the basis of patients' perceptions of their needs and of their reported actions in response to changes in measured glucose concentrations, recommended an analytical CV of 5%, with a bias ≤5%. As mentioned earlier, modeling of errors in insulin dose showed that to provide the intended insulin dosage 95% of the time, the bias and CV needed to be <1–2% (12). Finally, a quality specification for total allowable error (including both bias and imprecision) of 7.9% using biological variation criteria (2) is recommended, but with the caveat that additional studies are required.

Thus, for self-monitoring of blood glucose, quality specifications based on Levels 1 (12), 2A (18), 2B (17), 3A (22, 23), and 4A (20) strategies have been cited in recent guidelines (18). Moreover, at a number of these levels and at other levels of the hierarchy, including 3B, 4B, and 5A, recommendations for quality specifications for blood glucose have been published. Previous reviews have described these proposed numerical quality specifications (24, 25). Inspection and evaluation of these proposals clearly demonstrates the stated advantages and disadvantages of the strategies of the hierarchy. POCT users face a difficult decision in choosing which of the many published approaches to use. However, the hierarchy of models offers some clear guidance; the higher levels are preferred to the lower levels, but adoption of lower levels is preferred to none. The NACB/ADA guidelines advocated quality specifications based on biological variation. Previously, reviews on quality specifications (5, 26) have pointed out this quandary: In the many diverse locations that test results can be provided, why are different standards of analytical performance warranted? It seems widely accepted that quality specifications based on biological variation have so many advantages that these should be applied ubiquitously as the current, best-available, and general approach (27).

CONCLUSIONS

Analytical performance has many ramifications on clinical decision making, both in diagnosis and monitoring, irrespective of whether fixed numerical limits or population-based reference values are used as aids in interpretation of numerical test results. Imprecision affects the dispersion of the single test result and reference intervals, the number of samples needed to estimate homeostatic setting points, and the reference change value required to assess the significance of changes in results. Bias affects the location of the reference interval, causes more than the expected 5% to lie outside laboratory-defined reference limits, and affects clinical sensitivity and specificity. Quality specifications for imprecision, bias, and total allowable error are required for many purposes. Approaches to setting analytical quality specifications have been placed in a hierarchy, which offers up-to-date professional consensus. The hierarchy should be applied in practice. The approved models are appropriate for all situations in which test results are generated, including POCT; the models should be incorporated into quality management strategies everywhere. When in doubt, use of quality specifications based on biological variation is advocated, because they are widely supported by professionals everywhere, are directly related to the effect of analytical performance on clinical decision making, and are supported by readily available data.

Data from independent assessment of imprecision and bias should be readily available to all potential users of POCT devices, both patients and healthcare professionals. Guidelines and appropriate software should also be available for users to assess imprecision and bias; although quality appraisal is often best performed by professional staff (e.g., from a health technology assessment organization).

REFERENCES

1. Fraser CG, Hyltoft Petersen P. The importance of imprecision. Ann Clin Biochem 1991;28:207–11.
2. Fraser CG. Biological variation: from principles to practice. Washington, DC: AACC Press, 2001.
3. Ricos C, Alvarez V, Cava F, Garcia-Lario JV, Hernandez A, Jimenez CV, et al. Current databases on biologic variation: pros, cons and progress. Scand J Clin Lab Invest 1999;59:491–500.
4. Ricos C, Alvarez V, Cava F, Garcia-Lario JV, Hernandez A, Jimenez CV, et al. Biological variation database & desirable quality specifications. The 2001 update. http://www.westgard.com/guest21.htm (accessed October 2003).
5. Fraser CG. Optimum analytical performance for point of care testing. Clin Chim Acta 2001;307:37–43.
6. National Committee on Clinical Laboratory Standards. C28-A: How to define and determine reference intervals in the clinical laboratory; approved guideline, 2nd ed. Wayne, PA: NCCLS, 2000.
7. Hyltoft Petersen P, deVerdier CH, Groth T, Fraser CG, Blaabjerg O, Horder M. The influence of analytical bias on diagnostic misclassifications. Clin Chim Acta 1997;260:189–206.
8. Westgard JO. Basic QC practices. Madison, WI: Westgard QC, 1998.
9. Bonvicini P, Metus P, Pavón MA, Tocchini M. Requirements for reproducibility, trueness and error of measurement in internal quality control schemes. Clin Chem Lab Med 2003;41:693–9.
10. Fraser CG, Hyltoft Petersen P. Analytical performance characteristics should be judged against objective quality specifications. Clin Chem 1999;45:321–3.
11. Hyltoft Petersen P, Fraser CG, Kallner A, Kenny D, eds. Strategies to set global analytical quality specifications in laboratory medicine. Scand J Clin Lab Invest 1999;59:475–585.
12. Boyd JC, Bruns DE. Quality specifications for glucose meters: assessment by simulation modeling of errors in insulin dose. Clin Chem 2001;47:209–14.
13. Harris EK. Statistical principles underlying analytic goal-setting in clinical chemistry. Am J Clin Pathol 1979;374:72–82.
14. Gowans EMS, Hyltoft Petersen P, Blaabjerg O, Horder M. Analytical goals for the acceptance of common reference intervals for laboratories throughout a geographical area. Scand J Clin Lab Invest 1988;48:757–64.
15. Fraser CG. Judgment on analytical quality requirements from published vignette studies is flawed. Clin Chem Lab Med 1999; 37:167–8.
16. Thue G, Sandberg S, Fugelli P. Clinical assessment of haemoglobin values by general practitioners related to analytical and biological variation. Scand J Clin Lab Invest 1991;51:453–9.
17. Skeie S, Thue G, Sandberg S. Patient-derived quality specifications for instruments used in self-monitoring of blood glucose. Clin Chem 2001;47:67–73.
18. Sacks DB, Bruns DE, Goldstein DE, Maclaren NK, McDonald JM, Parrott M. Guidelines and recommendations for laboratory analysis in the diagnosis and management of diabetes mellitus. Clin Chem 2002;48:436–72.
19. National Academy of Clinical Biochemistry. http://www.nacb.org (accessed October 2003).
20. US Dept. of Health and Human Services. Medicare, Medicaid, and CLIA programs: regulations implementing the Clinical Laboratory Improvement Amendment of 1988 (CLIA). Final rule. Fed Reg 1992;57:7002–186.
21. American Diabetes Association. Consensus statement on self-monitoring of blood glucose. Diabetes Care 1987;10:93–9.
22. American Diabetes Association. Self-monitoring of blood glucose. Diabetes Care 1996;19(Suppl 1):S62–6.
23. National Committee for Clinical Laboratory Standards. Ancillary (bedside) blood glucose testing in acute and chronic care facilities; approved guideline C30-A. Wayne, PA: NCCLS, 1994.
24. Fraser CG. Analytical goals for glucose analyses. Ann Clin Biochem 1986;23:379–89.
25. Fraser CG. The necessity of achieving good laboratory performance. Diabet Med 1990;7:490–3.
26. Fraser CG, Hyltoft Petersen P. Desirable performance standards for imprecision in alternate sites. Arch Pathol Lab Med 1995;119: 909–13.
27. Fraser CG, Hyltoft Petersen P, Libeer JC, Ricos C. Proposals for setting generally applicable quality goals solely based on biology. Ann Clin Biochem 1997;34:8–12.

Part **Three**

Organization and Management

Chapter **9**

Whole-System Change, Pathology Services, and Point-of-Care Testing: A UK Policy Perspective

Sylvia Wyatt and Jeremy Wyatt

HOW IS HEALTHCARE CHANGING?

We live in a rapidly changing world. Many societies that industrialized in the 19th and early 20th centuries are now moving into a postindustrial phase. Service businesses and the knowledge economy far outweigh traditional manufacturing industries in their share of the gross domestic product and employment. A communications revolution is taking place with the convergence through information and communications technology of the Internet and digital TV. This is allowing the development of virtual communities of informed consumers. Increasingly, businesses in all sectors are responding to demands from customers for services to be available 24 h per day, 7 days per week.

As a result of these changes, the world of work is changing rapidly. Traditional hierarchies are breaking down. Demarcations are blurring, and the deference towards professionals once commonplace now seems a thing of the past. Those working in healthcare are part of this rapidly changing world but often find themselves trapped in institutionalized structures and job roles that hark back to an earlier age. The changes in healthcare delivery in the United Kingdom mean that more healthcare will be provided locally, more safely, and by fewer people and that patients' themselves will be taking more responsibility for their own care. A similar trend is seen elsewhere in the world.

Like many other countries, the United Kingdom has an aging population. This means that the burden of chronic diseases, in particular cardiovascular, respiratory, and neurological conditions, is set to increase even if advances in treatment lead to decreases in morbidity and mortality for these conditions. At the same time, developments in information and communications technology are supporting a paradigm shift in the way care can be delivered. Electronic patient records create the opportunity to provide more integrated care across organization and healthcare sectors. The application of information technology (IT) to healthcare presents the opportunity for considerable improvement in efficiency. In the United States, for example, physician order-entry systems in inpatient settings have been shown to reduce average length of stay by 12.5%, test expenses by 10.5%, and drug costs by 15.3% (1). At the

same time, new information technologies present challenges and difficulties for the healthcare team. New technologies create conditions in which information can more easily reside in the hands of the patient rather than those of the professional, altering the balance of power in their relationship.

In tandem with developments in IT, medical and technological advances are also significantly changing demand and service models. The miniaturization of medical and diagnostic equipment is likely to reduce the cost of some healthcare processes. It will also allow diagnosis and treatment much closer to the initial point of contact with patients or, indeed, even in their own homes. New pharmaceuticals based on our growing knowledge of genetics may reduce the requirement for inpatient care but increase the numbers of patients requiring long-term support for chronic conditions. Advances in surgery are likely to improve outcomes but also extend the range of eligible patients who may choose to opt for surgery.

This chapter examines how changes in the healthcare systems may affect pathology (laboratory medicine) services and how point-of-care testing (POCT) by patients outside hospital settings may become vital in modern healthcare provision.

WHERE ARE PATHOLOGY SERVICES NOW?

In the United Kingdom, diagnostic services, both pathology and imaging, are largely still concentrated in hospitals. Although there have been significant increases in the scope and the volume of the pathology tests provided, the way in which pathology services in hospitals are delivered has remained more or less the same. Pathology services are organized on a departmental basis and do not reflect patient pathways or help improve patient flow. There has been some development of onsite "hot labs" backed up by larger laboratories serving several acute care sites, but there has been little involvement of other provider (e.g., private sector) organizations. There have been some moves to get services (e.g., anticoagulant clinics) out of acute care hospitals.

In primary and community care, specimens are collected from general practitioner (GP) health centers and community clinics for analysis elsewhere, usually in hospital departments. Very little analysis is done in GP health centers because the equipment has been too expensive and quality control difficult. In addition, analysis is not easy to fit into the routine of the patient consultation. POCT is still unusual.

In contrast, home kits and monitoring are increasingly available to cover a range of tests, including pregnancy, diabetes, asthma, blood pressure, and cholesterol. This trend is likely to increase.

New Policy Directions

In the United Kingdom, there have been a number of recent policy initiatives that will affect the way in which pathology services are provided in the future. These include the following:

- Modernization of healthcare delivery—National Health Service (NHS) Plan (2)
- Decentralization of care—Keeping the NHS local (3)
- Choice of treatment at point of referral—choice, responsiveness, and equity (4)
- Development of expert patients, particularly those with chronic diseases (5)
- Investment into healthcare infrastructure and IT
- Changing the interface between industry and healthcare—Health Industries Task Force (6)

NHS Plan and Modernization. As part of the implementation of the NHS Plan, it has been recognized that improvements in pathology services are urgently needed in the NHS (2). Key to change is the development of clinical networks, which include pathology. For the first time, imaging and pathology are being considered together under the umbrella of a diagnostics strategy. The Department of Health (DOH) Access Directorate is working to support the modernization of diagnostic services across England for pathology, imaging, endoscopy, and physiological measurement. Common issues face these services, particularly workforce shortages and a lack of investment in equipment.

A new DOH policy, Modernizing Pathology Services, launched in February 2004, states that all managed pathology networks need to have a formal technology strategy in place, with a focus on getting maximum benefit from emerging technologies (7).

Keeping the NHS Local—A New Direction of Travel

In February 2003, the DOH published the first piece of acute care policy in nearly 10 years (3). This policy recognized the need to help health communities find solutions that command local support and fit with the modernization agenda, meeting technological, staffing and other challenges. There are three main themes that bring together policy reconfiguration and Working Time Directive change (8):

- Focusing on redesigning services rather than relocating them
- Taking a whole-system view
- Developing options for change *with* the public and patients, not for them

This has significant implications for pathology services in the future.

Choice, Responsiveness, and Equity

The national policy, *Choice, Responsiveness and Equity in Health and Social Care*, published in August 2003 (4) indicates that patients can expect to have wider and quicker access to services closer to home and in primary and community care settings, including pathology services. The full implications of this are still being worked out, but they will need to guide changes in the way in which pathology services develop.

Expert Patients

The development of e-health will empower patients to do more for themselves, safe in the knowledge that they are following best practice and becoming expert patients in the process (5). In June 2004, the Association of Clinical Biochemists launched a UK version (9) of the American Association for Clinical Chemistry's Lab Tests Online website (10), which will help the patient and the public understand the use of pathology investigations.

Investment in Health Infrastructure and IT

In the UK, there is currently unprecedented investment in new infrastructure (with >£10 billion being invested in infrastructure through Private Finance Initiative (PFI), Local Improvement Finance Trust (LIFT), and extra elective capacity in treatment centers over the next 10 years), supported by investment into process redesign through the NHS Modernisation Agency. An additional £2.3 billion is being invested in information technology, and more investment in a national procurement for diagnostic capacity outside acute care hospitals, to be implemented by 2006, will be announced in the summer of 2004.

Laboratory computing has often been at the leading edge of health information systems, but changes have often happened in isolation, leading to a patchwork of systems across the NHS. Improved information management, driven by the National Programme for IT (NPfIT) (11), will mean that laboratory matters can no longer be dealt with in isolation. There will be a need to address externally driven requirements such as integration across systems, integration of POCT, and clinical governance and service management. Pathology services will need to work closely with key stakeholders locally on the implementation of the NPfIT to ensure that new and more integrated ways of managing diagnostic and monitoring information are developed to meet the increasing needs of patients, clinicians, and pathologists.

Healthcare Industries Task Force

The establishment of the Healthcare Industries Task Force (HITF) (6) was announced on October 27, 2003. The task force brings together government and industry leaders to identify steps to develop and stimulate the growth and performance of the UK healthcare industry and maximize healthcare products' benefits to patients. The HITF is a year-long initiative jointly chaired by Lord Warner, undersecretary of state for health, and Sir Christopher O'Donnell, chief executive of Smith & Nephew. The task force is supported by four working groups bringing together experts on market access, research and development, regulation, and international export.

WHERE DO WE WANT PATHOLOGY SERVICES TO BE IN 5–10 YEARS?

Over the last 15 years, the horizons of pathology services have widened with the development of IT networks. This is illustrated in Figure 9-1, which also identifies how POCT has developed and will develop.

IT networks have expanded from internal laboratory-based systems, current until about 1990, through acute care provider intranet systems to a health economy internet that is becoming fully operational. The NPfIT and NHS Direct (12) are expanding this still further to provide each patient a safe and secure "Healthspace" portal for their clinical data on the World Wide Web. The following changes form the background against which pathology services need to develop to be fit for the future:

- Changing future capacity requirements and changing roles of professionals
- Patients taking more responsibility for their own health through e-health and chronic disease management

- Interconnected pathology information and clinical networks, and the changing location of services
- Technology integration with more emphasis on quality assurance and patient safety

Each of these will be discussed in turn next.

Changing Capacity Requirements and Changing Roles of Professionals

There is an acute shortage of trained specialists and technicians in most pathology services, in most parts of the UK; this picture is seen elsewhere in the world. NHS Trusts (health service provider organizations) are struggling to keep pace with the current levels of service, and it is very likely that the demand for tests will rise over the next 10 years. Any future plans based on more trained staff will almost inevitably fail as the available workforce dwindles.

The question is how much of a pathologist's role can safely and effectively be delegated. Assuming this can be quantified, workforce planners need to analyze how pathology professional and nonclinical roles can evolve, taking into account what can be computerized or automated, how much can be undertaken by patients and caregivers (using POCT and self monitoring), and how IT-facilitated clinical networks can help improve service quality by ensuring that the required skills and competencies are in the right place and available at the right time. This is illustrated by the four-tier role redesign model being adopted in imaging described in Figure 9-2 (13, 14).

This role redesign currently omits the role of the patient in providing care for themselves, which will increase capacity in the system significantly.

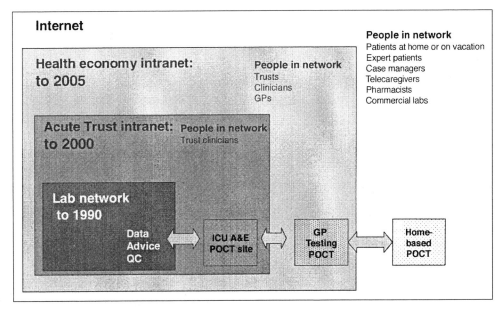

Figure 9-1 How pathology services horizons are changing.

The four levels represent escalating competencies and responsibilities within a multidisciplinary team and enable the team to review service requirements, determine who can do what, and identify the required skills and competencies. This model has been successfully developed and is now used in radiology.

The first (assistant practitioner) tier acts as a first rung on the ladder to a career in a health profession. The other tiers are designed to encourage clinical staff to delegate certain activities to others, while developing new and extended roles. The advanced and clinical tiers also reflect the requirements of clinical governance by contributing to the continuous improvement of the service.

- **Assistant practitioner.** Performs protocol-limited clinical tasks under the direction and supervision of a state-registered practitioner; undertakes less complex examinations or treatments under the supervision of state-registered colleagues.

- **Practitioner.** Autonomously performs a wide-ranging and complex clinical role; is accountable for his or her own actions and the actions of those directed; undertakes simple and complex imaging examinations or treatments on a full range of patient types and in a variety of settings. Works independently and may also supervise students and other clinical professionals.

- **Advanced practitioner.** Autonomous in clinical practice; defines the scope of practice of others and continuously develops clinical practice within a defined field; works in a specific area of expert clinical practice; is involved in delivering specialist care to patients. Also helps to develop other staff, leads teams, and contributes to service improvement.

- **Consultant practitioner.** Provides clinical leadership within a specialty; brings strategic direction, innovation, and influence within practice, research, and education; must have job descriptions developed as a response to service need, as outlined in "Meeting the Challenge: A Strategy for the Allied Health Professions" (14) and later guidance documents. Consultant posts are being developed or recruited at a number of development sites.

Figure 9-2 The four-tier role redesign model [UK Department of Health (13)].

Patients Doing More for Themselves Through e-Health

In the future, patients will want more information about themselves and better access to their health records. They will expect earlier certainty about their condition, giving them better prospects for successful treatment. Patients will be enabled to do this through the Internet, NHS Direct, Healthspace, and NHS Direct Online (12).

In addition, the range of products for self-testing and monitoring available without prescription is rapidly increasing. These products are rapidly becoming more sophisticated, with an intelligent IT-enabled user interface to allow patients to do more for themselves. Here are some examples of what may change:

- *Patients looking after themselves.* Expert patients will routinely use simple diagnostic devices themselves in the home without the help of caregivers or clinicians. This will include physiological monitoring of weight, lung function, blood pressure, and simple blood and urine testing through point-of-care self testing.
- *Care provided in the home.* Throughout the country, pilot projects in primary care trusts (PCTs; primary care provider organizations), led by the example of Kaiser Permanente and Evercare (15), are aiming to provide more care at home. Patients with complex co-morbidities are being looked after at home by case managers with the aim of preventing admissions to a hospital. This will require the use of POCT.
- *Intermediate tier centers for chronic disease management.* People want to be treated locally, and this will become possible through patient choice. They will want POCT to be used in local and intermediate-tier centers by clinicians, caregivers, and patients to support chronic disease management. Data interpretation by specialist acute care centers will need to be available 7 days per week and 24 h per day to support local-service development and avoid the need to admit people to hospitals unnecessarily.

Interconnected Pathology Information and Clinical Networks, and Changing Location of Services

Another major issue to be addressed in the next 5 years is how to interconnect information about individuals. Each health provider organization currently stores its own patient information in multiple systems. Clinical networks across hospitals, local care centers, and primary care will allow information to be moved around the system rather than patients having to move all the time.

It is crucial that pathology information be integrated into the overall network. The concept of Healthspace (12) will close the gap between where care is provided and where the results are generated, which will ensure that:

- Patients will receive test results more rapidly, wherever they are using Healthspace.
- Specialist pathology expertise, currently concentrated in a few centers, will be available more widely. IT connectivity will enable second opinions to be accessed rapidly, allowing time sharing and load sharing as well as access to the best experts anywhere in the world.
- Tests will only be performed once (rather than being repeated as the patient moves from the primary to the secondary and tertiary care sectors), and results will be available across the system, reducing duplication.
- Pathologists and clinical scientists will be much more involved in clinical decision making as they will be able to assess the test results in the context of the whole patient record.
- New kinds of data, e.g., results of home-based POCT, will be integrated and become part of a more complete clinical record and improved clinical decision.

The key to integrated chronic disease management may be for primary care clinicians to become managers of home-based disease monitoring services, using point-of-care and physiological monitoring systems.

Technology Integration, Quality Assurance, and Patient Safety

Over the last 10 years, there has been a move from internal laboratory-based quality-control systems to national, external quality assurance, training, and automated systems. There are, however, concerns from pathologists about assuring test and data quality in remote "uncontrolled" locations. These concerns may well be addressed by identifying the origin of the data. If a result has been generated by home POCT and seems not to fit the overall picture, there might be more reason to repeat it than if the result had come from a laboratory-based test.

Remote POCT will also depend on patients archiving the results of tests that they have undertaken themselves until POCT and monitoring provide automatic information integration mechanisms. The issue of POCT connectivity is discussed in greater detail in Chapter 20.

Increasingly, clinical standards and protocols will inform decision support systems, which will allow less highly trained staff and patients to take specimens and manage routine testing for both pathology and radiology to assure patient safety. This is already happening in many areas and will ensure a consistent approach.

Table 9-1   Examples of Old and New Planning Principles for Pathology

Old planning principle	New planning principle
All pathology is provided in acute care settings. Patients have to travel to acute trusts.	Information is moved rather than patients. Tests can be undertaken in a variety of settings—hospital, local care center, or home.
Tests are duplicated in different places.	Tests are done only once, and results are available across the system.
Separate diagnostic services for imaging and pathology are used.	*Routine* pathology and radiological services are integrated, with generic staff for taking routine specimens.
All results are checked by a pathologist	Interpretation of routine results is automated to help ensure that specialist expertise is used appropriately.
All tests must be requested by a clinician, usually a doctor.	Tests are nonclinician-based tests that patients can safely perform with minimum training, guided by protocol.
Laboratories provide analysis/interpretation.	Laboratories become information factories and libraries across the Internet.

SHOULD WE BE DOING THINGS DIFFERENTLY IN PATHOLOGY SERVICES?

To improve the way in which we are investing in infrastructure for the future, there needs to be some rethinking of the key principles in service redesign and environmental design to guide planners, designers, and project managers' investment decisions. Table 9-1 suggests a few ways in which future investment might be made into pathology.

There are many more design principles that underpin the planning of future pathology services. More work is needed to identify those that then need to be validated, disseminated, and incorporated into current guidance and investment.

REFERENCES

1. Tierney WM, Miller ME, Overhage JM, McDonald CJ. Physician order writing on microcomputer workstations. JAMA 1993;269: 379–83.
2. Department of Health. The NHS plan. London: Department of Health, 2000.
3. Department of Health. Keeping the NHS local: a new direction of travel. London: Department of Health, 2003.

4. Department of Health. Choice, responsiveness and equity. London: Department of Health, 2003.

5. Department of Health. Expert patients' programme. http://www.expertpatients.nhs.uk (accessed May 2004).

6. Department of Health. Healthcare Industries Task Force (HITF). http://www.advisorybodies.doh.gov.uk (accessed May 2004).

7. Department of Health. Pathology Modernisation Team. Modernising pathology services. http://www.dh.gov.uk/assetRoot/04/07/31/12/04073112.pdf (accessed May 2004).

8. Department of Health. European working time directive. http://www.dh.gov.uk/PolicyAndGuidance/HumanResourcesAndTraining/WorkingDifferently/EuropeanWorkingTimeDirective/fs/en (accessed May 2004).

9. The Association of Clinical Biochemists. LabtestsOnline. http://www.labtestsonline.org.uk (accessed May 2004).

10. American Association for Clinical Chemistry. Lab tests online. http://www.labtestsonline.org (accessed May 2004).

11. Department of Health. National IT programme. http://www.dh.gov.uk/PolicyAndGuidance/InformationTechnology/NationalITProgramme/fs/en (accessed May 2004).

12. NHS Direct, NHS Direct Online, and Healthspace. http://www.nhsdirect.nhs.uk (accessed May 2004).

13. Department of Health. A health service of all the talents: developing the NHS workforce. London: Department of Health, April 2000.

14. Department of Health. Radiography skills mix—a report on the four-tier service model. London: Department of Health, 2003.

15. Department of Health. NHS working with US healthcare provider to help cut hospital admissions. http://www.dh.gov.uk/PublicationsAndStatistics/PressReleases/PressReleasesNotices/fs/en?CONTENT_ID=4062742&chk=pBnb6/ (accessed May 2004).

Chapter 10

Research into Outcomes from Point-of-Care Testing

Christopher P. Price and Andrew St John

Since the development of point-of-care testing (POCT), one of the major controversies has been whether it can improve patient outcomes compared with testing performed in the central laboratory. In part, this debate has happened because the development of POCT coincided with the evidence-based medicine movement. Evidence-based medicine is now the standard of care and it is the responsibility of all those involved with patient care to ensure that the best evidence is used in the care of individual patients. Furthermore, the evidence has to be considered along with the benefits, risks, inconvenience, and costs of alternative strategies in clinical decision making (1–3). Evidence-based laboratory medicine (EBLM) is derived from the same principles, with evidence guiding decision making in all aspects of diagnostic medicine (4). This can include the following:

- Identifying the outcomes (and associated benefits) that can be achieved resulting from use of the diagnostic service.
- Producing guidelines on clinical practice.
- Determining the content of clinical protocols and care pathways.
- Establishing the quality specifications for the delivery of a diagnostic service.
- Determining the style of diagnostic service provided (e.g., offsite core laboratory, hospital central laboratory, laboratory network, satellite laboratory, point-of-care testing, self-testing).
- Providing a standard against which current practice can be audited.
- Informing a business case for investment in a particular diagnostic service and modality of delivery.
- Informing the education and training of healthcare professionals.

Adopting the principles of EBLM means that it should no longer be acceptable to adopt a new test or testing procedure without objectively assessing whether it will deliver clinical and/or economic benefits.

The main objective of POCT should be to achieve an improved health outcome through the timely delivery of the test result so it can be used in clinical decision making (1). Thus, to adopt an EBLM approach, POCT validation studies should be designed so they provide all the information that would be needed to decide whether to implement a POCT service.

THE CLINICAL QUESTION, DECISION, ACTION CASCADE

Prior to conducting research into the potential outcomes of POCT, it is important to understand the cascade of events in the diagnostic process from clinical question to outcome as shown in Figure 10-1. The cascade consists of the following:

- An explicit clinical question
- A decision being made upon receipt of the result
- An action taken such as a treatment or other intervention
- An outcome from the action or intervention

A diagnostic test may be used, primarily, to make one of four decisions: (*a*) rule in a diagnosis; (*b*) rule out a diagnosis; (*c*) monitor, and therefore, possibly change treatment; and (*d*) assess prognosis. A diagnosis means the support or rejection of an hypothesis (e.g., Did this patient with chest pain have a myocardial infarction?, or Does this pregnant woman have any evidence of a urinary tract infection?). Support for a diagnosis (rule in) might then lead to some form of action, whereas rejection (rule out) may lead to another diagnostic pathway and other hypotheses being pursued. Monitoring represents another type of diagnostic decision, which begins with ascertaining whether the treatment and the level of treatment (e.g., drug dose) have been adequate. If the answer to that question is negative, then the choice lies in increasing or decreasing the treatment level. A subset of the monitoring questions also relates more to the patient and his or her compliance with the established treatment protocol. Prognosis is an important issue for the clinician as it enables him or her to determine the course of action that might be taken in the particular circumstance for that patient.

The issue for POCT is whether a benefit will be gained from asking these questions, making the decisions, and taking action in a shorter time frame than will occur if the tests are performed in the central laboratory. Some examples of the question, decision, action cascade, and the potential outcomes from POCT are given in Table 10-1.

PATIENT

⇩ *test*

question ➔ decision ➔ action

⇩

OUTCOME

Figure 10-1   Cascade of events in the diagnostic process.

OUTCOMES FROM POINT-OF-CARE TESTING

Although the best quality of treatment for the patient is the goal of POCT, it is not always possible to measure the effectiveness of this modality of testing, in either an experimental or a real-life situation. Outcomes are typically seen in terms of benefit to the patient (clinical outcome), whereas there can also be a benefit in the delivery of care (operational outcome) as well as an economic benefit to the patient, healthcare provider, healthcare purchaser, and society (4, 5). As has been stated earlier in this book, the diagnostic performance of a test will invariably have been established, and thus the focus of any outcome study on POCT should address the impact of the alternative modality of testing.

Clinical Outcomes

The most objective measures of clinical outcome are morbidity and mortality indices. There are several problems with using these indices, and foremost, is the time that may be required to collect the relevant data. In addition, as has been pointed out by Rainey and others (1, 5–8) the mortality and morbidity endpoints depend on many more interventions after the provision of a test result. Indeed, the outcome is often seen solely in the context of the impact of the therapeutic intervention. It is therefore important to consider the use of surrogate outcome measures both in terms of attempting to study the unique impact of the test result and of finding an outcome measure that bears some relation to the objective indices of morbidity and mortality. The use of outcome measures should also be seen in the context of increasing the benefit to the patient while minimizing the risk. This introduces other features of the care pathway including ensuring compliance with therapy, reducing hospital stay (to minimize the risk of infection) and improving patient satisfaction. A number of surrogate clinical outcome measures are listed in Table 10-2. A quick appraisal of this list shows that several of the surrogate outcome measures are indices used in routine clinical practice, to monitor the effectiveness of the care pathway [e.g., hemoglobin A1c (HbA1c)].

Table 10-1   Clinical Question, Decision, Action, and Outcome Cascade Associated with POCT

Clinical question	Decision	Action	Outcome
Urinalysis in screening for early signs of renal disease	Refer to nephrologist	Monitor patient routinely and consider lifestyle change or use of ACE inhibitor	Reduce prevalence of end-stage renal disease
Urinalysis for detection of urinary tract infection	Rule out in low-prevalence patients; rule in in high-prevalence patients	Send urine to laboratory if positive, for confirmation; treat patient	More appropriate use of laboratory services and of antibiotics
Self monitoring of blood glucose	Alert to need for change in therapy if blood glucose outside defined limits	Maintain or change therapy regime depending on results	Better glycemic control, reduced rate of onset of complications
HbA1c result during clinic visit	Need for counseling of patient if level elevated	Review and change therapeutic regime and more patient education as appropriate	Better glycemic control, reduced rate of onset of complications, fewer clinic visits
Cardiac markers in emergency room	Direction of triage of patient with chest pain	Admit to coronary care unit, early intervention, monitoring, or discharge depending on result	Faster triage of patient, reduced length of stay in emergency room, fewer admissions to coronary care unit
Drug level in epilepsy clinic	Change of dose if subtherapeutic or toxic level found	Change drug level	Faster optimization of therapy, fewer clinic visits
First trimester Downs screening	Assessment of risk	Counseling of patient	Greater compliance with screening, higher rate of detection of affected fetus, greater patient satisfaction
Cholesterol result during clinic visit	Need for counseling if level not falling when statin given	Counseling of patient, checking with compliance	Improved compliance with therapy, more patients achieving treatment goal

Table 10-2   Examples of Surrogate Outcome Measures Used in Assessing Utility of POCT

Clinical outcome	Operational outcome	Economic outcome
Reduced HbA1c	Reduced operation time	Reduced blood product usage
Reduced cholesterol	Reduced clinic visits	Reduced drug usage
Reduced complication rate	Conversion to day-case surgery	Reduced length of stay
Reduced recurrence rate	Reduced length of stay	Reduced clinic visit
Improved mobility	Transfer of care to primary care sector	Lower cost per episode
Improved patient satisfaction	Rapid emergency room triage	Lower cost of staff and buildings

Operational Outcomes

Identification of changing practice that is associated with key outcome measures is the reason for specifically identifying operational outcomes. Thus operational changes should ultimately result in clinical and economic benefits. An example is reducing the time to treatment by the use of POCT, which is an operational benefit although it requires a change in the clinical process to deliver the benefit. There are many operational outcomes that may be achieved through the use of POCT, which include reduction in the length of stay, reduced clinic visits, transfer of care to the primary sector, and the use of diagnostic and treatment centers. These changes in practice may also bring improvements to the quality of care for both the patient and the caregiver, which are then translated into clinical benefits (e.g., greater compliance with a treatment protocol). Some surrogate operational outcome measures are listed in Table 10-2.

Economic Outcomes

It is important when considering an economic outcome to establish the perspective at the outset. This is important for a number of reasons, uppermost being the viewpoint of the evaluator and the potential for practical application of the information. Thus, one may view an economic benefit from the perspective of the payer of the test (e.g., individual, organization) at one extreme to the organization that pays for the care at the other end. This view extends from the rather narrow perspective of the cost of the test to the wider one of the societal benefit gained from the use of the test.

There are a number of ways of looking at the economics of diagnostic testing, from cost minimization to cost-benefit and from cost utility to cost effectiveness. Cost minimization is not worth any further consideration in relation to POCT as it focuses solely on the cost per test, which is quite inappropriate when one is trying to look at the benefits of different modalities of testing. All of the other approaches look at the costs against the benefits, which are expressed either in terms of money and natural units (i.e., life years, or a combination of quality and quantity of life gained) (9). As in the case of clinical outcomes, surrogate measures have an important place in economic analysis of the use of diagnostic tests, particularly in the case of POCT. Specifically, they enable an assessment to be made in relation to both the short- and long-term costs and benefits, with the shorter-term gains being most helpful at a local

decision-making level, whereas the longer-term gains will be of greater value in governmental health policy decision making. Some examples of surrogate economic outcome measures are given in Table 10-2.

QUALITY OF EVIDENCE AND STUDY DESIGN

It has already been pointed out in Chapter 1 that much of the early literature on POCT was concerned with the technical performance and the microeconomic considerations of cost per test (10, 11). Little of the early literature was concerned with the clinical impact of POCT, as reflected in the systematic review of POCT in primary care settings by Hobbs et al. (12), who found that although most of the papers did not meet basic quality criteria, few of the remaining papers addressed the clinical utility of POCT. However, in recent times studies of the clinical impact and benefits of POCT have started to emerge. In determining the quality of these published studies and in designing future ones, an understanding of how study design can affect the quality of the evidence is necessary.

There have been several papers that describe the quality of evidence for diagnostic tests, from the perspectives of the information that should be included in a study report as well as the design of the study itself (13–18). Thus, Reid et al. (13), in a review of all of the papers reporting on studies of diagnostic tests over a 15-year period in several major journals, found that there was poor reporting of key information in the majority of studies.

It is now accepted that the best study design to evaluate the effectiveness of an intervention is a randomized controlled trial (RCT), because this minimizes the bias and the effect of confounding variables (18–20). The randomized design is analogous to the trial of a therapeutic intervention, and in the case of POCT would involve randomization of patients to the usual testing approach (e.g., central laboratory) or POCT (18). Ideally, the trial should not only examine the testing process but also the steps afterwards, namely, the decisions and outcomes that follow. Comparing the POCT modality of testing against the central laboratory approach was used by Cagliero et al. (21) to assess the value of POCT for HbA1c in a diabetes clinic. They studied the effect of an immediate test result on counseling of the patient compared with the patient receiving the laboratory test result after leaving the clinic. This study was essentially a randomized trial of an algorithm, or protocol of care.

The RCT also enables the assessment of the impact of the test result on decision making, compared with a retrospective analysis of test result data. However, there are many problems associated with the use of an RCT, primarily because the result is only one part of a decision-making process that requires understanding and action on receipt of the result. The "understanding" may include education and ongoing counseling of the patient, which will be particularly relevant to the use of POCT in the context of chronic disease management (e.g., diabetes, anticoagulation therapy).

These problems associated with the RCT are exemplified by the metaanalysis of self-monitoring of blood glucose undertaken by Coster et al. (22), who found little evidence that frequent blood glucose testing led to improved clinical outcomes as shown by a reduction in HbA1c. However, the authors pointed out that the use of an RCT design (a key inclusion criteria for the metaanalysis) ignored the fact that glucose testing was only one part of an integrated-care package, which included patient education as a key component. The RCT design did not focus on the practice that it was seeking to investigate, and therefore, there was no assurance that the results had been interpreted correctly.

There are also difficulties with controlling other confounders of the POCT process (e.g., result is not accessed, result is not used, local clinical practice has not adjusted to the rapid receipt of the result). In the first example, although not specifically POCT, Kilpatrick and Holding (23) found that over 40% of results electronically transmitted to the emergency room were never accessed. An example of the second situation is described by Kendall et al. (24), who conducted a randomized controlled trial of POCT in the emergency room. They found no reduction in the length of stay, despite a significant reduction in the time taken to deliver the result. The authors concluded that the results may not have been accessed by staff as soon as they became available, because a change in practice had not been adopted. Nichols et al. (25) had a similar experience using POCT in an interventional radiology unit, reporting that improved outcomes were only delivered when changes in practice were instituted.

There are few RCTs of diagnostic tests, and fewer of POCTs; therefore, other study designs have been used. Lijmer and others (17, 26, 27) have reviewed studies on diagnostic tests, including outcomes studies, and found that some forms of study design could lead to significant bias in the results and to a poor quality of evidence for potential clinical and policy decision making. The most common form of bias comes from case-controlled study designs using a study population that is not representative of the clinical settings where the test will be used. Thus, the performance of a test will be compared in patients known to have the disease to those known to be free of disease. In reality, the test will be used in patients with unclear or borderline conditions; in this situation, the performance of the test will be different and inferior compared to the ideal test assessment conditions. Thus, test performance measures such

as the likelihood ratio will depend on the choice of patients being studied; consequently, this form of bias is sometimes called selection or spectrum bias. Sackett and Haynes (28) described this form of bias in relation to b-type natriuretic peptide tests and stated the importance of assessing any test in a cohort of truly consecutive patients.

Although the use of case-controlled studies and spectrum bias are the commonest problems with many diagnostic studies, there are additional examples of bias that must be considered in relation to study design (29). The use of a poor reference test or "gold standard" for comparison to the test or protocol under investigation will lead to underestimation of test accuracy, depending on the prevalence of the target condition being investigated (30). Review bias occurs when interpretation of the test results are affected by knowledge of the reference test or vice versa. This type of bias may be significant if the test method assessment is subjective, such as the visual reading of urinary dipsticks (31). There are several types of verification bias; however, all involve not applying the same reference test or protocol to all the subjects who undergo the index test or protocol (26, 32).

For studies of diagnostic accuracy, Bossuyt (33) has described randomized (described previously), paired, and before-and-after study design. The paired design involves undertaking both tests in the same patient, which can reduce one form of variability. However, it is not possible to use this design in an outcomes study, where the result is acted upon and the outcome is influenced by the test result. A special form of the paired design is the before-and-after study (34). In this approach, the outcome indices are collected initially for the routine approach to care, then, after a period of training, the study period begins with the adoption of the POCT strategy. This is the approach that has been used for a number of studies of POCT in the primary care setting. In the case of the study by Rink et al. (35), the before-and-after phase was then followed by another "before" period.

An alternative approach that has been used is that of an observational study. However, this type of study is regarded as providing evidence of inferior quality, because other factors besides the test result can affect the outcome. Furthermore, it is difficult to determine causality of any achieved outcome in an observational study. Although this is understandable, an observational study can provide a more holistic picture of the routine clinical process. The metaanalysis by Coster et al. (22) suggested that there was no evidence to support the use of frequent self-monitoring of blood glucose, whereas observational studies conducted by Karter et al. (36) and Schiel et al. (37), which involved large populations of diabetics, found that those who tested themselves more frequently had lower HbA1c results. However, these studies did not show that frequent testing was the unique feature that led to reduced HbA1c, only that a pattern of care, which included more frequent testing, led to a lower HbA1c. Furthermore, all of the patients were cared for in the same health program.

The use of an observational design makes it possible to study larger populations. However, there is a greater risk of encountering differences in the populations or the style of care, which could influence the final outcome data. Grieve et al. (38) studied two models of diabetes care within a similar locality. In one model, the HbA1c result was available at the time of the clinic visit (POCT provision), and in the other, the result was not available (central laboratory provision). The HbA1c results in the POCT cohort were lower, which suggested but did not prove that the POCT mode of delivery resulted in better outcomes for the patient.

Several key points emerge from this brief consideration of the impact of study design. First, the construction of a good study protocol is dependent on a careful consideration of the diagnostic decision and action cascade described at the beginning of this chapter. This consideration should involve the following:

- An explicit recognition of the patient group and the setting in which the patients will be studied
- A clear statement of the clinical question
- A clear understanding of the decision that would be made upon receipt of the test result
- An identification of the action(s) that would be taken upon the decision being made
- An identification of an expected outcome from the action being taken
- An understanding of any confounding factors that might lead to the interruption of the clinical question to outcome cascade

High-quality diagnostic studies have a number of key features, as shown in the checklist described in Table 10-3. Unfortu-

Table 10-3 Short Checklist of Features That Should Be Found in an Outcomes Study Associated with POCT

Clear statement of research question; namely, specific use of POCT

Identification of study population, including inclusion and exclusion criteria

Number of patients studied

Identification of characteristics of patients recruited (e.g., symptoms, severity of disease)

Identification of how patients were recruited (e.g., consecutive prospective)

Identification of trial design

Identification of decision made and action taken upon receipt of result

Identification of outcome measure used

Description of all methods used and their performance characteristics

Identification of whether operators were blinded to outcome measure

Documentation of results

Description of statistical methods used

Indication that attempts were made to ensure change of practice where required to deliver improved outcome

Documentation of confounding factors noted during study

Discussion of data and applicability of results

nately, few published studies contain all these essential features for ensuring high-quality evidence. The features shown in Table 10-3 can provide a template for designing a manageable and meaningful outcome study, in accord with the proposals of Rainey (6). These include the following:

- Use a prospective study, ideally with a randomized or crossover design.
- Minimize sources of variability (i.e., limit the study to a single service, diagnosis or procedure).
- Ensure that there are consistent interventions in response to test results.
- Choose outcome measures that can be quantified.
- Use outcome variables that are determined in close temporal proximity to the testing process.
- Use outcome measures that are good surrogates for long-term outcome measures (e.g., HbA1c).
- Use outcome measures that have intrinsic financial value (e.g., blood product usage).
- Identify local factors that might affect the results and therefore limit the application of the data.

The key objectives are to minimize the bias in the results reported and also to provide an explicit statement on the applicability of the data. The study has to be robust and reflect the clinical setting where the results might be applied.

ANALYSIS AND REVIEW OF DATA

The statistical analysis of data is beyond the scope of this chapter, and there are several good texts available on this subject Many of the data on diagnostic testing have been obtained from true and false, positive and negative observations (e.g., 2×2 tables), which have led to the generation of data on sensitivity and specificity and the construction of receiver–operator curves. However, as pointed out by Deeks (39), the receiver–operator curve is not easy to interpret in a routine clinical situation. In this context the use of the likelihood ratio is more meaningful, especially when linked to the use of the Fagan nomogram. The nomogram links the pretest and posttest probability to the observed likelihood ratio (40). At a glance, the clinician is able to identify whether a test result is helpful in ruling in or ruling out a particular course of action and to see how a particular result is associated with disease improvement and disease state.

When a number of studies are available on a particular subject, it is possible to perform a metaanalysis of the data (41). This has the benefit of enabling some assessment of the variability of the data between different studies as well as increasing the confidence in the data, especially when the variability (or heterogeneity) of the data is low. The construction of a Forest plot is a good visual means of assessing the variability as well as the overall quality of the data (42). Pooling of data can also indicate when the addition of further data is unlikely to improve its quality and when no further studies need to be undertaken.

Once the study is completed, it is important that the data are reported correctly. There are guidelines that provide a check on the quality of the reported data and provide continuity with the original objectives, design, and conduct of the study (43, 44).

IMPLEMENTING CHANGE

The crux of POCT is change in practice with the goal of improvement in outcomes. Thus, change in practice needs to be linked to implementation of POCT. In their study, Nichols et al. (25) stressed the importance of changing clinical practice to ensure delivery of outcomes. If POCT is considered as one part of a change in clinical management, then the effect of this new strategy on outcomes can be evaluated. Although this approach does not appear to specifically address the unique contribution played by the POCT element, it is more likely to lead to the identification of a clear benefit through a more robust study. There are difficulties in taking this approach as has been seen in the discussion on the self-monitoring of blood glucose. The Diabetes, Control, and Complications Trial (45) investigated the benefits of strict control of glycemia, using blood glucose testing as an element; however, the frequency of testing was not specifically addressed. Similarly, the optimal frequency of HbA1c measurement has not been studied, although the variation in practice indicates that this issue requires resolution. This is where observational studies and the use of audit to generate additional evidence may become of increasing value.

CONCLUSIONS

The use of POCT is associated with a style of clinical practice that demands the rapid delivery of the test result. The result should prompt a decision and action that will be implemented immediately. It is this speed of response that should deliver improved outcomes for the patient, caregiver, healthcare provider organization, and society. The study of outcomes from POCT should take into account the setting where the test is going to be used as well as the intervention that might be implemented upon receipt of the result. Table 10-3 provides a checklist that could be used for the design and implementation of the study as well as reporting of the results (43, 44). This checklist will also enable the reader to ascertain whether the study results are applicable to the clinical situation in which the reader is seeking to apply the results.

REFERENCES

1. Price CP. Point-of-care testing. BMJ 2001;322:1285–8.
2. Sackett DL, Haynes RB, Guyatt GH, Tugwell P. Clinical epidemiology; a basic science for clinical medicine, 2nd ed. Toronto: Little, Brown, 1991:1–441.
3. Guyatt G, Haynes B, Jaeschke R, Cook D, Greenhalgh T, Meade M, et al. Introduction: the philosophy of evidence-based medicine. In: Guyatt G, Rennie D, eds. User's guide to the medical literature. A manual for evidence-based clinical practice. Chicago: JAMA and Archive Journals, American Medical Association, 2002:3–12
4. Muir Gray JA. Evidence-based healthcare. How to make health policy and management decisions. Edinburgh: Churchill Livingstone, 1997:1–270.
5. Price CP. Evidence-based laboratory medicine: supporting decision-making. Clin Chem 2000;46:1041–50.
6. Rainey PM. Outcomes assessment for point-of-care testing. Clin Chem 1998;44:1595–6.
7. Price CP. Point of care testing. Potential for tracking disease management outcomes. Dis Manage Health Outcomes 2002;10:749–61.
8. St John A, Price CP. Measures of outcome. In: Price CP and Christenson RH, eds Evidence-based laboratory medicine: from principles to outcomes. Washington DC: AACC Press, 2003:55–74
9. Marshall DA, O'Brien BJ. Economic evaluation of diagnostic tests. In: Price CP, Christenson RH, eds. Evidence-based laboratory medicine: from principles to outcomes. Washington, DC: AACC Press, 2003:159–86.
10. O'Leary D. Global view of how alternate site testing fits in with medical care. Arch Pathol Lab Med 1995;119:877–80.
11. Roberts RR, Zalenski RJ, Mensah EK, Rydman RJ, Ciavarella G, Gussow L, et al. Costs of an emergency department-based accelerated diagnostic protocol vs hospitalization in patients with chest pain: a randomized controlled trial. JAMA 1997;278:1670–6.
12. Hobbs FD, Delaney BC, Fitzmaurice DA, Wilson S, Hyde CJ, Thorpe GH, et al. A review of near patient testing in primary care. Health Technol Assess 1997;1(5):1–230.
13. Reid MC, Lachs MS, Feinstein AR. Use of methodological standards in diagnostic test research. Getting better but still not good. JAMA 1995;274:645–51.
14. Mulrow CD, Linn WD, Gaul MK, Pugh JA. Assessing quality of a diagnostic test evaluation. J Gen Intern Med 1989;4:288–95.
15. Jaeschke R, Guyatt G, Sackett DL. Users' guides to the medical literature. III. How to use an article about a diagnostic test A. Are the results of the study valid? Evidence-Based Medicine Working Group. JAMA 1994;271:389–91.
16. Jaeschke R, Guyatt GH, Sackett DL. Users' guides to the medical literature. III. How to use an article about a diagnostic test B. What are the results and will they help me in caring for my patients? Evidence-Based Medicine Working Group. JAMA 1994;271:703–7.
17. Lijmer JG, Mol BW, Heisterkamp S, Bonsel GJ, Prins MH, van der Meulen JH, et al. Empirical evidence of design-related bias in studies of diagnostic tests. JAMA 1999;282:1061–6.
18. Bossuyt PM, Lijmer JG, Mol BW. Randomised comparisons of medical tests: sometimes invalid, not always efficient. Lancet 2000;356:1844–7.
19. Moher D, Schulz KF, Altman DG, for the CONSORT group. The CONSORT statement: revised recommendations for improving the quality of reports of parallel group randomized trials. JAMA 2001;285:1987–91.
20. Bruns DE, Huth EJ, Magid E, Young DS. Toward a checklist for reporting of studies of diagnostic accuracy of medical tests. Clin Chem 2000;46:893–5.
21. Cagliero E, Levina E, Nathan D. Immediate feedback of HbA1c levels improves glycemic control in type 1 and insulin-treated type 2 diabetic patients. Diabetes Care 1999;22:1785–9.
22. Coster S, Gulliford MC, Seed PT, Powrie JK, Swaminathan R. Monitoring blood glucose in diabetes mellitus: a systematic review. Health Tech Assess 2000;4:1–93.

23. Kilpatrick ES, Holding S. Use of computer terminals on wards to access emergency test results; a retrospective audit. BMJ 2001; 322:1101–3.

24. Kendall J, Reeves B, Clancy M. Point of care testing: randomised, controlled trial of clinical outcome. BMJ 1998;316:1052–7.

25. Nichols JH, Kickler TS, Dyer KL, Humbertson SK, Cooper PC, Maughan WL, et al. Clinical outcomes of point-of-care testing in the interventional radiology and invasive cardiology setting. Clin Chem 2000;46:543–50.

26. Begg CB. Biases in the assessment of diagnostic tests. Stat Med 1987;6:411–23.

27. Mower WR. Evaluating bias and variability in diagnostic test reports. Ann Emerg Med 1999;33:85–91.

28. Sackett DL, Haynes RB. The architecture of diagnostic research. BMJ 2002;324:539–41.

29. Horvath AR, Pewsner D, Egger M. Systematic Reviews in Laboratory Medicine. In: Price CP and Christenson RH, eds. Evidence-based laboratory medicine: from principles to outcomes. Washington, DC: AACC Press, 2003:137–58

30. Irwig L. Bossuyt P, Glasziou P, Gatsonis C, Lijmer J. Designing studies to ensure that estimates of test accuracy are transferable. BMJ 2002;324:669–71.

31. Moons KG, Grobbee DE. When should we remain blind and when should our eyes remain open in diagnostic studies? J Clin Epidemiol 2002;55:633–6.

32. Knottnerus JA. The effects of disease verification and referral on the relationship between symptoms and disease. Med Dec Making 1987;7:139–48.

33. Bossuyt PM. Study design and quality of evidence. In: Price CP, Christenson RH, eds. Evidence-based laboratory medicine: from principles to outcomes. Washington, DC: AACC Press, 2003:75–92.

34. Knottnerus J, Dinant G-J, van Schayk O. The diagnostic before-after study to assess clinical impact. In: Knottnerus J, ed. The evidence base of clinical diagnosis. London: BMJ Books, 2002.

35. Rink E, Hilton S, Szczepura A, Fletcher J, Sibbald B, Davies C, et al. Impact of introducing near patient testing for standard investigations in general practice. BMJ 1993;307:775–8.

36. Karter AJ, Ackerson LM, Darbinian JA, D'Agostino RB, Ferrara A, Liu J, et al. Self-monitoring of blood glucose levels and glycemic control: the Northern California Kaiser Permanente Diabetes Registry. Am J Med 2001;111:1–9.

37. Schiel R, Muller UA, Rauchfub J, Sprott H, Muller R. Blood-glucose self-monitoring in insulin treated Type 2 diabetes mellitus: a cross sectional study with an intervention group. Diabet Metab 1999;25:334–40.

38. Grieve R, Beech R, Vincent J, Mazurkiewicz J. Near patient testing in diabetes clinics: appraising the costs and outcomes. Health Technol Ass 1999;3:1–74.

39. Deeks JJ. Systematic reviews in health care: Systematic reviews of evaluations of diagnostic and screening tests. BMJ 2001;323:157–62.

40. Fagan TJ. Nomogram for Bayes theorem. NEJM 1975;293:133–4.

41. Irwig L, Macaskill P, Glasziou P, Fahey M. Meta-analytic methods for diagnostic test accuracy. J Clin Epidemiol 1995;48:119–30.

42. Boyd JC, Deeks JJ. Analysis and presentation of data. In: Price CP, Christenson RH, eds. Evidence-based laboratory medicine: from principles to outcomes. Washington, DC: AACC Press, 2003:115–36.

43. Bossuyt PM, Reitsma JB, Bruns DE, Gatsonis CA, Glasziou PP, Irwig LM, et al. Towards complete and accurate reporting of studies of diagnostic accuracy: the STARD initiative. Standards for reporting of diagnostic accuracy. Clin Chem 2003;49:1–6.

44. Bossuyt PM, Reitsma JB, Bruns DE, Gatsonis CA, Glasziou PP, Irwig LM, et al. The STARD statement for reporting studies of diagnostic accuracy: explanation and elaboration. Clin Chem 2003;49:7–18.

45. The Diabetes Control and Complications Trial Research Group. The effect of intensive treatment of diabetes on the development and progression of long-term complications in insulin-dependent diabetes mellitus. N Engl J Med 1993;329:977–86.

Chapter **11**

Training and Certification for Point-of-Care Testing

John F. Wood and David Burnett

Fifteen years ago a task force of the Scientific Committee of the Association of Clinical Biochemists in the United Kingdom published a review titled "Essential Considerations in the Provision of Near-Patient Testing Facilities" (1). This review acknowledged the growth in the numbers of tests being performed away from the central laboratory by nonlaboratory personnel and expressed concerns that the apparent simplicity of testing systems disguised their underlying complexity. It also stated that only properly trained staff should use the equipment, but anticipated difficulties caused by not only the large numbers of potential users but also by the frequent change of staff in the lifetime of the equipment. A statement by the Board of Governors of the College of American Pathologists (2) adopted a clear position in relation to point-of-care testing (POCT):

> Quality of patient care is the highest priority. Alternative-site testing must not introduce or augment clinically significant errors in the testing process. . . . Alternative-site testing requires adherence to the standards of good laboratory practice, including quality control, quality assurance, proficiency testing, and recording of results in the patient's medical record.

The need for POCT may develop because the laboratory gives a poor service, particularly with respect to turnaround times. Laboratory staff regard turnaround time (TAT) as the time interval between receipt of the specimen and the reporting of the result. The clinician regards the TAT as beginning when the need for the test is perceived and finishing when the result is received and interpreted (3). The requirement to minimize this "vein-to-brain" time for certain tests (4), together with significant improvements in POCT systems, (5) have led to an increase in the demand for POCT. Clinicians' attitudes to POCT are variable; they have demonstrated a need for rapid response testing, but many have held a preference for rapid specimen transport and central laboratory testing (6) or satellite laboratories providing a fast TAT service to specific areas (7). Within intensive care units patients are frequently ventilated and it is accepted that measurements of blood gases, electrolytes, and metabolites are performed by clinical staff using POCT systems (8). In other critical care areas such as emergency departments there is an increasing need for rapidity of results driven by clinical need for rapid diagnosis (9, 10).

Additional factors can influence the introduction of POCT, such as reduction in patient waiting times and admission rates (11, 12). For example, one of the UK government's targets for its National Health Service states that no patient should wait no more than 4 h in emergency departments from arrival to admission, transfer, or discharge (13). Along with increased usage of POCT in clinical areas, there has also been a rapid increase in the availability of home testing POCT devices. It is now commonplace for diabetic patients to monitor their own blood glucose levels, and with an ever-aging population it may be expected that there will be an increase in demand for these systems (14). These demands have led to a rapid increase in the global market for POCT, with worldwide costs increasing from $3 billion in 1997 to $5.4 billion in 2001 (15), and this is expected to double over the next decade (16).

QUALITY IN POCT

An extremely thoughtful paper on guidelines for POCT (17) presents them in terms of 15 objectives to be achieved in order to optimize the value of POCT and includes associated recommendations. Since then numerous professional organizations and learned bodies have contributed recommendations toward the POCT debate. Among these have been:

1997–1998   European Community Confederation of Clinical Chemistry (EC4) Working Group on Harmonisation of Quality Systems and Accreditation through a paper titled "Essential Criteria for Quality Systems in Medical Laboratories" (18). This was followed by a supplementary article, "Additional Essential Criteria for Quality Systems of Medical Laboratories" (19), making specific reference to POCT.

1999   The German Working Group on Medical Laboratory Testing (AML) (20).

2000   The Joint Working Group on Quality Assurance (JWGQA) and advisory committee to the UK's National External Quality Assurance Scheme (NEQAS) published guidance (21).

2002   The UK Medicines and Healthcare Products Reg-
            ulatory Agency (MHRA), formerly the Medi-
            cal Devices Agency, following a number of
            critical incidents, made recommendations re-
            garding the selection of equipment and use of
            POCT (22).

The UK government's white paper, "A First Class Service" (23) introduced the concept of clinical governance within
the NHS. Scally and Donaldson set out how clinical governance may be used as a framework on which quality improvement would be promoted and managed:

> Clinical governance is a system through which NHS organizations
> are accountable for continuously improving the quality of their
> services and safeguarding high standards of care by creating an
> environment in which excellence in clinical care will flourish. (24)

They identified areas in which clinical governance could be
used to establish a philosophy of quality improvement. These
included:

- Risk avoidance by developing well-trained staff who con-
  form to clear operating procedures
- Identification and elimination of poor performance by self-
  regulation, early detection, and decisive intervention
- Introduction of quality methods through evidence-based
  medicine and the spread of good practice
- Development of a culture of patient partnership and teamwork
- Improvements in infrastructure through increased learning
  and evidence resource
- Organizational coherence communication, partnership, and
  alignment of goals

Accrediting bodies have also provided standards:

- The College of American Pathologists (CAP) has produced
  a POCT checklist (25) based on the CLIA '88 standard.
- Within the United Kingdom, Clinical Pathology Accreditation
  (CPA) has defined "Standards for the Medical Laboratory"
  (26). These standards make no specific reference to POCT but
  there is an expectation that any laboratory-controlled POCT
  conforms to the general laboratory standards.

Facilities outside a hospital, such as primary care centers
and general practitioners' offices, are required in some countries to seek advice from the local hospital laboratory before
embarking on POCT. For example, in the United Kingdom,
Standard 13 of the Primary Health Care Standards and Criteria
of the King's Fund Organisational Audit Programme states:
"Near patient testing conforms to protocols developed with an
accredited pathology department" (27).

All of the preceding recommendations underline the importance of protecting the patient, the organization, and its staff
from errors caused by inappropriate use of POCT. The key
points of these recommendations and standards relate to issues

surrounding training, education, and certification of nonlaboratory POCT users and constitutes the rest of this chapter.

ORGANIZATION AND MANAGEMENT OF POCT

The overall responsibility for the provision should be with the
appropriate laboratory specialist from an accredited laboratory
(19). An essential prerequisite for a good POCT training program is the formation of a high-level multidisciplinary working
group. The title "working group" is chosen to emphasize that
people who are members of the group will have specific
responsibilities. The guidelines mentioned previously (19)
state that "There should be an interdisciplinary group on POCT
established to organize and manage the different aspects of the
service." The group should normally be chaired by a senior
member of the pathology laboratory and its membership should
consist of expert advisors such as intensive care staff, diabetic
nurses, nurse educators, pharmacists, and information technology professionals. Appropriate laboratory staff, together with
those with operational responsibility such as the POCT coor-
dinator(s) and area supervisors, should be identified. The College of American Pathologists Inspection Checklist for Point-
of-Care Testing (25) requires that "POCT programs MUST be
under the direction, authority, jurisdiction and responsibility of
the Director of Laboratories before the Commission on Laboratory Accreditation will consider inspection/accreditation."
The mandate of this group should be described in a management procedure, a suggested content of which is shown in
Figure 11-1 (28). Section 4 indicates that it is the responsibility
of this group to organize and oversee the training for POCT.

The group should be responsible for drawing up an organization-wide policy for the use of POCT. This policy should be a
statement of intent, defining the basic principles of how POCT is
carried out within the organization. Procedures should be written
and approved by the group and act as a mechanism for controlling
how the POCT policy is implemented. Procedures should exist for
all aspects of POCT including the specimen collection, the testing
operation, and reporting/recording of results. There should also be
detailed procedures relating to training of users together with
mechanisms for recording that an appropriate level of competence
has been attained.

LABORATORY SUPPORT FOR POCT

Laboratory staff will provide expert help and advice in many
areas, ranging from selection and siting of equipment to training,
quality control, and audit of device usage. Ideally, a service level
agreement should be in effect between the clinical area and the
laboratory that defines levels of support. Before deciding on the
use of POCT it is important to understand the users' needs and
expectations of the laboratory service. If a central laboratory is
failing to meet the users' needs, then problems must be investigated and where possible rectified. POCT should be targeted only
at patients and areas where it will prove effective and there should
be evidence of its efficacy. Tests should be targeted into clusters

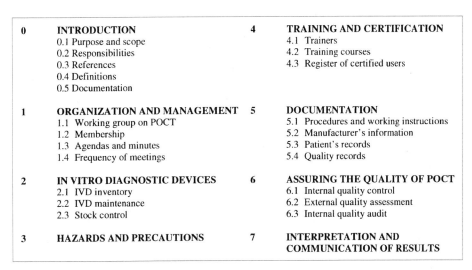

Figure 11-1 Content of a management procedure for POCT.

that are useful to the particular clinical need (29). There are many suppliers of POCT equipment and the quality of results may vary considerably. It is important that a full laboratory-based technical validation is carried out, taking into account robustness, accuracy and precision of results, potential interference from other substances, and concordance with existing laboratory methods in terms of correlation and reporting units. It is also important that POCT devices are evaluated by those staff who will be using them, within the proposed clinical area. Sometimes equipment may appear to be simple to use and robust in the hands of experienced laboratory staff yet create significant problems for nonlaboratory staff within the clinical environment. Where POCT is providing diagnostic data in the form of "rule-in" or "rule-out" tests, a full clinical evaluation of diagnostic sensitivity and specificity should be carried out comparing POCT with the accepted standard, usually the existing laboratory method. It is clear that if quality is to be promoted and maintained and the risk of erroneous results minimized, users of POCT devices must be appropriately trained to a high standard providing them with the requisite knowledge and practical expertise.

How Should Training Be Managed?

Before describing the process of training and certification for POCT it is useful to examine briefly the meaning of the words *training* and *certification*. In common usage (30), *training* is defined as "the process of bringing a person to an agreed standard of proficiency by practice and instruction." This is a valuable definition in that it emphasizes the need for an agreed standard of proficiency, and to attain that standard, both practice and instruction are required.

The term *certification* is distinguished from accreditation in international quality management definitions (31), but in practice the two words are used interchangeably in many texts. In medicine the term *accreditation* is used in three main ways, all of which impinge on POCT (see Table 11-1). In this chapter, training by instruction and practice is distinguished

from certification, the granting of a certificate of competence. The latter can be given only when training has been followed by a period of supervised testing.

Ideally training should be carried out within the ward area by POCT coordinators (32). As indicated in the introduction to this chapter, a major problem with POCT is the very widespread and diffuse nature of the operation. It is therefore important that individual responsibilities are clearly defined and that a management structure is created that enables people to understand their individual roles. The management structure for the delivery of POCT testing will be the backbone of the training, certification, and competence monitoring processes. Many models have been proposed, (32–34) and each model has to be tailored to the particular institution. Although articles are written from both laboratory and nursing standpoints, there is agreement that the designation of a person or persons as POCT coordinator(s) with substantial time allocated to the task will greatly enhance the success of any POCT activity. In a large or medium-size hospital, POCT activity in wards, clinics, or other designated areas might be represented on the working group by an area supervisor. In some cases the appointment of link nurses (or POCT liaison nurses) should provide a channel through which initial training sessions and updates can be organized. Figure 11-2 shows such a structure with examples of types of POCT indicated. It is through such an organizational structure that POCT training and certification should be managed.

Table 11-1 Usage of the Term *Accreditation*

Accreditation can recognize . . .
- The fitness of a person to carry out a specific task (certification in the context of this chapter)
- A health care facility or post in that facility as suitable for training purposes (accreditation of training)
- A health care facility as having reached the standard to carry out a prescribed function (accreditation of facility)

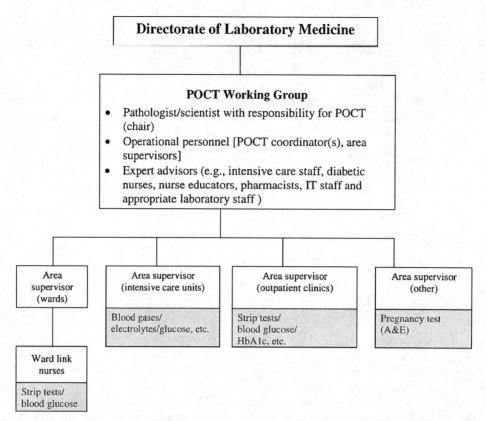

Figure 11-2   A suggested management structure for POCT training.

How Should Training Be Conducted and Organized?

Given the management model in the preceding section, the training would be organized by the POCT coordinator under the direction of the POCT working group, and ideally the coordinator and area supervisors would be trainers along with any other suitable staff in the hospital such as senior nurses and laboratory staff (35). A CAP study (36) showed that overall, nursing personnel were involved in 77.4% of training programs, manufacturer representatives in 51.6%, and laboratory personnel 36.9% of the time.

Some manufacturers, particularly of blood glucose measuring devices, offer to train staff as part of a package involving the use of their particular measuring device and disposables. It is important that this function is identified explicitly in the procurement contract as it will be an important and ongoing commitment. Before involving manufacturers in training, the amount paid for the training component of any package deal should be identified and a decision made as to whether the money could be better spent using in-house trainers. If the manufacturer's route is chosen, it is essential that the healthcare facility has a number of in-house trainers on its own staff to deal with day-to-day issues.

Experience shows that nurses and laboratory staff make good trainers but resources should be provided to enable them to develop good quality presentational skills. There is a growing trend to deliver healthcare through an integrated team

approach (37) allowing laboratory staff to have practical experience of issues faced by other healthcare professionals within clinical areas. Preferably these staff should be involved in quality audits, and be able to draw on that material to illustrate a point. Teaching material enlivened with practical examples is probably the most effective.

POCT training should be an ongoing process and initial training programs should be supplemented by mandatory attendance at regular (usually annual) updates. The majority of staff to be trained to do POCT will be nursing personnel with very heavy commitments to patient care. Finding suitable opportunities for training and for training updates is very difficult. The initial training of new staff must be part of their induction course, and certification of competence must follow quickly if they are to be carrying out POCT as soon as they take up their duties.

Key elements in the conduct and organization of training and certification are given in Table 11-2. The first three points concern the conduct of training; the content and form of the written material to be used is discussed in the following section. It is vital that the training has a high content of practical or hands-on instruction. The assessment on completion of training need not be elaborate but should be designed to check key issues; for example: What action do you take when the quality of sample is outside the set limits for acceptance? How should blood glucose test strips be stored? Travers et al. (38) give seemingly obvious but nevertheless practical advice on what not to do when using blood glucose

Table 11-2 Key Elements in the Conduct and Organization of Training and Certification

- Trainees should be given or have ready access to all written material used in training.
- Training must include theoretical and practical instruction.
- On completion of training, the theoretical and practical instruction must be formally tested.
- Before "flying solo" candidates must have a period of testing under supervision to check competence.
- Successful candidates should be given a "certificate of competence" which is dated and signed by the trainer and the competence supervisor and indicate the areas of POCT in which the candidate has achieved competence.
- Posttraining; competence should be checked at regular intervals.
- Attendance at regular updates should be mandatory.

test strips in a meter. For example, blood glucose strips must never be cut lengthwise, inserted in the meter backwards, blotted improperly, or washed in tap water. These bad-practice statements can be combined with statements of good practice and tested in a simple yes/no format.

What Should Be the Content of POCT Training?

The content of training will in part be determined by the nature of the POCT being undertaken in a particular facility and partly by the needs of the people receiving the training. It may seem obvious that the people who need the training are those who are to carry out the testing. It is equally important, however, that the clinical staff utilizing the results should have some instruction as part of their induction program in which the potential benefits and limitations of different types of testing are explained.

Irrespective of the nature of the POCT undertaken, training has two main objectives, both of equal importance. The first is to ensure that the testing is correctly performed and the second is to ensure that correct action is taken when the result of the testing is obtained.

Nurses and other nonlaboratory professionals who are entrusted with performance of laboratory testing within clinical areas are not likely to have a background in analytical process quality but this does not preclude them from performing acceptably (39). However, other issues need to be considered; in particular, there is a tendency for nonlaboratory personnel to have extreme overconfidence in the reliability of instrumentation and this may be reinforced by the presentation of POCT products as simply and easy to use.

The preparation of training material should take place in the context of the organization and management of a POCT service. The content of the training material must be informed by the contents of the management procedure (Figure 11-1), particularly with respect to (a) equipment, reagents and consumables; (b) procedures, instructions, forms, and records; and (c) quality assurance.

Prior to the introduction of any training program a risk assessment should be performed on the POCT system and the setting where it is to be used. This should take into account the type of user and the sample being handled and relevant information relating to the patients. Organizational health and safety procedures must be taken into account and any legislation adhered to.

Relevant staff should be formally trained in the use of the POCT device and any associated reagents, material, or equipment. The training should provide them with an understanding of the basic principles of the method and its limitations. By far the best basis for training will be the procedure (manual) that has been drawn up for a particular type of POCT in a particular setting. It has the singular advantage that when the trainee goes to the POCT location he or she will already have a familiarity with the written material. In a discussion on concepts of training (2) this is underlined with an ideal view that "each analyst-trainee would be provided at an early stage in their training with a copy of the policy and procedure manual for their own use and to retain for future reference." However, it is now commonplace for procedures to be controlled documents (26) and there should be a mechanism for updating individual copies to prevent risks associated with the use of out-of-date material. Some would argue that ownership of personal copies of a procedure or even notes should be actively discouraged or even prohibited. It is interesting that a CAP Q-probes study of program quality control documentation, program characteristics, and accuracy performance in 544 institutions in the United States showed that 98% of institutions had an organized training program and 98% had a written procedure manual (36).

The golden rule of any procedure is that it must contain all the information required to execute a particular task, and although a procedure may draw on manufacturers' material it is essential that such material is fully integrated in the procedure. Such procedures and associated forms used to record results will be subject to regular audit and review in any institution operating a quality system. Part of the procedure may consist of simplified instructions that are used on a day-to-day basis. Use of such material, which is often made available by manufacturers in a convenient laminated format, is acceptable providing the complete procedure is available for reference when required. Although preliminary drafts of procedures can be drawn up outside the POCT Working Group the final material must be scrutinized by other members of the group who have responsibility for equipment, reagents and consumables, quality assurance, and interpretation of results. Guidance on writing procedures has been published (28, 40), and a recent ISO standard provides guidance to manufacturers on the content of POCT manuals. The content should include, where appropriate, the items covered in Tables 11-3 and 11-4 (41).

Correct Performance of Testing

Correct performance of testing requires due attention to all the preanalytical and analytical factors that can influence the outcome of the testing as well as a demonstrable expertise in analytical skills (Table 11-3).

Table 11-3   Training for Correct Performance of Testing

Training for "correct performance of testing" requires . . .
- An awareness of preanalytical factors
  - Obtaining the correct specimen
  - The importance of clinical contraindications
  - Sample handling
  - Stability of sample
  - Stability of reagents, test strips, test devices
- A demonstrable expertise in analytical skills
  - Operation, calibration, and routine maintenance, together with, and understanding of, any analytical limitations of the instrument or test system
  - A recognition of instrument or test system malfunction and simple trouble shooting techniques
  - Principles, procedures, and documentation of internal quality control and external quality assessment (and patient results)
  - Cleaning, decontamination, and disposal procedures

Modified from a statement of the Council of the Institute of Biomedical Science on Near Patient Testing, 1996 (41).

Many of the preanalytical factors are of vital importance whether the specimen is being obtained for POCT or for laboratory testing. Obtaining the correct specimen involves not only using the correct procedure for collection but also the correct anticoagulant or preservative. The potential for substances to interfere with a test should be identified and brought to the attention of the trainee; e.g., sticky fingers may be useful for transferring sweets into one's mouth but they are not conducive to obtaining satisfactory fingerprick specimens for the measurement of blood glucose. When an invasive procedure (which can under certain circumstances constitute an assault) is required, it should be clear as to who is responsible for ordering the procedure. Certainly in many countries it would be unusual for nonmedical personnel to collect arterial blood for POCT for blood gases, and under certain jurisdictions it may be necessary for nursing or other personnel to be separately certified for venepuncture. Procedures should indicate methods of patient identification and specimen labeling with a view to minimizing the risk of error caused by specimen misidentification.

Clinical Contraindications to the Use of POCT

It is important to document in the procedure clinical contradictions to the use of POCT. The Veterans Administration's Sample Protocol for Whole Blood Glucose—suggested criteria for in-house fingerstick glucose monitoring (38)—includes criteria for requiring a serum glucose test to be performed in the clinical laboratory and not at the bedside. These include the situation in which the glucose value is <3.3 mmol/L (60 mg/dL) or >19.4 mmol/L (350 mg/dL), or the patient's packed cell volume (hematocrit) performed on the same day is <30% or >50%. Knowledge of the limitations of a POCT device in the presence of certain medications or diseases will obviate

crucial decisions being made on erroneous results. Recently a hazard notice was issued following three critical incidents including one fatality caused by a problem with bedside glucose meters overestimating glucose in patients whose treatment contained maltose (42).

Examples from testing for substance abuse in athletics have highlighted the importance of correct procedures for specimen handling and the importance of the stability of the specimen in relation to effects on the analyte of interest. As the purpose of POCT testing is to obtain a rapid result, the latter should not be a major issue. However, the problems caused by inadequate specimen mixing, by exposure to light in the case of analytes such as bilirubin, and evaporation caused by inadequate sealing of the specimen receptacle are legion and to be avoided.

In all procedures involving reagents, test strips, or other disposable test devices, ensuring the stability of these materials requires that they should be stored correctly (i.e., the desiccant retained in a strip test container) or if refrigerated brought back to room temperature as required before use. The batch number and expiration date should be checked as part of the procedure of recording results.

Demonstrable Expertise in Analytical Skills

Demonstrable expertise in analytical skills is a central issue in correct performance of testing, and the operation, calibration, and routine maintenance, together any analytical limitations of the instrument or test system, must be clearly described in the procedure manual as must the steps to be taken in recognizing instrument or test system malfunction and simple troubleshooting techniques.

The principles and procedures of internal quality control (IQC) are not familiar ground for personnel coming from a nursing background and it is essential that the concepts of minimum frequency, acceptance limits, and action be taken (whom to refer to) if results are outside those limits are carefully inculcated. In a CAP study (36) on blood glucose measurements, 99.4% of the participants reported that quality control specimens should be run for blood glucose monitoring, with 80.9% using two levels, 16.3% using three levels, and only 2.5% using one level of control material. Likewise the concept of external quality assessment (EQA) or proficiency

Table 11-4   Training to Ensure Correct Action is Taken When the Test Result is Obtained

Training to ensure that "correct action is taken when the result of the testing is obtained" requires . . .
- Action to be taken if result is outside the limits of the test system
- Action to be taken if the result is within or outside preprescribed action, critical, or alert limits
- Basic knowledge of the importance of abnormal results
- Accurate documentation of patient data

Modified from a statement of the Council of the Institute of Biomedical Science on Near Patient Testing, 1996 (41).

testing is best introduced in both an educational and a regulatory context to emphasize its importance in ensuring a quality service and also to provide an opportunity for self-improvement. The training must stress the importance of proper documentation of the IQC and EQA results in the context of troubleshooting. A useful training approach is to emphasize that for any individual patient result it should be possible to construct an audit trail that establishes who performed the test, with what IQC, where it was done and on what instrument (as appropriate), with what reagents, and at what time on a particular day.

Standards for cleaning, decontamination, and procedures for disposal of clinical waste should be endemic in any healthcare institution concerned for the welfare of its patients and staff but training should be aimed at instilling constant vigilance. Photographic evidence of poor practice obtained on audit visits to POCT sites, such as blood-contaminated instruments, unguarded needles, and overflowing sharps bins are sadly not difficult to obtain but provide valuable teaching material.

Correct Action Is Taken When the Result of the Testing Is Obtained

Having obtained the "correct" result, a further requirement to be taught is the correct action to be taken when the result of the testing is obtained. The key issues are shown in Table 11-4. Training to ensure that correct action is taken is as important as obtaining the test result itself.

Testing personnel must be trained to understand the limitations of different POCT equipment. If a result is outside the limits of the test system then the action to be taken must be a written part of the procedure. Such action would include sending a sample to the laboratory and notifying the requesting clinician. Similarly, if a result is outside preprescribed action, critical, or alert limits, then who to contact, clinician or a senior nurse, must be clearly documented. An assessment of a Critical Limit Protocol for glucose POCT (43) that requires all point-of-care glucose meter readings >22.2 mmol/L (400 mg/dL) and <2.2 mmol/L (40 mg/dL) be immediately confirmed by the laboratory showed 37% of such results were not followed. Furthermore, 77% of these results came from patients with multiple glucose meter readings in whom it may have been felt unnecessary to confirm such results. As a result the protocol now requires that after initial confirmation of a critically high/low result, these patients should be monitored by laboratory testing until levels are between 5.6 and 16.7 mmol/L (100 to 300 mg/dL).

Trainees must be carefully instructed in the procedure for recording POCT results and in particular the correct documentation of patient data. There are two aspects to this issue. First, it is for the healthcare institution to make the decision as to where the results should be recorded: in the patient's paper notes, in the nursing record, or on an electronic data record; but second, a decision must also be made as to what is recorded (44). A minimum data set for patient test results should include patient identification, date and time of specimen collection,

name of test performed (this should include an indication of the test method, i.e., blood glucose—Idealometer), reference (normal) values, test result, name of analyst, and location of the POCT.

It is now possible to connect POCT devices to central patient data management systems and upload information on patient identification and results (45). The use of automated methods of patient identification such as barcoded wrist bands has simplified this procedure, further reducing the risk of error (46).

A basic knowledge of the importance of abnormal results in relevant diagnostic situations should be an inherent part of the training given.

Finally, provision of information on the cost of procedures to users has been demonstrated to alter requesting patterns, producing a reduction in overall cost (47).

Certification of Training or Competence and Posttraining Surveillance

When the last steps in the training process having been completed the trainee must be assessed to check competence. *Competence* may be defined as an individual's ability to apply his or her skills and knowledge to carry out a particular task, and this may be assessed in numerous ways (48) ranging from self-assessment to written examination or mentor observation (see Table 11-5).

The purpose of competence assessment is to ensure that minimum standards of competence are defined and that those failing to meet the standard are provided with appropriate support. Assessment of competence is best carried out using multiple assessment techniques (49) in a real situations. When competence is proven, the certificate of training and competence (see Figure 11-3) may be issued. This certificate should carry a unique identifying number or alphanumeric (the certificate number), expiry date, and the name of the trainee, and indicate areas of competence in terms of tests and equipment. It is signed by the trainer and supervisor and dated. Finally, the certificate is valid until the expiry date, after which the holder will require a further test of competence. A register must be maintained of all certificated staff. This register should be structured in such a way that it is easy to identify the date of conclusion of the initial training and competence testing, what area(s) of POCT were involved, attendance at update sessions, and the date after which the analyst will require a further test of competence. Commercially available software packages are now available to make it possible to record and manipulate such data. Close liaison with human resource departments may

Table 11-5 Mechanisms for Assessing Competence

- Self-assessment
- Multiple-choice questionnaire
- Peer comparison
- Written examination
- Observation

St Elsewhere's Hospital Trust
**Certificate of Training and Competency
in Point-of-Care Testing**

This is to certify that .... has been trained and
certified competent in the following areas of Point-of-Care Testing in
accordance with the appropriate Hospital Trust procedures.

1. _____

2. _____

3. _____

4. _____

Signed...Date..........................
Point-of-Care Coordinator (Training)

Signed...Date..........................
Section Supervisor (Competency)

Certificate no......................Expiry Date......................

Figure 11-3 Certificate of training and competence.

assist in tracking the turnover of staff and identifying potential new users and the need for training courses.

It is now possible to monitor the use of POCT equipment continuously, (50) and compliance with procedures may be referenced by individual user (51). The use of in-house EQA schemes (52) is often viewed as an efficient method to monitor the performance of POCT devices. However, these systems are not without their pitfalls, as there is a tendency to concentrate on the device and not the user. It is common for there to be numerous users of each device and unless EQA samples are distributed to individual users the efficiency of detecting problems is questionable.

A continuous review process should be established to examine the competency standards on which evaluation procedures are based. This process must be sensitive to changes in the field and its technologies, and draw on research related to best practice (48).

Update Sessions and Continuing Education

The rationale for continuing education has been enumerated in four points (2). First, we know well those things that we do regularly and tend to forget knowledge and skills that we do not use. In point of fact, the skills taught will probably be underutilized, and thus frequent retraining will be necessary. Second, retraining will be necessary because of the continual technological advances in alternate-site testing. Third (in the United States) current federal regulations require a minimum annual certification of competence. Continual retraining is the only way to guarantee continual competence. Fourth, future state or federal regulations may actually mandate specific frequency or levels of continuing education for all analysts performing alternate-site testing.

Update sessions should be seen as a crucial part of any program and, in addition, imparting new information should

aim to cultivate a team spirit by which POCT operators feel that they have something to contribute to the ongoing process of ensuring a quality service. It is important therefore that the sessions involve participatory exercises such as the critical examination of quality control records and receiving and learning from the results of quality audits. It is now commonplace for healthcare professionals to keep a record of all training and education within a personal development portfolio. Such portfolios are a valid means of assessing an individual's knowledge and skills and provide a useful mechanism for identification of learning requirements, (53) and it would be appropriate for POCT training and certification requirements to be incorporated into such systems.

It is clear that realizing and maintaining high quality standards in POCT will prove to be a growing challenge for laboratory professionals in the foreseeable future. Serious consideration must be given to where limited resources are targeted in order to achieve maximum benefit.

REFERENCES

1. Marks V. Essential considerations in the provision of near-patient testing facilities. Ann Clin Biochem 1988;25:220–5.
2. Allred TJ, Steiner L. Alternate-site testing. Consider the analyst. Clin Lab Med 1994;14:569–604.
3. Green M. Successful alternatives to alternate site testing. Use of a pneumatic tube system to the central laboratory. Arch Pathol Lab Med 1995;119:943–7.
4. Azzazy HME, Christenson RH. Cardiac markers of acute coronary syndromes: is there a case for point-of-care testing? Clin Biochem 2002;35:13–27.
5. Crook MA. Near patient testing and pathology in the new millennium. J Clin Pathol 2000;53:27–30.
6. Gray TA, Freedman DB, Burnett D, Szczepura A, Price CP. Evidence based practice: clinicians' use and attitudes to near patient testing in hospitals. J Clin Pathol 1996;49:903–8.
7. Kilgore ML, Steindel SJ, Smith JA. Evaluating stat testing options in an academic health center: therapeutic turnaround time and staff satisfaction. Clin Chem 1998;44:1597–603.
8. Castro HJ, Oropello JM, Halpern N. Point-of-care testing in the intensive care unit. The intensive care physician's perspective. Am J Clin Pathol 1995;104(Suppl 1):S95–S99.
9. Olshaker JS. Emergency department pregnancy testing. J Emerg Med 1996;14:59–65.
10. Storrow AB, Gibler WB. The role of cardiac markers in the emergency department. Clin Chim Acta 1999;284:187–96.
11. Murray RP, Leroux M, Sabga E, Palatnick W, Ludwig L. Effect of point of care testing on length of stay in an adult emergency department. J Emerg Med 1999;17:811–4.
12. Stubbs P, Collinson PO. Point-of-care testing: a cardiologist's view. Clin Chim Acta 2001;311:57–61.
13. The NHS plan. A plan for investment. A plan for reform. London: The Stationery Office, 2000.
14. Lehmann CA. The future of home testing–implications for traditional laboratories. Clin Chim Acta 2002;323:31–6.
15. Freedman DB. Clinical governance: implications for point-of-care testing. Ann Clin Biochem 2002;39:421–3.
16. Bissell M, Sanfilippo F. Empowering patients with point-of-care testing. Trends Biotechnol 2002;20:269–70.

17. Kost GJ. Guidelines for point-of-care testing. Improving patient outcomes. Am J Clin Pathol 1995;104(Suppl 1):S111–S127.
18. Jansen RT, Blaton V, Burnett D, Huisman W, Queralto JM, Zerah S. Essential criteria for quality systems in medical laboratories. European Community Confederation of Clinical Chemistry (EC4) Working Group on Harmonisation of Quality Systems and Accreditation. Eur J Clin Chem Clin Biochem 1997;35:123–32.
19. Jansen RT, Blaton V, Burnett D, Huisman W, Queralto JM, Zerah S, et al. Additional essential criteria for quality systems of medical laboratories. European Community Confederation of Clinical Chemistry (EC4) Working Group on Harmonisation of Quality Systems and Accreditation. Clin Chem Lab Med 1998;36:249–52.
20. Briedigkeit L, Muller-Plathe O, Schlebusch H, Ziems J. Recommendations of the German Working Group on Medical Laboratory Testing (AML) on the introduction and quality assurance of procedures for point-of-care testing (POCT) in hospitals. Clin Chem Lab Med 1999;37:919–25.
21. Near to patient or point of care testing. The Joint Working Group on Quality Assurance. Clin Lab Haematol 2000;22:185–8.
22. Medical Devices Agency. Management and use of IVD point of care test devices. London: Medical Devices Agency, 2002.
23. Department of Health. A first class service quality in the new NHS. London: HMSO, 1998.
24. Scally G, Donaldson LJ. The NHS's 50 anniversary. Clinical governance and the drive for quality improvement in the new NHS in England. Br Med J 1998;317:61–5.
25. College of American Pathologists Commission on Laboratory Accreditation. Point of care testing checklist. Northfield, IL: College of American Pathologists, 2001.
26. Clinical Pathology Accreditation (UK). Standards for the medical laboratory. CPA UK website [1.0] 2001.
27. King's Fund Organisational Audit. Primary health care standards and criteria. London: King's Fund, 1993.
28. Burnett D. A practical guide to accreditation. London: ACB Venture Publications, 2002.
29. Kost GJ, Ehrmeyer SS, Chernow B, Winkelman JW, Zaloga GP, Dellinger RP, et al. The laboratory–clinical interface: point-of-care testing. Chest 1999;115:1140–54.
30. Collins English dictionary, 3rd ed. London: Collins Publishers, 1994.
31. International Organization for Standardization. Quality management and quality assurance—vocabulary. Geneva, Switzerland: ISO ANSI/ISO/ASQC A8402, 1994.
32. Miller KA, Miller NA. Joining forces to improve point-of-care testing. Nurs Manage 1997;28:34–7.
33. Hicks JM. Near patient testing: is it here to stay? J Clin Pathol 1996;49:191–3.
34. Lamb LS. Responsibilities in point-of-care testing. An institutional perspective. Arch Pathol Lab Med 1995;119:886–9.
35. Miller K, Miller N. Benefits of a joint nursing and laboratory point-of-care program: nursing and laboratory working together. Crit Care Nurs Q 2001;24:15–20.
36. Jones BA, Howanitz PJ. Bedside glucose monitoring quality control practices. A College of American Pathologists Q-Probes study of program quality control documentation, program characteristics, and accuracy performance in 544 institutions. Arch Pathol Lab Med 1996;120:339–45.
37. Wood J. The role, duties and responsibilities of technologists in the clinical laboratory. Clin Chim Acta 2002;319:127–32.
38. Travers EM, Wolke JC, Stitak MM. Consolidating ancillary testing in multihospital systems. Clin Lab Med 1994;14:493–524.
39. Handorf CR. Quality control and quality management of alternate-site testing. Clin Lab Med 1994;14:539–57.
40. National Committee on Clinical Laboratory Standards. Clinical laboratory technical procedure manuals, 2nd ed. Approved guideline. NCCLS document GP2–A2. Wayne, PA: NCCLS, 1992.
41. Near patient testing, a statement approved by the Council of the Institute of Biomedical Sciences. Biomed Sci 1996;April:165–7.
42. MDA. Blood glucose meter test strips: Roche Accu-Chek Advantage II. 16–4-2003. London: Medicines and Healthcare Products Regulatory Agency, 2003.
43. Lum G. Assessment of a critical limit protocol for point-of-care glucose testing. Am J Clin Pathol 1996;106:390–5.
44. Auerbach DM. Alternate site testing. Information handling and reporting issues. Arch Pathol Lab Med 1995;119:924–5.
45. Bissell M. Point-of-care testing at the millennium. Crit Care Nurs Q 2001;24:39–43.
46. Kost GJ. Preventing medical errors in point-of-care testing: security, validation, safeguards, and connectivity. Arch Pathol Lab Med 2001;125:1307–15.
47. Tierney WM, Miller ME, McDonald CJ. The effect on test ordering of informing physicians of the charges for outpatient diagnostic tests. N Engl J Med 1990;322:1499–1504.
48. Lysaght RM, Altschuld JW. Beyond initial certification: the assessment and maintenance of competency in professions. Evaluat Prog Plan 2000;23:95–104.
49. Norman IJ, Watson R, Murrells T, Calman L, Redfern S. The validity and reliability of methods to assess the competence to practise of pre-registration nursing and midwifery students. Int J Nurs Studies 2002;39:133–45.
50. Bernard D, Vanhee D, Blaton V. Implementation of an integrated instrument control and data management system for point of care blood gas testing. Clin Chim Acta 2001;307:169–73.
51. Dyer K, Nichols JH, Taylor M, Miller R, Saltz J. Development of a universal connectivity and data management system. Crit Care Nurs Q 2001;24:25–38.
52. Hortas ML, Montiel N, Redondo M, Medina A, Contreras E, Cortes C, et al. Quality assurance of point-of-care testing in the Costa del Sol Healthcare Area (Marbella, Spain). Clin Chim Acta 2001;307:113–8.
53. Neades BL. Professional portfolios: all you need to know and were afraid to ask. Acc Emerg Nurs 2003;11:49–55.

Chapter 12

Equipment Procurement and Implementation

M. Joan Pearson

Point-of-care testing (POCT) is now part of routine service in most hospitals and will continue to grow in the foreseeable future. A greater range of analytes; simpler, easier-to-use systems needing little expert maintenance; noninvasive systems; and developing possibilities for wireless connectivity; and improved data management and integration have also opened up more opportunities for POCT, especially after the agreement of the standard POCT1-A (NCCLS). Patient expectations and, for example, the "patient choice" agenda in the United Kingdom (http://www.doh.gov.uk/choice/index.htm) have helped to raise demand for test availability away from the hospital environment. At the same time, professional guidelines for the appropriate and safe implementation of POCT, plus regulation in some countries, have clarified the process and raised awareness of risks. POCT services are developing in:

- Outpatient services
- Community
  Decentralized services (e.g., diagnosis and treatment centers)
  Primary care: GPs (community physicians) and nurses
  Pharmacists
- Ambulances and other emergency services
- Patients' homes (self-testing in monitoring chronic diseases, e.g., diabetes mellitus)
- Workplace screening
- Retail and other outlets, health food shops, sports centers, catering for the "worried well" who may be happy to pay for screening tests

Quality, risk management, and clear lines of responsibility are of concern in all of these. Anyone involved in planning, evaluating, and implementing POCT should have a good strategic awareness, wide contacts with professional colleagues and industry, plus good communication and teamworking skills.

There may be different understandings around the world of the definition of POCT (see Chapter 1); all settings are included for consideration in this chapter.

MANAGEMENT STRUCTURES TO SUPPORT POCT SERVICES

Clinical users and general managers should be made aware of the importance and advantages of whole-system planning for POCT and should understand the professional expertise and the management structures necessary for efficient operation of the service. A senior member of the laboratory staff should have responsibility for directing the planning for implementation of new POCT systems within a strategic view of all diagnostic testing. Depending on the size of the organization there should ideally be a POCT manager, with strategic responsibility and supervising a POCT coordinator who has operational responsibility, probably one coordinator for each site within the institution. A POCT manager may work full-time on POCT, or have additional service responsibilities in the central laboratory. It is obviously advantageous to be closely involved with the service, organization, and strategy of the central laboratory when strategic decisions about POCT services are made.

A POCT committee and a POCT policy are essential in supporting this effectively. There is no single ideal format or constitution—what is optimal will vary with the organization. As a general principle, however, there should be wide representation from departments in the hospital that are likely to have an interest in POCT, encouraging a multidisciplinary approach to planning POCT. The typical composition for a POCT committee is given in Table 12-1 (see also Chapters 11 and 15).

The functions of the committee may include those listed in Table 12-2. A POCT policy, agreed upon and given authority by the committee, is likely to cover the points listed in Table 12-3 and should be widely accessible, such as on the hospital intranet.

An effective POCT committee and an up-to-date policy help prevent uncontrolled purchase and implementation of POCT, but the POCT manager and coordinator(s) will still have a significant responsibility for establishing and maintaining good communications with their clinical and management colleagues. They must also keep in touch with technological and analytical developments so as to be a source of up-to-date advice.

Many institutions now formalize the process of establishing the clinical need and evaluating proposals for implementation of POCT by issuing structured request forms to clinical staff via their POCT committees as a way of encouraging a systematic approach to the process from the start. These are likely to require clinical staff to specify:

- Test(s) required
- Indications of how this will improve patient care, including turnaround time (TAT) required and whether alternative solutions have been considered
- Whether it is a new test or an upgrade/replacement of a current system
- Estimated test number/frequency

Table 12-1 Typical Membership of a POCT Committee

POCT manager
POCT coordinator(s)
Medical physicist/engineer responsible for decentralized
    equipment maintenance
Information technology representative
Risk management/clinical governance (UK) representative
Finance manager
Planning representative
Nurse educator
Nurse manager
Clinical staff representatives from areas where POCT is
    employed, including primary care and community

- Data handling: entry of results to patient record
- Proposed users

Applications are then reviewed by the POCT committee for appropriateness and cost. Possible alternatives to POCT for meeting the clinical need should be considered (discussed later), but when POCT is approved, a list of suitable systems can be drawn up in cooperation with the POCT manager, followed by evaluation and option appraisal.

POCT Outside the Hospital

The amount and nature of advice and support for POCT outside the hospital is very variable depending on local factors as well

Table 12-2 Functions of a POCT Committee

Development of, and giving authority to, a POCT policy
Approval of all POCT devices before use in the hospital
Review of new POCT systems coming onto the market
Standardization of equipment and systems
Risk management, including compliance with all relevant
    legislation or national guidelines
Quality system (including proficiency testing) and
    arrangements for management and documentation
Approval of all POCT implementation and service
    development
Justification of POCT at a particular location by considering
    outcomes and evidence of clinical effectiveness
Audit of POCT services
Establishment of and support for a system for user training
    and certification, including link nurses at ward level, backed
    by documentation of contraindications and limitations of
    POCT systems in use
User competency: review of arrangements
Establishment of budgets for support of POCT or
    billing/charging systems
Integration of all POCT planning with the institution's IT policy
    and strategy
Coordination of connectivity planning and implementation,
    including interface with the laboratory information system
    and electronic patient record

Table 12-3 A POCT Policy

Compatibility with other policies where appropriate:
    Medical equipment management
    Infection control
Risk management and patient safety: procedures and lines of
    responsibility
Financial and management arrangements for procurement,
    operation and management of the equipment and any
    billing arrangements
Management of POCT by qualified (state-registered)
    laboratory staff
Accreditation of POCT, depending on national requirements
Training and competence of POCT users
Line of responsibility for patient results and any action taken
Standard operating procedures for POCT equipment and
    systems
Service-level agreements between clinical areas and
    laboratory
Equipment choice and coordinated procurement:
    standardization of equipment and systems
Connectivity: management, storage and use of patient data,
    unauthorized user lockout
Quality control and external quality assessment/proficiency
    testing
Health and safety
Audit
Record keeping
Existing POCT systems in the organization; ideally, a list of
    POCT equipment and systems in current use should be
    accessible along with the policy.

as national healthcare structures. In the United Kingdom, the increasing responsibility of primary care for managing chronic diseases and in commissioning and funding all healthcare, in addition to the patient choice agenda, will all tend to encourage greater use of POCT in GP offices and by patients who wish to monitor their own disease or therapy. Some community pharmacists in the United Kingdom are offering POCT for screening and monitoring diseases and drug therapies; development of such services are encouraged by the Department of Health (1).

These service providers may not be accustomed to using quality control (QC) and external quality assessment (EQA; proficiency testing) or developing user competency, so it is important that POCT staff in the nearest hospital are, whenever possible, proactive in offering advice and support to their community colleagues. POCT in leisure or retail environments is more problematic, as contact with the local hospital laboratory is unlikely to be considered.

Relationships with Suppliers (Vendors)

Maintaining good contacts and relationships with suppliers is important in preventing uncontrolled purchase and implementation of POCT in those institutions where formal structures for POCT management may not be in place. In the United Kingdom, the British In Vitro Diagnostics Association (BIVDA; http://www.bivda.com), which represents many suppliers, is developing a code of practice whereby members agree to inform the POCT manager or coordinator when marketing their products in a hospital. The NHS Purchasing and Supply Agency promotes best procurement practice for POCT by working with suppliers and customers. It has developed several procurement tool kits for NHS staff, including market information, standard procurement documents, and outline clinical and technical specifications. With BIVDA, it hosts a POCT managers contact database that can be accessed on its website (http://www.pasa.nhs.uk). Thus it is always recommended that suppliers deal with the relevant laboratory director rather than with the requesting physician.

ESTABLISHING THE CLINICAL NEED

Marks commented in 1988 (2), "It is important before accepting the need for NPT [POCT] on a particular site to define its purpose and nature and the benefits to be expected of it," and this is still relevant advice. The clinical need for POCT is most likely to be perceived by clinicians, who are now well aware of POCT and its potential advantages and who may initiate inquiries or proposals with their laboratory colleagues. Central laboratories may also see POCT as one option in planning service development or change, or dealing with a staffing or space problem. Should implementing POCT be primarily a decision for the clinician or on the laboratory's advice? The process is probably easier in the former case, because the interest and motivation are already there.

By adapting the current service, opinions about its usefulness still vary, however, with some laboratory staff still considering that the laboratory can provide an acceptable service in most cases where POCT is being considered. Similarly, many clinical staff, while seeing the potential benefits of POCT see it as an extra burden on clinical staff (3), or they (managers) may regard its cost, seen purely in terms of cost per test, as too high. The laboratory's responsibility is to establish a good working relationship with the clinical area so that the clinical and economic outcomes required can be realistically and jointly examined in the particular circumstances. Outcomes required may include patient length of stay (e.g., in an emergency department or intensive care unit), patient satisfaction (e.g., in an outpatient clinic) and reduced cost per patient episode.

POCT may be proposed for any of the purposes for which central laboratory testing is used: screening, diagnosis or monitoring patient treatment or progress. Most demand for POCT is based on its perceived convenience and immediacy, with an assumption that reduced TAT brings improved clinical outcomes. This is often true (4), but is not automatically the case (5), as laboratory TAT is not always the rate-limiting step in a care pathway (6) and simply moving testing from a central laboratory to the medical unit does not guarantee improved outcomes (7). Other studies have demonstrated real savings by implementing POCT, although this may require system reengineering (8).

These and other outcomes studies can give useful guidance, but each situation is likely to be unique (9). A rigorous outcomes approach is unlikely to be easy or possible in every case, but some attempt should be made to look critically at the whole patient pathway for any changes that may help to achieve the required outcomes, with POCT as one of various options. Clinicians and managers should therefore be made aware that a whole system view should be taken and that real improvements in clinical and economic outcomes may only be possible if systematic changes can be made and a way around "silo budgeting" can be found. The key is good communication and ensuring that evaluation, implementation and management of the POCT service are conducted as a partnership between the clinical service user and the laboratory service provider. Once it has been agreed that POCT is the optimum solution, it is necessary to consider:

- *The current service arrangements (if any), including any existing POCT.* An audit of tests done and existing costs and cost–benefit analysis allows comparison with a range of options for new POCT.
- *The menu of analytes required.* If there are other results required as part of the profile for clinical decision making which are not provided at point of care, then implementation of POCT may not improve the service to the patient.
- *Whether the analytes should be available all on one piece of equipment or more than one.* In a neonatal unit, for example, glucose or bilirubin results may be required alone far more frequently than as a profile along with blood gases. Separate availability may therefore limit the volume of blood to be drawn.
- *The expected test throughput and frequency, which will influence decision making about the most appropriate equipment.* For example, in a department with occasional or sporadic needs for blood gas and electrolyte analysis, a cartridge-based handheld analyzer such as i-STAT would cost nothing when not being used, while a conventional blood gas analyzer consumes reagents, quality materials and staff time even when not required for analytical use.
- *How the results will be used.* This will determine the performance characteristics (accuracy, imprecision) expected from the equipment.
- *Which staff will use POCT equipment.* In the United Kingdom, for example, while most POCT is conducted by nursing and junior medical staff, national initiatives to extend roles beyond traditional ones may result in other staff groups such as physiotherapists and dieticians performing POCT. They are unlikely to have the same familiarity with the central laboratory service as nursing and medical staff, which may affect the nature of training and competency programs for the new POCT system.

The National Academy of Clinical Biochemistry (NACB; http://www.nacb.org) develops and publishes Laboratory Medicine Practice Guidelines. Evidence-based guidelines for POCT implementation are in preparation, based on systematic review of the literature, and should be available some time in 2004. This will be a very important resource for POCT managers and coordinators.

ALTERNATIVE APPROACHES TO MEETING NEED

Much will depend on the nature of the clinical need, e.g., critical care and primary care. In the United Kingdom, the government has imposed patient waiting time targets, particularly in emergency departments, and clinicians or managers may see POCT as a way of meeting targets. POCT is almost always more expensive than the laboratory on a cost-per-test basis when considering the reagent or consumable costs, although a wider consideration of costs will often show lower costs per episode. Since most demand is based on a requirement for shorter TAT for pathology results, options for faster laboratory TAT should be examined first. The extent to which faster specimen transport, turnaround within the laboratory and issue of results to the clinical area are achievable will depend on local circumstances. Reducing test TAT will only bring about the improvement expected if it is the rate limiting step (6, 10); in this case, reengineering of other processes within the clinical area may bring about the required reduction in waiting time for the patient.

In one whole section of a hospital, possibly a group of departments on a remote part of the site, or those with similar acute needs (operating rooms, ICUs or neonatal units and delivery suites), the establishment of small satellite or stat laboratories, or expansion of existing ones, may be an option worth considering, although it is likely to be expensive. Some organizations may be able to staff such laboratories with laboratory staff; nurses or other health professionals (e.g. clinical physiologists) may be specially trained and accredited by the laboratory to have responsibility for conducting specific tests such as blood gases or clotting screens.

EVALUATING POCT EQUIPMENT AND SYSTEMS PRIOR TO PURCHASE

Regulation and Accreditation

The United States. All testing in the United States, whether in laboratories or decentralized (including POCT), is subject to the Clinical Laboratory Improvement Amendments (CLIA'88), with four designated categories of laboratory testing:

1. *Waived.* Tests that are simple to perform and require minimum interpretation (most POCT tests). The FDA website has a list of waived tests: http://www.accessdata.fda.gov/scripts/cdrh/cfdocs/cfClia/analyteswaived.cfm.
2. *Provider-performed microscopy (PPM).* Tests performed and interpreted by a physician or other provider.
3. *Moderate complexity.* Tests that require more complex equipment, judgment, and interpretation (e.g., conventional blood gas analyzers).

4. *High complexity.* Tests that require the most complex equipment, judgment, and interpretation and which would be performed in central laboratories.

CLIA imposes requirements for QC, EQA, user proficiency, quality management, and supervision for all POCT. There may also be state laws with further specific requirements. A CLIA certificate may be awarded to a laboratory to include all decentralized testing in that establishment or, alternatively, decentralized sites may be certified separately, and there are various possibilities for accreditation and inspection (11). The CLIA regulations continue to evolve as test systems develop, and these can be checked on http://www.phppo.cdc.gov/clia/default.asp and the Centers for Medicare and Medicaid Services website: http://www.cms.hhs.gov/clia.

The United Kingdom. POCT in the United Kingdom is subject to less regulation than in the United States. A number of guidance documents on management and conduct of POCT have been issued since 1989 by professional groups and the Department of Health. The most recent and comprehensive of these is from the Medical Devices Agency (MDA) (12), now merged with the Medicines Control Agency to form the Medicines and Healthcare Products Regulatory Agency (MHRA), an agency of the Department of Health. This guidance does not constitute a legal requirement. Accreditation of laboratory medicine services in the United Kingdom is now compulsory and is conducted by Clinical Pathology Accreditation (http://www.cpa-uk.co.uk), which includes any POCT services (13) supported by the central laboratory in its accreditation of the laboratory. POCT that is not managed or supervised by the central laboratory is therefore not accredited in any way.

Europe. The European Union (EU) issued "Directive 98/79/EC of the European Parliament and of the Council of October 27, 1998 on In Vitro Diagnostic Medical Devices." Its purpose is "to remove technical barriers to trade . . . and create a single market for medical devices within the EU. However, by harmonizing the regulations governing medical device manufacturers, [it] also aims to improve the level of protection of patients, users and third parties and ensure that devices perform as intended." A device is defined as "any reagent, reagent product, calibrator, control material kit, instrument, apparatus, equipment or system intended for use for the in vitro examination of specimens . . . derived from the human body." This directive (IVDD) requires manufacturers and other institutions placing in vitro diagnostic (IVD) medical devices on the market, or putting them into service after modification or in-house manufacture, to meet certain requirements concerning their safety, quality, and performance and to produce technical documentation that must be audited. Conformité Européene (CE) marking of devices indicates that they comply with the directive. There are transition periods within the directive and one of these ended on December 7, 2003. All new devices placed on the market must now be CE-marked. There is a further transition period, until December 7, 2005, during which existing systems already in service must be brought into compliance with the directive.

The IVDD is complex and requires interpretation and implementation within each member country of the EU. In the United Kingdom, the MHRA has taken legal advice on its interpretation, but how it will affect POCT is not yet fully understood. However, one condition of CE marking is that in order to be covered by its provisions, marked devices must be used strictly according to the manufacturer's instructions. Since POCT manufacturers generally specify that their equipment should be used only by appropriately trained personnel, this may be helpful to POCT managers when managing training programs for POCT users, who should be made aware that failure to comply with CE-marking requirements may constitute a criminal offense in the United Kingdom.

Meeting Performance Requirements

Evaluation of suitable equipment or systems must include a technical assessment of their suitability for the particular clinical need. This will include sample type and number, accuracy and precision required, patient population (including consideration of any therapy that may interfere with analytical methods) and comparability with the central laboratory method. Equipment marketed in any particular country is likely to comply with the relevant safety and regulatory standards, but this should be checked. Manufacturers generally provide technical data about their products for the use of laboratory personnel; clinical staff should follow the laboratory's advice with respect to such data. The technical performance of suitable equipment may be checked during trials in the clinical setting.

There are no specific national requirements for equipment or method evaluation prior to purchase or implementation in the United Kingdom, so practices vary considerably. The devices section of the MHRA (http://www.mhra.gov.uk) publishes evaluation reports on POCT equipment, free to NHS staff and organizations. Evaluations are conducted by independent specialist centers based at NHS hospital trusts and universities and include comparison with reference methods, error grid analysis, acceptance analysis, imprecision, linearity, and method interferences. Some aspects of these evaluations may be repeated by laboratory staff during trials of systems being considered for purchase.

In the United States, the Food and Drug Administration (FDA) Center for Devices and Radiological Health (CDRH) licenses in vitro diagnostic devices based on information provided by the manufacturer but does not evaluate devices or denote approval of licensed products. There are advisory committees, including a Medical Devices Advisory Committee, which provides independent expert professional advice and advises the commissioner of food and drugs on the safety and effectiveness of medical devices (http://www.fda.gov/cdrh/panel/index.html).

POCT committees may specify in their documentation the guidelines for technical evaluation and preimplementation validation in their institution. These may include within- and between-run precision, linearity, and comparison with reference methods by using split samples. NCCLS (http://www.

nccls.org) has published protocols for the technical evaluation of analytical equipment and systems that may be performed when considering options for purchase or after purchase and before implementation.

Table 12-4 Evaluation Criteria for POCT Systems

Compliance with regulatory standards
Connectivity: POCT1-A compliance for patient records and transfer of patient results to LIMS; potential for remote monitoring and management of equipment from the laboratory; compatibility with existing systems
Barcode recognition for operators, reagents (consumables), and patients
Analytes required (on separate analyzers or same—can be important in cases of small sample size)
Methodology; comparability with existing methods (in central or decentralized testing)
Any existing equipment standardization policy
Expected test number throughput; continuous or sporadic
Precision, accuracy, sensitivity, and specificity required, which should be appropriate for the clinical need
Specimen type and any special requirements or concerns about sample size or quality (e.g., neonates or fetal scalp specimens)
Comparability with the laboratory result, particularly with different specimen types (e.g., blood or plasma glucose) and different analytical methods
Degree of portability required
Cost: capital purchase, leasing, or "reagent rental"
Running costs: maintenance contract, consumables, analytical quality materials, staff, software licenses and connectivity costs (including any software upgrades)
Unauthorized operator lockout
QC:
   AutoQC and regulatory compliance
   QC lockout
Availability of external quality assessment (proficiency testing) materials
Space available: type of facilities required for the safe siting of equipment and any storage space needed (e.g., the consumables)
Particular siting needs (e.g., temperature or humidity), to be matched with availability in a clinical area
Maintenance requirements—clinical or laboratory staff time
Maintenance manuals supplied
Ease of use
Nature of any training material or sessions provided by the supplier (for clinical users or laboratory staff who will maintain the equipment)
Warranty (period of free attention and repairs after purchase)
Choice of service contracts, if appropriate
Supplier's engineer's availability and response times
Supplier's help line
Any backup (e.g., replacement equipment on loan) available from the supplier when equipment is out of service for repairs
Trial period available for equipment in proposed site
Safety features, e.g., regarding infection risk and decontamination

In addition to any detailed technical evaluation, the points in Table 12-4 may be considered—depending on the equipment or system—when making decisions to purchase. It can also be very useful to add to this list of objective information some feedback from professional colleagues with experience of equipment under consideration. Professional listservs (e.g., Association of Clinical Biochemists or American Association for Clinical Chemistry) can be a useful source of information, as can commercial POCT websites.

BUSINESS CASE AND PROCUREMENT PROCESS

Depending on the necessary formalities in a particular country or organization, a business case within the clinical department or directorate for the new system is likely to be necessary, to include details of the service development/equipment replacement proposed, together with purchase or leasing costs and running costs of the new system. The POCT manager has an important role in ensuring that the full costs of the system over its projected lifetime are understood, with all costs such as connectivity, quality, training, staffing, and accreditation included in the business case. Procurement will be prepared by the supplies or procurement department of the organization, in full consultation with the POCT manager. Depending on the equipment and system, other features and services from the supplier may be specified, such as free warranty period, staff training, audits, and supply and delivery arrangements for consumables.

In the United Kingdom and other EU countries, regulations apply to all contracts to supply goods with an overall value exceeding about £100,000 (subject to change). The contract must be advertised in the *Official Journal of the European Communities* (OJEC; http://www.ojec.com), with minimum prescribed times for suppliers to respond. The number of suppliers to be shortlisted and the criteria to be considered for shortlisting ("minimum economic and technical standards required of the supplier") can be specified in the OJEC advertisement. A contract award notice must be placed in the OJEC within 48 days of informing the successful supplier.

Equipment Standardization

Some test systems may be implemented throughout a hospital rather than in small numbers in specialized areas, so deciding on a standard may be part of an evaluation process. This may be a one-time decision for a batch of equipment (e.g., when implementing a new glucose testing system) or a standard for programmed replacement of equipment such as blood gas analyzers over a number of years.

Standardization has cost benefits, including dealing centrally with one supplier rather than several and negotiating of discounts on purchase and consumables costs by arranging central purchasing and stock control for reagents. It is also advantageous for staff training and competence—laboratory staff who maintain and supervise the equipment and clinical staff can be trained and retain competence on equipment even when they are transferred elsewhere in the organization. Comparability of results is another advantage; many users do not understand that there are differences between systems from different suppliers, and managing the implications of this may be time-consuming for the laboratory. A further advantage is connectivity; the POCT1-A standard will ensure that data transfer is possible across different suppliers' equipment, but the additional advantage of remote monitoring and management of analyzers is not generally possible in this case, and this can be an important feature of connectivity where there is networked equipment around an organization as it optimizes the use of support staff time.

Making a Choice

It is useful to have a subgroup, consisting of the POCT manager and/or coordinator, plus medical and nursing representatives of the clinical area concerned, and possibly finance and planning staff, to look systematically at a short-list of options that meet the requirements, with a formal checklist of the features to be considered, probably based on a subset of the evaluation criteria used for short-listing, any specific site-related requirements, and the experiences of colleagues elsewhere who use the system. When the equipment is evaluated, both the users and the laboratory staff who will maintain it should have an opportunity to contribute to decision making, and if the clinical staff can comment anonymously (e.g., via a book left next to the equipment), honest views are likely to be obtained. Even if laboratory staff have the main influence on the final decision, a degree of consultation and the maintenance of good communication will pay dividends later when the equipment is being used; clinical staff will feel ownership of the system and are then more likely to have a positive attitude toward it.

Contract with the Supplier

Formalities of such contracts will vary from country to country and will depend on whether systems are purchased or leased. Contracts should specify any agreement about costs and discounts; the free warranty period; response times for engineer visits, audits, and any contribution to user training and competency offered by the company, which may include training materials or the supply of dedicated trainers for intensive user training during the implementation period and follow-up/refresher training. Some companies will agree to fund an award system (e.g., retail gift vouchers for outstanding compliance by wards or clinical areas over a given time period) to encourage user compliance with training and quality procedures.

IMPLEMENTATION

Establishment of a service-level agreement (SLA) before implementation can work well so that everyone concerned knows

Table 12-5   Contents of a Service-Level Agreement

Ownership of the equipment: most likely to be the clinical area in which it is sited, but some POCT systems may be owned by the central laboratory, or there may be a separate budget for POCT

Lines of responsibility for:

Results and how these will be reported and integrated into the patient record; critical limits and action to be taken

Risk management

Health and safety, including infection control, disposal of blood and sharps, and maintaining the POCT equipment and surroundings in an uncontaminated condition

Equipment maintenance if not by laboratory staff

Management of regulatory compliance and accreditation of the POCT service (as required by the country or state concerned)

Connectivity: patient data management, interface with the LIMS

Maintenance: staff time for maintenance and any consequent costs

Contact details for maintenance problems or troubleshooting

Operating costs: reagents and other consumables, including QC and EQA

Billing (if applicable)

Stock control: storage and ordering arrangements

QC and EQA (proficiency testing):

Who will perform

Procedures to be followed when these are out of range

Staff training and competency; agreement and registration of key trainers if appropriate. Arrangements for regular checks and reaccreditation

Test protocol, covering patient preparation, sample preparation, and reporting and interpreting results

Standard operating procedure for the POCT system:

Analytical technique

Reference to QC and EQA procedures

Recording and reporting results

Records: what records will be kept, for how long, and who will have responsibility and access

Audit: what audits will be conducted and the line of responsibility and processes for implementing any system improvements deemed necessary from audit results

---

what is expected of them and the equipment; a generic SLA may be part of the POCT policy and can then be adapted according to the specific circumstances (Table 12-5).

Implementation of the new equipment or system should be conducted systematically, and many organizations have a formal process for doing this. In the United States, before a nonwaived test is used for patient results, CLIA regulations require it to be validated to demonstrate that performance specifications established by the manufacturer can be achieved. This is generally done by determination of inaccuracy or bias, imprecision, reportable range, and establishment of an appropriate reference range. This process is not obligatory for waived tests (http://www.westgard.com/cliafinalrule4.htm). In the United Kingdom, similar studies may have been done

during equipment trials before a choice was made, or on implementation of new POCT systems, but there are no formal regulatory requirements for preimplementation validation.

If the implementation is an infrequent single decision, such as a hospital-wide glucose testing system, then the group that managed the evaluation and choice of systems may wish to supervise implementation, or it may be the sole responsibility of the POCT manager or coordinator, working with the company. The likely time commitment for POCT staff for a successful implementation should not be underestimated.

The implementation starts with acceptance testing, which will include checking for completeness of equipment and components delivered and basic electrical safety, followed by installation and commissioning of the equipment (as appropriate) by the supplier, preferably with laboratory POCT staff available to oversee the process. Training for proposed clinical users of the system should be started as soon as possible after setting up the equipment.

The extent to which laboratory staff are involved in the ongoing operation of POCT equipment will vary depending on the nature of the equipment and local custom and practice, but it is always a good idea for an agreed individual in the clinical area to be responsible for ensuring that any necessary protocols are followed, the equipment is used only by accredited personnel, and analytical quality procedures are complied with, and to be the main point of contact with the laboratory. In high-population clinical areas, it can also be useful to appoint a key trainer, usually a nurse, who is trained and accredited by the laboratory to train staff locally and keep the list of persons having satisfactorily completed training.

PATIENT SAFETY AND RISK MANAGEMENT

This will have been considered in the preevaluation process as it should be explicit in the POCT policy and is likely to be part of the responsibility of the POCT manager. There is increasing awareness of the risks to patients of medical errors (14). Clinical governance, introduced into the UK NHS in the 1990s as a total quality system, specifies risk management as one of its components, and POCT managers have a clinical governance responsibility in their management of POCT (12). A more explicit emphasis on patient safety has followed in the United Kingdom with the publication of "An Organisation with a Memory" (15) and its implementation plan, "Building a Safer NHS" (http://doh.gov.uk/buildsafenhs). The United Kingdom has a Clinical Negligence Scheme for [Hospital] Trusts (CNST), which requires an annual subscription from members. This can be reduced if the member implements recommended quality and safety structures and procedures, including formal training for users of medical equipment and devices; CNST standards are published by the NHS Litigation Authority (http://www.nhsla.com).

The potential for medical error in POCT is well known (16–18). Analytical error is minimized by the simple-to-use, but not yet 100% foolproof, technology and increasingly sophisticated inbuilt QC systems. However, the pre- and post-analytical phases of testing are still prone to error and may be the major source of overall error (19). The potential for error in the whole POCT process is usually greatly underestimated by clinical users, so this should be explicit in planning and implementing a POCT service, including in SLAs between the laboratory and POCT users. Pre- and postanalytical error can be minimized by password protection and barcode access for users, although unauthorized exchange of passwords or barcoded badges is a common problem. The most effective way of preventing this is probably to agree to a disciplinary framework with the senior clinician and ensure that it is enforced.

POSTIMPLEMENTATION FOLLOW-UP

It is helpful if the POCT manager or coordinator can be present as often as possible during the few days or weeks following implementation so that any problems and concerns can be dealt with quickly and reassuringly. Ensuring that the POCT staff are seen as friendly and accessible can pay dividends later when clinical staff will see the laboratory as supportive partners rather than as remote and critical.

An audit should be conducted soon after the system is put into routine use and any shortcomings or problems dealt with quickly and constructively. These may include increased test throughput or untrained staff using the equipment.

Test Throughput

It should be appreciated by all concerned in the planning of new POCT systems that actual test throughput after implementation may turn out to be much higher than planned—with consequently higher costs than were first estimated. Whether this represents a real improvement in the service to patients or unnecessary extra testing because of increased access and availability, hence increased cost with no added value (20, 21), may not always be clear, but most POCT managers will be familiar with the phenomenon. Problems can be minimized if testing protocols are agreed before implementation and, if possible, which staff groups or individuals will have access to the system. This information should be incorporated into the user training process and documentation. Regular audits of workload and trained staff using the system will keep track of how effective this is. The implications of increased testing (mainly cost, but also staff time) should be discussed with the lead clinician, and any necessary management changes made.

Another occasional problem is double testing. There is some evidence that clinical staff may trust POCT less than results from the central laboratory (22), and so continue to send samples to the laboratory "just to make sure." There is an obvious cost concern here. It is best avoided by careful pre-implementation planning and evaluation, including some split sample testing; effective implementation and a supportive professional partnership should ensure that clinical users feel fully confident of their POCT system.

Compliance with a Service-Level Agreement

Complacence may set in after the initial implementation, with declining compliance with quality procedures or training and competency. It is important to work with the clinical area concerned to ensure that the risks are understood, and to encourage continuing local commitment to good standards as set out in the service-level agreement. This can form the basis of a continuing education and recertification strategy.

Change in Clinical Practice

Invariably, the availability of a rapid service will lead to the need for changes in the process of clinical care; indeed, that is one of the main drivers for use of POCT. When introducing a POCT service, it is therefore important to ensure that attention is given to the ways in which the test results are communicated and actions taken, in order that the benefits gained, compared with use of a laboratory-based service, can be realized (7). This will involve consultation with the clinical team, as well as identification of the clinical outcomes that are expected, when the effects of introduction of the service are audited at a later date.

CONCLUSIONS

Analytical and IT developments plus patient demand are widening the possibilities for POCT use, and POCT managers and coordinators need to keep up-to-date with these issues. National guidance and regulation of the management and conduct of POCT are developing in detail and complexity to meet the changing needs for service quality. POCT managers and coordinators need to be strategically aware and to ensure that planning, procurement, and implementation of POCT systems are effective, and establish good practice and constructive professional relationships from the start. High-quality POCT operates as a partnership between clinical and scientific staff.

REFERENCES

1. Moffat AC. Point-of-care testing in the community pharmacy. Pharm J 2001;267:267–8.
2. Marks V. Essential considerations in the provision of near-patient testing facilities. Ann Clin Biochem 1988;25:220–5.
3. Kilgore ML, Steindal SJ, Smith JA. Evaluating STAT testing options in an academic health centre: therapeutic turnaround time and staff satisfaction. Clin Chem 1998;44:1597–603.
4. Grieve R, Beech R, Vincent J, Mazurkiewicz J. Near patient testing in diabetes clinics: appraising the costs and outcomes. Health Technol Assess 1999;3:1–74.
5. Kendall J, Reeves B, Clancy M. Point-of-care testing: randomised controlled trial of clinical outcome. BMJ 1998;316:1052–7.
6. Parvin CA, Lo SF, Deuser SM, Weaver LG, Lewis LM, Scott MG. Impact of point-of-care testing on patients' length of stay in a large emergency department. Clin Chem 1996;42:711–7.
7. Nicholls JH, Kickler TS, Dyer KL, Humbertson SK, Cooper PC, Maughan WL, et al. Clinical outcomes of point-of-care testing in

the interventional radiology and invasive cardiology setting. Clin Chem 2000;46:543–50.

8. Lee-Lewandrowski E, Corboy D, Lewandrowski K, Sinclair J, McDermot S, Benzer T. Implementation of a point-of-care satellite laboratory in the emergency department of an academic medical center. Arch Pathol Lab Med 2003;127:456–60.

9. Foster K, Despotis G, Scott MG. Point-of-care testing: cost issues and impact on hospital operations. Clin Lab Med 2001; 21:269–84.

10. Scott MG. Faster is better—it's rarely that simple! [Editorial]. Clin Chem 2000;46:441–2.

11. Kost GJ, Ehrmeyer SS, Chernow B, Winkelman JW, Zaloga GP, Dellinger RP, et al. The laboratory-clinical interface. Point-of-care testing. Chest 1999;115:1140–54.

12. Management and use of IVD point of care test devices. MDA DB 2002(03); London: Medical Devices Agency, March 2002.

13. Burnett D. Accreditation and point-of-care testing [Comment]. Ann Clin Biochem 2000;37:241–3.

14. Kohn LT, Corrigan JM, Donaldson MS, eds. Committee on Quality of Healthcare in America, Institute of Medicine. To err is human: building a safer health system. Washington, DC: National Academy Press, 2000.

15. Department of Health. An organisation with a memory [Report of an expert group on learning from adverse events in the NHS, chaired by the chief medical officer, Department of Health]. London: HM Stationery Office, 2000.

16. Greyson J. Quality control in patient self-monitoring of blood glucose. Diab Care 1993;16:1306–8.

17. Kost GJ. Preventing medical errors in point-of-care testing. Security, validation, performance, safeguards and connectivity. Arch Pathol Lab Med 2001;125:1307–15.

18. Witt DL. Frequency of unacceptable results in point-of-care testing. [Editorial]. Arch Pathol Lab Med 1999;123:761

19. Plebani M, Carraro P. Mistakes in a STAT laboratory: types and frequency. Clin Chem 1997;43:1348–51.

20. Jahn UR, Van Aken H. Near-patient testing—point-of-care or point of costs and convenience? [Editorial]. Brit J Anaesthes 2003;90:425–7.

21. Sanehi O. Near-patient testing [Letter]. Brit J Anaesthes 2003; 90:608.

22. Gray TA, Freedman DB, Burnett D, Szczepura A, Price CP. Evidence based practice: clinicians' use and attitudes to near patient testing in hospitals. J Clin Pathol 1996;49:903–08.

Chapter **13**

Quality Control and Quality Assurance in Point-of-Care Testing

David G. Bullock

Though there are many definitions of quality, the most useful is *fitness for purpose*. In laboratory medicine this requires the right result for the right investigation on the right specimen from the right patient, available at the right time, interpreted using the right reference data, and produced at the right cost. The consequences of lack of quality include the following:

- Inappropriate treatment
- Inappropriate further investigation
- Failure to give indicated treatment
- Failure to investigate further
- Delay in clinical decision making
- Increase in costs

The quality of investigations, whether by point-of-care testing (POCT) or by conventional laboratory testing, must therefore be sufficient to permit reliable use of results to support patient care.

Quality assurance (QA) is a management approach that attempts to ensure the attainment of quality, enabling appropriate and timely clinical action. QA thus encompasses much more than analytical quality—"the right result."

POCT presents particular quality concerns. Surveys have shown that POCT, carried out by nonlaboratory staff outside conventional laboratories, is widespread in both the hospital sector and the community, with an increasing range of tests and number of testing sites. Systems used for POCT continue to develop, with more aspects of quality built in or controlled through manufacturing quality control. The equipment and procedures are increasingly sophisticated in design and seem easy to use, but quality is not provided automatically and effective QA is essential. Indeed, in some situations greater reliability of central laboratory investigations may outweigh the advantages of POCT (1).

Before POCT is introduced or extended there must be discussion and agreement of the pattern for service provision and its management (including quality assurance), based on clinical needs. Even where investigations are agreed to be appropriate for POCT, there should be an ongoing audit of the quality and effectiveness of testing in the interests of reliable patient care.

QUALITY SYSTEMS

The most effective management tool for ensuring quality in any situation is a quality system. A range of quality systems are in use, though there is increasing use of the International Organization for Standardization's (ISO) ISO 9000:2000 series of international standards. ISO 9001:2000 (2) may be used directly, with independent certification of compliance, or indirectly through incorporation in an accreditation body's standards (3) based on its medical laboratory counterpart ISO 15189:2003 (4). Accreditation and quality systems are, in principle, as applicable to POCT as to conventional laboratory services, though practice and legislation may differ from country to country.

Components of a Quality System

There are many components of a quality system, all of which should be in place and operating before the end product of quality services is likely to be fully achieved. Excessive attention to any of the individual components to the neglect of others will not achieve lasting improvements in quality, and a balanced approach is essential.

Quality Assurance (QA). QA is the total process to support the quality of the testing service, comprising all the various measures taken to ensure reliability of investigations. These measures start with the selection of appropriate tests; then obtaining of a satisfactory specimen from the right patient; followed by accurate and precise analysis, prompt and correct recording of the result with an appropriate interpretation, and subsequent action on the result. Adequate documentation forms the basis of a quality assurance system in achieving standardization of methods and traceability of results on individual specimens. Regular monitoring of equipment, preventive maintenance, and repair when needed are other important components of quality assurance.

Quality assurance must not be limited to technical procedures. All those who obtain specimens for analysis should contribute significantly to the reliability of the results through correct specimen collection, identification, and handling. Inappropriate specimen collection is a major source of variation, which must be minimized through careful training and adequate supervision.

Internal Quality Control (IQC).   IQC assesses, in real time, whether the performance of an individual testing site is sufficiently similar to its previous performance for results to be issued. Thus IQC controls reproducibility or precision, enhancing credibility in ensuring that sequential results are comparable and maintaining continuity of patient care. Most IQC procedures employ analysis of a defined control material and ascertain that the results obtained are within previously established limits of acceptability.

External Quality Assessment (EQA; Proficiency Testing).   EQA, by contrast with IQC, compares the performance of different methods and different testing sites. This is made possible by the analysis of an identical specimen at many sites followed by the comparison of individual results with those of other sites and the "correct" answer. The process is necessarily retrospective, and provides an assessment of performance rather than a true control for each test performed on patients' specimens.

Audit.   An audit is a process of critical review. An internal audit is a review of local processes conducted by senior staff. Such reviews are aimed at measuring various parameters of performance, such as timeliness, accuracy, and costs of reports, and identifying weak points in the system where errors can occur. An external audit widens the input by involving others in the evaluation of analytical services. The users of services (usually clinical colleagues) are asked how they perceive the quality and relevance of the service provided. Comparison of procedures, working practices, costs, and workloads between hospitals by regular discussion between department heads, forms a part of the external audit.

Accreditation.   Accreditation of laboratories is a process of inspection by a third party to ensure conformance to certain predefined criteria. Factors that may be considered include the following:

- Numbers and qualifications of staff
- Training and education of staff
- Competency assessment
- Facilities available
- Procedures used
- Evidence of effective quality assurance and IQC procedures
- Participation in EQA schemes
- Adequate documentation
- Reporting procedures
- Safety
- Communications within the laboratory and with users
- Management structure

Initially, accreditation is commonly based on written statements of conformity (or reasons for nonconformity), followed up by inspection to verify. Accreditation may be linked to a formal system of licensing, whereby only accredited testing sites are legally entitled to practice, or may be a voluntary system. In many cases accreditation of POCT sites is subsidiary to the accreditation of the laboratory that is responsible for them, though independent accreditation of a POCT site may be appropriate in some circumstances (particularly if a wide range of investigations is offered).

Validation of Results.   Validation is an attempt to measure quality by reexamination of specimens. This may be carried out by formal referral procedures, where results obtained with specimens submitted to a laboratory are checked against the POCT site's results; this may be for all or a sample of specimens. For qualitative tests, fixed percentages of negative and positive specimens reported may be selected for reexamination in a laboratory.

Good Manufacturing Practice (GMP).   GMP is the system by which manufacturers of reagents and equipment ensure the quality of their products. GMP is an element within the European Union Directive on in vitro Diagnostic Medical Devices (5). The component factors of GMP include the following:

- Traceability of components and processes
- Documentation
- Quality control of components and quality control of the product independent of the manufacturing procedures
- Adequate facilities
- Conformity with safety regulations
- Proper labeling, packaging, and product information

GMP is relevant to POCT in two ways. First, where alternatives exist, reagents and equipment should be purchased from manufacturers that can demonstrate that they follow GMP (or equivalent national regulations). Second, some laboratories act as manufacturers through production of reagents, control materials, or quality assessment materials, for internal use or for provision to POCT sites. Such laboratories must consider the application of GMP and related regulations to their manufacturing activities.

Training and Education.   This is probably the single most important component in any quality assurance program. Issues to be addressed include national policies and curricula for staff training, both during primary training and on an ongoing in-service basis. Professional status and career development are related factors. Training of medical students and nurses in the use of laboratory facilities and on where POCT may be appropriate is also important. Training needs should be continually monitored, and where new needs arise (such as, for example, introduction of new procedures), or where QA reveals the need for improvements, courses and workshops may be introduced.

Evaluation.   Evaluation of appropriate reagents and equipment for suitability for use may make significant contributions to overall quality. Choice of equipment and reagents requires considerable thought and coordination, and may be cost-effective in reducing duplication of effort and preventing repetition of expensive mistakes. It cannot be assumed that equipment and assays designed for use in one situation will perform well in another. In addition to analytical performance considerations, procedures should be selected according to rational practicability criteria that might include the following:

- Cost of purchase
- Cost per test (fully loaded)
- Revenue consequences
- The appropriateness of the technology
- Robustness under local operating conditions
- Level of skill required to operate
- Availability of spares and repair/support services

Likewise, choice of diagnostic assays must take account of similar factors, such as the effect of transport times and storage conditions, including humidity and temperature, and the degree of skill needed in reading the assay in the POCT setting. The predictive value of some tests (e.g., in microbiology) will depend on the sensitivity and specificity under local conditions with the population to be investigated, and these must be determined before valid interpretations can be made. Unfortunately, initial evaluation cannot guarantee the quality of subsequent batches of reagents, so some system of continual monitoring is advisable.

Documentation.   Documentation of all procedures is a universal accreditation requirement, and incorporation within a quality manual framework in accordance with ISO 9000:2000 standards is highly desirable.

QUALITY ASSURANCE TOOLS FOR POINT-OF-CARE TESTING

Three main tools are available for assuring quality:

- *Quality assurance (QA)* includes all measures taken to ensure the reliability of investigations, starting from test selection through obtaining a satisfactory specimen from the right patient, analyzing it, and recording the result promptly and correctly, to appropriate interpretation and action on the result, with all procedures being documented for reference.
- *Internal quality control (IQC)* assesses, in real time, whether the performance of an individual testing site is sufficiently similar to its previous performance for results to be used; it controls reproducibility or precision and facilitates continuity of patient care over time. Most IQC procedures employ analysis of a control material and compare the result with preset limits of acceptability—unsatisfactory sets of results may thereby be suppressed.
- *External quality assessment (EQA; proficiency testing)*, by contrast, looks at differences between testing sites, so that there can be continuity of care over geography (including among clinical units and between clinical unit and laboratory, in the case of POCT) and over time. Common mechanisms include analysis of identical specimens at many testing sites, and comparison of results with those of other sites and a "correct" answer; the process is necessarily retrospective.

The appropriate implementation and use of these tools, and appropriate support for quality in POCT, are reviewed in turn.

Quality Assurance

All laboratories apply QA procedures, but the requirements in POCT differ. Because results from POCT and laboratory investigations may be used interchangeably, the overriding need is for local comparability of results, which requires good IQC practices complemented by EQA. General quality assurance measures are essential in providing a secure basis within which this analytical quality control can be effective. In addition to the aspects mentioned above, any testing site must employ well-chosen, reliable procedures and equipment, carried out by trained, competent, motivated staff on correctly collected specimens in an environment which is safe, clean, well-lit, and appropriate to the task, and provide results that are recorded correctly.

QA is especially critical for POCT (Table 13-1). Staff must first have sufficient time to carry out the testing and all associated QA measures; otherwise they will be performed poorly and ineffectively. Responsibilities of staff should be clear, and testing should be included in their formal job descriptions. The overall responsibilities for POCT management must be clear, with active cooperation and collaboration among the various departments involved (e.g., 6–8). An overall institution (e.g., hospital) policy for POCT, based on relevant legislation and regulations, along with professional societies' guidelines and advice issued by the health authorities, should be in place; POCT can usually only be included in the scope of accreditation where it is carried out under such a policy. Identification of a lead individual, such as a link nurse, at each testing site (e.g., hospital ward or primary healthcare location) has proved to be helpful for liaison and communication.

Selection of test procedures and equipment has quality implications. In addition to stability, robustness, and reliability in the proposed situation, ease of use, acceptability to staff, and ease of training should be considered. In particular, the fewer operator-dependent steps are involved, the lower the chance of

Table 13-1   Major Quality Assurance Determinants in Point-of-Care Testing

Time to do the testing
Equipment/method selection
    System evaluation and performance assessment
    Operator-dependence
    Procedure harmonization
Operator training
    Specimen collection and identification
    Training and retraining
    Certification of competence
Good laboratory practice
    Maintenance
    Continuity of supplies
    Health and safety
    Patient identification and recording
    Results recording and information system implications
    Internal quality control (IQC)
    External quality assessment (EQA)

errors leading to unreliable results. Where staff are expected to carry out a range of investigations, mistakes are less likely if the operational procedures are all similar; the use of systems using conflicting procedures (e.g., one requiring wiping of reagent strips and another that is invalidated by wiping) should be avoided.

Staff must then be properly trained, by laboratory staff or by the commercial supplier, using a documented procedure. Training will include not only the test procedure (e.g., also any equipment maintenance) but also specimen collection. However good the testing (whether by POCT or in a laboratory), it cannot improve on a poor specimen, and the variability inherent in collection of the capillary blood used in much POCT can greatly outweigh test variability. Competence after training should be checked and certificated, with periodic verification and/or retraining to ensure continued competence; inclusion in the organization's retraining curriculum for nurses (which normally includes fire and safety training) may be helpful in ensuring release from duties for this to be carried out. Staff may be reminded that unauthorized use of POCT systems can leave them personally liable for incorrect results and could be a disciplinary matter.

Specimen collection is a major source of variation in POCT, and it is impossible to use IQC measures to control this; the variation must be minimized through careful training in the necessary procedures, with continuing supervision and vigilance.

In addition to the investigation itself, other aspects of good laboratory practice must be remembered. These include regular maintenance, health and safety implications, and accurate and accessible recording of all results and procedures. Results recording may have implications for information systems, since all results should be entered into the patient's record; accessibility from the laboratory for surveillance purposes may also be essential for microbiology data. Accurate recording requires reliable association of results and specimen with patient identity. Experience indicates that correct entry of patient identification is a continuing problem, with reported error rates of 1–3%; monitoring, auditing, and corrective action through education or retraining appear essential to maintaining this level of accuracy.

Ensuring continuous availability of within-date supplies without wastage due to expiry before use is a major problem, especially where usage is low, and such wastage can dramatically increase the cost of POCT. Good inventory control is essential. All these aspects can be included in a comprehensive support package for POCT from the laboratory, which may also include the pharmacy for consumable supplies and monitoring.

Internal Quality Control

IQC in laboratory medicine was developed by adaptation of control systems used in the manufacturing industry. However, clinical specimens are not expected to be identical, so quality control material must be included with each batch of patients' specimens to probe the performance of an analytical system.

Westgard (9) provides a comprehensive strategy for introducing quality control. Validated procedures have been evolved for the statistical interpretation of control data generated from quantitative (numerical) analyses, though these may not be directly transferable to establishments carrying out POCT (10). Some of the systems used in decentralized testing either do not require any calibration (standardization) by the user, as they are factory-calibrated, or require infrequent recalibration. Much of the variability of results from these methods originates from variations in operator technique. The analysis of an appropriate control material before starting and during analysis of clinical specimens can provide reassurance that the system and operator are working correctly.

It is essential that the results obtained with control materials are recorded and interpreted. Representation in graphical form is strongly recommended, and should be instinctive for nursing staff used to plotting and interpreting trends in observations on patients; experience, however, suggests that even these staff are resistant to plotting IQC data. For a quantitative analysis, control results must be compared with acceptance limits that have been determined from previous experience. The acceptance ranges quoted by manufacturers often include between-site and between-lot variability and are therefore inappropriately wide for control use at a single site; use of such ranges may lead to reporting of results that are unacceptable. Control limits must be realistic and based on within-site experience with the system, which is normally expressed in terms of the standard deviation (SD) obtained by repeated analysis on different days; the mean value provides the target value for a control chart.

For POCT use, results may conveniently be plotted on a control chart, with concentration as the y axis and batch number (usually day) as the x axis; this classical approach facilitates decision making if horizontal lines are drawn at the mean (expected) value and at 2 SD and 3 SD above and below the mean value, as shown in Figure 13-1. If the analysis is in

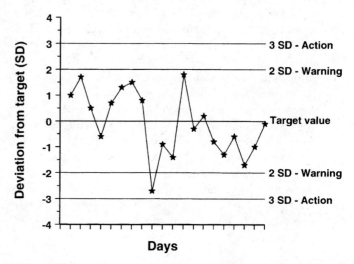

Figure 13-1   Shewhart control chart; daily analysis of one control material, with warning limits set at ± 2 SD and action limits at ± 3 SD from the target value.

control, results will be scattered randomly above and below the expected value, the distribution being such that only 1 in 20 (5%) will be more than 2 SD from the mean and only 1 in 100 (1%) more than 3 SD from the mean. Loss of precision, however, will yield a wider scatter of results, whereas loss of accuracy will cause a shift to higher or lower values; these changes can be seen on the graphical presentation (Shewhart control chart) and corrective action taken. It is common to set two limits, the first a "warning" limit indicating that the system is moving out of control and requires investigation, and the second an "action" limit indicating that the system is seriously out of control and that results from specimens in the batch should not be reported. These limits normally correspond to ± 2 SD (warning) and ± 3 SD (action).

More complex and effective control rules have been formulated, notably by Westgard and co-workers, who have validated their power (to reject unsatisfactory batches and accept satisfactory batches) using computer simulation studies. These "Westgard rules" for the interpretation of control data using two materials analyzed once in each batch have been published as a proposed selected method (10), and are given in Table 13-2. If both control results are within 2 SD from their target, the batch is accepted. If at least one control result is more than 2 SD from the target, the remaining rules are evaluated in turn, and the batch rejected if any one rule is satisfied. If none is satisfied, the batch is accepted, but the situation should be investigated before the next batch is analyzed.

If only one control material is analyzed in each batch, a simplified modification known as "Wheeler rules" (11) applies, with more stringent action rules. Whichever approach is adopted, written procedures must be prepared for the interpretation of control data and the action required. Most IQC procedures require a QC material, which must be stable and reliable. It is unwise to rely totally on control material provided by the manufacturer (particularly with an immunological assay) as part of a kit, as these are designed to control individual lots and do not provide continuity of control between reagent lots. Use of an independent control will allow comparison between lots and provide assurance of the reliability of the product. It must be noted that not all control materials are suitable for all systems—and may produce different results even if they are suitable—as they are essentially artificial, stabilized materials that are not necessarily compatible with the design features of all assays. It is important to ensure that the material used is compatible with the system used, by using either a material which the manufacturer states is suitable or a material which has been shown to give the same precision with the system as clinical specimens.

IQC must be run with appropriate frequency. Ideally, IQC should be run with every batch of clinical specimens, but this may not be practicable or necessary. In POCT specimens are often analyzed individually rather than in batches, and running IQC once per operator per shift (before analyzing their first clinical specimen) appears satisfactory in most situations. If staff are reluctant to carry out IQC due to "lack of time," then work practices should be reviewed to ensure they have sufficient time not only to perform assays on patients but also to implement this important safeguard for patient care.

POCT systems contain increasingly sophisticated data storage and manipulation elements. Through connectivity, for which standards are being developed, these enable download of IQC as well as patients' results (12), thus simplifying record keeping. Though useful for confirmation, subsequent analysis of the data cannot substitute for assessment at the time or the control function of IQC is lost.

For single-use devices without an instrument for reading the result, internal procedural controls may have been built in by the manufacturer. These are designed to ensure that results can only be obtained if the specimen has been applied properly and the reagents have worked correctly, and are particularly useful for nonquantitative, e.g., "positive or negative," investigations. Nevertheless, acceptance testing of each lot or container of devices with positive and negative controls may provide an invaluable quality control measure before issue to testing sites.

Some newer systems are equipped with electronic QC. Here a dummy device module mimics electronically the output from a real device, so that the reading instrument gives a valid reading; the same module may mimic several different concentrations. These modules are stable and provide an excellent validation that the reading instrument is working correctly for maintenance or troubleshooting purposes; they have been developed particularly for situations where valid specimens are difficult or impossible to provide, and their use is better than applying no IQC at all. However, they do not test either the operator's technique (e.g., for sample application) or the correct function of the measurement device (which may have deteriorated in shipment or through faulty storage or handling). Of course the specimen collection stage itself is excluded by

Table 13-2   Westgard Rules for Interpretation of IQC Data

Rules Apply Where Two Control Specimens Are Analyzed Each Day		
1_{2S}	Warning	1 result more than 2 SD from target
1_{3S}	Action	1 result more than 3 SD from target
2_{2S}	Action	2 consecutive results more than 2 SD from target in same direction
R_{4S}	Action	Difference between the two control results exceeds 4 SD
4_{1S}	Action	4 consecutive results more than 1 SD from target in same direction
10_{X}	Action	10 consecutive results same side of mean

most IQC and EQA procedures, but electronic modules must not be considered fully equivalent to effective IQC (13).

Much of the emphasis has been laid on the individual operator, who must be supported through education, training, and availability of advice. If problems occur, however, in almost all cases the system (a combination of the analytical system and work practices) rather than the individual is at fault, and the total system should be reviewed to try to avoid recurrence.

Performance Standards and External Quality Assessment

What standard of performance is required for POCT? The rapid turnaround time and other advantages of POCT may justify a management decision to implement it in specific situations and accept lower quality (although this may not always be the case) from POCT. The consequences for patient care must be assessed carefully, however, as the general principle is that the same quality standards should apply irrespective of testing site (14). Recent developments help assess the acceptability of performance against the "six sigma" approach to quality management (15).

Studies on glucose and other quantitative clinical chemistry tests in the United Kingdom have indicated that performance in a POCT situation gives a spread of 1.5–2 times that of laboratory assays when using similar equipment, and 2.5–3 times when using POCT systems such as glucose meters (16). Experience in the United States also confirms greater variability of analyses in a nonlaboratory situation (17). Though systems have improved and agreement for users of a single procedure is now tighter, this remains generally true. For cholesterol at least, the major contribution to between-laboratory variability comes from calibration differences, whereas for POCT procedures operator variability is the dominant contributor.

Many studies have also highlighted the problems of using artificial materials in EQA of a range of POCT procedures, due to matrix effects (e.g., 18, 19). Technological developments have increased rather than decreased dependence on the nature of the specimen, and their intended use is often for fresh blood without anticoagulant, still warm from the patient's finger. No ideal QC material has yet been developed, and studies have used a wide range of materials for blood glucose analysis, from colorless aqueous solutions through colored artificial materials with or without erythrocytes to stabilized whole blood preparations; some are available commercially. Colorless solutions give no assurance of sample application, and can thus present difficulties to operators. The selection of materials to be used may be dictated by the systems to be included, with in some cases different materials and in most cases different target values being required for different analytical systems (19).

Rather than distribute QC materials, some centers have used collection of a dried blood spot specimen for laboratory analysis and comparison with the POCT result (20). This approach avoids the material-related uncertainties by using clinical specimens, and should be capable of greater comparison frequency; indeed it may reduce the requirement for IQC. Though it requires more work by the laboratory in confirmatory analysis and does not provide a direct estimate of between-site variability, no specimens have to be prepared or distributed, and the problems of obtaining EQA results returns from participating sites should be minimized. Others have used the results of concurrent laboratory and POCT analyses, identified from the laboratory information system, to monitor and assess the comparability of POCT with the laboratory, with follow-up of discrepancies leading to improvement (21).

Though EQA provides assessment of the overall standard of performance and the influence of analytical procedures (methods, reagents, instruments, and calibration), its usual application is in the assessment of performance of individual sites.

External Quality Assessment Scheme Design

For an EQA scheme to be successful as an educational stimulus to improvement, participants must have confidence in the validity of the scheme design as well as reliability of operation, or they will not take action on information conveyed in reports. Experience with many schemes has indicated some essential design criteria for laboratory schemes (22):

1. Sufficient recent data, achieved through:
   - Frequent distributions
   - Rapid feedback of performance information after analysis
2. Effective communication of performance data, through:
   - A cumulative scoring system
   - Structured, informative, and intelligible reports
3. An appropriate basis for assessment, including:
   - Stable, homogeneous specimens which behave like clinical specimens
   - Reliable and valid target values

Specimens must be treated as near as possible to the way clinical specimens are dealt with, if the scheme is to provide an objective assessment of the participants' performance.

Scheme design for POCT may, however, differ from usual practice for laboratory participation. Reports should be predominantly graphical, containing no performance scores, with interpretation being performed by the organizing center to give helpful comments where performance appears inadequate; an example is shown as Figure 13-2. Participants with problems

Figure 13-2 Example of an external quality assessment scheme report for POCT cholesterol assay; data are presented graphically, with comments on performance where appropriate. Reprinted with permission from Wolfson EQA Laboratory, Birmingham, UK.

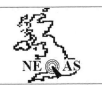

		WRL Extra-laboratory Cholesterol EQAS	Identity
	Distribution : 91	Date : 16-Jan-2004	Page 1 of 3
	Analyte : Cholesterol (mmol/L)		

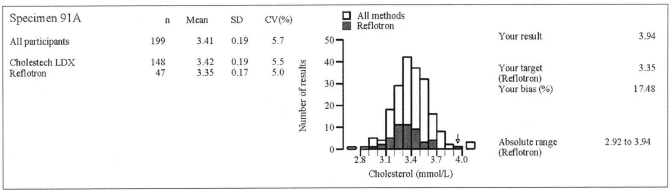

Specimen 91A

	n	Mean	SD	CV(%)
All participants	199	3.41	0.19	5.7
Cholestech LDX	148	3.42	0.19	5.5
Reflotron	47	3.35	0.17	5.0

Your result 3.94

Your target (Reflotron) 3.35

Your bias (%) 17.48

Absolute range (Reflotron) 2.92 to 3.94

Specimen 91B

	n	Mean	SD	CV(%)
All participants	207	7.06	0.39	5.6
Cholestech LDX	148	6.99	0.34	4.9
Accutrend GC	10	7.43	0.30	4.1
Reflotron	47	7.22	0.39	5.4

Your result 8.06

Your target (Reflotron) 7.22

Your bias (%) 11.61

Absolute range (Reflotron) 6.42 to 8.06

Specimen 91C

	n	Mean	SD	CV(%)
All participants	207	4.61	0.21	4.6
Cholestech LDX	148	4.57	0.20	4.3
Accutrend GC	10	4.68	0.18	3.8
Reflotron	47	4.73	0.23	4.8

Your result 4.92

Your target (Reflotron) 4.73

Your bias (%) 3.92

Absolute range (Reflotron) 4.26 to 5.57

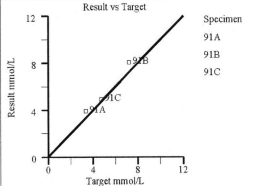

Specimen	Result	Target
91A	3.94	3.35
91B	8.06	7.22
91C	4.92	4.73

One of your results was more than 15% from the target value. The pattern of your results shows variability in their relationship to the target values. This suggests a problem of technique or possibly lack of care, and you should check the technique used against the instrument manual recommendations.

WRL Extra-laboratory Cholesterol EQAS, Wolfson EQA Laboratory,
PO Box 3909, Birmingham B15 2UE, U K
Phone (direct): 0121-414 7300;   FAX: 0121-414 1179

may be referred to the equipment supplier, who is often best placed to provide assistance (23). Similar schemes cover hematology as well as clinical chemistry assays (24).

National and Local Schemes

National EQA schemes can offer an assessment of the true standard of performance nationally and promote comparability. The number of POCT sites and the problems of communicating with them, along with the compromises inherent in stabilized specimens and selection of target values, may make such schemes impracticable. The lack of familiarity of many POCT participants with the concepts of EQA can lead to problems, and further uncertainties surround the issues of responsibility for the results and for performance surveillance. The main difficulty, however, remains the inability to contact and assist participants effectively if problems are seen.

EQA on a national scale therefore cannot be the complete solution for POCT. The systems used often require specimens of limited stability, the organizing center must carry out some of the interpretative role, and feedback must be fast and effective if problems are noted. These factors point toward the local provision of EQA, both in the hospital sector and in primary care. National EQA may still be preferable for specialized investigations, and essential where there is no access to local laboratory support, e.g., where laboratory staff are unwilling or the testing sites (e.g., occupational health units in industry and commerce) are outside the conventional healthcare system.

In the local situation EQA should be easier, particularly if there is agreement to use a single procedure. More important, the laboratory can contact the operator and visit if necessary. "Parallel" or "split-sample" testing (at both the POCT site and in the laboratory) can be a useful QA tool provided it is planned and the comparative data are recorded and scrutinized (25). Local schemes (e.g., 26) may form an integral part of a support system for POCT, including QA and maintenance.

As an example of a successful local scheme, Stahl et al. (27) used fresh, unstabilized, whole blood samples for EQA of blood glucose in primary care locations. These samples were prepared in the laboratory and taken to doctors' offices by a technologist; results were compared with an estimation performed in the central laboratory. Proficiency of testing was found to have improved (the proportion of results outside acceptable limits decreasing from 12% to 3%) after a program of consultation and assistance was instituted. It must be recognized that the costs of such schemes, including usage of staff resources, are not trivial.

The widespread implementation of local schemes, however, leads to fragmentation of data and loss of information. It is therefore difficult or impossible to draw reliable conclusions on the general standard of performance nationally. A partial answer is to use a national audit (e.g., Q-Probes), or to establish a network of local schemes with similar design and specimens so data can be collated to approximate a national picture (28).

SUPPORT SYSTEMS FOR POINT-OF-CARE TESTING

In any situation where investigations are required, it is essential to examine the circumstances and needs, then agree which should be carried out by a laboratory and which (if any) by POCT. This should ensure that all investigations are relevant and reliable, with appropriate resourcing to assure quality.

The optimal approach for POCT would thus be for a clinical laboratory (i.e., one which can support continuously and provide follow-up to resolve difficulties rapidly and effectively) to work with the departments and organizations as part of a multidisciplinary team to support the service (8, 26, 29). Such support should encompass assistance with system selection (standardization of products used can be helpful), site assessment, operator training, ongoing equipment maintenance, and an effective analytical quality control program including IQC and EQA. Designation of one individual, usually a laboratory professional, to take responsibility for quality as coordinator for POCT is helpful (e.g., 7, 29). The paramount need is for results from POCT to be interchangeable with laboratory results, to permit continuity of patient management (30). Support must be provided on a continuing and continual basis, including availability for consultation and personal visits to the testing site for consultation and maintenance. Such systems form the basis of many professional recommendations on POCT (e.g., 31, 32) and may be required for laboratory accreditation (3, 33, 34), and should improve the incomplete quality assurance systems found in many POCT situations (35). Indeed, it has been shown that guidelines and regulation have led to improved quality assurance practices in POCT (36).

Support in this manner must be costed realistically, and decentralized testing systems with appropriate quality assurance mechanisms are almost certain to require more resources than laboratory-based analysis (37).

CONCLUSIONS

Quality investigations are essential to support reliable patient care, and quality must be attained irrespective of who does the test and where it is carried out. The emphasis of QA measures, however, depends on these factors, and in POCT the emphasis must lie with general QA measures. The time to do the testing, operator training and monitoring, and reliable specimen collection are essential QA elements. IQC provides assurance of correct operation, increasingly through inbuilt procedural controls. Local EQA forming part of a support system is also desirable. Successful implementation of POCT requires a multidisciplinary approach to its management. The principles outlined here will remain valid as the scope and technology of POCT continue to develop, but the appropriate implementation requirements will require periodic reexamination to ensure continuing applicability.

REFERENCES

1. Kost GJ, Ehrmeyer SS, Chernow B, Winkelman JW, Zaloga GP, Dellinger RP, et al. The laboratory-clinical interface: point-of-care testing. Chest 1999;115:1140–54.

2. ISO 9001:2000. Quality management systems—Requirements. Geneva: International Organization for Standardization, 2000.

3. Jansen RT, Blaton V, Burnett D, Huisman W, Queralto JM, Zerah S, Allman B. Additional essential criteria for quality systems of medical laboratories European Community Confederation of Clinical Chemistry (EC4) Working Group on Harmonisation of Quality Systems and Accreditation. Clin Chem Lab Med 1998; 36:249–52.

4. ISO 15189:2003. Medical laboratories—particular requirements for quality and competence. Geneva: International Organization for Standardization, 2003.

5. Directive 98/79/EC of the European Parliament and of the Council of 27 October 1998 on in vitro diagnostic medical devices. OJ L 331, 7.12.1998, 1–37.

6. Jacobs E, Hinson KA, Tolnai J, Simson E. Implementation, management and continuous quality improvement of point-of-care testing in an academic health care setting. Clin Chim Acta 2001;307:49–59.

7. Freedman DB. Clinical governance: implications for point-of-care testing. Ann Clin Biochem 2002;39:421–3.

8. MDA DB2002(03). Management and use of IVD point of care test devices. London: Medical Devices Agency, 2002.

9. Westgard JO. Internal quality control: planning and implementation strategies. Ann Clin Biochem 2003;40:593–611.

10. Westgard JO, Barry PL, Hunt. A multi-rule Shewhart chart for quality control in clinical chemistry. Clin Chem 1981;27:493–501.

11. Wheeler DJ. Detecting a shift in process average: tables of the power function for charts. J Qual Technol 1983;15:155–70.

12. Searles B, Nasrallah F, Graham S, Tozer M. Electronic data management for the Hemochron Jr. Signature coagulation analyzer. J Extra Corpor Technol 2002;34:182–4.

13. Westgard JO. Electronic quality control, the total testing process, and the total quality control system. Clin Chim Acta 2001;307: 45–8.

14. Fraser CG. Optimal analytical performance for point of care testing. Clin Chim Acta 2001;307:37–43.

15. Westgard JO. From method performance claims to six sigma metrics: a POC chemistry analyser. Available at http://www.westgard.com/qcapp25.htm (accessed April 15, 2004).

16. Browning DM, Bullock DG. The quality of extra-laboratory assays: evidence from external quality assessment surveys. Ann Clin Biochem 1987;24(S1):171–2.

17. Hurst J, Nickel K, Hilborne LH. Are physicians' office laboratory results of comparable quality to those produced in other laboratory settings? JAMA 1998;279:468–71.

18. van den Besselaar AM. Accuracy, precision, and quality control for point-of-care testing of oral anticoagulation. J Thromb Thrombolysis 2001;12:35–40.

19. Wood DG, Hanke R, Meissner D, Reinauer H. Experience with an external quality assessment programme for point-of-care-testing (POCT) devices for the determination of blood glucose. Clin Lab 2003;49:151–9.

20. Burrin JM, Williams DRR, Price CP. Performance of a quality assurance scheme for blood glucose meters in general practice. Ann Clin Biochem 1985;22:148–51.

21. Kilgore ML, Steindel SJ, Smith JA. Continuous quality improvement for point-of-care testing using background monitoring of duplicate specimens. Arch Pathol Lab Med 1999;123:824–8.

22. Bullock DG. Proficiency testing of laboratories—methods and outcomes. Anal Proc 1992;29:189–90.

23. Broughton PMG, Bullock DG, Cramb R. Improving the quality of plasma cholesterol measurements in primary care. Scand J Clin Lab Invest 1990;198:43–8.

24. Woods TAL, Jennings I, Kitchen S, Preston FE. Near patient testing in blood coagulation: 18 months of UK National External Quality Assessment Scheme surveys. Br J Haem 1998;102: 260–4.

25. Novis DA, Jones BA. Interinstitutional comparison of bedside blood glucose monitoring program characteristics, accuracy performance, and quality control documentation: a College of American Pathologists Q-Probes study of bedside blood glucose monitoring performed in 226 small hospitals. Arch Pathol Lab Med 1998;122:495–502.

26. Hortas ML, Montiel N, Redondo M, Medina A, Contreras E, Cortes C, et al. Quality assurance of point-of-care testing in the Costa del Sol Healthcare Area (Marbella, Spain). Clin Chim Acta 2001;307:113–8.

27. Stahl M, Brandslund I, Iversen S, Filtenborg JA. Quality assessment of blood glucose testing in general practitioners' offices improves quality. Clin Chem 1997;43:1926–31.

28. Howanitz PJ, Jones BA. Bedside glucose monitoring. Comparison of performance as studied by the College of American Pathologists Q-Probes program. Arch Pathol Lab Med 1996;120: 333–8.

29. Kost GJ. Preventing medical errors in point-of-care testing: security, validation, safeguards, and connectivity. Arch Pathol Lab Med 2001;125:1307–15.

30. Cachia PG, McGregor E, Adlakha S, Davey P, Goudie BM. Accuracy and precision of the TAS analyser for near-patient INR testing by non-pathology staff in the community. J Clin Pathol 1998;51:68–72.

31. Anderson JR, Linsell WD, Mitchell FM. Chemical pathology on the ward. Guidelines on the performance of clinical pathology assays outside the laboratory. Lancet 1981;317:487.

32. Guidelines for near patient testing: haematology. Near Patient Testing Working Party. General Haematology Task Force of BCSH. Thrombosis and Haemostasis Task Force of BCSH. Clin Lab Haem 1995;17:301–10.

33. Laessig RH, Ehrmeyer SS, Hassemer DJ. Quality control and quality assurance. Clin Lab Med 1986;6:317–27.

34. Ehrmeyer SS, Laessig RH. Regulatory requirements (CLIA '88, JCAHO, CAP) for decentralized testing. Am J Clin Pathol 1995; 104:S40–9.

35. Hilton S, Rink E, Fletcher J, Sibbald B, Freeling P, Szczepura A, et al. Near patient testing in general practice: attitudes of general practitioners and practice nurses, and quality assurance procedures carried out. Br J Gen Pract 1994;44:577–80.

36. Binns HJ, LeBailly S, Gardner HG. The physicians' office laboratory: 1988 and 1996 survey of Illinois pediatricians. Arch Pediatr Adolesc Med 1998;152:585–92.

37. Lee-Lewandrowski E, Laposata M, Eschenbach K, Camooso C, Nathan DM, Godine JE, et al. Utilization and cost analysis of bedside capillary glucose testing in a large teaching hospital: Implications for managing point of care testing. Am J Med 1994;97:222–30.

Chapter 14

Unit-Use Quality Control
David L. Phillips

The following are the objectives of this chapter: (*a*) Provide an overview of the history and evolution of unit-use test systems; (*b*) review various quality control (QC) enhancements for unit-use test systems; (*c*) describe the development of the National Committee on Clinical Laboratory Standards (NCCLS) guideline, the Quality Management for Unit-Use Testing, EP18-A; and (*d*) outline a suggested method for establishing and managing a quality systems program.

HISTORY AND EVOLUTION OF UNIT-USE TEST SYSTEMS

History provides numerous examples of process controls applied to unit-use or single-test systems. Perhaps the most common is that of the *aca*® analyzer in the 1960s (DuPont, Wilmington, DE, USA), followed by the Ektachem® system (Johnson & Johnson, Rochester, NY, USA). A much older and nonautomated example of unitized testing methods is the use of commercially prepared microbiology blood agar plates, which are, by definition, unit-use single-test systems. Performing QC on each plate before use would contaminate the plates, thereby making them unusable for patient samples. In 1984, the NCCLS formed the Subcommittee on Media Quality Control to specify the requirements for quality assurance (QA) of culture media. This work resulted in the publication of M-22, "Quality Assurance for Commercially Prepared Microbiological Culture Media." The proposed standard was published in 1985, the approved standard in 1990, and the second edition of the approved standard in December 1996. The basic premise of M-22 is that retesting of commercially prepared media, which imposes a substantial financial burden on the clinical microbiology laboratory, might not be necessary, particularly for media of proven reliability (1). The subcommittee was able to gauge reliability by referring to College of American Pathologists (CAP) surveys (2). From a Microbiology Proficiency Testing Survey representing >350,000 lots and accounting for 67×10^6 plates, tubes, or bottles, the subcommittee set a failure rate of 0.3% as being acceptable. In other words, users of media plates that meet this level of failure, as documented by the manufacturer, do not have to retest QC measures.

Testing systems have continued to improve by incorporating microsampling techniques and microprocessors, but QA programs have essentially not kept up with these improvements. QC procedures were first widely used in the late 1950s and early 1960s, when it became necessary to check the analytical processes of instruments. One of the first devices to demonstrate the need for QC was the AutoAnalyzer® (the SMA6/60; Bayer Diagnostics, Tarrytown, NY, USA). QC was recommended for each batch, defined as the number of patient samples to be processed at one time. After many years and a great deal of discussion, a "run" began to be defined by time (i.e., the number of hours—either an 8-h or a 24-h shift).

James Westgard of the University of Wisconsin, well known for his development of the Westgard multirules, has described the evolution of laboratory statistical QC practices (3). As he points out, one reason the first generation of QC measures was put into general practice in the early 1960s and 1970s was to promote the fact that laboratories were performing QC. The primary tracking method was the Levey–Jennings chart for graphing analytical QC results. Westgard's multirules, which utilized the Levey–Jennings charts to maximize error detection and minimize false rejections, ushered in second generation of QC in the 1980s. The third generation, Westgard suggests, could be QC designed for individualized tests to ensure detection of medically important errors at the lowest cost; in other words, what is the allowable error? However, this practice has not been widely used.

Westgard has noted that even as QC procedures were changing, updates and innovations on the part of in vitro diagnostic (IVD) instrument manufacturers were leading to considerable changes in the test instruments themselves. These innovations continued through four generations of IVD devices (i.e., manual methods, continuous flow, multitest parallel continuous flow, and highly precise/highly stable instrumentation). According to Westgard, however, QC laboratory statistical models stalled somewhere after the second generation. Therefore, he suggests that QC procedures must evolve through three generations very rapidly, or alternative methods must be developed.

QC procedures in the clinical laboratory may be less relevant for unit-use test systems, because they detect process changes such as reagent lot changes or major instrument maintenance. The additional process that takes place in a conventional diagnostic analyzer at a clinical laboratory has already occurred in the manufacturing environment (assuming the manufacturer has implemented conventional QC throughout the manufacturing process), rather than in the clinical laboratory. Moreover, with unit-use tests, conventional QC materials and methods cannot provide the necessary assurance that good laboratory practice has occurred in the case of nonunitized test systems.

The attempt to apply conventional QA methods to unconventional testing methods has caused both controversy and concern among testing facilities, regulators, and manufacturers. QC for unit-use test systems has been an interesting area, particularly since 1992. It has been a controversial area, because the conventional methods and procedures that have been in place for decades are not directly applicable to the processes and procedures necessary for unit-use test systems, although these methods have nevertheless continued to be used. Even though there were no formal industry guidelines or regulations, manufacturers began to incorporate new types of QC methods into their test systems.

QUALITY CONTROL ENHANCEMENTS FOR UNIT-USE TEST SYSTEMS

The simplest and most straightforward devices are the true single-test systems (i.e., those devices that render only one test result per specimen) The best example of this is the fingerstick glucose test strip. A test strip is inserted into the meter, then a blood sample is placed on the strip and read by the meter. There is no way to obtain another test value for QC on that test strip. In order to determine the reliability of the test, several checks can be implemented in the test system. First, the strips are tested with reference materials upon receipt. Once the strips have passed, they can be placed into a controlled environment that is monitored for consistency. As long as the environment remains static and there is no other change in the test system (e.g., new reagent lot, change in storage conditions, or maintenance), it can be assumed that testing with these strips will be reliable. The other components of the test system in this example are the meter and the operator. Once the strips have been verified, a meter and/or operator can be tested at some frequency with a reference sample to ensure meter reliability and operator competence.

Many systems incorporate a single-test strip or cartridge and a meter/reader that utilizes electronic features to report results. These systems often provide an electronic check for the meter/reader. Electronic checks do not require the use of a strip and/or control material. This additional QC method is most often called an electronic simulator or electronic QC (EQC). "Electronic quality control usually involves the substitution of an electrical signal for the signal that would normally be generated by a sensor responding to an analyte in a specimen; sometimes an artificial nonliquid sample is substituted to cause the sensor to generate an electrical signal (4)." The EQC unit (simulator) can be used repeatedly to check the reader portion without having to reconstitute control solutions or use the disposable portion of the test system.

Electronic QC is not new. Photometer checks, filter balance checks, cuvette checks, blank (zero) checks, and a variety of electronic voltage checks have long been used as part of the monitoring system for laboratory instruments (5).

Even though electronic quality checks have existed for a long time, they took on greater importance after the passage of the Clinical Laboratory Improvement Amendments of 1988 (CLIA '88). CLIA '88 regulations specified that for most analytes, a minimum of two levels of QC was necessary every 24 h of operation. For certain exceptions, such as hematology, coagulation, and blood gases, QC was required every 8 h of operation. In addition, if the manufacturer specified more frequent QC, the operator was required to follow the manufacturer's instructions. In 1995, the Health Care Financing Administration [HCFA—renamed the Centers for Medicare and Medicaid Services (CMS) in 2002] issued a memorandum to the CLIA surveyors stating that "EQC monitored only the electronic circuitry . . . results obtained by these electronic simulator controls provide only a pass or fail of the analyzer and do not provide actual analytical QC test results" (6).

After much debate, HCFA issued the following letter to i-STAT on February 28, 1996 (7):

> We have reexamined our decision regarding CLIA compliance of the i-STAT test system and the current CLIA QC regulatory requirements. . . Accordingly, based on the change in manufacturer's instructions to users of the i-STAT, the requirements of 42 CFR 493.1202(c)(4) and 493.1245 for blood gases would be met, if the recommendation [EQC every 8 h] is followed by the laboratory.

Once HCFA accepted the electronic QC as meeting the two levels of QC for each day of testing, other deemed agencies such as the Joint Commission on Accreditation of Healthcare Organizations (JCAHO) and the CAP followed suit.

This precipitated the promotion and proliferation of EQC by many manufacturers, which was particularly evident with whole blood coagulation analyzers, including a relatively large installed base of activated clotting time (ACT) instruments and a growing installed base of prothrombin time/activated partial thromboplastin time instruments.

The large installed base of ACT devices was the more significant of the two reasons. First, by the time CLIA '88 was implemented in 1992, the ACT instruments had been in the marketplace for over 20 years and for the most part had not been managed by the clinical laboratory. Second, once CLIA '88 was implemented, the ACT instruments, which were very common in the cardiovascular operating room and other locations within the hospital, became the responsibility of the CLIA license holder, which was usually the clinical laboratory.

With the clinical laboratory's involvement and the obligation to meet the CLIA '88 requirement of two levels each day of use, management of these testing sites and their testing personnel became an area of concern for the clinical laboratory. QC for the ACT devices and other coagulation instruments was even more strenuous due to the CLIA requirement for two levels of QC per 8-h shift rather than two levels per 24-h day. For most hospitals, this meant that the cost of meeting this requirement could potentially be double or triple the current costs. The controversy continued because the testing sites were not provided with specific data as to the value or additional test reliability that these incremental costs would bring.

Even though the addition of EQC to the QC regimen represents a significant change to traditional QC processes, it provides a reliable and economical method to test many of the components. In the present generation of EQC or alternative QC methods, however, no system known to this author can meet the current guidelines of controlling the three main components: the test system, the operator, and the environment. Nevertheless, regulations and good laboratory practice must be flexible enough to allow innovation to continue in this area.

As unit-use test systems continued to evolve, many manufacturers began to introduce products with a control that was included as an integral part of the disposable component of the device. This is often called an onboard control (OBC) or internal control. With this method, some type of control is built into the disposable component and provides a QC result that is run simultaneously with the patient sample. Some of the early systems—most often qualitative tests (e.g., human chorionic gonadotropin)—included a procedural control to check sample type. Later versions included calibration checks and multiple channels for low and high controls, and in one system three levels of controls are run simultaneously with duplicate patient tests.

OBC can provide added assurances that the system is working properly, because it effectively combines the processes described previously in the glucose test strip example and the reader check by the EQC. The test strip or cartridge that has an OBC is effectively checking the entire system. In some instances, the OBC is also checking some of the preanalytical issues of testing, such as correct sample size or sample type.

DEVELOPMENT OF THE UNIT-USE TEST SYSTEMS GUIDELINE

Even with the checks and balances that have been incorporated into the systems discussed above, there remained a lack of QC standardization as in the traditional statistical QC. This lack of any standard method, coupled with the regulatory agencies' requirement to apply conventional QC methods to unit-use test systems, led this author to propose a project to NCCLS to develop guidelines for QC of unit-use test systems.

The project started as an industry initiative, including interested parties that represented users and industry. The first meetings were held in August 1995 to determine the feasibility of the project and the degree of interest on the part of the parties involved. The consensus was that the structure of NCCLS and the consensus process provided the best way to develop and implement a new QC process. After these informal meetings, a project proposal was drafted and submitted to NCCLS. It was subsequently approved, and the first meeting of the Subcommittee for Unit-Use Testing was held on March 29, 1996.

As the committee was being formed, it was imperative to have both diversity and balance among these three constituencies: industry, regulatory, and users. CMS had given deemed status to other organizations to perform laboratory inspections, provided their survey guidelines were equal to or more stringent than those of CLIA. Because of this, the NCCLS committee needed members from the four major regulatory agencies: CMS, JCAHO, CAP, and the CDC. Therefore, four members to represent industry and four users were needed to maintain balance. The committee was formed with 12 members. The subcommittee was assigned to the Area Committee on Evaluation Protocols, and this guideline was the 18th guideline from this area committee. Therefore, it was coded as EP18 and had the original name of "Quality Control for Unit-Use Tests."

The concept for the subcommittee evolved from two perspectives. The first was the desire to develop guidelines and standards in a collaborative rather than adversarial manner. Historically, IVD manufacturers have addressed QC in the design and labeling of their products but have left it to the users to implement QC—either adopting the manufacturer's system or developing their own. Neither user nor manufacturer worked with the accrediting agencies. It seemed logical, however, that the manufacturer, the user, and the regulator could work together to agree on how to produce quality testing with available resources. The manufacturer would then build the designated system into the product, the user would use it accordingly, and the regulator would inspect to verify the proper implementation of the process. This is a prospective, quality improvement process as opposed to a retrospective, punitive process.

The second perspective was a financial one. The resources required to meet the regulatory requirements added cost but not necessarily value and were therefore potentially prohibitive to innovation. This is not dissimilar to the catalyst for M-22, the plated media guideline. If unit-use test devices were to have an opportunity to be implemented, QC requirements and their cost would have to be addressed. An example of the financial issues involved was provided by Paula Santrach of the Mayo Clinic, for ACTs (8). Reviewing the QC material and number of employees necessary to meet the accrediting agency's requirements, Santrach discovered that her laboratory would spend 3.9 full-time employee equivalents (FTEs) and >$289,000 annually for reagents and control materials for 25 instruments measuring 43 channels to meet the requirement of "two levels per day of use" for 7 days per week. These data are based on ~$3 per QC test and 4 min per test. (The basic formula used for determining the FTE number was the number of channels × the number of control levels × the number of shifts × the number of days × 4 min/test.) The number of QC tests per day was thus 258, and at 4 min per test, would require >17 h each day. The calculation does not include the effects of logistics, which would be considerable for 25 devices located in 25 different locations, perhaps several minutes apart. Finally, no improvement in patient safety, increased accuracy, greater precision, or improved reliability was expected from this additional testing.

It may be a subtle point, and one not generally understood, but regulations can stifle innovation. If the regulatory agencies require a specific QC frequency (e.g., every 8 h), despite a stable, statistically verifiable test system, why would the manufacturer invest research-and-development dollars into developing a system that is stable for more than 8 h? If the regulators focus on what is necessary to provide reliable test results and not on completing checklists, innovation will be rewarded. Experts in the field have noted that laboratorians often lose sight of the true function of QC in the face of regulatory pressure. "The purpose of process control in the clinical laboratory is to ensure that patient results are correct, not to satisfy a bureaucratic demand or an artificial statistical need. Unfortunately, this view of QC is sometimes held by people who do not operate clinical laboratories and limit themselves to regulating them" (9).

The proposed objective of the NCCLS subcommittee was:

> To develop a guideline for unit-use test devices, which is practical to implement, applicable to various devices and settings, and scientifically based, so that device manufacturers, users, and regulatory and accrediting agencies can assure that correct results are obtained and that sources of error are identified, understood, and managed.

Other points to be addressed were identified, including:

1. A working definition for categorizing a test system as unit-use: A system is a unit-use system if the container where the test is performed is always discarded after each test, and the reagents, calibrators, and wash solutions are typically segregated as one test (i.e., there is no interaction of reagents, calibrators, and wash solutions from test to test).
2. The components of the testing process, which were defined as: specimen collection, sample presentation, instrument/ reagents, results/readout/raw data, preliminary review, integration/report in patient's chart, operator, and testing environment.
3. Sources of error. These are listed in the EP18-A matrix.
4. Management techniques for addressing the sources of error.

The subcommittee felt that it was imperative to broaden its thinking about the testing process and to cover more steps within the process rather than only the quality of the instrument and reagents. Therefore, the testing process (point 2) was defined to include both preanalytical and postanalytical steps.

According to the objective, the guideline was to apply to all testing systems. This flexibility can be provided only within a framework that permits innovation. Therefore, one focus of the subcommittee was to identify all potential sources of error in the testing process. The subcommittee identified as many sources of error as possible so that the list could be used as a points-to-consider document for both manufacturers and operators. The guideline recommends that management of the potential sources of error be addressed by each manufacturer in relation to a specific system. The manufacturer documents to

the users'—and ultimately, the regulators'—satisfaction that the source of error has been eliminated or controlled. If this is not possible, the user—with or without the manufacturer's assistance—will be charged with managing the source of error. This approach permits development of a quality system that includes review of all testing areas, identifies the potential sources of errors, and manages errors. The distinction is an important one. The subcommittee understood that, as a practical matter, not all errors can be eliminated, but all can be identified and managed appropriately.

Another area of discussion within the subcommittee involved the quality system methods and processes used in manufacturing. Beckham (10) noted many parallels between manufacturing and healthcare, even though hospitals (and by extension, laboratories) "don't appreciate their lineage to manufacturing. Few hospitals would describe themselves as being in the business of manufacturing care. Yet, the way they produce care suggests they are very much creatures of the manufacturing jungle."

The subcommittee's discussions uncovered many aspects of quality manufacturing that could potentially be utilized in the manufacturing of IVD tests, particularly in a unit-use format. These methods and processes, or good manufacturing processes, are utilized routinely by manufacturers and by the US Food and Drug Administration (FDA) as part of its onsite manufacturing inspections. Coincidentally, the FDA had just published the new Quality Systems Regulations (11), a revision to the Good Manufacturing Practices (published in 1990) to now include preproduction and design controls. FDA inspections implemented these regulations beginning in June 1997. The product life cycle, as defined by FDA, now includes product development, manufacturing, product handling (packaging, storage, and shipment), and product use. The subcommittee believed that a comprehensive quality system that built on existing methods and identified potential sources of error in each area would allow believable but erroneous test results to be identified and managed. This management component would enable innovation in both manufacturing and implementation and provide the necessary oversight and control of unit-use test systems.

The development of the proposed guideline was based on the following definitions and concepts:

- A unit-use test system is one in which reagents, calibrators, and wash solutions are segregated as one test—without interaction of reagents, calibrators, and wash solutions from test to test—and the container where the test is performed is discarded after each test.
- Unit-use test systems have diverse technology, designs, and functions.
- Unit-use devices are subject to error, and the relative importance and likelihood of these errors varies with the device, the specimen, the user, and the environment.
- A single QC/QA regimen cannot be developed to cover all unit-use test systems and to detect all errors.
- Principles of traditional statistical QC must be customized and adapted for each unit-use test system.

- QC/QA programs may evolve with increasing experience with the unit-use test system.

APPLICATION OF THE GUIDELINE

The guideline was based on a systems approach to quality management (12). It includes definitions of the phases of the testing process and identification of potential sources of error within each phase. It presents a generic sources-of-error matrix (see Table 14-1) that contains a list of possible errors in the preanalytical, analytical, and postanalytical phases of testing with unit-use devices. The sources-of-error matrix is the fundamental nucleus of the guideline. The subcommittee realized that it was impossible to create a comprehensive list, and even if it were possible, other systems could be developed that would make the current matrix obsolete, or at least outdated. Therefore, the subcommittee decided to develop the best list possible, but to position it more as a list of considerations for each audience: industry, user, and regulator. This list is not comprehensive but representative of areas to review. The purpose of the matrix is to aid the user and the manufacturer in considering and identifying sources of error applicable to a particular unit-use test system. It can be adapted for use in several environments:

- Manufacturers can use this matrix to identify potential failure modes and lessen the risk that they will actually occur.
- Clinical users can identify potential causes of erroneous results and develop individualized quality management programs.
- Regulatory and accreditation agencies can use both the generic and customized matrices to assess the appropriateness of a laboratory's customized quality management program.

The matrix contains seven columns:

1. *Potential sources of error.* Each of six categories in this column corresponds to a different phase of the testing process: specimen collection, sample presentation, instru-

Table 14-1   Potential Sources of Error

1. Specimen collection
   1.1. Contamination
   1.2. Inadequate sample
   1.3. Hemolysis
   1.4. Incorrect patient drawn
   1.5. Inappropriate sample
   1.6. Patient condition inappropriate for testing method
   1.7. Improper patient preparation

2. Sample presentation
   2.1. Incorrect procedure/technique
   2.2. Incorrect sample
   2.3. Delay from collection to analysis
   2.4. Sample inadequately mixed
   2.5. Sample inadequately mixed with reagents
   2.6. Inappropriate amount of sample presented
   2.7. Introduction of air bubbles
   2.8. Incorrect patient information entered into device

3. Instrument/reagents
   3.1. Adverse environmental conditions
   3.2. Outdated reagents
   3.3. Improper reagent shipment
   3.4. Improper reagent storage
   3.5. Incorrectly prepared reagents
   3.6. Incorrect use of reagents
   3.7. Reagent contamination
   3.8. Deterioration of reagent over time
   3.9. Lot-to-lot reagent variability
   3.10. Sample-related reagent failure
   3.11. Electronic simulator malfunction
   3.12. Improper control shipment
   3.13. Improper control storage
   3.14. Inadequate mixing of controls
   3.15. Improper calibration
   3.16. Poor precision

   3.17. Bias
   3.18. Incorrect analysis mode
   3.19. Sample carryover
   3.20. Instrument error
   3.21. Instrument failure
   3.22. Instrument/reagent performance not verified prior to use
   3.23. Improperly functioning instrument not removed from service
   3.24. Inadequate maintenance/handling
   3.25. Patient's personal equipment used
   3.26. Complicated procedure
   3.27. Incorrect technique

4. Results/readout/raw data
   4.1. Visual misinterpretation
   4.2. Incorrect setting for units
   4.3. Incorrect mode setting
   4.4. Accidental loss of data
   4.5. Calculation required

5. Preliminary review
   5.1. Improper interpretation of control results
   5.2. Outlier/nonsense result not recognized
   5.3. Result outside of linear range not recognized
   5.4. Alert value not recognized
   5.5. Need for a confirmatory test not recognized
   5.6. Effect of preanalytical variables not recognized
   5.7. Instrument malfunction not recognized
   5.8. Interference not recognized

6. Integration into patient record
   6.1. No result recorded
   6.2. Result recorded in incorrect patient chart
   6.3. Incorrect information recorded
   6.4. Information unreadable
   6.5. No aids for clinical interpretation
   6.6. Result difficult to find
   6.7. Result temporarily unavailable

ment/reagents, results/readout/raw data, preliminary review, and integration into the patient record.

2. *Applicability to system.* The identified source of error either applies or does not apply to the unit-use test system.

3. *Nature of impact.* This describes how the result is perturbed or impacted by the error.

4. *Device capabilities.* This describes how and when the device prevents or detects the error.

5. *Training/laboratory procedure requirements.* This describes requirements for the user in developing or modifying laboratory procedures and requirements for training to address error detection and elimination.

6. *Applicable quality monitoring.* This describes quality monitoring to minimize errors and/or detect errors that device design does not prevent.

7. *Frequency of monitoring.* The user ensures that the source of error is monitored at a frequency that optimizes error detection and meets all relevant regulations.

Completion of the sources-of-error matrix requires good communication between users and manufacturer. Tables 14-2 and 14-3 summarize responsibilities of manufacturers and users for completing the matrix. A separate matrix should be completed for each type of unit-use device utilized by each facility.

The goal of quality management is to prevent and detect problems in the testing cycle (13, 14). Based on information derived from the completed sources-of-error matrix, the user may revise, add, delete, or create facility policies as necessary depending on the nature of the error that needs to be detected. The following components should be included in such a policy:

- *Standard operating procedures.* Each unit-use test should have a written procedure that covers all aspects of the testing cycle. The procedure should include sources of error that are detected by the operator, dependent on proper technique, or managed by training.

- *Training and competency.* The subcommittee recommends that traditional liquid QC be used as a measure of operator competency. Frequent operators (those performing tests at least once per week) would perform liquid (i.e., not electronic) QC at least once per week. Infrequent operators

Table 14-2 Manufacturer's Responsibility for Completing the Sources-of-Error Matrix

Review items on the matrix.
Identify potential failure modes and include analyte-specific as well as system-specific sources of error that are not on the matrix.
Design the system to eliminate/minimize sources of error.
Disclose errors that remain.
Develop recommendations for managing these sources of error.
Summarize applicable information for the user.

Table 14-3 User's Responsibility for Completing the Sources-of-Error Matrix

Obtain the applicable error summary from the manufacturer.
Compare the manufacturer's summary to the sources-of-error matrix to determine compatibility with user's analytical/clinical needs and test setting.
Identify applicable training/laboratory procedure requirements, quality monitoring methods, and monitoring frequency.
Implement necessary procedures and monitors.
Periodically evaluate QMS to ensure sources of error are identified and managed at an acceptable rate.

(those performing tests less than once per week) would perform liquid QC with each day of testing. Each institution could modify these recommendations based on data and experience. Reagent stability determines the absolute minimum frequency: QC-testing intervals should be no longer than 0.1 of the stated reagent stability. In practical terms, QC testing should be performed no less than every 4 to 6 weeks.

- *Ongoing process control.* The goal of process control is to verify that system components (i.e., operator, instrument, reagents, sample, and environment) are performing as specified by the manufacturer and at a quality level acceptable to the user. Various forms of controls are available to test different parts of the process: acceptance testing, periodic QC (traditional liquid QC), split samples, other forms of QC (e.g., electronic QC), preventive maintenance, proficiency testing, delta checks, environmental monitoring, and clinical surveillance.

- *Error and incident reporting.* Retrospective review of variations, errors, and problems reported in the testing cycle may be used to improve product design and prevent errors (15).

- *Auditing.* Prospective searches for problems in the testing cycles can lead to quality improvement or corrective action.

The sources-of-error matrix may be used as a tool to help identify potential failure modes so that they can be addressed by the manufacturer or by the user. For example, the following errors identified for a point-of-care glucose device are used to illustrate completion of the matrix (*Note:* The numbers in the list refer to sections of the sources-of-error matrix.):

5.1. Potential source of error:
    2.6.1. Insufficient sample volume.
- Applicable to system (yes or no): Yes.
- Nature of impact: Insufficient sample volume gives falsely low results or no results.
- Device capabilities: Confirmation dot on back of reagent strip indicates sufficient blood application. Manufacturer claims that the device will detect insufficient blood volume, display an error message warning of low sample volume, and suppress test results.

- Training/laboratory procedure requirements: Procedure and training should include (*a*) instructions on required sample volume and error messages, (*b*) procedural step for visual examination of confirmation dot on the test strip, and (*c*) directions to repeat test.
- Applicable quality monitoring: Test traditional liquid QC materials. Review incident reports for cases of erratic/falsely low results. Perform operator competency assessment.
- Frequency of monitoring: Perform liquid QC daily. Review incident reports monthly. Assess operator competency annually.

5.2. Potential sources of error:

    3.6.1. Incorrect use of reagents: Reagent strip removed before result displayed.

    3.6.2. Incorrect use of reagents: Wrong lot of test strips used.

- Applicable to system (yes or no): Yes.
- Nature of impact:

    3.6.1. None.

    3.6.2. Possible QC failure or inaccurate patient results.

- Device capability? Device prompts operator to select test strip lot number.
- Training/laboratory procedure requirements: Provide instructions on correct use of test strips.
- Applicable quality monitoring/frequency: Test traditional liquid QC materials daily. Review QC logs weekly. Perform operator competency assessments annually.

5.3. Potential sources of error:

    5.2. Outlier/nonsense/critical result not recognized.

- Applicable to system (yes or no): Yes.
- Nature of impact: Possible incorrect therapy decision.
- Device capability: Device displays "critical high" or "critical low" warning messages; operators are required to select action comments.
- Training/laboratory procedure requirements: Instruct operators on handling critical/nonsense values (e.g., call MD). Confirm results with laboratory method if patient symptoms are inconsistent with bedside results.
- Applicable quality monitoring/frequency: Review error logs. Audit nursing records to verify appropriate procedures/policies are followed.

Construction of a quality management program for unit-use test devices requires identifying sources of error within each phase of the testing process. The sources-of-error matrix is a useful tool to identify, understand, and manage errors applicable to the device, operator, and setting. The key to the success of this proposed guideline is cooperation and open exchange of information among manufacturers, users, regulators, and accrediting agencies.

The US regulatory agencies, particularly CMS, have overseen hospital clinical laboratories since the original Clinical Laboratory Improvement Act of 1967, which was expanded by CLIA '88 to include all testing venues, including physician office laboratories. Draft QC regulations that became effective in 1992 remained in place until the final CLIA '88 regulation was published on January 24, 2003, with an effective date of April 25, 2003 (16). As to QC, the final rule establishes one QC standard for all nonwaived testing, combining the previous moderate-complexity and high-complexity testing into the same nonwaived category. In addition, the rule permits reduced frequency of some QC testing. These changes apparently were precipitated by the increase in the number of waived tests and the corresponding decrease in moderately complex tests. The logic was that this migration of simpler tests to the waived category effectively raised the bar for QC for all nonwaived tests.

The January 2003 Final Rule included a provision for a 2-year phase-in period; every laboratory would be allowed one inspection cycle that was characterized by CMS as educational. During an inspection, identified deficiencies based on the new regulations would not be enforced unless there were patient safety issues (17).

An additional major change is that the FDA will no longer review QC requirements for test systems for CLIA purposes. This responsibility will now belong to individual laboratory directors.

This movement to a more practical approach to QC from what had been a more prescriptive approach is beginning to evolve. It has been speculated that approximately 25% of a clinical laboratory's budget is spent on QA, QC, time, and materials. This is not to say that 25% is too much or too little; the question is whether it is the right amount. This author believes that since conventional QA/QC has been used to monitor unconventional (e.g., unit-use) test systems, resources have been spent not to add value or ensure patient safety—or even reliable test results—but rather to enable completion of a checklist that an inspector is required to complete.

With the new regulation, which lists EP18-A as a resource, CMS has taken a bold step in allowing laboratory directors to design a unique quality systems approach specific to their laboratory, their testing environment, and their staff. In other words, they are free to design a system that monitors the right things right, and to allocate resources in areas that need improvement and not on those that do not. This permits the development of a structure and format for improving efficiency, reducing costs, and maintaining—or perhaps even improving upon—current quality standards. It also provides an incentive for both laboratory directors and manufacturers to innovate continually in order to increase laboratory efficiency and potential profits.

As existing technologies continue to mature into fail-safe systems, highly trained laboratorians will be able to use their training and expertise on emerging tests and on evolutionary changes in QA/QC that have not occurred up to this point.

Laboratory directors should call upon the manufacturers with whom they do business to provide them with assistance in developing their unique quality systems approach. Collaborations between industry and operators with regulatory oversight will ultimately provide the best balance among patient safety, test reliability, and the necessary resources.

REFERENCES

1. National Committee on Clinical Laboratory Standards. Quality assurance for commercially prepared microbiological culture media, 2nd ed. Approved standard M22–A2. Wayne, PA: NCCLS, 1996;16(16):xiii.

2. MacLowry JD, Edison DC, Dreskin R. CAP Microbiology Resource Committee survey of commercially prepared media. In: Smith JW, ed. The role of clinical microbiology in cost-effective health care. Skokie, IL: College of American Pathologists, 1985:555–9.

3. Clinical Laboratory Improvement Advisory Committee. Summary report. Atlanta, GA: Centers for Disease Control and Prevention, May 29–30, 1996;6, addendum C.

4. Westgard JO. Electronic quality control, the total testing process, and the total quality control system. Clin Chim Acta 2001;307:45–8.

5. Phillips DL, Santrach PJ, Belanger A, Calvin V, Hinkel C, O'Neal WR, et al. Quality management for unit-use testing; approved guideline. NCCLS document EP18–A. Wayne, PA: NCCLS, 2002.

6. Letter from Health Care Financing Administration to field surveyors, October 1995.

7. HCFA letter to William S. Moffitt, i-STAT, February 1996.

8. Auxter S. Looking at laboratory quality control in a new light. Clin Chem News 1996;22:5.

9. Steindel S. Process control systems—a question to be answered. Pathologist 1984;38(8):465–6.

10. Beckham JD. Redefining work in the integrated delivery system. Clin Lab Manage Rev 1996;10:478–85.

11. FDA. Quality systems regulations. Final rule. Fed Regist 1996; 61:52601–62.

12. ANSI/ASQC Q90004–1-1994. Quality management and quality systems elements—guidelines I.

13. ISO 8402:1994. Quality management and quality assurance—vocabulary. Geneva, Switzerland: International Organization for Standardization, 1994.

14. National Committee on Clinical Laboratory Standards. A quality system model for health care: approved guideline. NCCLS document GP26–A. Wayne, PA: NCCLS, 1999.

15. Motschman T, Santrach P, Moore S. Error/incident management and its practical application. In: Duckett J, Woods L, Santrach P, eds. Quality in action. Bethesda, MD: American Association of Blood Banks, 1996.

16. Medicare, Medicaid, and CLIA programs; laboratory requirements relating to quality systems and certain personnel qualifications. Fed Regist 2003;68(16):3639–714.

17. Guidelines for quality systems to offer the labs. Clin Lab News 2003;29(12):28.

Chapter 15

Guidelines for Point-of-Care Testing

Robert Cramb

With the explosion in point-of-care testing (POCT), newly trained physicians may feel that they are pioneers in the use of tests near the bedside, but a review of the historical nature of medicine demonstrates that laboratory medicine and clinical pathology were both born at the patient's bedside (1–3). It is clear that in the 19th and 20th centuries the process of physical examination and evaluation of body fluids near to the patient was deemed perfectly natural, and standard textbooks of clinical chemistry used by medical students included a chapter on side-room testing (4). The side-room testing described referred to simple tests usually, for nonspecific urinary sugars, hemoglobin, or fecal occult blood. From the 1950s onward, there was an explosion in laboratory testing and the formation of more centralized laboratories that analyzed large numbers of samples for many different analytes. Because of their high throughput, there have been many comparisons with a factory environment. Most of the time, the more centralized laboratory paradigm has worked well to serve patients. Total quality management issues bound up with the requirements of accreditation in most countries have meant that the provision of services follows more rigidly set schedules, and the factory nature of the centralized laboratory is now highly organized and well controlled. The gain in the laboratory is the improvement in efficiency obtained through processing large numbers of specimens; the ability to purchase reagents in bulk and to efficiently use large, complex, expensive items of laboratory hardware. With high-speed data links, reports can be generated electronically and viewed on the wards, and with wireless networks the physician can see test results transmitted to a handheld wireless personal digital assistant (PDA).

Why has POCT therefore taken off? What pressures have lead to the reorganization of hospital laboratory services, including a significant amount of testing being directed at and near the patient's bedside? The answers are in some ways somewhat surprising. Subjectively, there is an historical precedent for laboratory testing at the bedside, and the feeling that some testing belongs close to the patient is in many ways not dissimilar to the views and the teaching that arise from decades of medical tradition. The second answer is that moving some hospital laboratory testing to the patient's bedside may have clear economic benefit (5). With 60–70% of patients' diagnoses and management dependent on laboratory investigations and the need for rapid throughput of hospital inpatients (6), there is little wonder that POCT has become an important issue in the overall management of patients. Despite the efficient factory nature of tests from the centralized laboratories, the time required for samples to reach the laboratories may exceed the time required for analysis and thus build into the testing equation delays that are unacceptable for the needs of patient turnaround (7).

Pathology has a key role in medical decision making and is not immune to changes in healthcare delivery. Some institutions have thought that pathology tests can be a rate-limiting step in achieving further clinical and cost improvements in patient care, particularly when delayed clinical management decisions and follow-up consultations are imposed by test turnaround times. The recognition that POCT can contribute to better healthcare and also create new commercial markets for diagnostic technology is reflected in the increasing range and availability of tests that can be used by patients, their caregivers, and the nonlaboratory community in general. POCT therefore can liberate the physician from delays and improve turnaround of patients with an aid to faster diagnosis. While this is a laudable aim of POCT, there is good evidence that this approach may not always yield the results that might be expected (8, 9).

The first issue that must be addressed is that of the quality of the result produced. Testing that does not meet quality standards may be misleading and contribute to erroneous clinical decisions and possible harm to the patient. The first rule of laboratory medicine is the same as the first rule of the rest of medicine: *Primum non nochere* (First do no harm). In a very real sense, to do no testing is better than to perform poor testing, and having a misleading erroneous test value is worse than having no answer at all (10). Part of the difficulty involves the operator who carries out the test. Operator dependence has been shown to be a critical factor in production of some results, particularly if older types of POCT devices are being used, and the seniority of the operator may be a factor in the production of the result (11). Those individuals involved in POCT must be given appropriate guidance to understand the concept of the analyses that they are undertaking. While large centralized laboratories turn over many hundreds of thousands or millions of tests per annum, POCT usually (but not always) is involved with small-scale testing (Table 15-1). Other authors in this book will outline the microeconomics and macroeconomics of POCT, but the benefits that can be accrued from its efficient use involve a necessary amount of education, training, and recertification to ensure that the quality of the service is maintained.

Table 15-1 POCT: Differences in Testing by Comparison to Centralized Laboratories

Number of tests performed by individual staff may be small.
General professional training does not cover formal technical training in POCT. Staff may not have the technical background in their specialist area.
POCT testing may be undertaken in environments not specifically designed for analytical work.
Unique health and safety issues may require review.

In POCT the majority of the errors occur prior to testing (i.e., in the preanalytical phase). The actual analytical technique is now becoming less operator dependent with new technologies. The choice of POCT should now be based on cost–benefit analysis. Arguments that still arise as a result of narrow vision from laboratories suggest that POCT is more expensive and therefore less cost effective. While it is true that individual tests are more expensive, the correct selection of tests is a much more pertinent argument that requires deeper thought into test characteristics and decision rules, a subject which is outside the boundaries of this chapter (12).

To apply POCT in individual settings, there has been a significant trend away from individuals setting up their own POCT either by moving to a regulated framework [Clinical Laboratory Improvement Amendment of 1988 (CLIA '88)] (13) or more practically by issuing guidelines of which individuals should take due account to meet the requirements of regulatory practice. Clinical guidelines are potential tools for standardizing care to improve its quality and cost-effectiveness. This chapter will therefore focus on guidelines that have been issued and the scope of their coverage.

GUIDELINES

A number of organizations and individuals have drawn up guidelines for POCT, and these are listed in Table 15-2.

Many of these guidelines have been adapted by individual healthcare providers to meet their own local needs. It is important to identify the critical areas in these guidelines that must be followed to ensure that POCT will meet the dual need of quality of measurement and enhanced clinical care (Table 15-3).

Assessment of Need

There will often be a perceived need for POCT in a clinical area, and individuals within that environment will drive the case for its introduction. The local hospital laboratory can play a supportive role in advice on POCT as well as lead a committee on the use of POCT (see later), and a standard set of questions should be posed to see what justification there is for the purchase of equipment. Standard questions found in the guidelines are detailed in Table 15-4. Posing these questions may identify problems with the current infrastructure. For instance, the analysis time in the department from receipt of the

specimen may be shorter than the time taken to transport the specimen from the patient (ward) to the laboratory.

Once these questions have been posed, investigated, and debated and the problem area that will benefit from POCT is identified, equipment selection can follow. Table 15-5 outlines the typical questions that must be considered before implementation of the service. The expected workload and the user of the instrument are important linked areas. If a device is situated in a busy clinical area, the equipment's ability both to cope with the expected workload and to do so within a short turnaround time are vitally important. Clinical staff will want equipment that analyzes samples within in a couple of minutes to achieve a rapid turnaround time. Longer analytical times may be unacceptable to clinical staff used to quick turnaround times, and they may question the reliability of results obtained.

Another issue with POCT devices is the lack of standardization that prevents comparison of results obtained in different laboratories from different devices (14). It is therefore vital that a dialogue between the laboratory and the end-user be estab-

Table 15-2 Major Publications on Guidelines for POCT

Association of Clinical Biochemists (UK). Guidelines for implementation of near patient testing 1993. Available from the Association of Clinical Biochemists 130-132 Tooley St London SE1 2TU.
Joint Working Group on Quality Assurance of Pathology (UK). http://www.acb.org.uk/docex/Docs/NPT/8.pdf
Medical Devices Agency (UK). http://www.medical-devices.gov.uk/mda/mdawebsitev2.nsf/
Guidelines for perfusionists in Canada. http://www.perfusion.ca/categ/poct.html
German Working Group on Medical Laboratory Testing. http://www.dglm.de/~Ziems/poct_engl.htm
National Committee for Clinical Laboratory Standards. Point of care in vitro diagnostic (IVD) testing; approved guideline. NCCLS Document AST2-A. Wayne, PA: National Committee for Clinical Laboratory Standards, 1999.
National Committee for Clinical Laboratory Standards. Point of care blood glucose testing in acute and chronic care facilities: approved guideline, 2nd ed. NCCLS Document C30-A2. Wayne, PA; National Committee for Clinical Laboratory Standards, 2003.
Department of Health & Aging (Australia). Introducing point of care testing in general practice. http://www.aacb.asn.au/pubs/poct_ps.pdf
Australasian Association of Clinical Biochemists. Point of care testing: position statement. AACB, 2002. http://www.aacb.asn.au/pubs/poct_ps.pdf
Department of Health (UK). Near-patient testing, a statement of best practice for Scotland. Edinburgh: Scottish Office
Department of Health, National Advisory Committee for Scientific Services, 1996.
Haeckel R. et al. Good medical laboratory services: a proposal for definitions, concepts and criteria. Clin Chem Lab Med 1998;36:399–403
Kost G.J. Guidelines for point-of-care testing. Improving patient outcomes. Am J Clin Pathol 1995;104(Suppl 1):S111–27.

Table 15-3   POCT Guidelines: Generic Areas Covered

Assessing the need for POCT
Procurement of POCT
Implementation of POCT
Risk assessment
Clinical governance
Standard operating procedures
POCT committee
Training and certification
Quality assurance
Maintenance
Stock maintenance
Accreditation
Data recording and IT

Table 15-5   Equipment Selection

What is the predicted workload?
Who is going to use the equipment?
What is the likely achievable analytical accuracy and
   imprecision required for the service to be workable?
Where will the equipment and consumables be sited?
Is there an appropriate area for POCT with services that may
   include power, water, and refrigeration?
Has the equipment been evaluated independently?
How comparable are the results with the local hospital
   laboratory?
What limitations are known with the equipment?
How will the POCT service integrate with the existing IT?
Have health and safety considerations been considered?

lished early to ensure that results are directly comparable. Instruments should be selected on these criteria and ideally should have had independent evaluation of their accuracy, precision, reliability, and comparability. Data handling and a record of results produced, including quality assurance data, are a vital part of the devolution of POCT to clinical staff. The question of IT compatibility is of increasing importance, but manufacturers are already engaged in a dialogue with end-users on connectivity protocols (15).

Procurement of POCT

Once there is agreement with the clinical users and local laboratory on the necessary equipment, a full business case must be constructed prior to purchase. The business case should demonstrate the clinical and economic benefits to back up the purchase of equipment that may duplicate items already available in a clinical pathology laboratory. The costs involved in submission of a business case are wide ranging; should take into account the costs of keeping patients in a ward, emergency room, or consulting area; and will require that clinical staff identify gains made through the use of the equipment. The costs associated with POCT alone are outlined in Table 15-6. It is vital that due account be taken of the clinical and economic benefits, and these must be wrapped up into a clear case. This is particularly important where

decisions on purchase of equipment may be hospital- or community-wide and where the rationalization of equipment can provide significant cost-savings benefits in reagent provision and clinical activity. Of paramount importance, however, is that the results provided are similar to those of the local main laboratory facility. It is inevitable that users will compare the laboratory and POCT results, especially when there is any uncertainty of the validity of POCT results. Dissimilar units of measurement or reference ranges will confuse clinical staff and may compromise patient management.

Implementation of POCT

The implementation of POCT will vary from country to country, but the majority of guidelines suggest that a local hospital pathology laboratory should be involved in the introduction of POCT.

Table 15-4   Assessing Needs for POCT

Identify the group of patients needing testing.
Identify the tests required.
Outline the current service and how closely it meets clinical
   needs.
If the clinical needs are not met, can these be done by
   conventional methods?
How easy is it to access the conventional laboratory service?
Has the laboratory service been contacted?
How will POCT enable more rapid or effective diagnosis or
   treatment?
Do you have the means to identify cost–benefit in the original
   service and new service?

Table 15-6   POCT Business Case Costs

Capital costs
   Equipment
   Accessories required for the equipment to function
   Health and safety requirements
   Site alterations
   Depreciation
   IT interfacing
Other fixed costs
   Routine and preventative maintenance (including servicing
      contracts)
   Internal and external QA
   Accreditation requirements
Variable costs
   Consumables
   Waste disposal
   Cleaning and disinfection
Professional costs
   Staff training
   Management of the program
   Indemnity and legal liability
   Operator time
Laboratory support

The local laboratory should take the key role in directing the users of POCT to any local or national guidelines that apply. It is significant that all of the guidelines issued by the various societies and regulatory bodies have identified that the single most important element in implementing a POCT program is to construct a business case based on service needs. Institutions that introduce a POCT program without consultation with their local laboratory show a lack of foresight by failing to review the current provision of service and the perceived and required clinical needs. Key questions that must be posed to identify the needs for POCT are detailed in Table 15-4. Failure to review these areas will miss the relevance of the economics of testing and will potentially encourage misuse of testing and duplication of tests and raise the potential for increased and perhaps unjustifiable costs. It is easier to provide POCT to satisfy clinical requirements where there is an evidence-based outcome. All POCT must be constantly audited and reviewed after introduction. This is necessary because clinical needs change with time. Thus the introduction of POCT may change working practices, leading to other efficiencies in the clinical area that may then negate or even extend the need for POCT.

While the laboratory should be the key to introduction of POCT, there must be a dialogue between all of the interested parties to ensure that there are no misunderstandings about the scope and limitations of POCT and the responsibilities that are required in the clinical area that is to use the system. By discussing these needs, the laboratory will be best placed to provide advice on the type of POCT that will best meet the needs of the clinical staff.

The array of systems available for POCT is extensive (Chapters 2 to 6) and can vary among the following:

- Noninstrumental systems, i.e., disposable devices that vary from reagent test strips for a single analyte to sophisticated multianalyte reagent strips incorporating procedural controls
- Small analyzers, usually handheld or "palmheld" devices (though the size may vary considerably), such as blood glucose meters
- Desktop analyzers, which are larger and include systems that are often designed for use in a clinic or small laboratory

In reviewing the type of equipment that is required, clinical staff need to have the details in Table 15-5 reiterated as many times as necessary to ensure that they have taken all points into account.

Risk Assessment

Risk assessment of POCT is one of the most neglected points within a POCT service. Clinical staff spend much of their time reviewing risks to the patient and discount the hazards of implementing POCT at their peril. The majority of issued guidelines on POCT identify that there are hazards that must be recognized, and these may not be immediately apparent in the enthusiasm to provide a service (16–18). They recommend appropriate controls and reviews to ensure that the equipment is safe to use and that it can be used safely within the environment where it is sited. These

areas have already been considered in Table 15-5. It is worth stressing that the ease of use of the instrument in the clinical area is of paramount importance. POCT instruments that require multiple procedural inputs from the operator or frequent manual intervention including recalibration are likely to be less successfully integrated into the clinical environment. While analytical performance is an important aspect of any POCT device, the time taken for analysis should not be overlooked. One of the major advantages cited for the use of POCT is the speed at which the result can be generated and subsequently influence clinical decision making. Blood gas analysis turnaround time is quick, but some of the immunoassay-based POCT tests may take up to 15 min to produce a result. Although this may be perfectly acceptable performance within a clinical laboratory, it may be unacceptable for clinical use unless this is clearly defined and identified before implementation. It is therefore important to specify the turnaround time on the instruments to take due account of any clinical timing issues. However, there is also a need to ensure that the correct infrastructure is in place to ensure that faster delivery of results means that clinical staff have readily available access to them, and that patient care may be changed in keeping with the new turnaround times.

Clinical Governance

In the United Kingdom, clinical governance is defined as "a framework through which NHS organizations are accountable for continually improving the quality of their services and safeguarding high standards of care by creating an environment in which excellence in clinical care will flourish" (19).

While this is a definition that has been adopted in the United Kingdom, it is applicable to all healthcare systems worldwide. Therefore, the process of clinical governance will include a number of processes for monitoring and improving service, such as:

- Doctor and patient involvement
- Risk management
- Audit, research, and effectiveness
- Staffing and staff management
- Education training and personal and professional development
- Use of information to support clinical governance and healthcare.

These are important issues, and individuals who are placed in management roles to support POCT should recognize these needs and keep them high on their priority lists (20). This is important because medicolegal aspects of medicine must be taken into account; it is therefore of some importance for managers of a service to maintain strict protocols and ensure that it is a high-quality service. Any organization of POCT should take due account of lines of accountability, and these must be properly written into local policies and procedures, which should cover the areas outlined in Table 15-7.

Table 15-7   Standard Operating Procedure

Information on the reason for testing
Information on the test methods employed
Hazards associated with the materials used in the test
Health and safety
Instructions for use
Quality assurance
Maintenance
Accreditation
Recordkeeping
Adverse incident reporting
Modifications to the standard operating procedure

Standard Operating Procedure

The standard operating procedure (SOP) is a document that provides all of the details required to undertake a test; the key headings are detailed in Table 15-7. The SOP should be readily accessible to all individuals who use the device and will be responsible for any tests measured by them. An SOP will require regular review and revision to ensure that it is kept up to date, particularly if manufacturers significantly change the reagents or other details applicable to the device, including software upgrades.

POCT Committee

Here guidelines and reality can often diverge significantly unless those who are in charge of the implementation of POCT make a very careful review of the way in which the business case is constructed and the progenitors of POCT envisage any testing to be undertaken. In reviewing this particular aspect of procedure there are specific points that require careful attention, and these include the following:

- Is the local laboratory involved in the provision of the POCT?
- Is the local laboratory providing active support for POCT?
- Is there a designated individual who will take responsibility for the test and act on the results?
- What procedures are in place to maintain quality of service?
- Are there clear instructions in the event of equipment failure or malfunction?

Although POCT management should be put within the remit of a single individual, there seems little doubt that this individual will have to interact with a number of other healthcare professionals and teams. Therefore, the introduction of POCT should be a collective decision-making process encompassing as many representatives as there are areas in which POCT will have benefit. It is recommended in the majority of the guidelines that there be a POCT committee on which all of the major specialties that have an interest in the outcome of POCT tests are represented. The role of a POCT committee will vary according to the establishment and country, but in general terms its role will be described by the headings noted in Table 15-8.

Training and Certification

Training and certification are important areas for POCT to be correctly utilized. It is important that individuals who are to use POCT equipment are aware of the performance limitations and the analytical steps involved in the production of any results. Many of the individuals who use POCT equipment will have no formal training in laboratory methods, and although the latest generation of POCT equipment can use disposable devices that are largely operator independent, this should not lead to a culture of brashness in their operation. There must be rigorous training accompanied by certification and backed up by performance review, whether by internal quality assurance (IQA) or external quality assurance (EQA) testing. Retraining and review of competency certification should be part of the standard program for these individuals. In the United Kingdom, this has been seen as an extended role of nursing and is also seen as an extended role of junior hospital staff, while in other countries this role can only be provided by staff who have the appropriate certification (as defined by local rules) and may not include the medical or nursing staff.

As already described above, the range of these devices can be considerable, and not all individuals may be able to operate them within their operating specifications. Therefore the correct selection of equipment is paramount, and due account of this selection should be taken within the business case. This cannot be emphasized enough because busy departments will not be able to cope with long turnaround times and the need for time-consuming steps such as measurement of accurate volumes of liquid (whether blood or serum) by means of a standard laboratory pipette. The use of POCT that involves complex preanalytical tasks may compromise the quality of the results obtained, and care in specimen sampling must become second nature if one wishes to avoid contamination with inappropriate blood or urine specimens.

Although preanalytical problems are well recognized, postanalytical problems are rarely reviewed, especially by clinical staff. Postanalytical documentation is a key area that has been neglected. Specific guidelines on the clinical use of POCT devices are now at the top of manufacturers' lists. In addition, some of the latest POCT equipment has the ability to ensure that the operator enters the correct ID prior to use of the device and before the result is displayed and printed. Moreover, some

Table 15-8   Role of POCT Committee

Review all requests for POCT
Establish continuing clinical audit of POCT
Ensure quality standards are met with POCT
Establish linkage with all POCT areas
Establish a certification and training program
Ensure that quality assurance programs are managed and
    provide feedback on performance

instruments will not display results unless appropriate QA (whether IQA or EQA) is utilized at specific set-points in the instrument cycle. Although laboratories are used to this type of data capture, individuals using POCT may not be familiar with it and will require training and education in order to understand its importance. Finally, all POCT operators should be known within any unit that is using a particular test. Ideally, no one should use POCT equipment without their due competency being recorded and/or appropriate access codes being allowed. With the advent of new recognition technology, whether by encoded swipe-cards or more sophisticated digital or retinal identification, it is possible to exclude individuals who are not trained in the use of the device from performing POCT.

Quality Assurance

Other areas within this book will deal more specifically with quality assurance, but once again careful attention should be paid to quality assurance and documentation of results. Clear areas within the SOP and the training of individuals should identify when the devices should be investigated fully. The appropriate QC results to obtain for any POCT device must take due account of the device, the individuals using that device, its demonstrated imprecision, and current operating performance. The IQC testing should satisfy a defined requirement for quality. At a minimum there will probably be a requirement to run at least one QA sample per shift, or an instrument check using dummy devices that interrogate the hardware and software of the device. These requirements should be defined by consultation with the laboratory and ensure that the appropriate procedures are documented, taking into account the number of patient samples that are processed and the number of individuals that use the device. EQA testing and proficiency testing are covered in more detail in Chapter 13.

Maintenance

All equipment needs regular routine maintenance, and this is as true of POCT as it is of any other laboratory instrument. As previously noted, the devices used for POCT can range from small disposable devices to larger desktop instruments. Some form of daily maintenance, however, is mandatory, and this must be properly undertaken and documented. The responsibility for routine maintenance should be agreed upon as part of the business case submitted for the POCT equipment. The instrument may be maintained by laboratory staff, nonlaboratory staff, or a combination of both groups. Because POCT may be an integral part of patient management systems, an immediate replacement may be necessary if any breakdown occurs. Duplicate instruments may therefore be considered available for immediate use in those situations, or, if the manufacturer is amenable and instruments readily available, exchange should be undertaken as soon as possible. These arrangements will be conditional on the proposed business case and regular audit of the service required. The repair of a device after breakdown may be a role of the pathology or other

department within an organization, but whatever is agreed, the needs of the service as described and agreed upon in the business case must be met at all times.

Stock Maintenance

Reagent replacement is an important part of POCT equipment maintenance, and an appropriate stock control system is mandatory, especially where the devices are disposable. Reagents must not be allowed to be used beyond their expiry date, and strict attention should be paid to the SOP for these reagents, some of which may have to be brought to an appropriate operating temperature (whether room temperature or otherwise) before use. Similar restrictions may occur for IQA and EQA materials.

Accreditation

Accreditation of laboratories may have different connotations depending on the part of the world in which it is based. In the United Kingdom, accreditation involves an external audit of the laboratory to demonstrate its ability to provide a service of high quality. All laboratories in the United Kingdom have been asked to register with Clinical Pathology Accreditation (UK) so that POCT can be inspected and included in external audited programs. In other environments, e.g., the United States, accredited laboratories have to participate in approved proficiency testing programs. The College of American Pathologists provides a POCT checklist for its laboratory accreditation program that covers all of the topics discussed in the guidelines above, because the mandatory CLIA '88 requirements define the conditions under which POCT can occur.

Recordkeeping and Information Technology

There has already been mention of the necessity for meticulous recordkeeping and the need for linking devices to information systems. There are key questions that should be reviewed when recordkeeping is undertaken, and these are detailed in Table 15-9. The eventual introduction of a common interfacing standard in all POCT devices will facilitate recordkeeping and many other aspects of clinical governance that have been outlined in Table 15-9 and the text above (15).

CONCLUSIONS

Pathology has a key role in medical decision making and is not immune to changes in healthcare delivery. Some institutions have thought that pathology tests can be a rate-limiting step in achieving further clinical and cost improvements in patient care, particularly when delayed clinical management decisions and follow-up consultations are imposed by test turnaround times. A modern pathology service will need to consider a wide range of technologies to provide its service, and this may be achieved by providing services in smaller, outlying labora-

Table 15-9 Recordkeeping—Key Questions

Are records kept of the current lot numbers of test kits, including date opened and use-by date?

Are results expressed in the same units with the same reference intervals as used by the hospital laboratory?

How are the patient results kept confidential?

Are operator ID and patient ID recorded when tests are undertaken?

Can laboratory staff access QA data?

What provisions are made for confirmatory results to be provided where POCT results are out of range of the device used?

How are results stored and for how long?

If the device is interfaced with an IT system, how long are the results stored and backed up, and how may they be accessed?

What procedures are there to record results in patient notes?

Are these stored in a written format, or in an electronic patient record?

Are results that are stored on an information system password protected?

tories through POCT and linking them remotely into the laboratory network. The recognition that POCT can contribute to better healthcare is tacitly confirmed by observing the changes in testing in hospitals in the United States. The large centralized laboratory still exists, but additional testing using POCT can now be found in emergency rooms and intensive care areas. The drive to greater centralization of laboratories paradoxically may enhance the use of POCT in some other areas of the hospital or primary practice. Commercial manufacturers have seen the opportunity, and this is reflected in the increasing range and availability of tests that can be used by patients, their caregivers, and the nonlaboratory community in general.

This chapter is a distillation of the guidelines that are commonly in use in the world and outline the key areas that require consideration before POCT is actively used. Guidelines vary around the world depending on the country and its regulatory agencies. In some countries there are mandatory requirements that must be fulfilled before using POCT; in others, guidelines are the only distributed source of POCT information and there are no mandatory requirements to consider prior to use of a device. Despite miniaturization of devices, increasing reliability, and greater precision and accuracy, devices are not foolproof, and their benefits are limited by their analytical performance and the skills and knowledge of the user. POCT is here to stay and will expand as new technologies are utilized, but its limitations must be explicitly stated, especially to users not schooled in laboratory techniques. Guidelines help to direct the user to the correct method for use of these devices, and clinical scientists need to actively promulgate protocols that allow the use of these systems, encouraging meaningful and timely care of patients.

REFERENCES

1. Foster W. A short history of clinical pathology. Edinburgh and London: E&S Livingstone, 1961.
2. Morman E. Clinical Pathology in America, 1865–1915: Philadelphia as a test case. Bull Hist Med 1984;58:198.
3. Rosenfeld L. Henry Bence Jones (1813–1873): the best "chemical doctor" in London. Clin Chem 1987;33:1687–92.
4. Whitby LG, Percy-Robb IW, Smith AF. Lecture notes on clinical chemistry, 1st ed. Oxford: Blackwell Scientific Publications, 1975.
5. Despotis GJ, Joist JH, Goodnough LT. Monitoring of hemostasis in cardiac surgical patients: impact of point-of-care testing on blood loss and transfusion outcomes. Clin Chem 1997;43:1684–96.
6. Pathology Modernisation Programme (UK). Pathology—the essential service. London: Department of Health, 2002. www.doh.gov.uk/patholgymodernisation.
7. Lee-Lewandrowski E, Corboy D, Lewandrowski K, Sinclair J, McDermot S, Benzer TI. Implementation of a point-of-care satellite laboratory in the emergency department of an academic medical center: impact on test turnaround time and patient emergency department length of stay. Arch Pathol Lab Med 2003;127:456–60.
8. Nichols JH, Kickler TS, Dyer KL, Humbertson SK, Cooper PC, Maughan WL, Oechsle DG. Clinical outcomes of point-of-care testing in the interventional radiology and invasive cardiology setting. Clin Chem 2000;46:543–50.
9. Scott MG. Faster is better—it's rarely that simple! Clin Chem 2000;46:441–2.
10. Handorf CR. Quality control and quality management of alternate-site testing. Clin Lab Med 1994;14:539–57.
11. Belsey R, Vandenbark M, Goitein RK, Baer DM. Evaluation of a laboratory system intended for use in physicians' offices. Reliability of results produced by health care workers without formal or professional laboratory training. JAMA 1987;58:357–61.
12. Barry HC, Ebell MH. Test characteristics and decision rules. In: Arron DC, Sowers M. eds. Endocrinology and metabolism clinics of North America: epidemiology and clinical decision making. Philadelphia: WB Saunders, 1997;26:45–65.
13. CLIA '88 final rules. Northfield, IL: College of Pathologists/American Society of Clinical Pathologists, February 1992.
14. Prisco D, Paniccia R. Point-of-care testing of hemostasis in cardiac surgery. Thromb J 2003;1:1–10.
15. National Committee for Clinical Laboratory Standards. Point-of-care connectivity; approved standard. NCCLS document POCT1-A. Wayne, PA: NCCLS, 2001.
16. Evidence-based guidelines for the prevention of hospital associated infection. J Hosp Infect 2001;47(Supp):S5–S9.
17. Guidance for healthcare workers: protection against blood-borne viruses. Recommendations of the Expert Advisory Group on AIDS and the Advisory Group on Hepatitis. HSC 1998/063. London: UK Health Departments, 1998.
18. Safe disposal of clinical waste. ISBN 0–7176-492–7. Health Services Advisory Committee, 1999.
19. Scally G, Donaldson LJ. The NHS's 50 anniversary. Clinical governance and the drive for quality improvement in the new NHS in England. BMJ 1998;317:61–5.
20. Gray T. Clinical governance. Ann Clin Biochem 2000;37:9–15.

Chapter 16

Regulatory Issues Regarding Point-of-Care Testing

Laurence M. Demers and Sharon S. Ehrmeyer

The advances in point-of-care testing (POCT) technology that have emerged in the past 10 years have significantly enhanced the ability to perform laboratory testing outside of the laboratory and closer to the patient. However, regulatory issues have been raised that are unique to this form of testing. The term *point-of-care testing* is rather broad in scope and covers any testing that is performed outside of the conventional clinical laboratory, whether it is a CLIA-waived test performed in a physician's office or complex testing performed in an ambulatory clinic. As defined by the 1988 Clinical Laboratory Improvement Amendments (CLIA '88), waived tests are laboratory examinations that use methods that are so simple to perform that an individual without specialist skills or formal laboratory training could produce an accurate result. It is the method and complexity of testing, however, that dictate the type of regulations that cover all forms of laboratory testing, whether performed in a central laboratory or outside the laboratory at the site of direct patient interaction. In the United States, all laboratory testing, both simple and complex, whether performed in a hospital laboratory, clinic, ward, physician's office, or emergency care center, is subject to some form of regulatory control. In the United States, the federal government mandates minimum standards for all laboratory testing and exerts control through regulatory policies, public law, and collaboration with professional organizations. Laboratory testing that is performed at the point of care most often includes simple or waived testing; however, this form of laboratory testing is still subject to minimal regulatory control in the United States. In contrast, very few countries outside of the United States have government regulations that mandate quality standards for POCT (Table 16-1). Many countries, however, have professional organizations that recommend specific guidelines for POCT that include quality assurance measures and proficiency testing.

CLIA '88

As mentioned previously, the most extensive government program in the world for clinical laboratory testing including POCT is in the United States. In 1988 Congress passed the Clinical Laboratory Improvement Amendments (CLIA '88), which require compliance with specific quality regulations and personnel standards for clinical laboratory testing. CLIA regulations were purposely written to be "site neutral," which means that all laboratory testing including POCT, regardless of where it is performed, would fall under the scope of the regulation. The US Department of Health and Human Services (HHS) assigned the Health Care Financing Administration (HCFA) the responsibility of implementing CLIA '88 and its regulations to ensure adherence to established CLIA regulatory standards. HCFA has since been renamed the Centers for Medicare and Medicaid Services (CMS). This agency provides CLIA certification of all laboratories performing testing for patient care and carries out inspections of laboratories that do not choose professional accreditation to ensure appropriate compliance. An oversight committee (CLIAC) was established at the Centers for Disease Control and Prevention (CDC) to review and update CLIA policies as new procedures and tests are developed. For many individual US states, CMS transferred the responsibility of laboratory inspection and quality assurance monitoring of clinical laboratory testing to the particular state. The bureau of laboratories in these states may have regulatory policies and guidelines for laboratory testing that are more stringent than the federal government's standards. The regulatory policies mandated by CLIA '88 for laboratory testing establish minimal standards for all laboratories performing testing for diagnosis, health assessment, and monitoring of patient care. However, several professional healthcare organizations with testing standards that are at least as or more stringent than those of CLIA have received so-called deemed status from CMS and participate in the regulation of clinical laboratory testing through voluntary accreditation. These include the Joint Commission on Accreditation of Healthcare Organizations (JCAHO), which inspects clinical laboratories as part of its accreditation of hospitals and healthcare organizations. The College of American Pathologists (CAP) is another organization afforded deemed status that also inspects laboratories through its Laboratory Accreditation Program. Another accrediting body that regulates laboratory testing is COLA, formerly known as the Commission on Office Laboratory Accreditation. Initially COLA focused on testing conducted in physician office laboratories. Now it accredits testing in a variety of settings including community, independent, and industrial laboratories.

Table 16-1   Guidelines and Government Imposed Regulations Regarding POCT

Country	Government regulations	Professional organization guidelines	PT[a]
Argentina	No	No	Yes
Australia	Yes	Yes	Yes
Belgium	No	No	No
Britain	No	Yes	Yes
Canada	Yes	Yes	No
China	No	No	No
Denmark	No	Yes	No
France	No	Yes	No
Italy	No	No	No
Israel	No	Yes	Yes
New Zealand	No	Yes	Yes
Norway	No	Yes	Yes
Sweden	No	Yes	Yes
United States	Yes	Yes	Yes

[a] PT, proficiency testing.

COMPLEXITY OF TESTING

The CLIA '88 quality standards for laboratories performing clinical testing are dictated by the complexity of the testing being performed.

CLIA '88 specifies three major categories of testing: high-complexity, moderate complexity, and waived testing. Provider-performed microscopy is a subset of moderate complexity and reserved for a specific group of clinical practitioners. Each category carries a different requirement for quality practices and personnel standards.

High-Complexity and Moderate-Complexity Testing

These two categories encompass about 80% of the testing performed in most laboratories. The high-complexity category is reserved for the most difficult test methods to perform, which usually are conducted only in large hospitals and reference laboratories. This category also includes tests that are either developed or modified by the laboratory from the original manufacturer's instructions. Under CLIA, the laboratory performing high-complexity testing must identify five positions: director, technical supervisor, clinical consultant, general supervisor, and testing personnel. The educational requirements and experience necessary for personnel are more stringent for this category of testing. For high-complexity testing, the director's qualifications range from a medical degree to a doctorate in chemical, physical, biological, or clinical laboratory science and board certification as of February 2003. The technical supervisor is the individual who establishes the quality standards of the laboratory through the selection and monitoring of test methods, verifying test performance, and documenting staff competency. The clinical consultant has

responsibility that relates to the clinical component of laboratory testing including appropriate test selection and the clinical interpretation of test result reporting, and if not the laboratory director, advises the laboratory director in those aspects of the laboratory operation that are clinical in nature. The clinical consultant qualifications include an MD or PhD degree. The general supervisor is responsible for the proper performance of all laboratory procedures and reporting of test results. Qualifications for this position range from a medical degree to education and training equivalent to an associate degree in clinical laboratory science plus appropriate experience. Testing personnel are responsible for specimen processing, test performance, and result reporting. The qualifications for testing personnel vary from a medical degree to an associate degree in clinical laboratory science. For moderate-complexity test methodologies, reagent systems are readily available and require fewer operator decision-making steps. CLIA stipulates that the operator must follow the manufacturer's instructions and the test method cannot be modified. In contrast to high-complexity testing, laboratories performing moderate-complexity testing need to identify only four positions—director, technical consultant, clinical consultant, and testing personnel—and these have less stringent personnel requirements. The laboratory director has overall responsible for all phases of the laboratory testing process and result reporting and can fill all of the roles simultaneously, provided the director has an MD or PhD degree. The laboratory director qualifications for a moderate-complexity laboratory also include individuals with a bachelor's degree in medical technology or clinical laboratory science or in the chemical, physical, or biological sciences plus appropriate experience. The technical consultant is the individual or group of individuals, depending on the size of the laboratory, who verifies test performance, establishes the quality control program, evaluates staff competency and performance, and resolves day-to-day technical problems. The minimum qualification to be a technical consultant is a bachelor's degree in the chemical, physical, biological, or clinical laboratory sciences and 1 year of laboratory training and experience in the designated area of responsibility. For the moderate-complexity category, testing personnel must at least have a high school diploma or equivalent and appropriate training for the tests performed.

Although the government still classifies test methods into one of the three complexity categories, the most recent revisions to CLIA make the quality control and quality assurance requirements the same for both moderate- and high-complexity testing. The specific requirements that must be in practice to monitor and evaluate the quality of the entire testing process including the preanalytical, analytical, and postanalytical phases of testing to ensure accurate and reliable patient test results are discussed in CLIA's new Subpart K—Quality Systems for Non-waived Testing. CMS uses the term *nonwaived* to reflect the combination of the moderate- and high-complexity categories for quality control and assurance purposes. These include daily assay control procedures, method and instrument validation, periodic calibration verification, accuracy assessment, and ongoing quality assurance and quality improvement activities. External proficiency testing is relied on as an indicator of the quality of testing service provided by the laboratory and is mandated for specified analytes.

Provider-performed microscopy is a subcategory of moderately complex testing that is reserved exclusively for physicians, dentists, nurse practitioners and midwives, and physician assistants performing the testing as part of a patient examination. This category was established primarily to control testing performed by the physician in his or her office and is limited in the scope of tests that are performed as the testing is primarily qualitative in nature (Table 16-2). The primary instrument for performing the testing includes those laboratory tests requiring use of a microscope to classify and identify cellular material present in the specimen. This category is limited to bright-field or phase-contrast microscopy and does not include other, more sophisticated forms of microscopy or tissue staining.

Waived Testing

This category covers the simplest level of testing and is the most common category used for testing performed outside of the central clinical laboratory in physician offices and clinics. Initially referred to as *dipstick testing*, this category has grown substantially. For a test method to fit in this category it must meet one of the following three statutory requirements: (*i*) The test must have been cleared by the FDA for home use; (*ii*) the test must be so simple and accurate to perform that the likelihood of erroneous results would be negligible; or (*iii*) if performed incorrectly, the test would not pose a reasonable risk to the patient. The list described in Table 16-3 includes all waived tests introduced since CLIA '88 regulations were first implemented.

Except to follow the manufacturer's instructions, this group of tests is considered waived from CLIA quality standards, and CMS surveyors do not inspect waived testing unless there is a complaint or fraudulent activity is expected. COLA also does not inspect waived testing but offers educational materials to assist sites performing tests in this category. In contrast, the JCAHO and CAP, as well as several individual states in the United States, require adherence to certain quality standards of practice to ensure quality test results for waived

Table 16-2 Provider-Performed Microscopy Testing under CLIA '88

Urine sediment examination
Semen analysis, limited to presence or absence of sperm and motility
Wet mount preparations of vaginal, cervical, or skin specimens
All potassium hydroxide preparations
Postcoital direct, qualitative examinations of specimens from the vagina or cervix
Fern testing
Pinworm examinations
Nasal smears for eosinophils
Fecal leukocyte examination

Table 16-3 CLIA '88 Waived Tests[a]

Microbiology/virology
  H. pylori
  Streptococcus Group A (direct from throat swab)
  Influenza A and B
Endocrinology
  Urine pregnancy tests (hCG) with chemistry analyzer
  Urine pregnancy tests (hCG) by visual color comparison
  Ovulation tests (LH) by visual color comparison
  N-telopeptides (for osteoporosis)
  FSH and LH
  Estrone-3-glucuronide
  Semen (for male fertility screen)
General chemistry
  Amines (Fern exam test card from vaginal swab)
  Cholesterol, total
  HDL cholesterol
  Creatinine
  Fecal occult blood
  Fructosamine
  Gastric occult blood
  Glucose
  Glucose monitoring devices (FDA cleared/home use)
  Glycosylated hemoglobin (HgbA1C)
  Microalbumin
  Triglyceride
  Vaginal pH
  Nitrazine pH paper for body fluid
  Ketones (blood and urine)
  Alanine aminotransferase
General immunology
  H. pylori antibodies
  Infectious mononucleosis antibodies
  Lyme disease antibodies
  Bladder tumor associated antigen
Hematology
  Erythrocyte sedimentation rate
  Hematocrit
  Spun microhematocrit
  Hemoglobin
  Hemoglobin by copper sulfate
  Hemoglobin, single analyte
  Prothrombin time (PT)
Toxicology
  Ethanol (alcohol)
  Nicotine and/or metabolites
  Cocaine metabolites
  Cannabinoids
  Opiates
  PCP
  Amphetamines/methamphetamines
Urinalysis
  Dipstick or tablet reagent for bilirubin, glucose, hemoglobin, ketones, leukocytes, nitrite, pH, protein, specific gravity and urobilinogen
  Urine catalase

[a] For the latest information and specific waived methodologies, see http://www.cms.hhs.gov/clia/waivetbl.pdf.

methodologies. These include minimum requirements for quality control, documented laboratory procedures, defined policies for reporting results, documented training for personnel responsible for performing the testing, and a listing of those personnel supervising waived testing. Personnel must have adequate training and orientation to perform the test but need not have had formal education in medical technology or laboratory testing. Policies must be in place to demonstrate satisfactory levels of competence for waived testing personnel. The waived laboratory needs to demonstrate that at a minimum, the manufacturer's instructions are followed for the testing and that quality control results and test records are properly interpreted and maintained. The written policies and procedures in a waived testing laboratory must address specimen collection issues, instrument calibration and performance practices, quality control and remedial action policies, and measures of test performance. The responsibility for determining the competence of personnel doing the testing is determined by the laboratory director and is based on how frequently the staff person performs the test and his or her technical background. In a physician office setting, the laboratory director is usually the lead physician in the practice and may or may not have had training in clinical laboratory testing. Nevertheless, the physician has overall responsibility for the test performance and result reporting in his or her office practice, and both JCAHO and CAP require that the personnel actually doing the testing possess a certain level of skill. Approaches to assessing the competence of personnel include the monitoring of quality control results, direct observation of the testing performed, and clinical correlation of the test result. Occasionally, sending a split sample to an established reference laboratory can provide assurance that the testing is being performed correctly. Often, for specific tests the manufacturer's representative will participate in the training of personnel on site. The quality control program in place for waived testing needs to specify how the methods are controlled for quality, the frequency of control testing, the stability of reagents being used, and the remedial action taken when the control results fail acceptable limits. Most reagent systems and devices carry explicit manufacturer's instructions for quality control monitoring. These instructions must be adhered to but JCAHO and CAP regulations may require more. Both accreditation agencies mandate maintaining quality control results and patient test results as well as linking these results to the instrument and operator. Quality control records and individual patient results are usually correlated and are a source of reference if and when a question arises either from the physician ordering the test or as required for accrediting agencies.

POCT REGULATIONS

As mentioned earlier, advances in available instrumentation for POCT has brought more testing, including moderate complexity testing, closer to the patient and into physician offices and small clinics. At one time, only waived testing was performed in the POCT setting. New advances in technology, however,

have allowed for much more sophisticated testing closer to the patient and thus personnel qualification and training considerations as well as adherence to more formal quality assurance practices have become issues not clearly recognized by POCT sites. When a method is classified in a nonwaived, complex category, it is subject to more stringent regulatory policies whether or not it is a POCT test. As noted in Table 16-1, the United States, Canada, and Australia are the only countries that have government regulations affecting POCT. A number of countries have guidelines for POCT quality control that come as recommendations from professional organizations in that particular country, but few have government regulations that dictate policy in the same manner as CLIA '88 in the United States. In the United Kingdom, guidelines exist on the organization and performance of POCT published by the Association of Clinical Biochemists. The Department of Health in the United Kingdom encourages but does not mandate the involvement of the laboratory in all aspects of POCT including training and quality control. As part of the recent consolidation efforts in Europe, there are discussions within the new European Union of establishing regulations for POCT in Europe akin to the CLIA regulations in the United States. In the United States, the personnel qualifications for performing POCT and for directing laboratories depend primarily on the type of testing performed (moderate complexity or waived), although CAP prefers that a pathologist or doctoral scientist be responsible for the testing performed under a POCT program. POCT personnel standards for JCAHO and COLA are identical to those specified by CLIA '88 for each test complexity level. The CAP generally follows the standards for personnel stated in CLIA '88 for the high-complexity level.

Tables 16-4 and 16-5 list the different quality control requirements according to test complexity and accrediting agency in the United States. Most of the requirements from CAP, JCAHO, and COLA are modeled after CLIA '88, but differences do exist. For example, CAP considers all testing equivalent in terms of its quality-control regulations, whereas CLIA, COLA, and JCAHO specify differences between waived testing and nonwaived complexity testing. There is no specific requirement by CMS for laboratories to use any one particular organization for regulatory control of laboratory testing. All laboratories must be CLIA certified but have the opportunity to use a regulatory organization such as CAP or COLA in lieu of CLIA to satisfy the requirements.

MANAGING POCT

Laboratory certification by CLIA also becomes an issue with POCT. POCT performed within an institution but outside the central clinical laboratory typically falls under the CLIA license of the central clinical laboratory. This requires the central laboratory to oversee the testing process as well as the personnel doing the testing and to verify the accuracy of all analytes performed outside of the central laboratory. The involvement of the central laboratory in the organization and management of POCT is also required in other countries. In the United Kingdom, for example, although

Table 16-4   Comparison of Waived Testing Requirements by Inspecting Organization

Requirement	CLIA and COLA	JCAHO	CAP
Daily QC	Follow manufacturer's recommendation.	Follow manufacturer's recommendation. If none are defined, the test site must define.	Two levels each 24 h of testing for most waived tests
Method verification *before* implementation	No, accepts manufacturer's data.	Accuracy, precision, reportable range, and appropriateness of reference ranges	Accuracy, precision, sensitivity, analytical interferences, reportable range (AMR) and appropriateness of reference ranges
Assessment of reportable range (AMR) every 6 months	No	No	Yes
Participation in proficiency testing	No	No	Yes, for all analytes tested when possible
Method correlations every 6 months (different instruments and/or different methods) as part of quality assurance	No	No	Yes, testing performed under the same CLIA certificate
Establishment of accuracy (twice each year) for analytes not in proficiency testing	No	No	Yes
Documented personnel training and annual competency assessment	No; however, good laboratory practice dictates personnel training and competency assessment.	Yes	Yes

formal regulation of POCT is not mandatory, the hospital accreditation program requires laboratory involvement in POCT.

POCT Certification and Proficiency Testing

In the United States, all physician offices and testing centers outside of an institutional clinical laboratory require their own CLIA certificate for POCT. From a proficiency testing (PT) perspective, CLIA '88 mandates participation in proficiency testing for specific analytes measured only by nonwaived test methods. The CMS recognizes and approves several PT programs that produce control materials, apply specified performance criteria, and provide feedback to the laboratory in terms of assay performance. For regulatory PT, CLIA '88 mandates three annual PT events with five specimens in each covering the dynamic range of the analyte being tested. The performance reports are sent both to the laboratory doing the testing and to CMS or a CMS designate such as the state in which the testing is performed. Table 16-6 lists the CMS- approved proficiency testing program providers in the United States. To successfully pass a proficiency test, the laboratory must obtain a score of at least 80% correct for each analyte. Failure to achieve a satisfactory score for the same analyte in two consecutive testing events or two out of three consecutive testing events can result in sanctions against the laboratory. For the initial unsuccessful performance, CMS may direct the laboratory to undertake training of its personnel or to obtain technical assistance, or both. Alternative or principal sanctions are applied when there is immediate jeopardy to patient health and safety, the laboratory fails to provide CMS or its agent with satisfactory evidence that it has taken steps to correct the problem, and/or the laboratory has a poor compliance history. These alternative sanctions include suspension of certification or limitation of testing. The laboratory must then demonstrate sustained satisfactory performance on two consecutive proficiency testing events, one of which may be onsite, before CMS will consider recertification.

When CLIA '88 was first implemented, surveyors exposed a number of deficiencies in POCT laboratories. According to CLIA surveyors, the rate and number of deficiencies were lowest in those institutions that had central clinical laboratories that provided oversight responsibility. POCT deficiencies were the highest in physician office laboratories, where there is typically a lack of experienced personnel who have had formal laboratory training. Nevertheless, the number and types of deficiencies originally cited by CLIA surveyors has decreased dramatically in all POCT laboratories since CLIA '88 was first enacted in September, 1992. Failure to follow the manufacturer's directions and to perform and document quality control are the more common deficiencies cited by CLIA surveyors. Table 16-7 lists the most common deficiencies noted in POCT laboratories. Because these deficiencies are

Table 16-5 Comparison of Nonwaived (Moderate-Complexity) Test Quality Requirements by Inspecting Organization

Requirement	CLIA and COLA	JCAHO	CAP
QC	Generally two levels each 24 hours of testing. Blood gases require one level each 8 h of testing; coagulation requires two levels each 8 h of testing.	Same as CLIA	Same as CLIA
Method verification *before* implementation	Accuracy, precision, reportable range and appropriateness of reference ranges	Accuracy, precision, reportable range and appropriateness of reference ranges	Accuracy, precision, sensitivity, analytical interferences, reportable range (AMR) and appropriateness of reference ranges
Assessment of reportable range (AMR) every 6 months	Yes, through calibration verification	Yes (beginning in 2005)	Yes (AMR only)
Participation in regulatory proficiency testing	Yes, for selected analytes	Yes, for selected analytes	Yes, for all analytes tested when available
Method correlations every 6 months (different instruments and/or different methods) as part of quality assurance	Yes	Yes	Yes
Establishment of accuracy (twice each year) for analytes not in proficiency testing	Yes	Yes	Yes
Documented personnel training and annual competency assessment	Yes	Yes	Yes

frequently found in physician office laboratories, it is often the lack of understanding of good laboratory practice by the physician responsible for the office laboratory that is the source of the problem. A license to practice medicine does not impart the training required for managing and performing quality laboratory

Table 16-6 CMS-Approved Proficiency Testing Providers[a]

American Association of Bioanalysts
American Academy of Family Physicians
American Proficiency Institute
California Thoracic Society
College of American Pathologists (two surveys): CAP and EXCEL
Medical Laboratory Evaluation
Commonwealth of Pennsylvania
Idaho Bureau of Laboratories
New Jersey Department of Health
Puerto Rico Department of Health
Ohio Department of Health
State of Maryland (cytology only)
State of New York (only for NY and NY state permits)
Wisconsin State Laboratory of Hygiene

[a] Not all programs offer PT for all analytes. For the most up-to-date list, see http://www.cms.hhs.gov/clia/ptlist.pdf.

testing and thus it is often a case of oversight rather than a deliberate means of averting regulatory policy. Another important factor that can influence POCT testing is the time it takes to implement and maintain the regulations required by certifying agencies such as CLIA. Studies have been carried out to assess the time required to perform POCT-related tasks. Typically, more than half the time spent implementing POCT regulations involves writing up the procedures, while less than 15% of the time is spent on quality assurance. Within institutions more than half of the staff time devoted to POCT is by nurses and less than 10% by laboratory staff. In contrast, in the physician office setting, nurses

Table 16-7 Most Cited Deficiencies in POCT Laboratories

Failure to following manufacturer's instructions
Failure to document patient results in patient record
Failure to include patient identification
Failure to perform and document quality control
Failure to document and take appropriate action for control outliers
Use of outdated/expired reagents
Failure to perform proficiency testing
Failure to have a procedure manual for testing
Failure to observe safety requirements
Failure to document personnel training and competency

constitute more than 80% of the staff performing POCT. This suggests that the vast majority of testing in the POCT setting is of the waived testing variety.

CLIA '88 is a self-funding law that requires certification and the payment of fees to the US government by all laboratory testing facilities regardless of the type of testing being performed. Laboratories must obtain either a certificate of waiver or certificate of accreditation to comply with CMS laboratory testing requirements. Laboratories certified by CMS or its designated state agency receive a registration certificate to begin performing testing, and once the laboratory is judged by CMS to be in compliance, a final certificate of compliance is issued. Those laboratories electing accreditation by an organization such as CAP, COLA, or JCAHO must begin by applying for a CMS registration certificate, and once the laboratory is inspected and found to meet the organization's standards it then receives a certificate of accreditation from the organization. As mentioned previously, these accrediting agencies are recognized by CMS as having regulatory standards equivalent to and usually more rigorous than CLIA.

As mentioned earlier, formal regulation of POCT is minimal in countries outside of the United States except for Canada and Australia. The quality assurance practices, when carried out, are usually performed because of the diligence of the individual laboratories involved and the influence of professional organizations in that country. As noted in Table 16-1, only a few countries have formal regulations for POCT although many countries have guidelines that come from professional organizations within that country. As POCT testing instrumentation expands beyond waived testing to include more moderate complexity testing, laboratories around the world might consider adopting the minimum standards required by CLIA '88 in the United States. Until then, the responsibility for quality laboratory testing in the point-of-care setting will reside in the hands of the clinical practitioner, who must weigh the importance and accuracy of a test result to patient care with the quality of the test result generated by the instrument or method his or her laboratory is using. The ultimate responsibility for a test result lies with the laboratory director. However, as POCT is practiced closer to the patient, the physician requesting the test must bear some of the responsibility in accepting the test result and acting on it.

SUGGESTED READING

1. US Department of Health and Human Services. Medicare, Medicaid and CLIA programs: regulations implementing the Clinical Laboratory Improvement Amendments of 1988 (CLIA). Final rule. Fed Regist 1992;57:7002–186.
2. CLIA final rule (2002 codification of all previous rules, 1992–2002). http://www.phppo.cdc.gov/clia/pdf/42cfr49302.pdf. CLIA final rule (January 24, 2003). http://www.phppo.cdc.gov/clia/pdf/CMS-2226-F.pdf.
3. Public Law 100–578, Section 353 Public Health Service Act (42 USC 263a) October 31, 1988.
4. US Centers for Medicare & Medicaid Services (CMS). Medicare, Medicaid, and CLIA programs: laboratory requirements relating to quality systems and certain personnel qualifications. Final rule. Fed Regist Jan 24 2003;16:3640–714.
5. CMS state operations manual. Appendix C. Regulations and interpretive guidelines for laboratories and laboratory services. http://www.cms.gov/clia/appendc.asp.
6. CMS website for CLIA '88. www.cms.hhs.gov/clia/.
7. CAP laboratory accreditation checklists. Northfield, IL: College of American Pathologists. http://www.cap.org/apps/docs/laboratory_accreditation/checklists/checklistftp.html.
8. JCAHO. Comprehensive accreditation manual for laboratory and point of care testing. Oakbrook Terrace, IL: Joint Commission on Accreditation of Healthcare Organizations, 2004.
9. COLA. Laboratory accreditation manual. Columbia, MD: COLA, 2004.
10. Ehrmeyer, SS. Regulatory affairs: quality assurance. Point of Care 2002;1:180–2.
11. Ehrmeyer, SS. Regulatory affairs: quality control. Point of Care 2002;1:104–6.
12. Ehrmeyer SS. Regulatory affairs. Follow manufacturer's directions to the T. Point of Care 2002;1:35–6.
13. Ehrmeyer SS, Laessig RH. Regulatory affairs: proficiency testing. Point of Care 2002;1:268–70.
14. Summers SH, Harmening D, Lunz ME. Who performs POCT. Lab Med 1998;29:85–8.
15. Goldsmith, BM. Point of care testing: how laboratorians can ensure quality beyond the lab. Clin Lab News April 2001;6–8.
16. Kost GJ, Ehrmeyer SS, Chernow B, Winkelman JW, Zaloga GP, Dellinger RP, Shirey T. Laboratory–clinical interface: point of care (POC) testing. Chest 1999;115:1140–54.
17. Ehrmeyer SS. Regulatory affairs: reportable range. Point of Care 2003;2:71–2.

Chapter 17

Clinical Governance—The Implications for Point-of-Care Testing in Hospitals: A UK Perspective

Danielle B. Freedman

Clinical governance has, for the first time, placed the quality of healthcare as a direct responsibility of the chief executive and therefore the board of all National Health Service (NHS) Trusts (hospitals), community providers and primary care trusts (primary care physicians) in the United Kingdom. The foundation for clinical governance was set out by the Department of Health in its document "A First-Class Service—Quality in the New NHS" (1). Much of this had been precipitated by the Bristol cardiac surgery cases and other series of medical disasters in the United Kingdom relating to cervical screening, breast screening, psychiatric care, and misdiagnoses emanating from the pathology laboratory.

Clinical governance has been formally defined as "a framework through which the NHS organizations in the UK are accountable for continuing to improve the quality of the service and safeguarding high standards of care by creating an environment in which excellence in clinical care would flourish" (2–6). Clinical governance provides an umbrella under which all aspects of quality can be gathered and continuously monitored.

One of the aims of the NHS in the United Kingdom is to ensure continued improvement in the overall standard of clinical care, reduce variation in outcomes, offer access to services, and ensure that clinical decisions are based on the most up-to-date evidence of what is known to be effective.

Clinical governance is central to that strategy and is a systematic approach to quality assurance (Table 17-1). Furthermore, it provides a framework for accountability for total quality management. The responsibility of clinical governance involves guaranteeing quality through a number of processes, many of which are currently in use and should be familiar to clinicians, laboratory personnel, and managers. They include clinical effectiveness and optimization of clinical care, clinical risk management and accountability, clinical auditing and monitoring, commitment to learning from complaints and ensuring the competence of staff and continuous professional development, implementation of good quality clinical data systems, and, importantly, involvement of patients and care providers. The interpretation of clinical governance for laboratory medicine is illustrated in Table 17-2, which describes the elements of a clinical governance plan. Table 17-3 shows an agenda for a laboratory's clinical governance meeting, which occurs on a monthly basis.

This commitment is part of the wider statutory responsibilities of any NHS healthcare organization and includes that of financial probity, accountability, and ensuring value for public money on behalf of the taxpayer or, indeed, for a private payer. Therefore, in the specific context of laboratory medicine, clinical governance provides an integrated framework of accountability for the highest standard of service and maintenance of high quality in the context of patient outcomes, embracing all of the clinical teams involved in patient care. This can be challenging because in many instances, to give one example, the laboratory medicine budget is managed as an isolated entity, whereas resource allocation and clinical outcomes are viewed within the whole context of patient care. Thus clinical governance extends beyond the boundaries normally encompassed by total quality management initiatives in laboratory medicine.

The Healthcare Commission (HcC), an independent inspection body for the NHS, regularly inspects clinical governance arrangements in all NHS healthcare organizations and identifies any significant system failures with subsequent serious implications for that organization. How does clinical governance apply to point-of-care testing (POCT) in hospitals or in the community?

POINT-OF-CARE TESTING

It is over 20 years since Marks (7) suggested that advances in technology might bring biochemistry nearer the patient. However, it is only in the last few years that this has become a reality, due to a variety of factors. These include technological advances, increasing pressure to shorten hospital length of stay (LOS), increased clinician efficiency and decreased turnaround times, the consolidation of laboratories, and, importantly, public expectation, including the desire for self-management of chronic disease, such as oral anticoagulation treatment.

In 1997, POCT was a $3 billion market worldwide, and by 2001 this had almost doubled to exceed $5.4 billion (8). Enterprise Analysis Corporation (EAC) has forecast that sales in the POCT market will increase up to 50% over the next 5 years (9).

Table 17-1   Clinical Governance Involves Guaranteeing Quality

Leadership and accountability
Clinical effectiveness and practice with evidence-based medicine
Optimization of clinical care
Risk management
Learning from adverse events/incidents and complaints
Continual professional development
Good quality clinical data systems
Involvement of patients and care givers

Both the clinical and cost-effectiveness benefits of POCT continue to be debated. Although there may be weaknesses in laboratory services, this in itself cannot justify potentially expensive technologies like POCT unless there is clear evidence that the patient will benefit.

EVIDENCE

Clinical governance is about practicing evidence-based medicine and ensuring clinical effectiveness. The evidence for the use of POCT, particularly in hospitals to improve clinical outcome, is often conflicting. In addition, in the primary care setting the health technology assessment by Hobbs et al. (10) found very few papers providing evidence of the effectiveness of POCT—primarily be-

cause few studies actually addressed the clinical requirements for undertaking the test. They also recognized the point made in a recent editorial in the *British Medical Journal* that "the absence of evidence is not evidence of absence" (11).

In a review of POCT cardiac markers (12), the authors postulated that in situations in which treatment and monitoring decisions are based on time-sensitive diagnostic results, POCT linked with improved triage and treatment strategies may lead to improved resource utilization and clinical outcome. Ng et al. and McCord et al. (13, 14) showed this to be the case in evaluations of a 90-min chest pain protocol, in which they found it was possible to implement an effective rule-out strategy. This led to a significant reduction in admissions to the coronary care unit without significant risk to the patients. However, Kendall et al. (15), in a randomized control of POCT for blood gas and electrolytes in the accident and emergency department, demonstrated that POCT had no impact on a number of outcome measures. These included the amount of time patients spent in the emergency department, length of stay in the hospital, admission rates, and mortality.

In contrast, Murray et al. (16) recognized that previous studies in clinical settings had failed to demonstrate a reduction in patient LOS associated with the use of POCT. However, in their randomized control study they demonstrated that patients randomized to the POCT group had a shorter LOS in the emergency department. This shorter stay was thought to be

Table 17-2   Example of a Clinical Governance Annual Plan

Clinical Governance Plan 2003–2004

Area for development	Actions	Key staff	Date of review or completion
Leadership and accountability			
Clinical governance is well understood in the department. Leadership and accountability is clear.	This will continue.	Clinical director and lead clinicians	Ongoing
The clinical governance meetings in all departments are well structured.	The agenda for each department's clinical governance meetings will be reviewed to ensure that all aspects of clinical governance are addressed.	As above	Ongoing
Clinical audit			
Progress with clinical audit programs and progress with recommendations and actions agreed as a result of audit and effectiveness projects is discussed systematically in all departments.	Progress with clinical audit will be a standing agenda item within each department's clinical governance meetings.	Leads for clinical audit	Ongoing
Risk management			
The risk management process is well established. All incidents are discussed at clinical governance meetings.	Continue to build on this strength, ensuring that all departments take the same rigorous approach.	Leads as outlined under Leadership and Accountability and general manager, clinical support services	Ongoing

Table 17-2 Continued

Clinical Governance Plan 2003–2004			
Area for development	Actions	Key staff	Date of review or completion
Human resources, continuing professional development, and individual performance Consultants in pathology have been appraised for many years as part of the CPA process. Consultants are appraised using the portfolio approach.	Consultant appraisal will continue.	Clinical director	Ongoing
All staff (nonmedical) are appraised within the department in line with CPA accreditation.	This will continue	Departmental managers and general manager	Ongoing
Patient/user consultation and involvement The main method for involving patients and users is through questionnaire surveys. Other methods are less well understood.	The hospital's lead manager for Patient Advocacy Liaison Service (PALS) will be asked to attend a directorate meeting to discuss patient/user involvement. Training opportunities will be sought.	Clinical director	June 2003
Use of patient/user surveys is good with actions resulting. Recommendations and actions agreed as a result of patient/ user surveys are not always actioned.	Continue to ensure that action results from patient/user surveys by always developing specific action plans with assigned responsibilities and timescales. These will be assessed in directorate meetings and action taken when inadequate progress is being made.	Departmental heads	Ongoing
Use of information The approach using information routinely to evaluate quality is well developed through Datix* reports, the directorate information pack, and monthly external quality assurance (EQA) reports.	Continue the development of using information routinely to evaluate the quality of care and services.	Departmental leads	Ongoing
The use of information gained through surveys will be used to further develop services.	This will continue.	As above	Ongoing
Research and effectiveness The process used to receive and respond to evidence from national and professional bodies is well developed.	This will continue.	Department leads and general manager	Ongoing

* Datix is software used for incident reporting.

primarily due to the fact that the "normal" test results from POCT led to an earlier discharge. These authors also recognized that many of the triage decisions were delayed because the clinician had to wait for some results to arrive from the laboratory. In other settings within hospitals, e.g., with outpatients, Grieve et al. (17) demonstrated that mean glycated hemoglobin was significantly lower for patients in the POCT cohort compared with a conventional testing cohort. A recent

Table 17-3   Example of a Clinical Governance Meeting Agenda for Clinical Biochemistry

All staff are expected to attend
CLINICAL GOVERNANCE MEETING
AGENDA

1. Minutes of last meeting
2. Matters arising
3. Risk management Datix summary
4. Recent incidents/complaints
   4.1 Bilirubin reference range
5. Audit
   5.1 Progress with forward plan
   5.2 Forward plan 2004–2005
   5.3 Cardiac rehabilitation cholesterol
   5.4 C-reactive protein
   5.5 Ongoing audit—request card completion
   5.6 Inappropriate request
6. Guidelines
   6.1 Progress with National Institute for Clinical Excellence (NICE) guidelines
   6.2 Progress with National Service Framework (NSF) guidelines
   6.3 National Sweat Test guidelines
   6.4 National/regional/professional guidelines
   6.5 Creatinine clearance
   6.6 PSA
7. Professional development and training
   7.1 EQAS interpretative comments
   7.2 WEQAS November 2003 guidance
8. Patient/user involvement
9. CPA accreditation—horizontal and vertical audits
10. Review in hospital—feedback from POCT committee
11. EQA performance
12. Any other business
13. Date of next meeting

study by Lee-Lewandrowski (18) demonstrated that test turnaround time (TAT) declined an average of 87% after institution of POCT. The emergency department LOS decreased for patients who received pregnancy testing, urine dipstick testing, and cardiac-markers testing. Although these differences were not significant for individual tests, when the tests were combined, the average LOS was 41.3 min ($P = 0.006$ compared with the conventional testing approach). Another part of the study demonstrated clinician dissatisfaction with the central laboratory TAT and increased satisfaction with the TAT of the POCT program ($P < 0.001$).

However, in the primary care setting, the evidence for improving clinical outcome in the use of POCT remains substantially underresearched, mainly because of a lack of focus on the clinical impact of the test (19).

ECONOMIC CONSIDERATIONS

It goes without saying that the cost of performing a test at the point of care will be more expensive in terms of the consum-

ables than that which can be provided from the central laboratory. The POCT device is a complex product engineered to minimize the risk of operator error, and, furthermore, POCT cannot take advantage of the economies of scale possible with a central laboratory service. Costs of the numerous analyzers that need to be provided in different clinical areas, specially formulated reagents, sample tubes, specimen containers, QC material, and the like are in addition to the underlying central laboratory expenses. It has to be realized that implementation of POCT devices either in hospitals or in primary care settings will not entirely replace measurement in the central laboratory on a cost per item basis and therefore does not necessarily reduce central laboratory costs. More important, if there is to be any benefit from POCT, then it will be seen predominantly outside of the laboratory, whether it be in the short term through fewer clinic visits, in the longer term with reduced hospital admissions, or another ways.

The quality of the literature is poor and sometimes contradictory regarding the cost–benefit of POCT. There are enormous problems with POCT studies and the data can be utilized to benefit either advocates of POCT, those against POCT, or those with neutral views regarding POCT. Crucially, few studies to date have taken a holistic view of the economic benefit of POCT. There is an urgent need for research comparing the cost for the entire patient episode of care in patients with POCT versus the same care in patients without POCT. In order to effectively assess the cost–benefit ratio of POCT, each clinical situation has to be evaluated in its own unique circumstances (20).

ACCOUNTABILITY AND RISK MANAGEMENT

Over 9 billion laboratory tests are performed annually by clinical laboratories in the United States. These tests provide up to 80% of the information contained in patients' records and used by physicians to make important medical decisions. There have been many studies concerned with laboratory testing mistakes. A study of primary care physicians revealed that laboratory testing mistakes occurred in 34 out of 100,000 patient visits; 27% of these mistakes were considered to have an effect on patient care; and mistakes were most likely to occur before or after actual specimen analysis (21). Demers (22) has listed the 10 most cited deficiencies in POCT (see Table 17-4).

A review of some 50 studies on errors in laboratory medicine found that most studies focused on analytical errors; thus, the incidence of inappropriate test ordering and interpretation are more difficult to detect (23). However, all studies report a similar distribution of errors, with most occurring the in the pre- and postanalytical steps in the total testing process.

From the point of view of POCT, focusing only on the analytical process, some of the state-of-the-art instruments used today demonstrate de facto that the traditional quality characteristics, namely, accuracy, precision, reliability, and the like, are now primarily the responsibility of the device manu-

Table 17-4   The 10 Most Cited Deficiencies in POCT Laboratories

Failure to perform quality control testing

Failure to document QC activities

Failure to follow manufacturer's instructions explicitly

Failure to document personnel training and competency

Failure to document and take appropriate corrective action for control outliers

Failure to perform proficiency testing

Failure to have a procedure manual for testing and result reporting

Failure to perform and document calibration verification at least every 6 months

Failure to verify accuracy of analytes not included in a PT program

Failure to provide for continuing education for testing personnel

Source: Demers (22).

facturer. In the context of today's testing, the search for improved quality is appropriately shifting to both preanalytical and postanalytical variables, together with ensuring operator competence. The need to attend to these nonanalytical issues is emphasized in the CLIA 2003 and ISO 15 189: 2003 regulations (see Chapters 11 and 16).

Clinical governance is about accountability and leadership. This means that local laboratories must get involved in POCT to protect the patient. Poor management and the lack of appreciation of the requirements for reliable POCT have led to some disastrous incidents, and such incidents could lead to large legal claims against hospital trusts. Clinical governance includes having a robust risk management strategy and thus a POCT policy, which must be adhered to by all staff. POCT is always presented as easy to use and capable of producing accurate results. However, problems occur particularly when procedures for training and quality assurance are poor. Guidance from the Joint Working Group on Quality Assurance (24) categorically states, "To ensure reliable performance and manage the risks associated with POCT, the pathology laboratory must have a central role in the management of these devices." This guidance has been reinforced by the Medical Devices Agency (MDA) publication (25) that was brought to the attention of all healthcare professionals involved in POCT in the United Kingdom, including managers. The MDA has now been subsumed by a larger organization in the United Kingdom—the Medicines and Healthcare Products Regulatory Agency (MHRA), which was established in April 2003 and is an executive agency of the Department of Health. It is committed to safeguarding public health and ensuring that medicines, healthcare products, and medical equipment meet appropriate standards of safety, quality, performance, and effectiveness and are used safely. In addition, the MHRA ensures that medical devices meet appropriate standards of safety, quality, and performance and comply with the relevant directives from the European Union.

In 2001, the Department of Health published the document "Building a Safer NHS for Patients" (26), and as a result of this document a newly formed agency was established—the National Patient Safety Agency (NPSA), which is a special health authority created to coordinate the efforts of the entire country to report and, more important, to learn from mistakes and problems that affect patient safety. Besides making sure that errors are reported in the first place, the NPSA is trying to promote an open and fair culture within the NHS and to report "near misses" when things almost go wrong. The culture of the NPSA and the emphasis on the government's agenda with patient safety is more about the "how" rather than the "who." It also aims to prevent recurrence of such incidents and, in the past, incidents involving POCT equipment have led to MDA warning publications (hazard notices) on blood glucose meters (27), blood glucose test strips (28), blood gas analyzers (29), and sweat testing devices (30). Any adverse incidents relating to POCT must be reported to the newly formed NPSA as well as the MHRA.

It has been estimated in the United Kingdom that the number of errors within the NHS could be as high as 6 million per annum. The NPSA was launched in February 2004 as a new management system that will draw together reports of patient safety errors and systems failure from health professions across England and Wales. The National Reporting and Learning System (NRLS) is an international first in healthcare. It will help the health service to understand the underlying causes of problems and act quickly to introduce practical changes to prevent mistakes.

The patient safety movement is gaining momentum not only in the United Kingdom, but also in the United States, as healthcare professionals begin to design processes that minimize the potential for human error and to implement nonpunitive ways in which to deal with human error. As with laboratory testing, one must consider the pre- and postanalytical steps for potential mistakes in POCT.

In the United States, the newly created Joint Commission on Accreditation of Healthcare Organizations (JCAHO) has launched its national patient safety goals for 2004, and, indeed, the JCAHO has newly created guidelines (31). They refer to highlighting the importance of having proper identification of patient samples, as mistakes in labeling can lead to critical medical errors, such as giving medication to the wrong patient, and are of similar relevance to POCT. Other measures must be developed and employed to reduce the potential for mistakes, such as the need for POCT to be linked with a central laboratory's information system to assist not only documentation of test and quality control results but, importantly, interpretation. Guidelines are directed mainly at central laboratories but must encompass POCT.

SUCCESSFUL IMPLEMENTATION

An essential prerequisite to good, successful delivery of a POCT service is that a multidisciplinary group must be established with recognized accountability, management support, and appropriate resources (32). Ultimately, the director for laboratory medicine must be responsible. In addition, final responsibility for POCT results must be defined, and there must be a continuing assessment, auditing, and appraisal of the need for POCT in any institution (33).

Specific pro forma procedures for application of POCT have to be established and be part of the hospital POCT policy. The pro forma procedure requires background information such as clinical benefits; workload costs; the ability to provide more rapid effective diagnosis and/or treatment; equipment requirements, including location and responsibility; staff and personnel requirements, including who will be the users and who will do the training; information on the reports and results, e.g., reference ranges, documentation, external quality assurance (EQA) and its interpretation, and, finally and importantly, the continual auditing and appraisal of the POCT.

Clinical Pathology Accreditation (CPA) Ltd., the UK national laboratory accrediting body both for the NHS and the independent sector, has taken a stance with its new standards, which were implemented in the autumn of 2003. POCT in hospitals should be under the control of laboratory management; it should be included in the medical laboratory repertoire and inspected to the same standards by CPA inspectors as the medical laboratory. The position now taken by CPA is that if the above does not comply with the standards, the chief executive of the trust in question is informed that there is a local clinical governance issue and patients may be at risk. Part of HcC's remit is not only routine inspection of clinical governance arrangements, but also investigation of serious service failures. HcC's inspection process concerns the "whole patient journey," and POCT may be part of that journey, thereby reiterating the importance of both the pre- and postanalytical stages of POCT.

CONCLUDING REMARKS

To ensure successful implementation of POCT, including pre- and postanalytical phases, there has to be ownership of a pragmatic POCT policy (see Chapters 11, 12, and 15).

Laboratories are familiar with monitoring quality through EQA, which obviously applies to POCT. As part of clinical governance, continual professional development must be supported and all staff involved in POCT must be monitored. There needs to be formal individual performance assessment procedures in place to remedy poor performance.

In addition, clinical auditing will assess the continual need for POCT and, importantly, affect patient outcome, and this should be incorporated as part of the clinical governance plan.

Quality, clinical governance, and patient involvement are high priorities on the UK healthcare agenda. Clinical governance encompasses setting delivery and monitoring standards of healthcare. This applies to all aspects of healthcare, including POCT. With the growth of POCT worldwide, it would be negligent if the laboratories did not make it one of their high priorities.

APPENDIX

Evidence for Improvement of Quality of Healthcare:

Case studies from the NHS Modernisation Agency clinical governance support teams. Website: www.cgsupport.nhs.uk/Resources/Case_studies/default.asp.

REFERENCES

1. Department of Health. First-class service: quality in the new NHS. London: HMSO, 1998.
2. Department of Health. NHS Executive Clinical Governance. Quality in the new NHS. London: HSC, 1999:65.
3. Freedman DB. Clinical governance—bridging management and clinical approaches to quality in the UK. Clin Chim Acta 2002; 319:133–41.
4. Taylor G. Clinical governance and developments of a new professionalism in medicine—educational implications. Educ Health [Addendum] 2002;15:65–70.
5. Campbell SM, Sweeney GM. The role of clinical governance and strategy for quality improvement in primary care. Br J Gen Pract 2002;52:S12–7.
6. Pickard S, Marshall M, Rogers A, Sheaff R, Sibbald B, Campbell S, et al. User involvement in clinical governance. Health Expect 2002;3:187–98.
7. Marks V. Clinical biochemistry nearer the patient. BMJ 1983; 286:116–7.
8. Felder RA. Distributed laboratory: point of care services with core laboratory management. In: Price CP, Hicks JM, eds. Point-of-care testing. Washington, DC: AACC Press, 1999.
9. Hughes M. Market trends and point of care testing. Point of Care 2002;1,2:84–94
10. Hobbs FD, Delaney BC, Fitzmaurice DA, Wilson S, Hyde CJ, Thorpe GH, et al. A review of near patient testing in primary care. Health Technol Assess 1997;1:1–230.
11. Alderson P. Absence of evidence is not evidence of absence. BMJ 2004;328:477–9.
12. Hudson MP, Christenson RH, Newby LK, Kaplan AL, Ohman EM. Cardiac markers: point of care testing. Clin Chim Acta 1999;284:223–37.
13. Ng SN, Krishnaswamy P, Morissey R, Clopton P, Fitzgerald R, Maisel AS. Ninety-minute accelerated critical pathway for chest pain evaluation. Am J Cardiol 2001;88:611–7.
14. McCord J, Nowak RM, McCullough PA, Foreback C, Borzak S, Tokarski G, et al. Ninety minute exclusion of acute myocardial infarction by use of quantitative point of care testing of myoglobin and troponin I. Circulation 2001;104:1483–8.
15. Kendall B, Reeves B, Glancy M. Point of care testing: a randomised control of clinical outcome. BMJ 1998;316:1052–7.
16. Murray RP, Leroux M, Sabaga E, Palatnick EM, Ludwig L. Effect of point of care testing on length of stay in adult emergency room. J Emerg Med 1999;17:81–6.
17. Grieve R, Beech R, Vincent R, Mazurkiewicz J. Near patient testing in diabetic clinics: appraising the costs and outcomes. Health Technol Assess 1999;3:1–74.
18. Lee-Lewandroski E, Corboy D, Lewandroski K, Sinclair J, McDermot S, Benzer TI. Implementation of a point of care satellite laboratory in the emergency department of an academic medical centre:

impact on test turnaround time and patient emergency department length of stay. Arch Pathol Lab Med 2003;127:456–60.

19. Hobbs R. Point of care testing in primary care. In: Price CP, Hicks JM, eds. Point-of-care testing. Washington, DC: AACC Press, 1999.

20. Jahn UR, Aken H. Near patient testing—point of care or point of costs and convenience. Br J Anaesth 2003;90:425–7.

21. Nutting PA, Main DS, Fischer PM, Pontius M, Siefert M, Booned DJ, et al. Towards optimal laboratory use. Problems in laboratory testing in primary care. JAMA 1996;275:636–9.

22. Demers LM. Regulatory issues in point of care testing. In: Price CP, Hicks JM, eds. Point-of-care testing. Washington, DC: AACC Press, 1999.

23. Bonini P, Plebani M, Ceriotti F, Rubboli F. Errors in laboratory medicine. Clin Chem 2002;48:691–8.

24. Joint Working Group on Quality Assurance. Near-patient or point of care testing guidelines. Han 1999 [available from D. Kilshaw, Joint Working Group on Quality Assurance Guidelines on NPT/POCT, c/o Diagnostic Services Ltd., Mast House, Derby Road, Liverpool, L20 1EA, UK].

25. Management and use of IVD point of care test devices. MDA DB 2002 (03). London: Medical Devices Agency, 2002.

26. Department of Health. Building a safer NHS for patients: implementing an organisation with a memory. London: HMSO, 2001.

27. Department of Health. Hazard notice HN (87) 13 for glucose analyzers. London: HMSO, 1987.

28. MDA safety warning: One-touch—blood glucose test strips—lot number 925722A: Recall. HN 2000 (02). London: Medical Devices Agency, 2000.

29. Department of Health. Hazard notice HN (89) 31 for blood gas analyzers. London: HMSO, 1989.

30. Medical Devices Agency. Prevention of burns during iontophoresis (sweat testing). Safety Notice MDA SN 1999(05). London: Medical Devices Agency, 1999.

31. JCAHO. Laboratory-specific national patient safety goals [NPSG 2004]. www.jcho.org.labfocus.issue1.2004 (accessed February 2004).

32. Burnett D. Accreditation and point of care testing. Ann Clin Biochem 2000;37:241–3.

33. Freedman DB. Guidelines on point of care testing. In: Price CP, Hicks JM, eds. Point-of-care testing. Washington, DC: AACC Press, 1999.

Chapter 18

Health Economic Aspects of Point-of-Care Testing

Joseph H. Keffer

Clinical economics involves three key elements: costs, benefits, and point of view, as succinctly described by Eisenberg (1). Economics has been described, briefly, as "The study of choice" by Shiell (2) and, more elaborately by Paul Samuelson, as "the study of how men and society end up choosing, with or without the use of money, to employ scarce productive resources that could have alternative uses"—as quoted by Shiell (2) who provides a useful glossary for those interested in further study of the field.

The challenge, for the health economist and for those attempting to assess new technology, lies in the capture and intelligent, unbiased assessment of all of the relevant costs and benefits with clear discernment of the point of view, or "perspective," as it is known in the economics literature. These may differ depending on the point of view of the physician, the patient, society, the government, or the ultimate payer. Fleisher, an experienced and respected clinical chemist, has assessed point-of-care testing (POCT) (3). He admonishes us, as do others, to ensure that "testing is cost-effective." While this is a common and seemingly reasonable expectation for the laboratorian and the clinician, one must ask if this directive is appropriate and valid counsel, and whether it can be anticipated to permit guidance to laboratory management in making the decision to implement a new POCT service. Can POCT be proven to be cost-effective and has the evidence been presented and accepted? This chapter addresses these questions and acknowledges the limitations of the answers. A key issue is whether a technology itself, in isolation, can be formally assessed as cost-effective or whether the application of that technology to a specifically defined group is essential to an attempted formal assessment. For example, should the POCT test for hemoglobin, per se, be proven cost-effective, as opposed to its use in an emergency setting to benefit an actively bleeding patient? Those who generically categorize a particular test method or device as cost-effective, in isolation from the application and the clinical benefit, are too narrowly focused. Assessment of cost-effectiveness is about comparisons and about benefits as well as costs. Recently published studies firmly establish that such efforts must measure the global impact of the innovation on the total economics of the institution (4). The effects must be assessed beyond the factors inherent in the technology of the test system (5).

When considering the economic aspects of POCT, several generally useful concepts immediately come to mind. Evidence-based medicine teaches us that we should seek the highest level of data available in adopting new technology, preferably randomized, prospective, and blinded studies. In this era of limited resource availability, the choice of a medical modality is essentially the choice of one among several competing alternatives for investment. As such, we also seek formal cost-effectiveness analysis (CEA) or cost–benefit analysis (CBA) to assist us in our decision making. "A cost-effectiveness analysis determines the difference in total costs and the difference in health outcomes between an intervention and an alternative" (6). So-called patient-focused care is a notably extreme form. Although originally highly touted in anecdotal reports (7), this strategy proved to involve reduplication of the substantial capital-intensive laboratory equipment in multiple wards and has lost favor (8). In this discussion we focus on the more modest and typical applications of POCT. What is the available evidence for POCT and what is the status of cost-effectiveness studies in this field?

EVIDENCE-BASED MEDICINE

Although addressed in a separate chapter, I introduce the concept of "evidence-based medicine" (9) into the present discussion to acknowledge the strong influence of this teaching. It is conceptually sound, emphasizing deliberation with regard to both expensive technologies and low-cost but highly prevalent applications. Both result in large and significant aggregate costs. POCT clearly should be studied in light of the latter consideration. Growing rapidly, the trend to bedside or near-patient testing deserves consideration with regard to value. What evidence exists to validate the contribution of POCT? Very few studies have attempted to perform randomized and controlled investigations. In a study of the emergency room application of stat electrolytes using a portable device, Parvin et al. (10) reported no impact of the periodic availability of POCT on the throughput of patients, and no reported improvement in patient outcomes compared to the testing performed in the central laboratory. Illustrative of the defects of such putative studies, most study subjects also had additional central laboratory testing for other analytes not available by POCT, which delayed their disposition and confounded the analysis. Application of POCT to this entire group may have been inappropriate. In contrast, the most valuable study to date performed for the United Kingdom's National Health Service reported significant changes in medical decision making and resultant management due to more timely result reporting in 59 of 859 emergency room patients (11). The cost analysis of this process change has subsequently been published and confirms the assessment of significant savings (12). By virtue of being a prospective and randomized study, this is the most robust systematic evidence available to date to support the value of POCT. In terms of outcomes, no change in mortality or measurable morbidity could be shown. Collinson performed a disciplined, prospective, randomized study of the effect on chest pain management of POCT for cardiac markers that demonstrated the cost-effectiveness and efficacy of this innovation (4). In Boston, at a large university-affiliated hospital emergency room, the introduction of POCT had a dramatic effect on patient throughput, physician and patient satisfaction, and the total economics of the institution (13).

The evidence is growing, though still limited, that selective application of POCT not only is economically feasible and attractive, but also can be a boon to a health care system. In addition, the limitations of evidence-based medicine as a source of answers to all questions has been recognized (14, 15).

Recently, an evolving consensus has stated that there are a series of parameters that permit decisions regarding introduction of POCT to be a "no-brainer" decision. These include decreasing length of stay (LOS) in the emergency department by 15–30 min, decreasing empty operating room waiting time by 30 min, decreasing LOS in the intensive care unit by 1 day, decreasing blood product usage by 2 units per patient, or enabling an inpatient procedure to be performed as an outpatient procedure (16–18). An apt statement attributed to Rainey is that "medical intervention may directly alter medical outcomes, but laboratory tests do not—[because] a test result is always filtered through the change in medical management it engenders" (19).

To address the question of introduction of POCT further, we should review general cost-effectiveness literature and studies of costs associated with this technology.

COST STUDIES OF POCT

In previous reviews of this subject (20, 21), I have noted the limitations of the available works in relation to cost analysis and cost-effectiveness rigors. There are few studies of note. Most POCT reports omit significant data and identify only partial costs when comparing central laboratory costs with POCT. Typically, the studies favor one or the other of the alternative interventions with obvious deletions of data such as cost of labor, capital investment or, indirect costs of the preferred technology that bias the report. As is always wise practice, the serious reader is advised to carefully review the detailed methods employed by the investigators to evaluate a particular investigation. Claims of cost-effectiveness reports typically consist of reagent cost-comparisons of the analytical tests without assignment of values for the entire set of data required for the formal cost-effectiveness study. More elaborate and complete lists of cost elements are well reported by

DeCresce (22) and Howanitz (23), in representative publications. Recently, a review of the subject by Baer (24), a particularly knowledgeable and objective authority on POCT, brings us up to date on issues of cost analysis. He summarizes the deficiencies in published cost analyses as follows:

1. Only incremental costs of labor and consumables are included, with many assumptions about the costs of nonlaboratory personnel.
2. They do not differentiate between fixed and incremental costs as they affect the central laboratory and POCT.
3. They do not consider the costs of the episode of care or the patient's long-term follow-up costs.

From reviewing all of the available cost literature for the POCT field, I conclude several summary comments:

First, testing at the point of care is generally and arguably more costly than batch testing performed in the central laboratory. Second, pneumatic tube transport of specimens can optimize the delivery of specimens for centralized testing with minimal delays if operating under ideal conditions (25, 26). This includes constant surveillance of the terminus of the tube, an aspect not consistently and economically achievable in my own hospital practice experience. Few would argue that POCT is less expensive as measured in terms of producing a single data point. Rather it is clearly a consensus view that performance of central laboratory testing to generate the same data point is usually at a lower cost per test result. However, the assignment of costs for central testing is frequently underestimated, including training, certification, quality assurance, quality control, method duplication to support the perceived need for backup capability, proficiency testing, and other less obvious factors that are significant cost burdens and have led to mandated regionalization of laboratories and downsizing with increasing referral of testing volumes to outside laboratories. Third, not assessed in studies of costs solely focused on the analytical test are additional "negative and positive costs" associated with the use of POCT as listed in Table 18-1, modified from an earlier publication (21). Many of these costs are sometimes approximated as "indirect costs employing a formula." They are expressly listed here to emphasize the significance in comparing and contrasting institutions and applications not adequately addressed by standard formulas. A more recent study, worthy of emulation, reported a detailed assessment of the introduction of extensive POCT replacing traditional central laboratory functions and analyzed the costs in detail. This report provides a useful template for cost comparison and decision making as well as the introduction of process change (27).

It is important to recognize that one should take a more holistic approach in assessing cost-effectiveness of the introduction of POCT to a particular setting in view of savings to be gained for another budget in the health care system, for example, reduced numbers of follow-up visits to clinic. This is the "global budget" perspective that must take precedence over the focus on a laboratory budget impact in isolation (22). The improvement in management can be facilitated, e.g., in diabe-

Table 18-1   Negative and Positive Costs Associated with POCT

1. Cost of performing a CEA/CBA study
2. Cost of the intervention of proposed technology and comparison with another
   a. Preanalytic costs: specimen acquisition to include order entry, phlebotomy/fingerstick, transportation, centrifugation, breakage in centrifuge, pouring off, distribution, and storage of residue
   b. Analytic costs: production costs including capital equipment (purchase or lease disguised as reagent rental or encompassing actual deferred purchase), space, disposables, reagents, operator time, training time, supervision time, troubleshooting, and professional review.
   c. Quality component or prevention costs including training and retraining, continuing education, quality control, quality assurance, proficiency testing, preventive maintenance, service contracts, costs of repeat testing, and dilution of high values
   d. Postanalytic costs: the costs of data capture and transmission to the recipient including documentation in the medical record, as well as the STAT report, and long-term storage of laboratory reports to fulfill regulatory requirements
   e. Variable costs associated with unique institution/site/proposed intervention
      i. Indirect costs for overheads including heat, electricity, and institutional support
      ii. Institutional debt costs (vary as debt-free or debt-laden institution)
      iii. Alternatives for resource investment, e.g., to include the revenue stream that could be generated by an alternative investment of dollar resources
      iv. Variable associated costs depending on who performs the test, e.g., physicians, nurses, clerks or baccalaureate-level medical technologists, costs for "base staffing" the laboratory for 24 h, 7 days and to cover vacations and illness with relevance to changing test volume in these times
3. The costs, or the avoidance of costs, of the morbidity and mortality consequent from the introduction or deferral of intervention A or B
4. Induced costs associated with additional healthcare, or support for individuals who benefit from the technology including costs associated with prolongation of life, and the attendant continuing costs of care not experienced if death occurs
5. Negative costs consisting of costs that are averted, e.g., by effective diabetic control diminishing progression to renal failure
6. Cost of discounting for current dollars versus inflationary dollars in the cost–benefit mismatch of time and cost of lost opportunity for alternative investment and revenue stream
7. Impact of economy of scale resulting in marginal test cost changes; e.g., by decentralizing blood glucose testing, the unit cost for glucose in the central laboratory will inevitably increase

tes, epilepsy, coagulopathy, and others, as discussed by Price (28), and in testing for glycated hemoglobin, glucose, urine nitrite and esterase, *Helicobacter pylori*, cardiac markers, urine drugs of abuse, as a reported consensus among symposium participants by Hicks et al. (29). Although these indications are approved by a consensus on their face value, it is difficult to assign numerical financial value to these applications.

What then are the compelling reasons for the surge in this enabling technology viewed from a total economic perspective? Precisely because POCT *enables*, as discussed below, and the value associated with the result.

POCT As an Enabling Technology

In reviewing the reasons for using POCT, one can identify these as benefits and that they are suitable for entry into formal cost-effectiveness analysis. They include a variety of categories from the perspective of the several individuals affected by its use: the laboratorian, the nurse, the physician, the hospital, the payer, and, most important, the patient. If genuine economic assessment is to be introduced beyond the simplistic assessment of the costs per analytical result, then one must consider all perspectives and the total economic impact on the healthcare delivery system. To illustrate, while serving as Director of Clinical Laboratories for the Parkland Hospital System in Dallas, Texas, I introduced proven and recommended testing for HbA1c to be performed in the primary physician's offices so that we might empower the physician and the patient to monitor diabetic status together at the time of the encounter. The goal was to achieve a higher compliance rate. The effect of this intervention on both physicians and patients was immediate, dramatic, and best characterized as enabling.

Although it may seem self-evident that this anecdotal report should be bolstered by a detailed cost-effectiveness analysis, we simply did not have the resources to invest in such a study. Consider that the indication for the test is self-evident and established, the implementation is readily accomplished, and performance of a formal CEA, while desirable, would appear unnecessary for the decision by an individual institution. Although numerous funded studies establish monitoring of HbA1c levels as the key element in tracking glycemic control of diabetes to minimize adverse outcomes, there are no studies that prove the cost-effectiveness of providing POCT for this critical data, as contrasted with the availability of the data several days later. Cagliero et al. (30) demonstrated the improved outcomes (as a decrease in HbA1c) when using POCT for HbA1c, while Grieve et al. (31), in a preliminary costing study, identified a reduction in clinic visits associated with POCT for HbA1c.

The substantial funding required for the rigorous validation of the POCT aspect of such policies has not been provided by available sources such as the National Institutes of Health. Other areas of obvious medically based need include the POCT testing for antibodies to streptokinase prior to thrombolytic therapy with this pharmaceutical enzyme therapy, cardiac markers in chest pain triage, and emergency room screening for pancreatitis markers. Although it would be desirable for the diagnostic companies to fund such cost-effectiveness studies and others, the economic reality of the limited market size differs from that facing the pharmaceutical industry. In performing randomized, prospective, double-blind studies of drugs, the pharmaceutical industry places a wager on the potential for large revenues of future sales to ensure the return on investment. The total profit yield even for a successful diagnostic test is insufficient to underwrite such expensive projects, and patent protection is not protective. As a consequence, one should not anticipate an answer to such questions of cost-effectiveness to be promptly forthcoming.

Other motivating benefits derivable from POCT, which would require formal validation in an authentic CEA, are listed in Table 18-2, adapted from an earlier report (21). Again, although some would combine many of these in generic terms, they are explicitly listed to convey the impact of each at the level of the perspective of the beneficiary. Each has been cited in prior literature.

While often implicit under the global use of the term "turnaround time," each of these items is worthy of independent assessment and valuation. The contribution of each is difficult to validate in a formal cost-effectiveness study, as discussed below. The so-called intangible costs of an economic

Table 18-2   Benefits Derived from POCT

1. Improved turnaround time
2. Improved patient management, e.g., waking the diabetic hospital patient at 0700, rather than 0500 for fasting glucose status
3. Improved patient satisfaction, gratitude for immediate disposition, e.g., pregnancy testing or early discharge from the emergency clinic
4. Improved productivity resulting from throughput of the clinic
5. Improved laboratory–clinic relations due to better support
6. Improved job satisfaction of the physician and nurse empowerment
7. Improved clinic reputation resulting from word-of-mouth compliments and managed care organization's assessments
8. Decreased errors from transcription, clerical transfer, transportation of patients, breakage in centrifuge, repeats, and dilution of lab samples
9. Improved communications: result transfer, immediacy of report, barcoding on site, decreased phone time waiting
10. Decreased physician mental switching on/off from patient to patient with immediate disposition opportunity
11. Decreased transfusion in surgery and reexploration
12. Decreased operating room time
13. Decreased dietetic services awaiting early morning glucose testing
14. Improved outcomes, morbidity, and mortality
15. Overcome shortage of professional medical technologists
16. Investment of capital in alternative yield opportunities
17. Decrease from comprehensive laboratory profiling to targeted essential test needs

analysis are acknowledged to be difficult or impossible to value. Pain, suffering, and fear (of illness and adverse diagnoses) may be promptly alleviated by POCT and should be weighed in these evaluations (32). Decisions to implement or reject innovation in medical practice must be made in day-to-day practice in concert with numerous other management decisions. The evidence is often lacking for scientific guidance of the sort offered by formal cost-effectiveness or cost–benefit studies. Well-intentioned economic analysis may inappropriately legitimize both suboptimal health production and discrimination on the basis of illness (33). In such an instance, the preservation of the status quo is bolstered by a CEA, which is incomplete and not truly comprehensive in dealing with all-important values. While abuse of laboratory testing is a constant threat, failure to act is another vice when good though imperfect evidence favors action. The failure to establish policy creates a vacuum that supports abuse of clinical care. At times, a pragmatic decision to support POCT applications may be mandated based on professional judgment exercised by taking into consideration not only laboratory operational issues but also clinical implications. Will the patient clearly benefit from the availability of POCT or will they be adversely affected by denial of access to POCT?

Recently, the concept of a hospital "core laboratory" for essential critical functions has been fostered to permit closure of esoteric laboratory functions and satellite laboratories. This supports referral of low-priority noncritical testing to a single large, batch-oriented, automated laboratory, often some distance from the hospital. In this sense, POCT is also an enabling strategy that can augment centralization and automation by providing immediate essential laboratory testing to support critical medical decision making while transferring less time-critical testing to an offsite or central laboratory. This concept was recently reported in terms of downsizing of clinical laboratories in Japan, a trend seen also throughout North America (34). The need for a far-reaching vision of the economics of health care is emphasized. Clearly, contrasting the direct costs for testing a single analytical result performed by central testing, or POCT, is an insufficient assessment. They are different services. The more comprehensive benefits and costs must be included.

Cost-Effectiveness Analysis

In a classic 1977 publication, Weinstein and Stason (35) set forth the "Foundations of Cost-Effectiveness Analysis for Health and Medical Practices." This has served as the premier reference for the field and remains highly regarded in the relevant expert literature of the day. Prompted by the growing awareness of the limits of healthcare resources apparent even at that time, they made an effective case for thoughtful assessment of alternative choices for investment of scarce funding resources. While emphasizing the disciplined approach to cost studies, they also reminded us of the persistent realities we still face today. Some of their cautions are worthy of reemphasis as they clearly state the premise, "for any given level of resources available, society (or the decision-making jurisdiction involved) wishes to maximize the total aggregate health benefits conferred." Furthermore, "the principal value of formal cost-effectiveness analysis in health care is that it forces one to be explicit about the beliefs and values that underlie allocation decisions." Realistically, they also provide advice that has subsequently been borne out by experience. They caution: "The tendency among health professionals to demand objective, scientifically valid proof, though laudable, begs the necessity to use the best available evidence, however uncertain, to make today's resource-allocation decisions." In addition, "the choice [among allocation decisions] is often between relying upon a responsible analysis, with all its imperfections, and no analysis at all" because "current decisions must inevitably be based on imperfect information." Subsequent to the publication of this primer, numerous publications appeared purporting to provide CEA. As reviewed in 1992 (36), a thoughtful analysis of 77 articles attempting to present formal CEA yielded only three that accurately reflected the six key principles laid down by Weinstein and Stason in the earlier teaching (35). Those principles are listed in Table 18-3.

Most studies dealt with only three of these six principles. The most notable omissions were failure to make the underlying assumptions explicit and therefore available for verification, and failure to test the assumptions such as cost estimates with sensitivity analyses. These defects permeate the POCT cost studies that are not truly CEA studies. Further, it is apparent that the thorough performance of this disciplined allocation approach is an intense investment of resources in and of itself. The collection of all the necessary data and the valuation of all the positive and negative costs is time- and labor-intensive. Few institutions, as yet, have comprehensive cost-oriented information systems, regrettably, even in this new millennium; yet these are essential to the collection of real cost data in a comprehensive fashion. While evolving, such systems are still being progressively implemented and will provide more detailed data in the future. For the present, many institutions retain global departmental (silo) budgets, or charge-based, rather than true cost-based accounting, and in

Table 18-3 Principles of Cost-Effectiveness Analysis

1. A summary measurement of efficiency, such as a cost-benefit or cost-effectiveness ratio, should be calculated and preferably expressed in marginal or incremental terms unless one alternative or strategy is dominant.
2. An explicit statement of a perspective for the analysis should be provided.
3. An explicit description of the benefits of the program or technology being studied should be provided.
4. Investigators should specify what types of costs were used or considered in their analysis.
5. If costs and benefits accrue during different periods, discounting should be used to adjust for the differential timing.
6. Sensitivity analyses should be done to test important assumptions.

From (35).

these institutions, the charges are more often fantasy than true. As a consequence of the limitations in available data and the quality of the cost data, the first issue necessary to decide whether to attempt CEA is a judgment as to whether it is cost-effective to do so. If the data are extremely difficult to seek out, and if the data are not reliable, then the conclusion is obvious. This may explain the paucity of published studies. Indeed, in a review of costing in published studies, Jacobs and Bachynsky (37) emphasized precisely these points: the case-mix variations, the site differences, and particularly the bias of the studies. They stated: "We concluded that biases occurred in most studies and in most categories." Further, they emphasized that these studies, being from Canada, were less relevant to the United States, "where costing based on charges is the most common method."

Other reviews of cost-effectiveness literature have been equally disappointing. Hillner et al. (38), seeking information regarding cost evaluation of stem cell transplantation as an alternative to bone marrow transplantation, summarized the costing literature, especially the Canadian guidelines proposed by Laupacis et al. (39) and the principles of cost-effectiveness. He found very little that was credible and applicable to the subject of their quest. However, they did conclude with wise advice that "it is insufficient to simply compare the cost of (one procedure) traditional bone marrow transplantation with one using [stem cells—the alternative procedure]." They emphasized that one must assess "the incremental benefits of the strategy" alternatives. This is akin to our observation that one cannot simply assess the cost of testing to achieve one analytic result, but rather, must assess the cost of POCT in light of the economic impact of the patient encounter on the entire health-care delivery system. More recently, Yin and Forman reported that they found 3200 studies purported to be CEA and CBA publications from 1979–1990 (40). This paper provides an excellent update to the theory and details associated with such tools, including the elements of formal analysis, its shortcomings, and its advantages. They conclude with cautions regarding ethical issues raised for policymakers by CEA and CBA, including the fact that the methods are still under development, the use of quality adjusted life years (QALYs) is still controversial as an outcome measure, and the reality that clinicians are, first and foremost, advocates for the individual patient. Clinicians, including clinical laboratorians, should maximize each individual patient's outcome. At the same time, these studies raise ethical issues of equity for society. When practically applied, however, the aggregate literature is disappointing. Seeking guidance for cost-effective decision making in critical care, Heyland et al. (41) screened 4187 papers "to determine the extent to which economic evaluations published in the critical care literature provide information to improve the efficiency of [the] unit." Only 29 papers met the inclusion criteria for their formal study. Of these, only 14 described competing interventions adequately, 17 provided sufficient evidence of efficacy, 6 dealt with costs adequately, and only 3 performed sensitivity analysis. Their conclusion with regard to the enormously resource-intensive critical care area is the same as mine with regard to useful data for assessing the economics of POCT: There is very little that is useful. Another consideration in reviewing published studies is whether the analysis is subjective and unique to an institution or whether it can be applied to other situations.

SUBJECTIVITY AND GENERALIZABILITY OF COST-EFFECTIVENESS STUDIES

Inherent in all CEA is significant subjectivity. The first element to be assessed prior to cost analysis is whether the desired result is efficacious, i.e., does the intervention get the job done? To the laboratorian, the question may be whether POCT produces a result analytically comparable to the central laboratory. To the clinician, efficacy may be more softly defined in terms of turnaround time, rule-out of a considered diagnostic possibility, or throughput of patients. A precise and accurate test result received too late to affect clinical assessment is often perceived as devoid of value by the clinician. While professional laboratorians operate in a data-driven world of quality control, the clinician involved with POCT is often subjectively influenced by less quantifiable yet valid factors. Subjectivity actually is recognized to permeate all CEA, even in the most rigorous studies. Consider that values must be assigned for all benefits including life extension, quality of life, and estimates of reduced or increased long-term expenditures. It is for this reason that sensitivity analysis is a key requirement of these studies recalculating on the basis of extremes of actual projections. Significant limitations exist even with regard to measurement of outcomes such as QALYs, commonly employed in CEA. Conversion of all values to dollars is the basic distinction in CBA. Recently, Gafni and Birch (42) have suggested an alternative in a sophisticated economics discussion. They propose the substitution of "healthy year equivalents," which they define in a complex fashion. Further limiting such studies, site- and time-specific data are often a reality in CEA. In terms of POCT studies, the presence or absence of pneumatic tubes for sample transfer, the salary scale employed, the use of personnel with lower degrees as opposed to baccalaureate and postgraduate credentials, the cost of credit to the particular institution for the purchase or deferral of capital equipment investment, and many other factors influence every study. The foregoing considerations may partially explain the lack of generalizable studies of POCT in the literature. By far, the most profound and universal objection to the assessment of a POCT device or other near-patient test by formal CEA is that such a property does not reside in the test but rather in the application, the case-mix selected for testing, and the clinical site. By way of analogy, performance of an electrocardiogram on all young healthy males in a secondary school would probably not be cost-effective; however, in middle-aged patients who present to the emergency department with chest pain, it is not arguable. It is the selection of patients and application of the technology that determines cost-effectiveness, not the device itself. So too, with POCT for electrolytes, blood gases, glucose or hemoglobin, or cardiac markers of ischemic injury. The key is not the

cost per analytical result but the application of the test to a clinically defined need in which laboratory data empower or enable a critical medical decision in which time is relevant. For CEA studies to be the basis for management decisions to support or defeat initiatives for POCT, it is necessary to assess the full clinical relevance and application. In a controlled and randomized study, Kendall et al. (11) report the effective use of POCT in the emergency room. The notable result reported was that in 59 out of 859 patients in the POCT arm of the study, the earlier availability of test data resulted in changes in patient management based on time-critical decisions, which may be the greatest value. However there were no measurable differences in outcomes, including length of time spent in the emergency department.

While outcomes are a desirable endpoint, they are not the only measure of value and may be confounded by the numerous unidentified elements that also contribute in both a positive and negative manner to the surrogate measure of outcome. The value of these findings is not contradicted by the report of Parvin et al. (10), which failed to produce reportable affirmative findings. The design of the Kendall and Parvin studies are different in that they are site-specific and subjective variables also influence the outcome of the assessment. Parvin et al. (10) did not attempt to assess the impact on medical decision making.

Dealing With Uncertainty and Lack of Formal Studies

As anticipated by Weinstein and Stason (35) and others, decisions must be made in the daily course of events in spite of the lack of hard data. A valuable practical contribution to this dilemma is the paper by Laupacis et al. (39), which provides guidance and a proposed semi-quantitative approach to the adoption of new technology. In this model, summarized in Table 18-4, two categories of information are developed: cost and quality impact of the proposed technology.

The intent is to encourage the use of good judgment incorporating both medical and management judgment. This creates a framework for the categories combining better or worse, cost and quality, and the relative degrees of each. Laupacis et al. divide the border categories by cost per QALY and the cost breakout at $20,000 to $100,000 per QALY. Such data are not available without elaborate studies. I foster the use of judgment in the absence of hard data to counter the abuse by those who would obstruct the introduction of useful care in the

Table 18-4 Means of Decision Making Based on Effectiveness—Cost and Benefit

Category	Benefits	Cost	Conclusion
1	Better	Lower	Implement
2	Better	Higher	Judgment
3	Lower	Lower	Judgment
4	Lower	Higher	Reject

absence of hard data. A case in point was recently emphasized in the editorial previously cited regarding evidence-based medicine, which addresses the denial of coverage for services not proven to be cost-effective. The authors (9), in discussing perinatal practices, comment regarding discharge after delivery of a newborn: "In the case of early discharge, science does not and probably cannot supply airtight evidence that longer stays are more effective (let alone cost-effective) compared with other approaches." The subsequent commentary is relevant to the assessment of the economics of POCT and the analogy is clear. They emphasize that "during a period of heavy pressures for cost containment, payers could stand to gain substantially from insisting that medical practice and reimbursement policies be based on rigorous comparative studies of outcomes and costs." Countering this, they provide wisdom that we can relate to the void of data proving cost-effectiveness of POCT. "We need to reflect on where the burden of proof should be when definitive studies have not been conducted and cannot be conducted quickly if at all, but good judgment based on available knowledge tells us that a service is needed." They also observed that "scientists and the policymakers who depend on science to guide public policy must be aware of the potential consequences of unquestioning devotion to the outcomes movement without adequate consideration of science (including limitations of statistical power), and ethics (beneficence, nonmalfeasance, and distributive justice)." The issue of ethics is increasingly crucial as the deprofessionalization of the medical profession is pursued by those who wish to deal with wellness and disease only in financial terms. Often, one may have a duty to a patient to advocate the use of a technology not yet proven to the satisfaction of CEA/CBA and evidence-based medicine studies. The same editorial (9) concludes with a similar note: "In the absence of an adequate base of scientific knowledge about what is most effective and efficient to achieve the best health outcomes, it appears rational and ethical to be guided by a combination of good judgment, caution, and compassion in weighing the best evidence available." It is in this sense that the choice of employing POCT must be decided. In summary, simply declaring a position that holds that each form of testing must be shown to be cost-effective reveals a lack of understanding of the complexity of CEA, the associated costs and difficulty, the limited generalizability, and the reality that it is the application of a technology and not the technology itself that can be shown to be cost-effective.

CONCLUSIONS

While it would be desirable to have formal CEA studies to guide our decisions, these do not exist with regard to POCT, nor are they likely to appear in the near future. Limited resources are available to provide systematic and rigorous detail required for such studies. Available cost-containment studies have limited applicability to the many diverse settings and applications that govern both the costs and benefits associated with the setting rather than the technology itself. Indeed, Fleisher, as noted in the introduction (3), specified the desir-

ability of cost-effectiveness data and yet he also wisely acknowledged that each hospital may be unique in the diverse circumstances which present. Subsequent experience has proven him to be correct as reflected by the limited utility of the published studies of POCT relating to cost-effectiveness. While it is axiomatic that the POCT must be shown to be "effective," the overall utility of testing, short of formal CEA, must be undertaken in terms of comprehensive assessment of clinical and operational benefits, not merely as a comparison of laboratory and POCT delivery costs. It remains a reality that the laboratorian, in conjunction with professional colleagues, physicians, nurses, and administrators in the medical enterprise must make reasoned judgments to achieve best practices.

REFERENCES

1. Eisenberg JM. Clinical economics. A guide to the economic analysis of clinical practices. JAMA 1989;262:2879–86.
2. Shiell A, Donaldson C, Mitton C, Currie G. Health economic evaluation. J Epidemiol Community Health 2002;56:85–8.
3. Fleisher M. Point-of-care testing: Does it really improve patient care. Clin Biochem 1993;26:6–8.
4. Collinson PO. The need for a point of care testing: an evidence-based appraisal. Scand J Clin Lab Invest Suppl 1999;230:67–73.
5. Briggs A, Gray A. The distribution of health care costs and their statistical analysis for economic evaluation. J Health Serv Res Policy 1998;3:233–45.
6. Loening-Baucke V. Prevention and medicare costs. N Engl J Med 1998;339:1158–9.
7. Jenner EA. A case study analysis of nurses' roles, education and training needs associated with patient-focused care. J Adv Nurs 1998;27:1087–95.
8. Heymann TD, and Culling W. The patient-focused approach: a better way to run a hospital? J R Coll Physicians Lond 1996;30:142–4.
9. Braveman P, Kessel W, Egerter S, Richmond J. Early Discharge and Evidence-based Practice. JAMA 1997;278:334–6.
10. Parvin CA, Lo SF, Deuser SM, Weaver LG, Lewis LM, Scott MG. Impact of point-of-care testing on patient's length of stay in a large emergency department. Clin Chem 1996;42:711–7.
11. Kendall J, Reeves B, Clancy M. Point of care testing: randomised controlled trial of clinical outcome. BMJ 1998;316:1052–7.
12. Kendall JM, Bevan G, Clancy MJ. Point of care testing in the accident and emergency department: a cost analysis and exploration of financial incentives to use the technology within the hospital. J Health Serv Res Policy 1999;4:33–8.
13. Lee-Lewandrowski Lee-Lewandrowski E, Corboy D, Lewandrowski K, Sinclair J, McDermot S, Benzer TI. Implementation of a point-of-care satellite laboratory in the emergency department of an academic medical center. Impact on test turnaround time and patient emergency department length of stay. Arch Pathol Lab Med 2003;127:456–60.
14. Feinstein AR, Horwitz RI. Problems in the "evidence" of "evidence-based medicine." Am J Med 1997;103:529–35.
15. Grahame-Smith D. Evidence-based medicine: challenging the orthodoxy. J R Soc Med 1998;91(Suppl 35):7–11.
16. Scott M. Faster is better—it's rarely that simple! [Editorial]. Clin Chem. 2000;46:441–2.
17. Rainey PM. Outcomes assessment for point-of-care testing. Clin Chem 1998;44:1595.

18. Foster K, Despotis G, Scott MG. Point-of-care testing. Cost issues and impact on hospital operations. Clin Lab Med 2001;21: 269–84.

19. Giuliano KK, Grant ME. Blood analysis at the point of care: issues in application for use in critically ill patients. AACN Clin Issues 2002;13:204–20.

20. Keffer JH. Economic considerations of point-of-care testing. Am J Clin Pathol 1995; 104(Suppl 1):S107–10.

21. Keffer JH. The economic aspects of new delivery options for diagnostic testing. In: Kost GJ, ed. Handbook of clinical automation, robotics, and optimization. New York: John Wiley & Sons, 1996.

22. DeCresce RP, Phillips DL, Howanitz PJ. Financial justification of alternate site testing. Arch Pathol Lab Med 1995;119:898–901.

23. Howanitz PJ. College of American Pathologists Conference XXVIII on alternate site testing: what must we do? Arch Pathol Lab Med 1995;119:979–83.

24. Baer DM. Point-of-care testing versus lab costs. MLO Med Lab Obs 1998;September:46–56.

25. Nosanchuk JS, Keefner R. Cost analysis of point-of-care lab testing in a community hospital. Am J Clin Path 1995;103:240–3.

26. Winkleman JW, Wybenga DR. Quantitation of medical and operational factors determining central versus satellite laboratory testing of blood gases. Am J Clin Path 1994;102:7–10.

27. Bailey TM, Topham TM, Wantz S, Grant M, Cox C, Jones D, Zerbe T, Spears T. Laboratory process improvement through point-of-care testing. Jt Comm J Qual Improv 1997;23:362–80.

28. Price CP. Medical and economic outcomes of point-of-care testing. Clin Chem Lab Med 2002;40:246–51.

29. Hicks JM, Haeckel R, Price CP, Lewandrowski K, Wu AH. Recommendations and opinions for the use of point-of-care testing for hospitals and primary care: summary of a 1999 symposium. Clin Chim Acta 2001;303:1–17.

30. Cagliero E, Levina E, Nathan D. Immediate feedback of HbA1c levels improves glycemic control in type 1 and insulin-treated type 2 diabetic patients. Diabetes Care 1999;22:1785–9.

31. Grieve R, Beech R, Vincent J, et al. Near patient testing in diabetes clinics: appraising the costs and outcomes. Health Technol Assess 1999;3:1–74.

32. Meltzer MI. Introduction to health economics for physicians. Lancet 2001;358:993–8.

33. Oliver A. Unintended consequences of applying economic evaluation. J Health Serv Res Policy 2002;7:129–30.

34. Hasahara Y, Ashihara Y. Simple devices and their possible application in clinical laboratory downsizing. Clin Chim Acta 1997; 267:87–102.

35. Weinstein MC, Stason WB. Foundations of cost-effectiveness analysis for health and medical practice. N Engl J Med 1977;296: 716–21.

36. Udvarhelyi S, Colditz GA, Rai A, Epstein AM. Cost-effectiveness and cost-benefit analyses in the medical literature. Ann Intern Med 1992;116:238–44.

37. Jacobs P, Bachynsky J. Costing methods in the Canadian literature on the economic evaluation of health care. A survey and assessment. Int J Technol Assess Health Care 1996;12:721–34.

38. Hillner BE, Smith TJ, Desch CE. Principles of cost effectiveness analysis for the assessment of current and new therapies. J Hematother 1993;2:501–6.

39. Laupacis A, Feeny D, Detsky AS, Tugwell PX. How attractive does a new technology have to be to warrant adoption and utilization? Tentative guidelines for using clinical and economic evaluations. Can Med Assoc J 1992;146:473–81.

40. Yin D, Forman HP. Health care cost-benefit and cost-effectiveness analysis: an overview. JVIR 1995;6:311–20.

41. Heyland DK, Kernerman P, Gafni A, Cook DJ. Economic evaluations in the critical care literature: do they help us improve the efficiency of our unit? Crit Care Med 1996;24:1591–8.

42. Gafni A and Birch S. Preferences for outcomes in economic evaluation: an economic approach to addressing economic problems. Soc Sci Med 1995;40:767–76.

Chapter 19

The Patient Interface and Point-of-Care Testing

John D. Piette

Point-of-care testing (POCT) has the potential to improve patient care by enriching the information base available for clinical decision making. Discussion of point-of-care test results also can provide "teachable" moments in which patients begin to understand the connections between their behavioral health choices and health status. Unfortunately, primary care practitioners often are inundated with clinical information and may have difficulty incorporating additional data from point-of-care tests into their practice. Moreover, most physicians face daunting time pressures associated with high expectations regarding the number of patients they see and the preventive services they deliver during illness-related visits (1). Most diseases treated in primary care have a strong behavioral component (2), and even the best POCT information cannot improve outcomes if patients have difficulty adhering to recommended treatment plans. For all of these reasons, point-of-care tests may have only a limited impact on patient outcomes unless the patient interface is carefully considered when conducting tests, interpreting their results, and using those results in disease management.

The focus of this chapter is on the characteristics of the patient–provider dynamic that influences the impact of POCT in real-world practices. Some of these factors (e.g., the time allotted to primary care visits) may be difficult for clinicians to influence, at least in the short term. However, the emphasis here is on practical strategies for improving patient–provider communication in the context of POCT that can be useful in most healthcare settings.

Examples in this chapter focus on the care of patients with chronic health problems. Outside of pediatric medicine, chronically ill patients comprise the bulk of all healthcare visits, and chronic illness care is particularly complex. Because most chronically ill patients visit multiple providers, coordination of their health monitoring and care planning is especially important. Moreover, most chronically ill patients must engage in an array of self-care behaviors, such as monitoring changes in their health status, adhering to medication plans, and sustaining changes in lifestyle behaviors such as diet and exercise. Unfortunately, most health systems are poorly equipped to meet the challenges of chronic illness care (3). Patients frequently fall short of self-care goals, and clinicians often provide services that are uncoordinated and suboptimal from the perspective of treatment guidelines. POCT can improve chronic illness care if appropriate attention is given to the context of these tests and how they are used in clinical decision making.

PATIENT–PROVIDER COMMUNICATION

Importance of Effective Communication

Effective patient–provider communication is essential to chronic illness care as well as to the care of almost all patients treated in ambulatory settings. Without the ability to elicit reliable information from patients regarding their self-care (e.g., medication adherence) and health behaviors, it may be difficult for clinicians to identify appropriate responses to POCT findings. POCT results often suggest changes that patients should make in the way they manage their illness, and effective communication is essential to ensure that they understand the implications of test results for their treatment. Clear communication also is essential to ensure that patients appreciate the connections between their health status as indicated by point-of-care tests, necessary changes in health behaviors, and how they can make those changes in the context of the barriers they face in their daily lives. Rigorous research has shown that effective patient–provider communication can lead to increased patient satisfaction, better self-care behavior, and improvements in health outcomes (4–10).

Factors Influencing Communication Regarding Point-of-Care Testing

The characteristics of patients, providers, and health systems influence the quality of patient–provider interactions. Patients' culturally derived health beliefs and behaviors provide an important context for discussing test findings, although providers often fail to fully appreciate cultural differences (11, 12). Female physicians often engage in more patient-centered communication than their male counterparts (13), and patients often are more satisfied with female providers (14–17). Continuity of care has been associated with better communication among asthma patients (18) and greater patient satisfaction and quality in general (19, 20). Some health systems facilitate enhanced patient–provider communication by allowing for more time during critical outpatient encounters or by improving the information base available to clinicians about patients' preventive health needs.

Interactions between patients and clinicians often incorporate multiple goals, including eliciting information from patients; explaining objective findings (e.g., the results of POCT); decision making and treatment planning; and strengthening the relationship bond between the clinician and patient that fosters respect, honesty, and cooperation (21). Both instrumental (information giving) and affective dimensions of the communication dynamic are important determinants of patient outcomes (22), and discussion of POCT results should include a recognition of their meaning for patients beyond the objective measure itself. For example, some diabetes patients may experience consistently elevated glycosylated hemoglobin (HbA1c) levels despite their sincere concern about diabetic complications and their best efforts to follow self-care regimens as prescribed. For such patients, reporting these HbA1c values without attention to their emotional impact may lead to discouragement, anxiety, and an increase in adherence problems.

Importance of General and Disease-Specific Communication Dynamics

Point-of-care test results necessarily focus the clinician's attention on specific issues related to the patient's health or the progression of his or her disease. Until recently, no studies have examined whether intensive disease-specific education is sufficient to motivate behavioral change or whether other general characteristics of the patient–provider encounter (e.g., the extent to which the patient feels he or she has input into decision making, receives a thorough explanation of his or her health status, and is respected by clinicians) are important regardless of the type of focused information patients receive. We examined the relative importance of disease-specific and general communication dimensions as determinants of diabetes patients' self-care (23). As with many chronically ill patients, people with diabetes must integrate information from multiple test findings over time and are responsible for a variety of self-care activities. As such, diabetes patients provide an ideal population within which to determine the relative importance of improving disease-specific education around specific point-of-care tests or improving the dynamic of patient–provider communication more generally.

A total of 752 patients was recruited from three health system types, and all participants completed detailed telephone interviews that included ratings of their interpersonal processes of care using a previously validated methodology (24). Patients also reported whether they had received various forms of diabetes-specific education from their clinicians about issues such as diet (e.g., "how to adjust your eating to improve your blood cholesterol"), foot care ("how to care for your feet"), physical activity ("how to exercise properly"), and the benefits of controlling blood sugar.

Using multivariate techniques, we examined the independent influence on patients' self-care of diabetes-specific communication and a measure representing the foundational aspects of patient–provider communication more generally (25). We found that *both* diabetes-specific and general communication processes were independent predictors of patients' self-care adherence, even when controlling for their sociodemographic characteristics, health status, and characteristics of their healthcare setting (Figure 19-1). For example, the probability that patients reported taking their diabetes medications as prescribed increased from 75% when they received poor

diabetes-specific and poor general communication to 97% among patients who reported the best scores on both dimensions. Among patients with consistently poor general communication ratings, improvements in diabetes-specific communication were associated with a 14% improvement in medication adherence (from 75% to 89%). Among patients with the worst diabetes-specific communication scores, regression models predicted a 16% absolute improvement in adherence across the range of general communication scores (from 75% to 91%). Dietary behavior and exercise also were independently associated with both diabetes-specific and general communication measures. For example, patients' predicted probability of following their recommended diet increased from 3% among patients with both poor diabetes-specific and general communication to 28% among patients with the best possible combination of communication scores.

The results of this study suggest that patients' self-management is influenced both by the extent to which they are given specific information about their self-management as well as by the more general communication dynamics between them and their clinicians. In the context of POCT, patients' behavioral response to test results may be improved by emphasizing these general interpersonal care processes, such as whether patients feel respected by their clinicians, even if disease-specific information transfer remains consistently poor. However, as illustrated in Figure 19-1, improving both disease-specific communication and more general characteristics of the communication exchange is the ideal strategy for improving patients' self-care following a point-of-care test.

THE IMPORTANCE OF COLLABORATIVE GOAL SETTING

Many patients with chronic illnesses have multiple health problems simultaneously, and POCT results must be considered in the context of the complexity of their clinical status. For example, depression is twice as common among diabetes patients as in the general population, with 15% to 30% of diabetes patients meeting depression criteria (26). Patients with heart failure often are obese, and many have comorbidities, including hyperlipidemia, hypertension, back pain, and osteoarthritis. The medication regimens of chronically ill patients often reflect this complexity, especially when they are elderly. Most older adults (73%) who use prescription medications use more than one, and 29% use four or more (27).

POCT may improve the care of patients with multiple health problems by providing timely and accurate information on a number of health status indicators while patients are meeting with clinicians and available for discussion about possible treatment changes. However, patients with multiple health problems often have several test results out of range simultaneously, and it is important that the additional information from POCT be used to develop a clearly articulated set of treatment goals. For example, many patients with diabetes have inadequate glycemic control, as well as poor blood pressure control and dyslipidemia (the so-called metabolic syndrome)

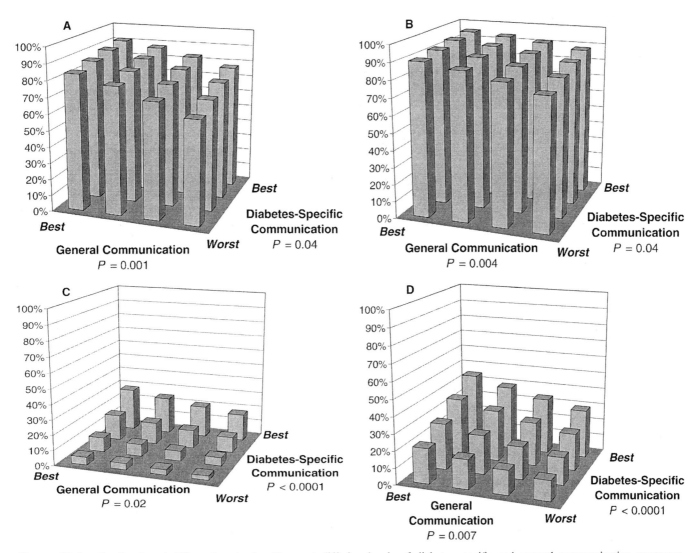

Figure 19-1 Predicted probability of optimal self-care at differing levels of diabetes-specific and general communication processes. Probabilities were calculated based on multivariate, ordinal probit models controlling for patients' sociodemographic characteristics (race, language, gender, age, and educational attainment), clinical characteristics (insulin use, A1c level, hypertension, history of MI, and number of diabetes complications), and characteristics of the treatment context (whether the primary provider provides most of the diabetes care, provider gender, length of the primary care relationship, and site of care): (A) the probability of "daily" or "almost daily" foot checks, (B) the probability of "always" taking diabetes medications as prescribed, (C) the probability of "always" following a recommended diet, and (D) the probability of "daily" exercise. Reprinted with permission from (23).

(28). It is probably unreasonable to expect them and their care teams to focus on improving all of their physiological outcomes at the same time. Focusing too broadly may cause patients to become confused and frustrated—factors that can hamper adherence to care plans. If POCT is used in multiple specialty clinics visited by the same patient, various providers may complicate this process further by emphasizing different health problems. Even if patients have a clear picture of their health and treatment goals at one point in time, it is critical that those goals be maintained across visits in order to reinforce educational messages and keep both patients' and providers' efforts focused. POCT can facilitate this process, but only if providers develop a coherent set of treatment priorities and patients' health targets are clearly documented in their medical records.

Most patients want to have an active role in setting priorities for their care (29), and research suggests that involving them in the process of defining treatment goals improves outcomes (10, 30). Involving patients in decision making about behavioral changes increases their sense of personal control and ensures that the goals are realistic—an important factor in determining patient compliance (31–33).

Unfortunately, patients often do not have an active role in their care planning, and many go through treatment with goals that are different from those of their clinicians. In one recent study (34), 127 pairs of diabetes patients and their physicians were surveyed about goals for the patient's diabetes-related health status as well as their preferred strategies for achieving those health improvements. The investigators found that agreement between patients and their physicians was low. Nineteen percent of patients agreed with their providers on none of their health-related goals, and an additional 40% agreed with their providers on only one of their three top health priorities. Moreover, 13% of patient-provider pairings disagreed on all of their top three preferred strategies for attaining health goals, and 56% agreed on only one of three strategies. Importantly, patients who reported less collaborative decision making with their physicians were especially likely to report priorities that differed from their clinicians. Primary care physicians who reported discussing more areas of diabetes care with their patients were more likely to agree with those patients regarding the course of their treatment. Greater agreement between patients and their physicians about treatment goals was associated with greater patient confidence (i.e., self-efficacy) in their ability to adhere to self-care plans. This study suggests that POCT can improve patient care if the results are used as the basis for collaborative goal setting but will be less beneficial without such discussions.

USING THE FIVE *A*'s TO STRUCTURE BEHAVIORAL COUNSELING

Collaborative goal-setting is both possible and beneficial in the context of busy primary care practices (35, 36). However, goal setting represents only one element of effective behavioral counseling about POCT results. Extensive research has identified specific interventions to assist patients in changing health behaviors via counseling in primary care settings, and many of these strategies are relevant to patient counseling about point-of-care tests (31). Unfortunately, the literature on behavior counseling is so vast that clinicians often have difficulty identifying the components of successful techniques. To address this problem, the Counseling and Behavioral Interventions Work Group of the US Preventive Services Task Force (USPSTF) systematically reviewed the literature on behavioral counseling strategies and developed a framework for understanding the most potent elements (37). The result of their efforts was the Five *A*'s framework: Assess, Advise, Agree, Assist, and Arrange (Table 19-1).

Assessment. Assessment is the most immediate goal of POCT. Point-of-care assessment can identify individuals who would benefit from behavioral intervention and allow practitioners to tailor their counseling efforts according to the unique needs of patients. As noted by the USPSTF working group, ideal assessments are brief, accurate, able to be scored and interpreted easily, and enhance intervention appropriateness. Although POCT often has these attributes, the results only provide an outcomes-based indication of patients' behavioral risk factors. In most cases, clinicians should follow up with assessments of relevant behaviors directly, through clinical interviews or the use of structured surveys. As later described, assessment of patients' functional health literacy levels may also be important (38).

Advise. Some clinicians provide POCT results to patients only with general advice to "do something" about the value. However, the results of POCT alone will seldom be

Table 19-1   The Five *A*'s as an Organizational Framework for Behavioral Counseling

Assess.   Ask about behavioral health risks and factors affecting the choice of behavioral change goals/methods.
Advise.   Give clear, specific, and personalized behavioral change advice, including information about personal health harms and benefits.
Agree.   Collaboratively select appropriate treatment goals and methods based on the patient's interest in and willingness to change the behavior.
Assist.   Using behavioral change techniques (self-help and/or counseling), aid the patient in achieving agreed-upon goals by acquiring the skills, confidence, and social/environmental supports for behavioral change.
Arrange.   Schedule follow-up contacts (in person or by telephone) to provide ongoing assistance/support and to adjust the treatment plan as needed, including referral to more intensive or specialized treatment.

Reprinted with permission from (37).

sufficient to motivate clinically important and sustained behavioral changes. Tailoring behavioral change advice to the health concerns of patients, past experience and sociocultural context are more effective than giving pamphlets or other standard forms of educational messages (39, 40). Many physicians lack the training and time to be the primary facilitator for making behavioral changes. Often their role is to highlight for patients what changes are especially important, and these brief messages can be critical motivators. Physicians also should link patients with more comprehensive and coordinated follow-up, such as that provided through nursing or health education services. A respectful and nonjudgmental approach to advising patients is more likely to result in patient receptivity, while a dictatorial interpersonal style may lead to passive resistance (41).

Agree. As noted above, collaboration with patients is essential to facilitate sustained behavioral changes in the context of POCT findings, and providers must be willing to share responsibility with patients for creating the treatment plan. Collaboratively identified goals should be clearly documented in clinical records so that they are available to facilitate the coordination of care across providers and the continuity of behavioral change efforts over time.

Assist. Providers should use "behavioral change techniques to aid patients in achieving agreed-upon goals by acquiring the tools they need to be successful, such as the skills, confidence and environmental supports for making behavioral adjustments" (37). Taking extra steps to assist patients is important, since general recommendations for making changes in diet, physical activity, smoking, or other health behaviors often are ineffective. Patients who are willing to make behavioral changes often confront unexpected barriers that require assistance from their providers to address effectively. For example, patients may have difficulty avoiding smoking when faced with powerful environmental pressures. For such patients, specific advice regarding strategies such as stimulus control (42, 43) may be important. For other patients, practical advice (e.g., where to purchase healthy food) or specific techniques such as contingency contracting (44, 45) may be beneficial. While a detailed description of behavioral change techniques is beyond the scope of this chapter, pragmatic approaches to brief counseling in primary care settings are available (31), and many health systems provide clinicians with access to professionals who can implement more intensive interventions or educate them about specific behavioral change tools.

Arrange. Providers and patients should agree on a specific schedule for follow-up contacts to provide ongoing support and adjustment in treatment plans. For POCT, direct person (face-to-face) follow-up will be required. However, intermediate contact via telephone (46) or email (47, 48) are effective strategies for monitoring patients' progress toward behavioral goals and responding to new challenges. Aside from the actual content of these follow-up interactions, the simple knowledge that follow-up is planned may be a powerful motivator. Arranging these follow-up contacts gives patients the message that their behavioral targets are important and that clinicians plan to work with them to resolve problems identified via point-of-care tests so that they can reach their optimal state of health.

USING POINT-OF-CARE TESTING WITH PATEINTS WHO HAVE HEALTH LITERACY PROBLEMS

Epidemiology and Consequences of Low Functional Health Literacy

Functional health literacy (FHL) consists of a number of skills that are important in the healthcare environment, including the ability to perform basic reading and numerical tasks (49). Poor FHL is common among patients with low educational attainment, those from racial/ethnic minority groups, older patients, and individuals whose primary language is not English. As many as one-third of all Medicare patients have low FHL, and the majority of patients treated in public health care settings have this problem. Although low FHL is correlated with other sociodemographic characteristics that make patients especially vulnerable, FHL is more than just a proxy for these characteristics, and it affects patients' health, health behavior, and health care costs even when these other factors are controlled. Medicaid patients with low FHL have annual health care costs that are more than four times those of other patients (50). One study found that only half of diabetes patients with low FHL knew the symptoms of hypoglycemia, compared to more than 95% of demographically similar patients with adequate FHL (51). In another study (52), diabetes patients with low FHL had 2.3 times the odds of retinopathy (a serious diabetes-related complication) relative to patients with adequate FHL, and 2.7 times the odds of cerebrovascular disease. These differences were observed even when controlling for differences between the groups in age, sex, race, education, insurance, language, social

support, depression, hypoglycemic regimen, years with diabetes education, hypertension, and smoking.

Unfortunately, patients with low FHL experience problems with a range of interpersonal care processes, including verbal communication during encounters with clinicians. Patients with low FHL are less likely to report that their providers' instructions are clear, that they understand their providers' explanations of their health conditions, and that they understand their providers' explanations about processes of care (53).

Meeting the Needs of Patients with Low Functional Health Literacy

Patients remember as little as 50% of what they are told during outpatient visits (54–56), and those with the greatest need for health education (e.g., individuals with a new diagnosis or a change in treatment) are often the least likely to absorb, process, and retain information (51, 53, 57, 58). Information about physiological parameters provided via POCT during a busy clinic visit may be especially difficult to convey. For individuals with low FHL, communicating the significance of these tests and suggestions for treatment changes can pose significant challenges. Fortunately, there are strategies that clinicians can use with low FHL patients to improve communication when discussing test results.

One useful technique for improving patients' understanding of POCT findings is to ask patients to restate information or instructions in their own words so that clinicians can assess the effectiveness of their own explanations. This technique, termed the *interactive communication loop* (see Figure 19-2) checks for lapses in recall and understanding. This technique also can uncover health beliefs, reinforce messages, and alert

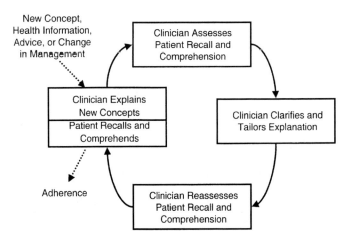

Figure 19-2 The interactive communication loop in clinician–patient education. Only by assessing recall and comprehension can the clinician ensure that a key concept has been understood and remembered. The clinician should repeat, clarify, or tailor information about point-of-care test results that the patient has difficulty understanding and reassess the patient's recall and comprehension until a common understanding has been achieved. Reprinted with permission from (57).

patients by opening a dialogue about their self-care goals and values (59, 60). Enhancements in recall and comprehension that are made possible via this communication strategy have been shown to improve subsequent adherence (61).

Recent research has shown that physicians rarely use this communication technique, although it may lead to better health outcomes. Schillinger and colleagues audiotaped clinic visits between 38 physicians and 74 English-speaking patients with diabetes and low FHL (57). They found that physicians rarely assessed patients' recall and comprehension when a new concept was presented. Only 20% of visits included any instances of using this technique, and the technique was used for only 12% of new concepts. Patients whose physician did assess recall and comprehension were nine times as likely to have HbA1c levels below the overall sample mean of 8.6% (i.e., to have better glucose control). After multivariate adjustment, the two variables most strongly associated with adequate glycemic control were higher FHL (odds ratio = 4.0; 95% CI = 1.1–14.5), and physicians' application of the interactive communication strategy (odds ratio = 15.2; 95% CI = 2.1, 110.8). Most POCT results represent new information, and many signal the need for changes in treatment plans. This study suggests that it is therefore critical for clinicians to have their patients reflect back their understanding of the test findings, the significance of the result, and the changes required in medical management or self-care.

CONSIDERING PATIENTS' TREATMENT COSTS

Many chronic illnesses require ongoing medication administration, and medication nonadherence is a major barrier to treatment effectiveness. The reasons patients fail to take their medications as prescribed include difficulty managing complex medication schedules, beliefs about potential efficacy of the treatment and its side effects, mental health challenges such as depression, and other problems.

In countries such as the United States, in which many patients lack adequate insurance coverage for prescription drugs, out-of-pocket drug costs represent a particularly important barrier to adherence that may not be considered by clinicians when monitoring patients' progress via POCT. Because the drug costs for chronically ill patients may be particularly high, many restrict medication use in response to cost pressures (62, 63). One recent survey found that 14% of heart failure patients with prescription drug coverage chose not to fill a medication prescription in the prior year because of the cost, and 25% of those with no medication coverage failed to fill one or more prescriptions (64). As many as 1 million diabetes patients and 2.9 million patients with asthma in the United States may cut back on medication use due to cost pressures (65). Not surprisingly, cost-related medication underuse is especially common among individuals with low incomes (62), although even moderate-income patients may face significant out-of-pocket medication costs if they are in treatment for multiple chronic conditions. Chronically ill patients who un-

deruse their medication due to cost often restrict essential medications such as hypoglycemics, diuretics, bronchodilators, and antipsychotics (66–69). This underuse has been associated with serious health consequences, including increased emergency department visits, nursing home admissions, acute psychiatric hospitalizations, and decrements in self-reported health status (66, 69–72).

POCT results should be interpreted in the context of accurate information about the patients' adherence to the medication protocol, including adherence problems due to cost pressures. However, one recent study found that chronically ill adults often fail to tell clinicians about cost-related medication underuse (73). In this study, two-thirds of chronically ill respondents who reported underusing their prescription medication due to cost never told a clinician in advance, and 35% never discussed the issue with clinicians at all. The reasons patients failed to talk about cost-related adherence problems with clinicians were varied and included feeling that there was not enough time during visits to discuss medication costs (31%), feeling embarrassed (46%), and believing that health care providers could not help them with medication cost problems (58%). Two-thirds of patients reported that they did not discuss cost-related adherence problems with clinicians because their clinicians never asked them about medication costs.

These findings have important implications for the use of POCT in clinical practice. When POCT results indicate that a patient is not improving on his or her current medication regimen, typical clinician responses may include increasing the patient's dose, adding augmentation therapy, or changing to a different agent. If the source of the patent's nonresponse is underuse due to cost pressures, clinicians may inadvertently exacerbate the underlying problem by discarding the patient's prescription before all of the medication is used in order to try another drug—a waste that many patients can ill afford. Moreover, clinicians may misinterpret "medication failures" as an indication of patients' lack of commitment to the treatment plan and lose motivation for treating patient' health problems aggressively. Identifying adherence problems resulting from cost pressures may lead to more effective remedies, such as switching to generic or lower-cost-branded drugs, providing more doses in order to lengthen the time between refills, or providing information on medication payment assistance programs. Even if treatment costs cannot be reduced, clinicians should explicitly inquire about potential adherence problems due to out-of-pocket costs when point-of-care test findings indicate inadequate improvement. More generally, the problem of cost-related medication underuse provides another example of the ways in which the meaning and response to POCT is fundamentally dependent on the information base available to clinicians through candid conversations with their patients.

SUMMARY AND RECOMMENDATIONS

Although POCT provides exciting opportunities to improve patient care, the potential benefits can only be achieved through a concerted effort to address barriers both patients and their clinicians face in using this new information. Fortunately, pragmatic strategies are available to improve the usefulness of POCT through relatively simple changes in the way care is delivered and an effort to communicate with patients effectively in the context of their socioeconomic and clinical circumstances. Table 19-2 summarizes the questions that clinicians should consider when using POCT in their practice.

Understanding the Test Result

From the clinician's perspective, understanding POCT results requires a familiarity with relevant treatment guidelines and the epidemiologic literature documenting the relationship between the measured physiological parameter and desired health outcomes. In many cases, guidelines regarding physiologic targets will need to be modified in the light of patients' age, competing health demands, and other factors. POCT results will only be useful in understanding the trajectory of patients' condition when viewed in the context of prior test values. Thus, documentation of POCT results and access to medical records that include all previous findings are critical if testing is to enrich the information base available for clinical decision making.

Patients may not understand their POCT results unless clinicians make a concerted effort to explain the test and its significance within a framework that reflects the patients' personal view and values. General communication processes, such as the extent to which patients have input into decision making and their providers recognize the emotional impact of test findings, can influence patients' receptivity to behavior change in light of POCT. A significant number of patients have functional health literacy problems, and these patients may require added attention using established techniques, such as "closing the informational loop," in order to confirm that they understand a point-of-care test's findings. Several strategies for identifying patients who have inadequate functional health literacy have been developed, including the use of validated brief screening texts that can be administered in primary care (38).

Developing an Etiologic Explanation

Understanding the reasons for POCT is critical in order to develop a treatment plan that will lead to improvements in the health status of patients. For some patients, unacceptable test findings may indicate that their current medications are inadequate and therefore a change in pharmacotherapy is warranted. However, other patients may respond to a given treatment but fail to take it as prescribed because of barriers to adherence, including out-of-pocket cost pressures. Still other patients may be achieving maximum benefit from medications or may be able to make further improvements through lifestyle interventions. In many cases, a frank ongoing dialogue will be essential to identify the behavioral factors influencing patients' POCT findings. Research suggests that these discussions are most likely to be fruitful as part of a trusting relationship between the patient and their clinicians (74).

Table 19-2   Important Questions for Clinicians Using Point-of-Care Tests

Understanding the Test

1. Is the result in normal limits? If not, how bad is it?
2. What does the result say about the trajectory of the patient's condition? Is he or she improving or getting worse?
3. Does the patient understand what the test measures, what the normal range is, and where he or she stands?
4. How do the patient's sociodemographic characteristics and functional health literacy level influence his or her understanding of this test and its significance?

Developing an Etiologic Explanation for the Patient's Test Result

1. Does the test result suggest a change in the patient's regimen?
2. How do the patient's self-care and lifestyle behaviors affect this result?
3. Are there significant financial access barriers preventing the patient from improving this result (e.g., the ability to purchase medication or healthy food)?
4. What other perceived barriers to improving self-care exist (e.g., the patient's beliefs regarding a medication's importance or comorbidities that preclude increasing physical activity levels)?
5. Is the patient confused or frustrated by the lack of a coherent process of treatment planning across providers or from one visit to the next?

Developing a Plan for Action

1. What is a realistic goal for improving the test result over the near term (e.g., 3–6 months)?
2. Do the patient and all of his or her treatment providers agree that the treatment goal is meaningful and realistic, given other clinical problems and barriers to care?
3. What are the primary strategies for meeting this goal through clinician action (changing medications) and patient behavioral change (e.g., increasing physical activity levels)?
4. What are the barriers to achieving behavioral changes, and how can they be addressed?
5. What is the strategy for monitoring the patient's progress and addressing new barriers to behavior change that may arise?

Developing a Plan of Action

Once patients and providers share an understanding of a point-of-care test result and a causal model to explain its value, the next step is to develop a plan for making needed changes in treatment and self-care. Treatment goals that are defined in terms of unrealistic targets or those that will take more than 6 months to achieve likely will result in patient frustration, while more realistic and short-term targets can lead to better adherence and improvements in patients' health. Health goals should be defined with all of the patient's health concerns in mind, and should reflect their preferences. Although providers may be concerned about the long-term consequences of patients' cholesterol levels, patients may have different priorities, such as back pain or impotence that must be addressed in order to agree on overall treatment strategies.

Some of the factors limiting adherence to self-care regimens are complex and may require extended discussions to identify barriers to change. Research has shown that patients can overcome barriers to self-care with providers' assistance and the use of structured approaches such as the Five A's framework. Other barriers to success may reflect problems in coordination and treatment among providers that make it difficult to identify and pursue a coherent strategy for improving test results. It is essential that patients receive a clear and consistent message regarding their POCT results that carries over across clinicians and over time. For that to happen, clinicians must make efforts to coordinate their understanding of patients' status and agree on what is and is not working to maximize patients' health.

Overarching Importance of the Nontechnical Dimension of Point-of-Care Testing

The primary message from research described in this chapter is that POCT must be conducted in recognition of the important role that patients themselves play in implementing treatment plans and determining their health outcomes. POCT can improve patient care if it is delivered as part of a patient-centered approach in which patients collaborate with clinicians to identify treatment goals and formulate a plan for reaching those goals. Strategies such as the Five A's approach provide clinicians with clear guidelines as to how to assist patients in this process. Given these advances in our understanding of how patient–provider communication and behavioral counseling can be most effective, POCT can play an important role in monitoring patients' progress and motivating needed treatment changes.

REFERENCES

1. Yarnall KS, Pollak KI, Ostbye T, Krause KM, Michener JL. Primary care: is there enough time for prevention? Am J Pubic Health 2003;93:635–41.
2. McGinnis JM, Foege WH. Actual causes of death in the United States. JAMA 1993;270:2207–12.
3. Wagner EH, Austin BT, Von Korff M. Organizing care for patients with chronic illness. Milbank Q 1996;74:511–44.
4. Heisler M, Bouknight RR, Hayward RA. The relative importance of physician communication, participatory decision making, and patient understanding in diabetes self-management. J Gen Intern Med 2002;17:243–52.
5. DiMatteo MR. The physician–patient relationship: effects on the quality of health care. Clin Obstet Gynecol 1994;37:149–61.
6. Greenfield S, Kaplan S, Ware JE. Expanding patient involvement in care: effects on patient outcomes. Ann Intern Med 1985;102:520–8.
7. Sherbourne CD, Hays RD, Ordway L, DiMatteo MR, Kravitz RL. Antecedents of adherence to medical recommendations: results from the Medical Outcomes Study. J Behav Med 1992;15:447–68.
8. Kaplan SH, Greenfield S, Ware JE. Assessing the effects of physician-patient interactions on the outcomes of chronic disease [published erratum]. Med Care 1989;27:S110–27.
9. Stewart MA. Effective physician–patient communication and health outcomes: a review. CMAJ 1995;152:1423–33.
10. Anderson RM, Funnell MM, Butler PM, Arnold MS, Fitzgerald JT, Feste CC. Patient empowerment. Results of a randomized controlled trial. Diabetes Care 1995;18:943–9.
11. Robins LS, White CB, Alexander GL, Gruppen LD, Grum CM. Assessing medical students' awareness and sensitivity to diverse health beliefs using a standardized patient station. Acad Med 2001;76:76–80.
12. Resnicow K, Baranowski T, Ahluwalia JS, Braithwaite RL. Cultural sensitivity in public health: defined and demystified. Ethn Dis 1999;9:10–21.
13. Roter DL, Hall JA, Aoki Y. Physician gender effects in medical communication: a meta-analytic review. JAMA 2002;288:756–67.
14. Sprague-Jones J. Gender effects in physician–patient interaction. In: Lipkin M, Putnam SM, Lazare A, eds. The medical interview: clinical care, education, and research. New York: Springer-Verlag; 1995:163–71.
15. Arnold RM, Martin SC, Parker RM. Taking care of patients—does it matter whether the physician is a woman? West J Med 1988;149:729–33.
16. Zare N, Sorenson JR, Heeren T. Sex of provider as a variable in effective genetic counseling. Soc Sci Med 1984;19:671–5.
17. Linn LS, Cope DW, Leake B. The effect of gender and training of residents on satisfaction ratings by patients. J Med Educ 1984;59:964–6.
18. Love MM, Mainous AG III, Talbert JC, Hager GL. Continuity of care and the physician–patient relationship: the importance of continuity for adult patients with asthma. J Fam Pract 2000;49:998–1004.
19. Howie JG, Heaney DJ, Maxwell M, Walker JJ, Freeman GK, Rai H. Quality at general practice consultations: cross sectional survey. BMJ 1999;319:738–43.
20. Hjortdahl P, Laerum E. Continuity of care in general practice: effect on patient satisfaction. BMJ 1992;304:1287–90.
21. Ong LML, DeHaes JCJM, Hoos AM, Lammes FB. Doctor–patient communication: a review of the literature. Soc Sci Med 1995;40:903–18.
22. Molleman E, Krabbendam PJ, Annyas AA, Koops HS, Sleijfer DT, Vermey A. The significance of the doctor–patient relationship in coping with cancer. Soc Sci Med 1984;18:475–80.

23. Piette JD, Schillinger D, Potter MB, Heisler M. Dimensions of patient–provider communication and diabetes self-care in an ethnically-diverse population. J Gen Intern Med 2003;18:1–10.

24. Stewart AL, Napoles-Springer A, Perez-Stable EJ. Interpersonal processes of care in diverse populations. Milbank Q 1999;77: 305–39.

25. Lipkin M; Putnam SM; Lazare A. Three functions of the medical interview. The medical interview: clinical care, education, and research. New York: Springer-Verlag, 1995:3–19.

26. Anderson RJ, Freedland KE, Clouse RE, Lustman PJ. The prevalence of comorbid depression in adults with diabetes: a meta-analysis. Diabetes Care 2001;24:1069–78.

27. Centers for Disease Control and Prevention. National health and nutrition examination survey: patterns of prescription drug use in the United States, 1988–94. http://www.cdc.gov/nchs/data/nhanes/databriefs/preuse.pdf (accessed May 2004).

28. Ford ES, Giles WH. A comparison of the prevalence of the metabolic syndrome using two proposed definitions. Diabetes Care 2003;26:575–81.

29. Little P, Everitt H, Williamson I, Warner G, Moore M, Gould C, et al. Preferences of patients for patient centered approach to consultation in primary care: observational study. BMJ 2001;322: 468–72.

30. Olivarius NF, Beck-Nielsen H, Andreasen AH, Horder M, Pedersen PA. Randomised controlled trial of structured personal care of type 2 diabetes mellitus. BMJ 2001;323:946–7.

31. Rollnick S, Mason P, Butler C. Health behavior change: a guide for practitioners. Edinburgh and New York: Churchill Livingstone, 1999.

32. Lerman CE, Brody DS, Caputo GC, Smith DG, Lazaro CG, Wolfson HG. Patients' perceived involvement in care scale: relationship to attitudes about illness and medical care. J Gen Intern Med 1990;5:29–33.

33. Donovan JL, Blake DR. Patient non-compliance: deviance or reasoned decision-making? Soc Sci Med 1992;34:507–13.

34. Heisler M, Vijan S, Anderson RM, Ubel PA, Bernstein SJ, Hofer TP. When do patients and their physicians agree on diabetes treatment goals and strategies, and what difference does it make? J Gen Intern Med 2003;18:893–902.

35. Von Korff M, Gruman J, Schaefer J, Curry SJ, Wagner EH. Collaborative management of chronic illness. Ann Intern Med 1997;127:1097–102.

36. Bogardus ST, Bradley EH, Tinetti ME. A taxonomy for goal setting in the care of persons with dementia. J Gen Intern Med 1998;13:675–80.

37. Whitlock EP, Orleans T, Pender N, Allan J. Evaluating primary care behavioral counseling interventions, An evidence-based approach. Am J Prev Med 2002;22:267–84.

38. Davis TC, Michielutte R, Askov EN, Williams MV, Weiss BD. Practical assessment of adult literacy in health care. Health Educ Behav 1998;25:613–24.

39. Skinner CS, Streecher VJ, Hospers H. Physicians' recommendations for mammography: do tailored messages make a difference? Am J Public Health 1994;84:43–9.

40. Kreuter MW, Streecher VJ, Glassman B. One size does not fit all: the case for tailoring print materials. Ann Behav Med 1999;21: 276–83.

41. Emmons KM, Rollnick S. Motivational interviewing in health care settings: opportunities and limitations. Am J Prev Med 2001;20:68–74.

42. Brownell KD, Cohen LR. Adherence to dietary regimens. 2: components of effective interventions. Behav Med 1995;20: 155–64.

43. Foreyt JP, Poston WS. The role of the behavioral counselor in obesity treatment. J Am Diet Assoc 98(10 Suppl 2):S27–30, 1998.

44. Janz NK, Becker MH, Hartman PE. Contingency contracting to enhance patient compliance: a review. Patient Educ Couns 1984; 5:165–78.

45. Boehm S, Schlenk EA, Funnell MM, Powers H, Ronis DL. Predictors of adherence to nutrition recommendations in people with non-insulin-dependent diabetes mellitus. Diabetes Educ 1997;23:157–65.

46. Wasson J, Gaudette C, Whaley F, Sauvigne A, Baribeau P, Welch HG. Telephone care as a substitute for routine clinic follow-up. JAMA 1992;267:1788–93.

47. Tate DF, Jackvony EH, Wing RR. Effects of internet behavioral counseling on weight loss in adults at risk for type 2 diabetes. JAMA 2003;289:1833–6.

48. Tate DF, Wing RR, Winett RA. Using internet technology to deliver a behavioral weight loss program. JAMA 2001;285: 1172–7.

49. Ad Hoc Committee on Health Literacy for the Council on Scientific Affairs AMA. Health literacy: report of the Council on Scientific Affairs. JAMA 1999;281:552–7.

50. Weiss BD, Blanchard JS, McGee DL, Hart G, Warren B, Burgoon M, et al. Illiteracy among Medicaid recipients and its relationship to health care costs. J Health Care Poor Underserved 1994;5:99–111.

51. Williams MV, Baker DW, Parker RM, Nurss JR. Relationship of functional health literacy to patients' knowledge of their chronic disease: a study of patients with hypertension or diabetes. Arch Intern Med 1998;158:166–72.

52. Schillinger D, Grumbach K, Piette JD, Wang F, Osmond D, Daher C, et al. Association of functional health literacy with diabetes outcomes among public hospital patients. JAMA 2002; 288:475–82.

53. Schillinger D, Bindman A, Stewart A, Wang F, Piette JD. Functional health literacy and the quality of physician–patient communication among diabetes patients. Patient Educ Couns 2004; 52:315–23.

54. Rost K, Carter W, Inui T. Introduction of information during the initial medical visit: consequences for patient follow-through with physician recommendations for medication. Soc Sci Med 1989; 28:315–21.

55. Rost K, Roter D. Predictors of recall of medication regimens and recommendations for lifestyle change in elderly patients. Gerontologist 1987;27:510–5.

56. Crane JA. Patient comprehension of doctor–patient communication on discharge from the emergency department. J Emerg Med 1997;15:1–7.

57. Schillinger D, Piette JD, Grumbach K, Wang F, Wilson C, Daher C, et al. Closing the loop: physician communication with diabetic patients who have low health literacy. Arch Intern Med 2003; 163:83–90.

58. Williams MV, Baker DW, Honig EL, Lee TM, Nowlan A. Inadequate literacy is a barrier to asthma knowledge and self-care. Chest 1998;114:1008–15.

59. Bertakis KD. The communication of information from physician to patient: a method for increasing patient retention and satisfaction. J Fam Prac 1977;5:217–22.

60. Schwartzberg J. Health literacy introductory kit. Chicago: American Medical Association, 2000.
61. Ley P. Communicating with patients: improving communication, satisfaction, and compliance. New York: Croom Helm, 1988.
62. Steinman MA, Sands LP, Covinsky KE. Self-restriction of medications due to cost in seniors without prescription coverage. J Gen Intern Med 2001;16:793–9.
63. Hwang W, Weller W, Ireys H, Anderson G. Out-of-pocket medical spending for care of chronic conditions. Health Aff [Millwood] 2001;20:267–78.
64. Safran DG, Neuman P, Schoen C, Montgomery JE, Li W, Wilson IB, et al. Prescription drug coverage and seniors: how well are states closing the gap? Health Aff [Millwood] 2002;Suppl Web: W253–68.
65. Piette JD, Heisler M, Wagner TH. Cost-related medication underuse among chronically-ill adults: what treatments do people forego? how often? who is at risk? Am J Public Health [in press].
66. Soumerai SB, Avorn J, Ross-Degnan D, Gortmaker S. Payment restrictions for prescription drugs under Medicaid: effects on therapy, cost, and equity. N Eng J Med 1987;317:550–6.
67. Martin BC, McMillan JA. The impact of implementing a more restrictive prescription limit on Medicaid recipients. Med Care 1996;34:686–701.
68. Federman AD, Adams AS, Ross-Degnan D, Soumerai SB, Ayanian JZ. Supplemental insurance and use of effective cardiovascular drugs among elderly Medicare beneficiaries with coronary heart disease. JAMA 2001;286:1732–9.
69. Tamblyn R, Laprise R, Hanley JA, Abrahamowicz M, Scott S, Mayo N, et al. Adverse events associated with prescription drug cost-sharing among poor and elderly persons. JAMA 2001;285: 421–9.
70. Melfi CA, Chawla AJ, Croghan TW, Hanna MP, Kennedy S, Sredl K. The effects of adherence to antidepressant treatment guidelines on relapse and recurrence of depression. Arch Gen Psychiatry 1998;55:1128–32.
71. Soumerai SB, Ross-Degnan D, Avorn J, McLaughlin TJ, Choodnovsky I. Effects of Medicaid drug-payment limits on admission to hospitals and nursing homes. New Eng J Med 1991;325: 1072–7.
72. Soumerai SB, McLaughlin TJ, Ross-Degnan D, Casteris CS, Bollini P. Effects of limiting Medicaid drug-reimbursement benefits on the use of psychotropic agents and acute mental health services by patients with schizophrenia. New Eng J Med 1994; 331:650–5.
73. Piette JD, Heisler M, Wagner TH. Cost-related medication underuse: do patients with chronic illnesses tell their doctors? Arch Intern Med [in press].
74. Dibben MR, Morris SE, Lean ME. Situational trust and cooperative partnerships between physicians and their patients: a theoretical explanation transferable from business practice. QJM 2000;93:55–61.

Chapter **20**

Informatics in Point-of-Care Testing

Richard G. Jones and Andrew St John

Several of the earlier chapters in this book have focused on the measurement or sensing technologies used in various point-of-care testing (POCT) devices. Crucial as these technologies are to the success of any device, the processing and management of information within the device is of equal importance. Consequently, advances in information technology (IT) have also greatly facilitated the development of novel POCT instruments. Miniaturization would not be possible without IT, and the ability to package instrument control and analysis functions into the current range of devices is largely as a result of the increasing information handling power and the availability of low-cost computing devices. Similarly, the recent rapid advances in computer communications have allowed distribution of such devices to occur without them necessarily existing in total isolation.

Recent attention has focused on how information technology can affect events downstream from the analytical process, and to some extent the processes that take place before the analysis. Table 20-1 lists the steps involving informatics in carrying out a POC test on a typical system, and it can be seen that informatics is the glue that integrates the whole process into a coherent diagnostic activity. This chapter will also consider the contribution of IT to the environment in which POCT is practiced, describing some of the software products that are now available as part of POCT devices.

INFORMATION TECHNOLOGY INFRASTRUCTURE AND POCT

It is assumed that readers are aware of the generic issues involved in laboratory applications of IT, and the following sections concentrate on technological issues specific to POCT instrumentation in the context of the wider laboratory computing environment. It is important to draw a distinction between IT and informatics. IT refers specifically to technologies such as computers, connections, and software, whereas informatics, which will be defined in more detail later, refers to the way in which these are harnessed to enable data and information exchange. As technology has developed, the challenges of the former have diminished and the challenges of the latter have increased largely because our expectations of what should be possible continuously run ahead of what is actually possible. Information technologies have been classified as disruptive technologies (see Table 20-2) and our understanding of the potential impact of these technologies on human or corporate

behaviors lags behind our ability to introduce them to clinical environments (1).

Information technology has played a vital role in enabling the development of instrument interfaces that encompass a wide range of functionality as well as being relatively easy to use (2). New POCT devices are now available that use the touch screen as the standard type of interface, and this trend will continue, with a wide range of functions being incorporated. This reflects the trends in consumer products such as mobile or cell telephones. The adoption of standard interfaces of this type is of economic benefit to manufacturers and consumers alike as development costs on nonstandard platforms are high. The use of standard platforms allows many functions to be incorporated at marginal cost. This will be of particular significance in relation to the integration of devices into networked solutions where easy and economical access to the communications capabilities of modern PC devices will be of great significance.

A disadvantage of this simplification is that manual data entry is more difficult as the traditional keypad or keyboard is displaced. Furthermore, while the use of check digits can overcome the potential errors from manually typing patient identifiers into an instrument, many hospitals have abolished these error checks for various reasons, including the lack of standardized algorithms (3). Barcodes are now being widely used for both patient and sample identification, and coupled with barcoded test selection menus, these can obviate the need to use keyboards for typed data entry. Thus, some POCT instruments come with a barcode reader and wand as a standard attachment. Although barcoded wristbands for patient identification are not acceptable in certain countries, with the recent focus on medical error (4), including the US Institute of Medicine report, it is likely that the use of this type of patient identifier will increase. In conjunction with networked access between clinical databases, laboratory information management systems (LIMS), and POCT devices, the use of barcoded data entry systems is likely to expand. Their benefits in terms of ensuring that all patient data is correctly identified are summarized in Table 20-3 (5).

At this stage, although handwriting recognition systems are common in personal digital assistant (PDA) devices, they have not yet appeared in POCT devices. One consequence of the effort to combat terrorism is major investment in various biometric identifiers, such as iris and fingerprint recognition. It remains to be seen whether these will be used in the medical environment. The use of radio frequency identification tags

Table 20-1 Functions of IT in POCT Devices

Instrument control—pumps, samplers, etc.
Signal transduction
Calculation and data reduction
Data capture and storage
Provision of decision support
Remote communication and control
Display of system states and data
Test selection
Online instruction

(RFIDs) is increasing in the logistics and supply-chain businesses, and these tags are certainly small enough to be incorporated in armbands and specimen tubes, and they have been implanted under the skin for veterinary purposes (6). As the name implies, RFID systems are based on radio waves, and each tag is equipped with a tiny radio transmitter. When it detects a special radio signal from a reader, the tag responds by sending its own unique serial number through the air. At this stage their cost is still relatively high, and they may not offer significant advantages over barcodes, particularly as the latter become more sophisticated and capable of containing ever more information. However, whichever identification system is used, it still remains difficult to convince many operators of POCT systems to identify the patient and the specimen to the device.

NETWORKING TECHNOLOGY

Intranets and the Internet

Many, if not most, hospitals in the developed world now have some form of IT network (7). Driven by what is now relatively inexpensive networking technology, local area networks (LANs) have now extended across complete health regions and are linked externally to create private, secure wide area networks (WANs), spanning in some cases many institutions and laboratories, and commonly referred to as *intranets* (8). Consequently, many POCT devices are now either linked to information systems directly or via intermediate data managers through IT networks. This has all but replaced the concept of linking a single device to a PC via an RS232 serial port. In the meantime, the Internet has continued to expand, and in most situations intranet and Internet networks are contiguous, with their separation maintained only at a logical level through the use of secure gateways and firewalls. The degree of physical continuity varies from country to country, largely determined by the differences in the legal framework surrounding the regulation of data transmission over the networks and whether the state concerned has the resources available to develop parallel, private health networks (9). There will be some regional convergence, as indicated by European legislation aligning member states of the European Union, but elsewhere, especially in countries that do not support centralized health programs, use of the open Internet is likely to prevail.

These days, most if not all network connections are via Ethernet, which can carry data at rates of 10–10,000 MB/s or more, depending on the volume of competing traffic on the network. In such an arrangement, devices can be moved at will between network ports without recourse to rewiring, and any number of devices can be flexibly connected to a network, the bounds being set only by the size. More recent trends include the convergence of data and voice communications, as more and more organizations also use the local network and Internet for telephony as well as data traffic. This will facilitate the distribution of data points to be as widespread as that of the ubiquitous telephone system.

The cost of digital cameras, including intranet-ready digital cameras (webcams), continues to decrease, and they have been used in a number of remote monitoring applications, including 24-h surveillance of the actions of analytical robots in a large pharmaceutical laboratory (10). Although one can think of possible uses in relation to POCT, such as assessing the degree of tidiness of a POCT location or to create a timed video audit trail of the use of instruments by members of staff, no commercial or published applications have appeared to date. However, several manufacturers commonly use modems or networks to remotely access a wide variety of analytical instrumentation, including POCT devices.

Wireless Communication and Networks

Many hospitals and other medical institutions have augmented or replaced their existing networks with wireless devices that provide POCT users with greater mobility. For example, downloading results from a handheld device to an information system can take place at any location within the range of the access point or base station and obviates the need for the user to return to a central docking station (11). The best-developed example of this type of connectivity is the i-STAT™ clinical chemistry analyzer (i-STAT Corporation, East Windsor, NJ, USA), which uses infrared signaling to connect the handheld device to the base station PC. This allows data from multiple devices to be consolidated into a single PC and enables online, real-time data control, logging, and display. The base station may itself be a network node allowing data to be forwarded to a LIMS or to a clinical information system such as an intensive care unit (ICU) database.

The most common wireless network is, of course, that provided by mobile telephony, where devices in any one area or cell can operate up to several miles from the access point, and individual cells are linked to form a network. Figure 20-1 illustrates the use of wireless or telemetry links as the method of network device connection. In contrast, Infrared Data As-

Table 20-2 IT as a Disruptive Technology

Disruptive technologies have three important characteristics:
1. Initially underperform established products
2. Enable new applications for new customers
3. Rapidly improving performance

Table 20-3 Improvement in Patient Identification Rates and Better Retention of Data Following Barcode Identification

Result	Samples per month, mean ± SD		Significance
	Before barcoding (22 months)	After barcoding (36 months)	
Correct identification	123 ± 34	149 ± 44	$P = 0.001$
Incorrect identification	2 ± 2	11 ± 7	$P < 0.001$
Lost data	37 ± 14	2 ± 2	$P < 0.001$
Total samples	163 ± 44	162 ± 43	NS[a]

[a] NS, not significant.
Data from (5).

sociation (IrDA) devices—which, as the name implies, rely on infrared transmission— may only operate a few meters from the access point. A typical application is in a critical-care area where a POCT device can communicate information to a data management station and all that is required is a line of sight between the device and the access point. Many infrared devices operate under Institute of Electrical and Electromechanical Engineers (IEEE) Standard 802.11 (12). There are also IrDA standards, and because IrDA-related devices are commonly used in laptop computers and mobile phones, and can be made at low cost, they have been incorporated into the NCCLS POCT Connectivity standard (discussed later). A modification of Standard 802.11 (802.11b) allows higher transmission speeds, but because transmission power remains low, interference from other devices is minimized, thus making it an ideal standard for POCT devices (3). It is likely that remote network connectivity of analytical devices will increase, with the potential for it to be used to provide real-time decision support and integration of patient data into electronic medical records.

Security and Confidentiality

In recent years, there has been growing concern about security of patient data. While networks facilitate access to information

for all patient care providers, they can also result in patient data being passed on to those who might use it for inappropriate or even malicious purposes. The United States recently enacted the Health Insurance Portability and Accountability Act (HIPAA), a significant part of which concerns patient privacy (13). The law substantially increases the responsibility of providers, including those involved with POCT, to ensure the privacy of patient information. Other countries are adopting or about to adopt similar measures, many of which are encompassed within the area of clinical governance (see Chapter 17).

Security measures include separating hospital and laboratory intranets from the main Internet with firewalls or electronic barriers. The latter have assumed even greater importance with the increase in computer viruses. Passwords, although relatively easy to circumvent, are an important measure for securing data as well as for preventing untrained personnel from using POCT equipment. Data transmission across the Internet can be safeguarded through encryption and is a stated requirement under the HIPAA. All these pose challenges for the laboratory, but the process may be helped in situations where security issues are resolved at the institutional rather than individual laboratory level. A continuing problem is that the technology is continually changing, computing is be-

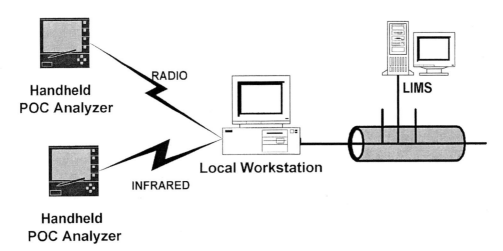

Figure 20-1 Using infrared and radiotelemetric links to connect handheld devices to a central workstation, where they are linked into the clinical network.

come more powerful, and more sophisticated measures are required to safeguard information.

INFORMATICS AND THE ORGANIZATION OF POCT

An appreciation of how informatics affects POCT requires some understanding of the terms *data, information,* and *knowledge.* These terms are often used interchangeably, but they should be considered in terms of a hierarchy of meaning (14). This is illustrated in Figure 20-2 which shows raw data at the bottom of the hierarchy, moving up to information, with knowledge at the top. Each layer adds to the one before, so that meaning increases as one moves up the hierarchy. A patient's glucose result of 7.0 mmol/L (126 mg/100 mL) is an example of data that becomes information when it is considered in relation to a reference range; by comparing the result, the clinician can see that the glucose result is abnormal. Knowledge is about the relationships between different sets of data, so if the patient in this example had an abnormal nonfasting glucose on more than one occasion, then the patient may have diabetes. This is an example of knowledge. Thus, from a piece of knowledge being applied in a particular context, data are interpreted to produce information (14).

In the central laboratory, most analytical devices are directly linked or interfaced to laboratory information systems (LIS); if there is no direct interface, data from the device is input manually. The purpose of the LIS is to combine data with information, and in some cases even provide knowledge through expert systems. The end result is to produce useful and accessible clinical information. This information process goes hand-in-hand with other LIS processes that are designed to ensure the quality of all the transactions that take place and to provide evidence of this, such as audit trails and other quality statistics. The LIS also plays a major role in extracting maximal efficiencies from automated and semirobotic equipment, which itself has high demand for rapid, reliable access to the databases containing information on the orders to be processed and samples to be analyzed. All of these procedures, such as real-time quality control, are now an accepted part of laboratory practice and processes, and are demanded by organizations such as the US Joint Commission on Accreditation of Healthcare Organizations. Similar regulations exist in other countries (15).

A major concern of clinical scientists about POCT is that in most cases the above goals in relation to quality are rarely achieved. Furthermore, the caregiver who is using POCT is unaware of the significance of the issues involved and is unwilling to accept the costs, both managerial and operational, that are needed to achieve them. These costs can be substantial and must be taken into account when considering business cases for POCT (16). Table 20-4 lists some informatic, or data-processing, principles applicable to any clinical analytical process. It can be seen that there are examples in every case where many current POCT systems fail to meet these criteria either because of potential errors due to human factors or because economic constraints conflict with the ideals.

A prime example is a POCT device without a database, or a device that cannot easily interface with an information system. Data will have to be entered manually into such a device, with the potential risk of transcription error. More likely, the data will in fact not be entered, not reach the clinical record, and never have a clinical effect on patient care. One consequence for the laboratory is that failure to record data often leads to unnecessary repetition of testing, which adds to costs and reduces the clinical cost-effectiveness of POCT systems. Table 20-5 lists the dataset that has traditionally been used to form a laboratory report. When comparing POCT with traditional methods, it is unlikely that this dataset will be available in full for the majority of POCT results generated. Thus, it follows that the information available from POCT devices is likely to be inherently inferior to that arising from more traditional routes, assuming that the traditional best-practice applies in these circumstances. A challenge to professionals responsible for the design, development, and deployment of information systems must be to attempt to harness the technologies previously mentioned to appropriately control these systems. Above all, users should insist that POCT devices capture data in ways that allow their meaningful analysis, especially with regard to the clinical quality of the information generated, if the benefits of testing are to be realized as improvements to the care of patients.

The development, management, and organization of such POCT systems within the clinical environment presents many challenges, not least because the scenario envisaged will be very different from that in which we work today. The cost/complexity/convenience equations are changing dramatically as a result of the development of informatics. Previously, the costs of POCT could be easily justified for complex instruments required for rapid turnaround of results in critical care situations. Because, in relation to these costs, the additional costs of IT equipment to provide remote access support were marginal, these developments could also be justified without undue difficulty. In contrast, with the newer, low-cost instruments, especially those providing results based on disposable chemistries such as the unit-device immunoassay systems, the additional costs of information capture are high compared to the base instrument cost. Thus, paradoxically, as the ability to distribute testing becomes easier, there is a tendency to relax the degree of control over the information generated. This is

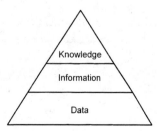

Figure 20-2   Informatic hierarchy relationship among data, information, and knowledge.

Table 20-4 Principles of Information Management

Principle	Problem with POCT
Patient samples should be positively identified to the system.	Strip devices do not carry identification and meters do not read IDs.
Operator access to the system should be password protected.	Not true of many handheld meters.
A hard-copy record of the results, positively identified, should be generated.	Many meters do not carry printers and results must be manually transcribed.
Data should be stored in a local or remote database.	Not available on the majority of devices.
A log of events and of access should be maintained.	Not available on the majority of devices.

occurring at a time when the potential benefits from informatics are increasing and when, in a litigious society, the requirements to capture and record information are increasing. There is, of course, no reason that nontechnical approaches cannot be taken to solve this conundrum. For example, the insistence that human users manually log all data could overcome the potential for data loss. However, as previously discussed with regard to sample identification, attempts to enforce best practice by this means have generally proven that humans are unreliable at such tasks and, furthermore, that such demands undermine much of the perceived convenience of POCT.

An alternative paradigm would be to reduce the computing power of individual devices and concentrate control back into a common base station. Welch-Allyn has initiated a multivendor project to look at the possibility of treating POCT devices merely as transducers that interface back to a common informatics platform, where common functions of patient identification, user control, and decision support can be shared (17). The benefits of this are both financial and clinical. Expensive hardware is not duplicated, and software development costs can be spread across many functions. Clinical data is automatically consolidated, further reducing costs by minimizing the need to interface between multiple data sources. An additional perceived benefit is that the physical size and complexity of instruments and supporting systems can be reduced. To achieve such a situation, much work will be required to develop a suitable hardware interface protocol, similar to and possibly derived from the medical information bus (MIB; formerly known as the IEEE-1073 interface) already implemented for plug-and-play medical devices in the area of critical care (18, 19).

In addition to concerns about the mechanics of data capture and data quality, it is important to understand the context in which information will be handled downstream. With the increasing use of electronic record systems, diagnostic data will be viewed by the majority of clinicians through electronic portals that consolidate information from a multiplicity of databases. This will include the LIMS and POCT systems. It is highly likely that as data passes forward the knowledge of its precise origin will be lost, and all results will effectively become equivalent. Thus, for example, all glucose results might be merged to a single data type to simplify storage and presentation functions. If such results are not exactly equivalent, apparent changes in glucose concentration that are merely artifacts might become visible. Clinicians viewing a table or graph of such results could therefore be misled about the true clinical picture and make erroneous diagnostic and therapeutic judgments. This problem already exists in situations where patient samples are analyzed in multiple laboratories using poorly standardized methods (e.g., in testing for tumor markers such as prostate specific antigen). As complex tests such as this move out into the POCT arena, there is a danger that the electronic patient records will be degraded through contamination by poor-quality and poorly standardized information. One answer will be to ensure that results are always transmitted using formally agreed-on codes such as LOINC or SNOMED-CT and that these code schemes include method-specific elements to allow data to be selectively retrieved and displayed.

CONNECTIVITY STANDARDS

As previously indicated, there are many significant problems with POCT processes, some of which can be addressed by linking POCT devices to information systems. As POCT has become more widespread and the growing need for informatics support has been highlighted, the difficulties and costs of interfacing devices to information systems have received considerable attention. The term *connectivity* is now widely used to describe this interfacing or linking process. In the late 1990s, the lack of connectivity was extensively discussed at meetings organized by the Industry Liaison Division of the American Association of Clinical Chemists (AACC) POCT Division. An accompanying survey conducted by the Enterprise Analysis Corporation for the AACC in 1999 showed that in >500 US hospitals, only 17% of POCT data was sent to the LIS electronically, while 67% never reached the LIS (20).

Although manufacturers introduced data management software systems for critical care analyzers and glucose de-

Table 20-5 Minimum Dataset That Should Be Applied to Clinical Results

Patient ID
Patient demographics
Sample ID
Date and time of specimen collection
Type of specimen
Clinical diagnosis (ICD-9 coded in US)
Clinical reason for testing
Date and time of analysis
Analytical test
Numerical/qualitative result
Reference range if appropriate
Derived values

vices at the end of the 1990s, these systems were often not compatible with each other and therefore required separate interfaces with all the attendant costs (21). In addition, these proprietary data management systems usually could not incorporate the products of other manufacturers. In the late 1990s, these were seen as major problems hindering the implementation of POCT, and in 1999 manufacturers involved in the POCT sector took the unique step of forming the Connectivity Industry Consortium (CIC) (20). Several key members of the consortium have written an excellent account of the activities of the CIC and the development of the standard (22).

The CIC was an open, not-for-profit, industry-based organization, comprised of over 30 members from device manufacturers, information system vendors, and healthcare providers. The vision of the CIC was as follows: "To expeditiously develop, pilot and transfer the foundation of a set of seamless, plug-and-play POC communication standards ensuring fulfillment of the critical user requirements of bi-directionality, device connection commonality, commercial software intraoperability, security and QC/regulatory compliance" (22).

Connectivity between POCT devices and information systems can be simply represented as two interfaces, as shown in Figure 20-3. The device interface involves passing patient results and quality-assurance or quality-control (QA/QC) information between the POC instrument and devices such as docking stations, concentrators, terminal servers and POC data managers. The latter have to be linked to a variety of information systems via the electronic data interface for transmission of ordering information and patient results. The CIC approach was to standardize both these interfaces via a technical team responsible for each interface. Both interface teams used similar guiding principles to develop the architecture. These included the following:

- Basing the process on a proven approach and architecture in a standard notation.

- Using existing standards and architectural patterns wherever possible.
- Minimizing what needed to be standardized.
- Focusing on services that would enable software interoperability and add value to the overall functionality.
- Reducing the complexity of device communications.

The team developed the architecture proposal to the stage of workable interface specifications, prototyped the interfaces under development, and planned the pilot demonstrations to validate the entire architecture and approach.

After agreement on the specifications and architecture of the connectivity standard by all the members of the CIC, the proposed standard was handed over to three accredited US standard development organizations—the National Committee for Clinical Laboratory Standards (NCCLS), Health Level 7 (HL7), and the Institute of Electronic and Electrical Engineers (IEEE). In 2001, the connectivity standard was approved by the NCCLS as the POCT1-A standard (23). Essentially, if a POCT device incorporates this standard, it should easily communicate with laboratory and hospital information management systems, allowing exchange of data and information in a standardized format irrespective of vendor, location, or interface.

In addition to publication as an NCCLS standard, the relevant parts of the connectivity standard will also be integrated into the appropriate chapters of the HL7 and IEEE standards. The purpose of the CIC in seeking the involvement of these organizations was not only to obtain implementation of the current specifications, but also to ensure that the standard is developed further as user requirements change and technology develops. In addition, there is the need to create an internationally recognized standard by working with other standards bodies, such as the International Organization for Standardization (ISO) and the European Committee for Standardization (CEN), in Europe and elsewhere.

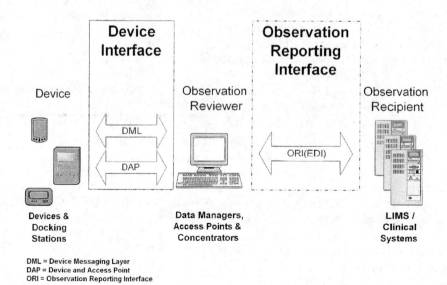

DML = Device Messaging Layer
DAP = Device and Access Point
ORI = Observation Reporting Interface

Figure 20-3   POCT interfaces in the CIC connectivity standard.

Manufacturers are now likely to base competitive features of devices around these applications, and in future years the introduction of the standard may well be seen as a watershed for the development of both POCT and clinical informatics. The full informatics benefits of connectivity may be some years away, since the standard is likely to be included only in new products. However, in recent years manufacturers have also provided more open architecture to their device management systems, so many of them can now incorporate a range of devices as well as competitors' products. Pressure from laboratory scientists and users will encourage this approach, as well as adoption of the CIC standard, just as it helped with the formation of the Connectivity Industry Consortium.

While the CIC standards should greatly simplify the process of integrating POCT systems, there will still be some challenges linking the POCT process into the conventional LIMS. Some of the approaches by manufacturers to these problems will be addressed under the specific applications described next.

INFORMATIC APPLICATIONS IN POCT

Informatics plays a central role in automating POCT testing processes and enriching the value of clinical data generated to provide useful clinical information. Apart from the physical control of the instrumentation and management of patient data, there are various ancillary functions associated with the testing process in which informatics also plays a role. These include various quality management functions, training and decision support, and their relationship to the POCT delivery process, as shown in Figure 20-4. Examples of these different roles will be discussed below in relation to specific clinical applications.

Critical Care Testing

In several countries, such as the United Kingdom and Australia, POCT and critical care testing have gone hand-in-hand for several decades, which is one reason why IT and informatics applications are well developed in this area. With increasing numbers of POCT users working in distributed sites and looking to laboratories for support, the focus of the laboratory scientist is increasingly outward (16). Thus, many laboratories now support critical care testing outside of their central laboratory, with instruments being located in a wide variety of locations including adult and neonatal intensive care units, emergency departments, and operating rooms. Some of these may be located in hospitals located some distance from the central laboratory. This technology still requires regular quality management procedures such as measurement of QC samples and monitoring of results, replenishment of reagents, and monitoring of calibration and patient data together with the monitoring and implementation of maintenance procedures. To perform these procedures requires daily visits from laboratory staff in order to ensure that the quality of testing is maintained. If multiple instruments are located long distances from the central laboratory, then the demand on laboratory resources is

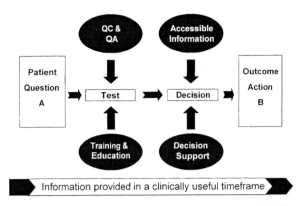

Figure 20-4   Effect of informatics on the delivery of POCT.

considerable and providing support outside of normal working hours is particularly difficult.

Serial interfacing of multiple blood gas instruments to a single controller has been available for many years (24). This was done primarily to ensure that patient data reached the patient record, but serial connections could only be used for instruments that were close to each other in the same unit or laboratory. To meet the quality management needs previously described for multiple devices spread over a geographically wide area, blood gas and critical care instrument manufacturers have taken advantage of the ubiquitous IT network and devised sophisticated software packages such as RapidLink (Bayer Diagnostics, Medfield, MA, USA) and Radiance (Radiometer Copenhagen, Bronshoj, Denmark). Similar systems are available for other blood gas instrument manufacturers (25).

A key component of many of these remote monitoring and control packages is hardware that automatically samples internal QC test material at times programmed by the operator. This solves a major problem of local users forgetting to perform QC tests at the appropriate times. The automated QC systems can also set the QC rules for interpretation of the results and warn the operator if they are not within appropriate limits. The software component, which is located on a PC server in the central laboratory, is built around a relational database containing details of machines, users, sites, and QC materials. Typical features include the operator in the central laboratory having a real-time display of the status of the analyzer, such as the reagent and waste levels, without any local user intervention. Remote operations include cleaning functions, filling of electrodes, and aspirating solutions. There are many benefits to this approach—a single technician can potentially monitor many POCT systems simultaneously and control access to individual analyte channels without the need to physically visit the POCT site. Consequently, the productivity of staff can be increased with less loss of time on unnecessary visits to outlying work stations. Furthermore, staff can be better prepared for such visits, since faults can be diagnosed prior to a visit and appropriate spares prepared. It also means that visits can be more easily scheduled, with a reduction in emergency calls to repair failed equipment (26). The key benefits of information systems such as these are shown in Table 20-6.

Critical care instruments now also include many other informatic features that operate in conjunction with connectivity to the LIS or other information systems. Many of these features are concerned with patient data management, but they also include simplifying preanalytical processes. One of the latter relates to a problem that differentiates POCT from conventional laboratory testing. In the laboratory, the test order or request is generated in advance of the test, and the information flow through the LIS allows a requisition or sample number to be generated in advance of the sample being presented to an instrument for processing. In POCT, the test result is generated simultaneously to the test order. Different approaches are used to solve this problem, ranging from the preallocation of requisition numbers to two-stage data interchanges in which a pending request is made by the POCT system to obtain a requisition number, which is then transmitted back to the LIS with the result (Figure 20-5).

Most patient data will be transmitted to the LIS for eventual inclusion in the patient record, whether as hard paper copy or an electronic record. Whatever the destination for the patient data, there are usually options in the information management software to allow operators to review the data before transmission. However, in the case of critical care testing, patient data may be transmitted to bedside monitors and clinical information systems that reside in critical care units. These systems integrate data from various sources, including vital signs as well as diagnostic results, and in conjunction with clinical guidelines and expert systems can produce critical care maps to be used in the management of the critically ill patient (27). The necessity for links to these information systems and repositories unique to the critical care unit highlights the importance of easy connectivity and common interfacing standards.

Glucose Testing in the Hospital and Clinic

The vast majority of critical care testing instruments are benchtop devices that perform a relatively large number of analyses

Table 20-6 Benefits of Automated QC and Remote-Control Software

1. Overall improvement in quality of analyses
   QC samples are always analyzed.
   Operator variability associated with QC analysis is removed.
   QC results are always interpreted according to rules set by operator and, if necessary, warnings are indicated.
2. Labor savings
   Daily visits to analyzer are no longer required.
   90% of problems can be fixed remotely.
   Visits to analyzers can be planned.
3. Overall improvement of service
   Problems can be fixed before ward staff become aware of them.
   Out-of-hours problems can be more easily fixed.
   Parameters can be selectively deactivated, leaving remaining ones available.

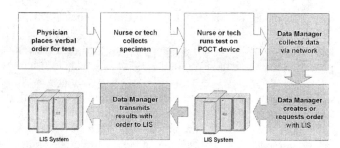

Figure 20-5 Process to automate the generation of a POCT order and combine it with a result.

in batch mode to the extent that QC processes occur on a regular basis. In contrast, glucose meters are single-use devices that are not amenable to conventional QC approaches. Furthermore, they are deployed in large numbers over wide areas with a high number of users. At the worksite of one of the coauthors of this chapter, there are nearly 200 meters in use in 150 locations by 4000 potential users. In the United States, complaints about glucose meters represent the largest number received by the FDA for any medical device (28). Thus, the task of quality management for these devices is very different and more demanding than that of critical care testing and could not be done without IT and informatic approaches.

Until recently, the tendency was for suppliers to provide complementary analysis packages either onboard or on companion PCs to which QA data could be exported. While highly sophisticated, the features of some of these packages were overwhelming, particularly to the average clinical end-user, who is unlikely to have been schooled in the art of quality management. However, such skills are now starting to be taught to nursing staff as POCT grows and errors in such systems continue to be documented.

Consequently, in the United Kingdom, all POCT glucose systems are now sold alongside software for the administration of QA, and its use is recommended by professional guidelines and encouraged as part of the laboratory accreditation programs (16). Similar conditions apply to glucose meters in the United States (15). One of the coauthors has developed a QA system, MediQAL, that automates the distribution of test samples and allows customized performance reports to be printed for individual users. Evidence from this scheme did show measurable improvements in analytical performance for samples distributed, but hard evidence that overall performance has improved is difficult to find. However, the system did enable improved dialogue with end-users and an ability to track the many meters in use.

The informatic features of glucose meters are improving, and a minimum requirement for use in the hospital or other clinical areas outside of the home is computerized data capture with linking of the result to date, time, meter, strip lot number, QC data, and operator, thereby providing a complete audit trail for the patient result. Manufacturers now offer systems that link these devices to information systems, and although these were proprietary even to the extent of different types of connection cables, the implementation of the POCT-1 connectivity standard will ensure greater commonality and ease of interfacing.

With the implementation of these newer glucose data management systems, evidence is starting to appear as to their usefulness. This is important because the cost of such systems is significant. Klein et al. (29) have shown a number of important clinical outcomes by bidirectionally linking the glucose meters used at the bedside to the LIS and combining the glucose results with other pertinent patient information. The outcomes include time savings from rapid availability of results, accuracy of data due to elimination of transcription errors, and a decrease in possible treatment errors by easily identifying suitable insulin regimens.

Aside from the challenges of tracking QC and patient data, the widespread distribution of glucose meters means that staff training is a significant requirement. Besides sheer numbers, there is also the issue that training has to be tailored to nonlaboratory users, mainly nurses, although once again, aspects of POCT are now appearing in nursing education curricula. IT can provide new opportunities for training support. Incorporation of POCT systems within multimedia medical workstations allows for not only the inclusion of a high degree of instruction directly into the instrument interface, but also provides the potential access to other multimedia materials on the desktop at the point of care. Documentation such as training and procedure manuals and clinical guidelines can be presented very easily in this multimedia format. This can be stored locally on the instrument PC or made available from a central server, either privately through an intranet or across the World Wide Web. From a laboratory perspective, this approach has the attraction of allowing the creation of a single, centrally controlled resource of support material that can be made directly available to all users. Exploitation of interactive features of this software provides more functionality. Interactive training systems have been developed that provide background information as well as step-by-step procedural instructions on instrument use. Such training support can be extended to aspects of data interpretation, and programmable elements can allow automated expert interpretation of results. By combining elements of the system with database-controlled access, auditable logs of individual training can be created, thereby enabling improved management of users and POCT systems.

Such systems are already in daily use and provide full tutorials on the use of the local range of POCT instruments. Making them available across the hospital intranet allows them to be accessed by ward staff when appropriate. Such tutorials may contain formative assessments in the form of multiple-choice questions, and performance can be monitored both to control local reinforcement of learning and to regulate certification of end-users. One such tutorial takes approximately 40 min to complete, and a recent audit of its use showed not only that users appreciated it as a convenient and valuable form of initial training, but also returned to it voluntarily to refresh their skills (30). The ease with which such tutorials can now be developed allows simple customization to local needs such that a wide array of instruments can be easily encompassed within a standard learning framework. Such modules can cover not only theory but also the practicalities of each instrument's use and training in any relevant local policies and procedures.

Home Testing

The volume of testing that will take place in the home is predicted to increase significantly as healthcare providers take further steps to reduce the patient's length of hospital stay. Although released from hospital early, some patients will still require medical assistance, including diagnostic tests that can be carried out at the point of care. At the present time the majority of home testing involves diabetics performing self-monitoring of blood glucose (SMBG) and, to a much lesser extent, patients taking anticoagulants who monitor their own prothrombin times.

SMBG is a major portion of the total glucose testing market and has involved IT and informatics applications similar to those previously discussed for hospital glucose testing. A major advance in meter design for the home user was the incorporation of memories in the devices for storage of results. These have largely replaced log books for hand recording of data, which was often incomplete and inaccurate (31). When the patient attends the clinic, data from the meter can be downloaded into a PC for interpretation by the caregiver. This process can also take place in the home when the patient links the meter to a modem and transmits the data to the physician's office or clinic. Fresh impetus is being given to similar telemedicine applications for home testing of a wider group of patients as data such as vital signs, results of respiratory function tests, and glucose levels can now be easily transmitted by modem or via the Internet (32).

Many applications of telemedicine to the management of diabetes have been described in the literature. The success of these depends on a number of aspects, including accurate collection of the data in digital format, incorporation of the data into an electronic record that may be transmitted without alteration, protocols for distant analysis, and communication tools to permit effective dialogue among caregivers and patients (33). A major goal of such programs is to reduce the costs of managing diabetes and provide more satisfaction and convenience for the patient. Outcome data from early studies was not convincing, but more recent data has demonstrated at least reductions in clinic visits and costs (34).

The number of patients taking warfarin and performing self-monitoring of prothrombin time is far less than of those performing SMBG, but it is growing as the clinical indications for warfarin therapy increase. This type of POCT is significant for being one of the few areas of diagnostic medicine where decision support has had a demonstrably positive effect. While commercial expert systems are now available for central laboratory testing (35) they have had only limited effects on POCT applications, such as blood gases, despite the latter being amenable to such an approach through a well-researched mathematical framework of interpretation based on the classical Henderson–Hasselback equation and other derived parameters (36).

In the case of prothrombin time measurements, patients use commercial decision support software to self-manage their warfarin therapy in conjunction with small POCT devices to measure prothrombin time (37). As in the case of diabetes management, this type of service and support can be delivered in the home a telephone or via the Internet (Figure 20-6). Several studies in primary care and at home, including randomized controlled trials, have shown that the level of care provided by such a system is at least as good as routine hospital follow-up (38). Further studies are determining whether this application of informatics and POCT can be transferred to the wider population. Similar efforts have been applied to self-managing routines for diabetics by using glucose meters designed to hold serial data and programmed to provide insulin dosing regimes, but there is little evidence that they have been suitable for routine and widespread use (39). However, software support for diabetics is likely to grow following recognition of the importance of the education and training of the diabetic patient in relation to glucose testing (40). It is possible that informatics and/or telemedicine may be the means to deliver such support (41).

CONCLUSIONS

The effects of IT and informatics on POCT continue to grow as computing and network technologies continue to extend through the clinical domain. However, the utilization of IT in

medicine, and diagnostic medicine in particular, has not yet reached the same stage as that in the wider business world, where some commentators believe that IT no longer matters and is now so commonplace that it is just another commodity, like electricity (42). Many clinicians still doubt the value of IT to the clinical process, but this is just one factor in the chronic underinvestment of IT in medical care.

One barrier to investment that has disappeared in relation to POCT is the adoption of a common interfacing or connectivity standard. Adoption of the NCCLS POCT-1A standard is a significant step forward, and one of its most important benefits will be to facilitate the transfer of patient and quality-related data into a permanent record. This is timely because more and more institutions are moving to electronic record-keeping, the value of which is now beginning to be demonstrated (43). However, these records will be degraded if they do not encompass all patient data, including that generated outside the central laboratory.

Significant challenges with POCT still remain. Connectivity is obviously important, but the importance of thinking beyond it was demonstrated in a recent study that showed that many test results transmitted to an acute care ward electronically, instead of by the usual telephone calls, were never accessed for use in the clinical care process (44). One might argue that by performing the test at the point of care, one overcomes a major problem of central laboratory testing. While this is true, there remains a significant portion of POCT that is not performed right at the patient's side, and therefore the result still has to be integrated into the clinical process. A

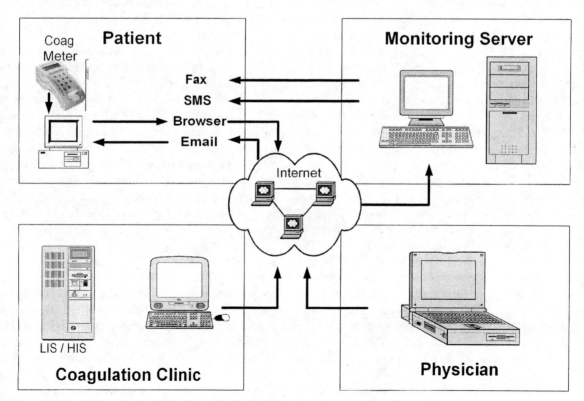

Figure 20-6   A typical telemedicine application to deliver POCT and self-management for patients on anticoagulant therapy.

greater understanding of this process is required if the real benefits of POCT are to be delivered in the future.

Other challenges for informatics and POCT are making devices easier to use and building in forms of process control that prevent or minimize errors but are not seen as arduous by the operator. The lack of effect of decision support in POCT is perhaps surprising, given that it is being performed by relatively inexperienced users. Linking POCT systems to the wider network through connectivity and making other pertinent information available in the decision-making process may be one less barrier to development in this area.

REFERENCES

1. Christensen CM. The innovator's dilemma: when new technologies cause great firms to fail. Cambridge, MA: Harvard Business School Press, 1997.
2. McClelland I, Adamson K, Black ND. Information issues in telemedicine systems. J Telemed Telecare 1995;1:7–12.
3. Chou D, Aller R. Informatics and data management. In: Kost GJ, ed. Principles and practice of point-of-care testing. Philadelphia: Lippincott Williams & Wilkins, 2002:487–97.
4. Kohn LT, Corrigan JM, Donaldson MS, eds. To err is human: building a safer health system. Washington, DC: National Academy Press, 2000.
5. Bernard D. Laboratory supervision of point-of-care blood gas testing. http://www.bloodgas.org/4C15D5D2–B4A0–4D40–B68D-5789A2B84BFD.W5Doc (accessed April 2004).
6. Want R. RFID. A key to automating everything. Sci Am 2004; 290:56–65.
7. Elevitch FR. Multimedia communications networks: patient care through interactive point-of-care testing. Clin Lab Med 1994;14: 559–67.
8. Neame R. The crucial roles of standards and strategy in developing a regional health information network. Int J Biomed Comput 1995;40:95–100.
9. Neame R. Privacy and security issues in a wide area health communications network. Int J Biomed Comput 1996;43:123–7.
10. Benn N, Jefferies B, Wheable J, Hall R, O'Connell J, Binnie A. Local and remote operation/monitoring of fully auto mated high throughput screening systems: proceedings of Eurolabautomation98. Oxford, England, September 1998. http://labautomation.org/ConferencePDFs/EL98Book.pdf (accessed May 27, 2004).
11. Jacobs E. Information integration for point-of-care and satellite testing. In: Kost GJ, ed. Handbook of clinical automation, robotics and optimization. New York: John Wiley & Sons, 1996;620–030.
12. ISO/IEC 8802-11: 1999 (ANSI/IEEE Std 802.11, 1999 ed.). Information technology—telecommunications and information exchange between systems—local and metropolitan area network specific requirements. Part 11: Wireless LAN medium access control (MAC) and physical layer (PHY) specifications. Piscataway, NJ: IEEE, 1999. http://standards.ieee.org/catalog/olis/lanman.html (accessed May 27, 2004).
13. Standards for privacy of individually identifiable health information. Final rule (45 CFR, parts 160 and 164). Federal Register 2000;65:82461–829.
14. Coiera E. Guide to health informatics, 2nd ed. London: Arnold, 2003.
15. Ehrmeyer SS, Laessig RH. Regulatory requirements [CLIA '88, JCAHO, CAP] for decentralized testing. Am J Clin Pathol 1995; 104:S40–9.
16. Seamonds B. Medical, economic, and regulatory factors affecting point-of-care testing: a report of the conference on factors affecting point-of-care testing. Clin Chim Acta 1996;249:1–19.
17. Allyn E. The office of the future: A Welch-Allyn project for an integrated vision of the healthcare system. Proceedings of Eurolabautomation98. Oxford, England, Sept. 1998. http://labautomation.org/ConferencePDFs/EL98Book.pdf (accessed May 27, 2004).
18. Kennelly RJ, Gardner RM. Perspectives on development of IEEE 1073: the medical information bus (MIB) standard. Int J Clin Monit Comput 1997;14:143–9.
19. Kennelly RJ. Improving acute care through use of medical device data. Int J Med Inf 1998;48:145–9.
20. Stephens EJ. Developing open standards for point-of-care connectivity. IVD Technology 1999;10:22–5.
21. St John A, Jones RJ. Connectivity: the key to point-of-care testing. Med Dev Technol 2000;July/August:35–8.
22. Perry J, Anders B, Boecker D. Point-of-care testing integration and connectivity. In: Kost GJ, ed. Principles and practice of point-of-care testing. Philadelphia: Lippincott Williams & Wilkins, 2002;507–15.
23. National Committee for Clinical Laboratory Standards. Point-of-care connectivity; approved standard. NCCLS Document POCT1-A. Wayne, PA: National Committee for Clinical Laboratory Standards, 2001.
24. Scott P, Andrews DJ, Gosling P. Laboratory control via telecommunications of analysers in critical care areas. J Clin Chem Clin Biochem 1985;23:607.
25. Blick KE, Halpern NA. Information systems for point-of-care testing in critical care. In: Kost GJ, ed. Principles and practice of point-of-care testing. Philadelphia: Lippincott Williams & Wilkins, 2002;498–506.
26. Hirst D, St. John A. Keeping the spotlight on quality from a distance. Accred Qual Assur 2000;5:9–13.
27. Halpern N. Point of care diagnostics and networks. Crit Care Clin 2000;16:623–39.
28. Clarke W, Nichols JH. Bedside glucose testing: applications in the home and hospital. Clin Lab Med 2001;21.305–10.
29. Klein E, Barglowski M, Stanley E, Dean H. Clinical application of point-of-care testing informatics. http://www.lifescan.com/pdf/hospital/058–658A.pdf (accessed April 2004).
30. Hirst AD. An intranet-based tutorial for ward-based blood glucose testing. In: Kost GJ, ed. Principles and practice of point-of-care testing. Philadelphia: Lippincott Williams & Wilkins, 2002;528–9.
31. Stone AA, Shiffman S, Schwartz JE, Broderick JE, Hufford MR. Patient non-compliance with paper diaries. BMJ 2002;324: 1193–4.
32. Lehmann CA. The future of home testing—implications for traditional laboratories. Clin Chim Acta 2002;323:31–6.
33. Klonoff DC. Diabetes and telemedicine: is the technology sound, effective, cost-effective, and practical? Diabetes Care 2003;26: 1626–8.
34. Chase HP. Modem transmission of glucose values reduces the costs of and need for clinic visits: response to Perlemuter and Yomtov. Diabetes Care 2003;26:2969–70.
35. Edwards G, Compton P, Malor R, Srinivasan A, Lazarus L. PEIRS: a pathologist-maintained expert system for the interpretation of chemical pathology reports. Pathology 1993;25:27–34.

36. Larsen VH, Siggaard-Andersen O. The Oxygen Status Algorithm on-line with the pH-blood gas analyzer. Scand J Clin Lab Invest Suppl 1996;224:9–19.

37. Fitzmaurice DA, Hobbs FD, Murray ET, Bradley CP, Holder R. Evaluation of computerized decision support for oral anticoagulation management based in primary care. Br J Gen Pract 1996; 46:533–5.

38. Fitzmaurice DA, Murray ET, Gee KM, Allan TF. Does the Birmingham model of oral anticoagulation management in primary care work outside trial conditions? Br J Gen Pract 2001;51:828–9.

39. Holman RR, Smale AD, Pemberton E, Riefflin A, Nealon JL. Randomised controlled pilot trial of a hand-held patient-oriented, insulin regimen optimiser. Med Inf [London] 1996;21:317–26.

40. Nattrass M. Improving results from home blood-glucose monitoring: accuracy and reliability require greater patient education as well as improved technology. Clin Chem 2002;48:979–80.

41. Price CP. Point-of-care testing in diabetes mellitus. Clin Chem Lab Med 2003;41:1213–9.

42. Carr NG. IT doesn't matter. Harvard Bus Rev 2003;81:41–9.

43. Chin HL, Krall MA. Successful implementation of a comprehensive computer-based patient record system in Kaiser Permanente Northwest: strategy and experience. Eff Clin Pract 1998;1:51–60.

44. Kilpatrick ES, Holding S. Use of computer terminals on wards to access emergency test results: a retrospective audit. BMJ 2001; 322:1101–3.

Chapter 21

Successful Implementation of a Multisite Point-of-Care Testing Program

Lou Ann Wyer and Richard P. Moriarty

It has always been the responsibility of the laboratory to provide the highest quality laboratory data for patient care. Point-of-care testing (POCT) has enabled healthcare professionals to provide that level of care at the patient's bedside. The demand for faster turnaround times of critical test results has driven the growth of POCT over the last decade. Surveys estimate that one in four laboratory tests is done at the point of care, and this number is growing at an annual rate of 12% (1).

Sentara Healthcare, a premier integrated healthcare network in southeastern Virginia and northeastern North Carolina, serves over 2 million residents and has over 15,000 employees. More than 70 care sites constitute the Sentara network, including six acute care hospitals as well as nursing homes, acute care clinics, and private physician groups.

Sentara's multisite POCT program is one of the most mature and nationally recognized programs in the United States. The comprehensive POCT program includes >5000 operators who perform >1 million tests annually in the hospital setting. The hospital-based POCT programs and testing menus are shown in Table 21-1. In addition, extensive testing is performed at other care delivery sites outside the hospital.

VISION

In the early 1990s, Sentara launched a large-scale reorganization and laboratory services reinvention. The laboratory was asked to address service issues, gain financial efficiencies, and improve quality; Sentara endorsed the vision that laboratory testing performed at the bedside could be one component of the redesign and POCT could fulfill all of these objectives.

Originally, the POCT plan was designed to address service issues at Sentara's largest facility, Sentara Norfolk General Hospital. Laboratory service objectives were to improve cycle time (turnaround time) measurements and to reduce specimen handoffs and collection requirements. Upon implementation of the POCT program, these objectives were achieved. Additional cost reductions, secondary to more rapid clinical decision making (e.g., more rapid movement to step-down units and even decreased length of stay), were among the long-term effects of incorporating an extensive POCT program. Ultimately, the program was implemented at other Sentara facilities, with similar results.

PLANNING

The introduction of new processes and technology in any setting is always unsettling and disruptive, and in many cases can represent a significant culture shock. Therefore, the planning stage for a multisite POCT program is not only complex and extensive, but also critical to the success of the program.

Administrative Support

Unwavering support from upper-level management is crucial in facilitating the process changes that are required of both laboratory and nonlaboratory staff as a POCT program is implemented. In addition, the cross-disciplinary nature of POCT requires upper-level administrative support to ensure that a consistent message is communicated to all groups involved in this testing, such as nursing and respiratory care.

Support from senior managers is also needed to affirm technology and implementation decisions, through the empowerment of a project leader and a POCT committee. Technology planning starts with a clinical and fiscal evaluation of the current technology and practice. Second, a comprehensive needs analysis must assess the clinical and fiscal impact of the newly proposed technology (2). Program decisions must be made regarding whether to use handheld instruments at the bedside, a strategically placed small laboratory among patient care units, or a mobile cart with equipment that moves to the patient. Potentially, up-front costs as well as per-test costs may be higher than those of central laboratory testing. These costs must be weighed against the benefits of more timely results, diagnosis, and treatments. Consideration can be given to potential benefits in the form of decreased length of stay in the emergency department or intensive care unit. However, POCT proponents must recognize that strong political and financial pressures may be brought to bear on the decision makers as they assemble the data required for POCT implementation. With adequate data, the administrative team will be able to support the decision to implement POCT.

Another issue for many laboratories is how to handle governmental regulation and accountability for the POCT program. Whether agency certification comes from the Clinical Laboratory Improvement Amendment of 1988 (CLIA '88), the College of American Pathologists (CAP), the Joint Commission on Accreditation of Healthcare Organizations (JCAHO),

Table 21-1   Multisite Hospital POCT Program

Variable	Hospital					
	1	2	3	4	5	6
Beds	644	250	158	274	194	139
POCT FTEs	4.0	1.0	0.8	1.0	1.0	1.0
POCT units	42	20	14	30	33	25
ABGs	X	X	X	X	X	X
Ionized calcium	X		X	X	X	
Na	X	X	X	X	X	
K	X	X	X	X	X	
CL	X	X	X	X	X	
BUN	X	X	X	X	X	
Creat	X	X	X	X	X	
Hgb	X	X	X	X		
Hct	X	X	X	X	X	
PT INR	X	X	X	X	X	X
ACT	X	X	X	X	X	
Glucose	X	X	X	X	X	X
Hemoccult	X	X	X	X	X	X
Gastroccult	X	X	X	X	X	X
pH	X	X	X	X	X	X
sO$_2$	X	X	X	X	X	X
Urine dip	X	X	X	X		
Pregnancy					X	X

or another accrediting agency, a decision must be made regarding the line of responsibility and accountability for the accreditation. In most programs, the clinical laboratory holds the certificates and accepts the accreditation responsibilities as well as the ultimate accountability for POCT. However, prior to the onset of a program, the administrative body should decide whether the POCT units will hold separate certificates or whether the units fall under the same certificate as the laboratory. Again, a clear line of authority, responsibility, and accountability must be established.

Ultimately, there must be a commitment from administration to provide all the resources necessary to implement POCT correctly and thoroughly. POCT must meet the same rigorous standards to which any hospital laboratory adheres.

POCT Committee

Once the decision to implement a multisite POCT program is made by administration and the laboratory leadership, a POCT coordinator should be chosen and a POCT committee formed. Representatives should include: physicians, nurses, respiratory care practitioners, laboratorians, finance advisors, materials management consultants, and information technology (IT) support personnel. All disciplines involved in the implementation, use, monitoring, and evaluation of the POCT program should be represented. This committee must understand and support the goals of the project, identify key resources, develop relationships with key staff members, and help develop a plan for implementation. The committee members with clinical roles will eventually become the experts and contacts for each unit.

They must have the authority to make changes on those units. Through their continued support, these committee members become champions for the program.

The POCT committee will gather workflow ideas and determine how the proposed new processes will modify current operating procedures. The members of a carefully chosen committee will know what works best in their areas or disciplines, thereby identifying and addressing roadblocks to design changes and improving efficiencies in care delivery. In addition, committee members should be the frontline communicators, who are able to address potentially disruptive rumors immediately.

The POCT committee can also help to develop policies and procedures for POCT and ensure that the procedures are written in language that will be understood and well received. Members can develop both general and unit-specific educational materials for training and ongoing communications as well as the corresponding competency and performance improvement programs.

The POCT committee can remain active even after program implementation. The extent of the committee's activities will depend upon the size of the program and the number of assigned staff. Some institutions may dissolve their committees after continued monitoring indicates program stability; ad hoc committees can be formed to address issues as needed. This latter approach can be more time-efficient, especially if team members must travel from outlying sites to attend committee meetings. Selecting the right people to work together to achieve a common goal is a key requirement (3).

Assigned POCT Staff

The majority of programs designate a POCT coordinator to oversee the entire POCT program, usually a laboratorian. However, some systems assign associate coordinators so that a nurse or respiratory care practitioner can also take a lead role in program administration. It is important to choose the right type of individual to oversee the POCT program, one who is an especially strong communicator and a team player, as well as someone able to embrace creative change. The POCT coordinator will be interacting most often with nonlaboratorians, and must be comfortable working with a variety of healthcare staff, including physicians, nurses, respiratory care practitioners, and nursing assistants. As a team player, the POCT coordinator will be required to facilitate teams for program development and ongoing POCT activities such as quality control (QC).

Responsibility for the oversight of specific portions of the overall POCT program must be assigned to specific POCT staff. The number of POCT staff needed for a multisite program is dependent on the extent of the program and the geographical distance between facilities. Assigning POCT staff for each facility is optimal; staff do not have to be full-time employees if the program is small, but must be dedicated POCT personnel. This continuity of support leads to better compliance and a stronger commitment to the program by all involved departments. If geography and POCT instrumentation and technology permit, one person can monitor POCT at more than one facility. Today, IT enhancements allow more freedom to monitor POCT data through network channels at any location in the system.

At Sentara, the POCT program is administered by a clinical specialist from the main clinical laboratory who oversees the POCT staff at each outlying facility. For the program, there is an assigned medical director, who is a pathologist. The ultimate responsibility for efficient program operations and compliance lies with the administrative and medical leadership of the clinical laboratory.

Information Technology

Efficiencies can be gained for any POCT program when the testing devices have electronic data management and connectivity. Additional efficiencies are realized when the multisite program utilizes the same laboratory information system (LIS). This common LIS allows the database for bedside test parameters to be built just once, for all tests used across the system. New tests may easily be added, and current tests changed, in an environment with a single LIS. Electronic data management systems for automated POCT devices offer not only QC performance statistics, but also the information needed to assure medical and administrative laboratory directors that quality testing is being performed according to policies and procedures.

All procedures performed by POCT staff (e.g., calibration verification, linearity, and acceptance testing) are posted on a network shared drive, which only they can access. These procedures are password protected as part of the document management process so that they cannot be altered. This shared drive also stores the myriad of forms and competency tests that are used for the POCT program. In addition, each facility has site-specific information entered on this shared drive so that it is accessible to the POCT staff. This information includes a listing of unit managers and contact persons, the operator databases, and the testing performed on each unit. Everything is at the fingertips of those responsible for the POCT.

Connectivity to a central workstation allows patient results and operator data to be transmitted to the laboratory and/or hospital computers, allowing automated ordering of point-of-care tests as well as automated result entry, charting, and billing. Therefore, nurses and clerks no longer need to enter orders for each test—a significant time savings.

Patient identification, operator identification, lot numbers of reagents and QC material, date and time of testing, location of testing, operator performance rates, recertification dates, and transmission activities—all these are captured for monitoring from any identified workstation. These workstations can be placed in the laboratory for regular monitoring and reconciliation by the POCT staff or can even be web-based so that nurses or other nonlaboratorians at any site can have access to reports and employee databases.

Integrating connectivity and the respective electronic data management systems for a multisite program into the organization's LIS requires a great deal of IT support. POCT coordinators become increasingly dependent on the IT department for maintaining connectivity, pulling network lines, and assigning transmission control protocol/Internet protocol addresses. Maintaining software upgrades and customizations on a single client-server personal computer (PC), rather than on multiple PC workstations, simplifies IT's work and helps maintain standardization (4).

Adequate time should be allotted for IT work prior to POCT program implementation. Database building, testing, billing, and charting all are time-consuming and usually beset by delays. If testing devices are connected to an electronic network, additional computer connections and lines may also be necessary. It is wise to build in extra time for this phase of the project.

When selecting a solution for POCT data management and integration, it is important to look for a platform that allows for program expansion. Several vendors have connectivity solutions that not only streamline workflow but also address compliance and economic issues of POCT. These solutions can connect multiple vendor-provided POCT data management systems—especially important because multiple devices from multiple vendors are used within a large, comprehensive, multisite POCT program. A well-chosen system can provide both a single interface to the LIS and tools for operator and device compliance. All these benefits allow improved efficiency for the POCT program, which can, in turn, reduce labor costs.

Standardization

The standardization of instruments, policies, and procedures across multiple sites can result in economic efficiencies for POCT, just as it does for the clinical laboratory. Achieving standardization takes time and effort, but is justified by the resulting benefits.

The following processes and systems, when standardized, offer the greatest benefits:

1. Policies
2. Procedures
3. Instrumentation
4. Reagents
5. Training
6. Quality program

When there is standardization of instrumentation, POCT policies and procedures can become uniform across a multisite program. Within the Sentara organization, a multidisciplinary group selects new POCT technology. Materials management consultants negotiate contracts, and IT representatives review the infrastructure needed for integrated electronic data management systems. Laboratory personnel perform extensive precision, linearity, and method comparison studies for correlation with the laboratory's main analyzers.

A multisite POCT program utilizes numerous device operators who must be trained by the POCT staff. POCT operators from each facility are included in the assessment process for each new test method, device, or technology. Their involvement ranges from attending a vendor demonstration to conducting a pilot study. Pilot studies are conducted on patient care units so that the POCT operators themselves have input into the final decision. Each pilot study includes a staff critique of the device. Critique scores are weighted and contribute to the decision making process.

Orientation and training of these operators at the multiple sites is simplified with instrument standardization. Because of uniform operator training, flexible scheduling of assigned POCT operators is possible, and individuals' vacations and sick leave do not hamper workflow. With instrument standardization, uniform cost-effective reagent choices and similar multisite QC procedures are also possible.

Although these efforts may be time-consuming, Sentara has discovered that the process of involving staff leads to a win–win outcome. Building consensus is important to achieve success.

Quality Program

A primary motivation for the laboratory to become involved in managing the POCT program is quality—not only to ensure that QC is being performed at the frequency required, but also to ensure that the POCT operators truly understand the importance of performing a test correctly at the bedside. A comprehensive quality program for POCT can be developed to cover all aspects of preanalytical, analytical, and postanalytical testing. National Committee for Clinical Laboratory Standards (NCCLS) Document GP-26-A2 is a good resource for preparing such a program (5).

Review of QC, maintenance of operator training and competency records, and monitoring results for performance improvement—all of these require the ability to capture critical POCT information and to transmit this data to a database where statistical manipulations can be performed and summary reports compiled. The ability to monitor these quality indicators is enhanced by an effective information management system. Benefits are realized when the devices can electronically capture both operator and patient identifiers, link these data to the date and time the tests are performed, monitor QC of the device, and evaluate training and competency of the operator (6).

QC components of a POCT program should be established prior to program implementation and continually reviewed and modified with the addition of each new method, device, or procedure. Although many technical procedures can be established that are identical to those of the clinical laboratory, often the POCT device and/or technology is altered (i.e., geared toward decreasing the complexity of procedures that are used by nonlaboratory staff). For example, electronic QC (EQC) testing does not require the dilution of traditional liquid QC testing. Therefore, decisions as to the type of QC and the frequency of QC measurements must be established prior to the implementation of these devices or technologies. Regulatory and/or accrediting agencies often dictate these parameters, but it is the responsibility of the program leadership to establish a comprehensive QC program.

Most electronic data management systems now offer QC lockout features that prevent instrument operation unless a valid QC result is obtained. In addition, an operator lockout function can ensure that only valid, trained, and certified operators can use the POCT device. A transmission lockout function can ensure that the test data are uploaded to the electronic data management system, so that charting and billing can take place in a timely manner. These lockout features also provide data for the regular review of operator activities; the assigned POCT staff can therefore identify training and competency issues that may need attention. These lockout functions can be turned on or off as determined by the needs and goals of the program.

The POCT program at Sentara accepts operator-performed EQC as one component of the QC program. Acceptance studies for incoming reagents and control materials are evaluated by the POCT staff prior to release for patient testing. Similarly, supplemental liquid QC materials are tested at defined intervals by the same staff so that trends and shifts in reagents are detected quickly. They are responsible for establishing in-house QC ranges, monitoring daily QC activities, and investigating any discrepancies. Operator lockout and transmission lockout features ensure compliance with established procedures. Indicators are in place for the prompt detection and resolution of issues resulting from noncompliance.

All QC data are analyzed for trends and shifts by the POCT coordinator and assigned POCT staff. Reports are reviewed by the clinical pathologists, and then stored on an electronic shared disk drive on the intranet, eliminating the need for paper copies.

Specific POCT indicators have been selected to monitor and assess the program on a regular basis. The goal is to work toward an error-free environment. Emphasis on the standardization of methods, procedures, and instrumentation will allow the POCT operators to recognize errors and defects easily and to troubleshoot effectively. Whatever decisions are made regarding the QC program, QC strategies must be in place to maximize the chances of detecting operator and test system errors.

A standard template for documentation of all QC activities and statistical analysis should be developed. All staff members use this template even when they substitute at other sites. Detailed compliance reports can be provided to the testing unit managers to keep them informed on the status of each operator and of overall testing performance. A calendar of system-wide POCT activities outlining the assigned duties for each month (e.g., calibration verification, linearity, maintenance schedules, and proficiency surveys) is mapped out annually to help staff complete their assignments.

In summary, a quality POCT program must be multidimensional, with involvement of all individuals engaged in POCT. The POCT committee and associated staff approve procedures for standardization and ensure that the operators are competent to perform each test. POCT staff monitor daily performance of testing from each patient care unit. Electronic or liquid QC testing is performed at defined intervals. POCT results are uploaded to the LIS, then electronically transferred into the hospital information system for retrieval anywhere in the system. The duties of assigned POCT staff are the following: (*i*) Perform all linearity, calibration verification, and reagent acceptance procedures; (*ii*) establish in-house QC ranges; and (*iii*) work with each patient care unit to ensure ongoing compliance (3).

The POCT program administration and medical directorship must be empowered to insist that all POCT operators adhere to the quality program as outlined. The medical director should have the authority to withdraw testing privileges at any site when adherence to the quality program does not meet the established criteria.

Implementation

Incremental. Institutions will adopt different approaches when planning an implementation of a POCT device. Some will distribute hundreds of analyzers to multiple nursing units. Others will opt for incremental program implementation, which may be more manageable for institutions with minimal staffing. The disadvantages of an incremental implementation are that two testing processes will be in place simultaneously at the same site, and the process of training operators on the new procedures will be prolonged—possibly jeopardizing the momentum of the project.

Global. Global implementations tend to be more successful, when sufficient personnel are available. Global implementations introduce a new POCT device or process to several testing units, or to an entire facility, at one time. Training can be conducted within a concentrated time period, communication for all parties involved will be simultaneous, and all IT databases and instrument procedure changes can be implemented on the same day.

Sentara's implementation of a multisite POCT program began at Norfolk General Hospital, the tertiary care facility for the Sentara Healthcare system. The vendor strongly advised that the program be implemented across the entire facility at once—a global implementation. Although initially reluctant, Sentara did so, with tremendous success. Sentara has continued to apply global implementation with subsequent devices and processes. Global implementation has made optimal use of both time and resources.

Whether the implementation is incremental or global, continued support by the laboratory and direct contact with each new operator are required for at least a few weeks; this arrangement helps new operators to work through the training curve. If the implementation is incremental, this follow-up phase may stretch onsite resources—resources that might have been saved up front by the use of global implementation.

Training. A detailed training program must be in place prior to any implementation. Training should address the introduction of new procedures, competency assessment, and remedial instruction.

It is preferable to train, upon hiring, any new employee who will be assigned to a hospital site where POCT is performed. This practice allows the employee, after orientation, to report to the patient care unit with all the skills necessary to function as a certified POCT operator. Facility educators and/or laboratory staff usually provide the training. Trainers should provide testing procedure instruction as well as the theory supporting the procedures. They must allow time for practice and return demonstrations to ensure that trainees are comfortable performing each procedure. It is best to provide initial training sessions away from patient care units, so that distractions are kept to a minimum (3). Training schedules should provide frequent and timely training opportunities for new employees. Online enrollment can facilitate scheduling, as it is helpful in predicting the completion dates for certification of POCT operators.

The vendor often provides training for the introduction of new devices. It is advised to take advantage of these offers, but be certain that all operators on all shifts receive the training. Although vendors may balk at providing this training over the course of a 7-day, 24-h hospital week, successful implementation depends on training all personnel, regardless of assigned shift or day.

Competency requirements should be outlined prior to an implementation. If these requirements are not predetermined by regulatory agencies (CLIA, CAP, etc.), then the POCT committee must develop the requirements. Issues to consider include employee needs, laboratory needs, complexity of the testing procedure, frequency of testing by each operator, and type of module needed to prove competency. (For example, if the nursing staff performs competency certification via a computer-based training program, then the IT department should be enlisted to provide all POCT competency certification on the same platform. A shared platform enables the achievement of high rates of competency completion.) Competency of all operators must be ensured.

Within the Sentara organization, employees undertake an initial standardized orientation to POCT devices at the time of hiring. Annual competency certification for each point-of-care test is required. Competency requirements are developed and distributed each year for recertification in POCT procedures for all operators. A variety of teaching methods is used to facilitate adult learning. Trainers use unique themes to reinforce skills, while allowing some fun in the process. The POCT staff maintains a database of all active POCT operators, which is updated with each completed competency and is readily available to regulatory assessors.

Medical Staff Issues. Working with individual medical staffs at each site throughout the organization can be an extremely challenging and frustrating, yet rewarding, experience. If the organization is fortunate enough to have a single medical staff across its facilities, the challenge becomes manageable. If not, standardization of the above processes and systems will prove surprisingly time consuming. Through experience, Sentara has learned that physician agreement on policies, procedures, and instrumentation is no easy task. All physicians, including pathologists, have their own ideas about what will work best in their facilities. They often hesitate to compromise, especially if they were not the initial proponents of the changes under discussion. Timing is important, and both patience and persistence are required. It is critical to marshal all the necessary supporting documentation for presentation and discussion with members of the medical staff. Physicians closest to the POCT product should be involved at the appropriate phases of project development and implementation. Inclusion encourages cooperation.

An important element for successful POCT implementation is single-pathologist leadership. A single pathologist leader within a multisite program is preferable, in order to prevent pathologists with dissident opinions from derailing the progress of the program. Multiple, equally empowered pathologists who serve as medical directors at different sites may impede the process. Even some pathologists have difficulty accepting changes in the testing culture of their laboratories.

Communication. Throughout the course of any multisite POCT project, communication is a key factor in establishing an effective and successful program. At Sentara, regular updates on the progress of each project are provided to senior administrators, prospective POCT operators, and clinical laboratory staff. Before, during, and after implementation, it is to be expected that both laboratory and patient care staff will worry about their future roles. Sentara laboratorians feared that their jobs would be taken by nonlaboratory staff unqualified to perform the tasks; patient care staff initially presumed they would be overburdened with new responsibilities. Through careful communication, both disciplines learned to redefine patient care, and the POCT program currently functions with notable efficiency (3).

As part of Sentara's ongoing POCT program, the POCT staff remains highly visible on each testing unit, and participates in interdepartmental collaborative groups—thus earning respect as content experts. POCT operators recognize that the assigned POCT staff at each site has expertise in technology, QC, and laboratory support services. Information on POCT is communicated via newsletter, e-mail, and memo as well as through staff meetings held during regular visits to the units by POCT staff.

POCT staff meet monthly to discuss current issues and new projects and to network with colleagues. In addition to these workgroup sessions, educational sessions and preparation for regulatory assessments are also scheduled. Occasionally, crowded staff schedules mandate the use of conference calls, and more teleconferencing is anticipated in the future—although face-to-face interaction has its own benefits.

The sophisticated electronic resources at Sentara provide the POCT staff the means to communicate effectively across all of the Sentara facilities. All procedures performed by non-laboratory staff are posted to the organization's intranet, allowing all POCT operators to have access to the most current procedures at all times. Paper manuals are no longer needed, which eliminates the associated costs of the material and of the labor that was required to distribute the manuals to >100 patient care units. For easy retrieval, all QC logs for manual tests are also posted on the intranet.

No matter the size of the POCT program, communication is the most crucial element in its success. Whether it is with nurses, physicians, or other staff, one can never communicate enough. The methods of communication that work best in your organization should be decided on (e.g., e-mail, telephone, written correspondence and documentation), and consensus on their use should be obtained. Information will therefore be received in a timely manner by all parties involved. Barriers to success should be prevented and avoided. The right people for the job should be enlisted and strong relationships built. Sentara discovered that the most vocal resistors eventually became the strongest supporters.

Celebrate. Whether it is the implementation of a new POCT device or the completion of a regulatory assessment, any success is dependent on the entire professional healthcare team and the POCT team. Success should be celebrated. Banners, flyers, letters to administration, or a meal and/or movie tickets—all are inexpensive methods to show the POCT operators appreciation for a job well done.

CONCLUSION

At Sentara, POCT has simplified testing procedures and decreased turnaround times. Financial benefits have been significant. Successful implementation of a multisite POCT program requires a collaborative effort by the entire professional healthcare team. Although the journey to design and implement a multisite POCT program is lengthy and tedious, the benefits are extensive and far-reaching.

REFERENCES

1. Nichols JH. Management of remote laboratory data. Lab Med 2001;32:532–4.
2. Halpern N, Pastores S. Technology introduction in critical care: just knowing the price is not enough! Chest 1999;116:1092–9.
3. Wyer L, Spingarn S. Standardization of POCT in an integrated health care system. In: Kost G, ed. Principles & practice of point-of-care testing Philadelphia: Lippincott Williams & Wilkins, 2002:93–5.
4. Jones J. Challenges of the post connectivity era. Clin Lab News 2003;29:10–2.
5. National Committee for Clinical Laboratory Standards. Application of a quality system model for laboratory services; approved guideline, second edition. NCCLS document GP26-A2. Wayne, PA: NCCLS, 2003.
6. Taylor M, Nichols JH, Saltz J. POCT connectivity: opening the door to a laboratory without walls. Am Clin Lab 2000;19:12–3.

Chapter 22

Ethics and Responsibility in Point-of-Care Testing

Jocelyn M. Hicks

Ethics is described as a system or set of moral principles, or the rules of conduct governing a particular group, or the branch of philosophy dealing with values relating to human conduct or moral principles (1). *Responsibility* is defined as the state of being accountable or a particular obligation upon one who is responsible (accountable) (1). This chapter will attempt to deal with these two issues as they pertain to point-of-care testing (POCT).

The very phrase "point-of-care testing" sounds attractive. What better idea than that patients or clients should have their tests performed right where they are, or when they want them? It is clearly incumbent on all laboratorians to see that the requesting physician gets an accurate result that is delivered within a time frame that is of greatest benefit to the patient and his or her care team and that can also be interpreted for the patient's well-being or benefit. While it might appear self-evident that all results should be delivered rapidly and therefore at the point of care, there are factors which must be taken into account before boldly stating that it is clearly ethical to perform such testing in this way.

Two of the most important issues are quality and cost. The quality of any diagnostic test encompasses preanalytical and postanalytical issues as well as the analytical quality of the result itself. Therefore, quality embraces ensuring that the correct test is requested, the patient is prepared correctly, the test is performed correctly, and the result is interpreted correctly. It would be unethical merely for the purposes of speed or convenience to favor either testing in the central laboratory or POCT, with any potential risk of an inferior quality of service. Similarly, it would not be ethical to perform testing at the bedside if it were exorbitantly more expensive than performing the test in the central laboratory, particularly if it could be demonstrated that medical outcomes were not improved in a particular diagnostic or treatment situation. It would also be unethical to choose the central laboratory testing modality purely on the basis that it appeared to "cost less."

While these may appear to be very simple statements, they allude to some extremely fundamental and challenging issues in the field of laboratory medicine, and indeed the practice of medicine as a whole. While there are many publications that in the past have cast doubt on the quality of the results produced by POCT, there are very few data that actually demonstrate the link between analytical quality and health outcome (2, 3).

There is a plethora of papers that show that the costs of the consumables for POCT are greater than for central laboratory testing (e.g., 4–6), and yet there are studies that show that, if all costs are taken into account, a POCT-based service is generally not more expensive than testing in the central laboratory (7). One of the challenges is that the benefits (savings from an economic perspective) are always gained outside of the laboratory.

Ethical conduct is described as "taking the organization, or in this case testing, to the next level at which decisions are made not to just comply with the law, but to do the right thing" (8). It is important to consider the ethical question from the perspective of both the healthcare providers and the patients.

ETHICS AND THE PHYSICIAN

It is incumbent on any physician to do the right thing for the patient, whether that is in diagnosis, therapy, or disease prevention. This includes establishing the balance between benefit and risk in relation to every clinical decision (9). Within the hospital setting the physician generally needs rapid results so that the patient's diagnosis or treatment can begin and be followed up expeditiously. This is particularly so in critical care units such as the emergency room, the intensive care unit, the neonatal unit, and the operating room (10). If a clinical decision is going to be made and an intervention implemented based upon a set of results, then it could be argued that it is unethical to perform the important tests such as electrolytes and blood gases in any other way other than by POCT in these areas, unless there is a very reliable pneumatic tube system between the unit and the central laboratory. In the emergency room it is important that drugs of abuse testing be done onsite, so that a rapid decision may be made as to the course of treatment. Also, to rule out an ectopic pregnancy, pregnancy testing must be readily available (11).

In the outpatient setting there are clearly tests that should be undertaken by POCT. These include, but are not limited to, glucose, microalbumin, HbA$_1$C for diabetic patients, and prothrombin time/international normalized ratio (PT/INR) for patients such as those with congestive heart failure who are taking Coumadin® (warfarin). There are 16 million diabetics in the United States and approximately 125 million worldwide, which illustrates the clinical and economic responsibilities associated with this condition.

The physician who is caring for the diabetic patient has an ethical responsibility to (*i*) maintain professional competence to practice, which includes keeping up to date with the current best evidence on the care of the patient (12); (*ii*) ensure that all the services are available for the care of the patient to comply with any guidelines emanating from the best evidence; (*iii*) ensure that the patient understands and (as far as is possible) complies with the planned care pathway; and (*iv*) identify the benefits and risks associated with the personalized treatment strategy adopted. Intuitively, the most ethical thing to do therefore is to obtain test results at the time of the patient's visit to counsel the patient if any dietary or medication changes are needed, as well as to provide objective evidence of the progress of the personalized treatment strategy. There is considerable observational data to support this contention, although there is little formal experimental evidence (13). Does this create another ethical challenge, both for the physician and the healthcare purchaser and provider organizations?

Another area in which POCT tests are becoming used more frequently is in the area of infectious diseases. Over the past 10 years many tests have been developed for the diagnosis of streptococcus, and these are much more reliable than in the past. The reliability of a positive test is about 99%, whereas the reliability of a negative result is ~90–93%. These tests are very suitable for a pediatrician's office. A child who has a positive result can be treated with antibiotics. If the test is negative, the child will generally not be given antibiotics unnecessarily unless the clinical symptoms are severe. If this is the case, a rapid DNA test can be done. There are many more examples of infectious disease testing in POCT, but these are well described in Chapter 36.

Congestive heart failure (CHF) is found in 5 million Americans, and 500,000 cases are added annually. Patients with CHF visit the physician frequently, and it is much better to be able to obtain the result of the PT/INR at the time of the clinic visit. If tests are not provided at the point of care, much time may be wasted on the part of both physician and patient. The physician will have to obtain the result from the central laboratory, and then one of the staff must call the patient with the result and let them know if the dose of Coumadin must be changed or if there is a need to get a follow-up test. This may also cause inconvenience to the patient, although perhaps of greater concern is the risk that the more distant relationship between the patient and his or her caregiver may result in poor compliance with the care program.

In the home setting, again the right thing is to have the patient be able to self-test for glucose in the case of the diabetic patient and PT in the case of the CHF patient. This prevents frequent visits or even telephone calls to the physician. However, there is an implicit responsibility to ensure that the patient is able to use the POCT device such that the results are reliable, understood, and acted upon correctly.

ETHICS AND OTHER MEMBERS OF THE HEALTHCARE TEAM

Other healthcare providers are also bound to make ethical decisions regarding POCT. The point was made earlier that the benefits of POCT are seen outside of the laboratory and have an impact on many members of the clinical team. It is clear that one of the major challenges of implementing a POCT program is making the changes in clinical practice to ensure maximization of the health benefit, both clinical and economic (14). It is obvious from the studies discussed in the various chapters of this book that there are considerable benefits to be gained from the use of POCT. However, as Nichols et al. (14) showed, practice must be changed to realize the benefit. It might be considered that testing at the bedside could interfere with other duties. However if it is in the patient's best interest to get the testing done quickly, then it is right to be undertaken in this way. Although there may originally have been resistance by nurses to performing POCT at the bedside, this has now changed as it has been realized that the nurse spends less time actually performing the testing than checking up on results from the central laboratory. It has also created a large improvement in the relationship between nurses and laboratory staff. Performing POCT has given nurses a sense of empowerment because they get results quickly and can discuss them directly with the requesting physician or act upon them directly. Respiratory therapists have often become part of the POCT program, especially in some intensive care units and neonatal nurseries. This is obviously advantageous to all because their training gives them a good knowledge of respiratory function and they can quickly recognize any problem with pH and blood gas results, especially in the ventilated patient. POCT instruments are gradually being integrated into the battery of diagnostic devices available on the wards that include the thermometer and the sphygmomanometer!

Ethics and Laboratory Staff

At the beginning of POCT programs, the clinical pathologist or laboratory medicine specialists had considerable concerns about this approach to testing. They were concerned about loss of control, loss of jobs, and of course, about quality. It soon became apparent that the role of the laboratory director has changed over the past two decades and that one of the important aspects of the job is now to make sure there is a rapid flow of information with regard to testing. The laboratory professional is an important resource for the clinical team in relation to POCT because of the training and competence in the use of analytical devices as well as the knowledge of how they should be used in the care of patients.

Ethics and the Healthcare Purchaser and Provider Organizations

Organizations have the same responsibilities and accountabilities toward the patient as do the healthcare professionals themselves. This may be observed at a societal level through the actions taken by governments in terms of laws regulating professional practice and legislation regarding resources committed to healthcare provision. Regulations are perhaps the most transparent of these actions, as they protect the patient against harm, which in many respects appears to be easier to achieve than ensuring benefit!

Thus, in relation to POCT the delivery is regulated, insofar as the assurance for the delivery of an accurate analytical result is maximized through practice guidelines covering training and certification (see below). However, the commitment to ensuring that the most appropriate modality of delivery is chosen, namely central laboratory testing or POCT, is not adequately covered in terms of the evidence required to enable explicit policymaking. Hobbs et al (15), in a systematic review of POCT in primary care, found very few articles dealing with health outcomes, the majority of studies focusing instead on technical and economic issues. In a more recent review, Price (16) found a similar situation, pointing to the problems of performing robust studies in this area of healthcare provision. However, there is an ethical requirement to determine whether, and to what extent, POCT can improve health outcomes. Intuitively, the evidence that does exist would indicate that there are many other opportunities to implement POCT. Interestingly POCT has proliferated in some areas of medicine to become the standard of care without robust outcomes-based evidence, such that it would be unethical to embark on any formal studies to evaluate whether the current standard of care is appropriate.

RESPONSIBILITIES

The ethical challenges identified highlight a number of issues regarding responsibility and accountability for POCT. The most important issues that must be addressed are:

- Who has the overall responsibility for the POCT program?
- How is the equipment chosen?
- Where should testing be offered?
- Who is responsible for the testing?
- Who is responsible for quality control?
- Who will train the staff?
- How will competency of the testing personnel be assessed?
- What proficiency testing and accreditation will be done?
- Who is responsible for inventory control?
- Who is responsible for connectivity of equipment?

These issues are addressed in detail in Chapter 11 (training and certification), Chapter 12 (equipment procurement), Chapter 13 (quality control and quality assurance), Chapter 15 (guidelines on POCT), Chapter 16 (regulation and POCT), and finally, looking at the holistic picture, Chapter 17 (clinical governance).

PATIENT RESPONSIBILITIES AND ETHICS

So far, the emphasis in this chapter has been directed toward the healthcare professional and the purchaser and provider organizations, but the patient also has certain ethical rights and responsibilities that should be considered.

Patient Ethics

Patients have the ethical right to be informed about any form of testing that might be offered, its benefits, and its limitations. They also have the ethical right to be informed of their test results and how these are interpreted by the physician. If a patient has read about self-testing at home, he or she should feel comfortable discussing it with the clinician and deciding whether it is appropriate. Good examples would be an informed discussion about measuring one's own blood pressure and the quality of monitors or the efficacy of performing one's own ovulation testing. In many cases, the patient may elect to self-test without first discussing it with a physician. Is this ethical? In certain instances such as pregnancy testing, there is little problem. If the result is positive, there will generally be immediate follow-up with a physician. In other cases, the patient may elect not to follow up because of being frightened. An example of this could be a positive occult blood test. It is certainly incumbent on the manufacturers of self-testing kits to warn the patient about follow-up with the doctor.

We are embarking on an era of "patient choice" supported by an information revolution that will enable the patient to find more out about his or her health and well-being. Patients are already far better informed than they were a decade ago, including having a greater knowledge about laboratory tests, in part as a result of successful initiatives such as LabTests Online (www.labtestsonline.org). This will undoubtedly change the relationship between the healthcare professional and the patient; but if anything, it will accentuate the need for a patient or any individual member of society to have access to support from a healthcare professional. This then raises a whole raft of questions: What is the nature of the new relationship? What will be the form of the contact or consultation? How will knowledge be stored and made available? How will the patient be protected against harm (which in theory could be self-inflicted if the opinion of a healthcare professional is not sought at the appropriate time)? These are important issues that pertain to POCT and specifically extend to self-testing; they must be debated so that the patient's interests are protected.

Patient Responsibilities

The patient's responsibilities become particularly important with home testing. It is incumbent on the patient to keep records and inform the physician of any unexpected results. This is particularly important for diabetics monitoring their glucose, as well as for patients measuring their INR on a routine basis. Results that are not good should not be swept under the carpet or ignored, nor left out of the recording document. This issue has been resolved to a degree by the introduction of glucose meters with onboard memory, which record all measurements over a defined period, then use mobile phone communications to download the data to a central computer for review by a healthcare professional. It is very important that the physician make patient responsibilities very clear to the patient.

THE FUTURE

Two areas of major interest for POCT in the future are cancer testing and genetic testing. As molecular diagnostics moves closer to the area of DNA chip technology, one can imagine handheld analyzers that determine the presence of genes indicating, for example, increased risk of colon cancer, breast cancer, or Huntington's disease. This poses tremendous ethical problems. If patients can be shown to carry genes for diseases such as the aforementioned, one can imagine employers avoiding such individuals as candidates for job positions or, even worse, insurance companies denying them medical coverage. Patients are already beginning to request tests off the Internet; what might be available in the future is exciting, challenging, and somewhat frightening.

POCT is a rapidly growing and advancing field, and we must all understand the ethical issues and responsibilities that are associated with it. There is no doubt that the advances in POCT technology, our knowledge of health and disease, new diagnostic tests and interventions, and the empowerment of individuals will provide many challenges to the relations among the laboratorian, the patient, and the patient's caregiver.

REFERENCES

1. Random House Webster's college dictionary. New York: Random House, 1999.
2. Boyd JC, Bruns DE. Quality specifications for glucose meters: assessment by simulation modeling of errors in insulin dose. Clin Chem 2001;47:209–14.
3. Roddam AW, Price CP, Allen NE, Ward AM. Assessing the clinical impact of prostate-specific antigen assay variability and nonequimolarity: a simulation study based on the population of the United Kingdom. Clin Chem 2004;50:1012–6.
4. Lee-Lewandrowski E, Laposata M, Eschenbach K, Camooso C, Nathan DM, Godine JE, et al. Utilization and cost analysis of bedside capillary glucose testing in a large teaching hospital: implications for managing point of care testing. Am J Med 1994;97:222–30.
5. Parvin CA, Lo SF, Deuser SM, Weaver LG, Lewis LM, Scott MG. Impact of point-of-care testing on patients' length of stay in a large emergency department. Clin Chem 1996;42:711–7.
6. Greendyke RM. Cost analysis: Bedside blood glucose testing. Am J Clin Pathol 1992;97:106–7.
7. Hicks JM. Near patient testing: Is it here to stay? J Clin Path 1996;49:191–3.
8. Cohan R. Compliance and ethics: A critical interdependence. Healthcare Exec 2004;19:32–4.
9. Montori VM, Guyatt GH. Evidence-based medicine and the diagnostic process. In: Price CP, Christenson RH, eds. Evidence-based laboratory medicine. Washington, DC: AACC Press, 2003; 1–37.
10. Castro HJ, Oropello JM, Halpern N. Point-of-care testing in the intensive care unit: the intensive care physician's perspective. Am J Clin Path 1995;104(Suppl 1):595–9.
11. Olshaker JS. Emergency department pregnancy testing. J Emerg Med 1996;14:59–65.
12. Sackett DL, Haynes RB, Guyatt GH, Tugwell P. Clinical epidemiology: a basic science for clinical medicine, 2nd ed. Toronto: Little, Brown, 1991;1–441.
13. Piette JD, Glasgow RE. Education and home glucose monitoring. In: Gerstein HC, Haynes RB, eds. Evidence-based diabetes care. Hamilton, ON: BC Decker, 2001;207–51.
14. Nichols JH, Kickler TS, Dyer KL, Humbertson SK, Cooper PC, Maughan WL, et al. Clinical outcomes of point-of-care testing in the interventional radiology and invasive cardiology setting. Clin Chem 2000;46:543–50.
15. Hobbs FD, Delaney BC, Fitzmaurice DA, Wilson S, Hyde CJ, Thorpe GH, et al. A review of near patient testing in primary care. Health Technol Assess 1997;1:1–230.
16. Price CP. Point of care testing: Potential for tracking disease management outcomes. Dis Manage Health Outcomes 2002;10: 749–61.

Part **Four**

Application of Point-of-Care Testing

Chapter **23**

Point-of-Care Testing in Patient Transport Settings

Robert W. Hardy and Glen L. Hortin

There are many potential settings for medical care delivery outside of traditional hospitals and outpatient facilities. Some of these settings include ambulances, helicopters, and other aircraft used for transport of patients in emergencies and for tertiary care; sites of field responses to emergencies; and remote sites such as spacecraft. In the past, the answer as to whether we should perform any laboratory testing in these settings generally was a very simple no; it was impossible or impractical to perform most tests in these settings. Chemistry and blood gas analyzers were too large and expensive and their use required extensive utilities, careful environmental control, and highly trained operators. It was unthinkable to pack typical laboratory instruments into an ambulance or airplane to perform testing during patient transport. However, progressive technological advances, miniaturization of analyzers, and simplification of operation have made it possible to perform an increasing array of tests in mobile settings. Consideration of whether to offer testing in mobile settings has become much more complicated. Now, rather than presenting a simple clear-cut impossibility, the question of point-of-care testing (POCT) in transport settings requires careful evaluation of multiple factors related to cost and benefit.

EVALUATING WHETHER TO PERFORM TESTS IN MOBILE SETTINGS

As outlined in Table 23-1, three major questions need to be considered in evaluating whether to offer testing in a mobile setting.

1. It technically possible to perform tests accurately within the desired setting given the limitations of specimen types, testing environment, and personnel available within the planned site of testing?
2. Are the financial resources available to buy the necessary equipment and supplies, and does the cost–benefit ratio favor testing?
3. Will the testing result in improved patient care and medical outcomes?

Some of the factors considered in evaluating whether to offer POCT in a mobile setting are similar to those in other healthcare settings. However, the major factor that distinguishes POCT in a mobile setting is the lack of any other testing alternative. The decision to offer testing is not one of POCT versus laboratory testing but rather a choice of POCT versus no testing at all or testing that is delayed until a medical facility is reached. In the case of a brief ambulance trip to a hospital, the delay in access to testing may not be a significant factor, but in other situations no other testing alternative may be available for hours or days. The following sections discuss in greater detail factors that need to be considered for mobile testing and that may distinguish testing in this environment from other forms of POCT.

Technical Factors

The mobile testing environment poses a number of challenges for POCT, as summarized in Table 23-2. One of the greatest challenges is the space constraints in a number of transport settings. The limited space for POCT in jet transport is clearly illustrated in Figure 23-1. One example of an effort to address space limitations during critical care transport is a self-contained stretcher-based miniature intensive care unit containing a blood gas and blood chemistry analyzer that has been developed for the US Army (1). Termed the Life Support for Trauma and Transport (LSTAT), it is designed to fit into the size constraints of a North Atlantic Treaty Organization (NATO) stretcher. It has been favorably evaluated in a postoperative environment; however, data on field performance are not yet available

Helicopters are used for the transport of critically ill patients in several situations. Prehospital POCT in a helicopter transport program for the critically ill indicated that measurements of sodium, potassium, glucose, hematocrit/hemoglobin, and urea nitrogen showed no significant unexplained differences from the laboratory analysis of parallel samples (2, 3). Although the correlation studies were necessarily performed when the helicopter was typically <20 min away from the hospital, these studies indicate the potential usefulness of POCT in a helicopter transport setting. Imprecision studies at 10 to 27 days indicated coefficients of variation (CVs) comparable to laboratory CVs for control specimens. Nevertheless, two control values exceeded specified limits, underlining the importance of operator training in troubleshooting and documenting corrective action in transport settings.

Table 23-1   Evaluating Whether to Provide POCT in a Mobile Setting

Technical factors
   Specimen type
   Test menu
   Adequate test performance
   Environmental suitability
   Required operator expertise
   Quality assurance
Financial factors
   Capital expense
   Costs for licenses
   Labor costs
   Supply costs
   Income
Medical considerations
   Time and distance from medical facilities
   Physician support/communication
   Detection of problems not apparent by clinical monitoring
   Need for immediate treatment
   Ability to treat newly diagnosed problems
   Potential impact on patient outcomes

Table 23-2   Potential Factors Affecting Performance of POCT Devices in a Mobile Setting

Limited space
Lack of utilities
Vibration
Changes in barometric pressure
Temperature variation
Humidity (decreased humidity at high altitudes even in pressurized aircraft)
Unpredictable motion (bumps, air pockets, etc.)
Acceleration and deceleration
Lack of personnel expertise in laboratory testing and quality assurance procedures
POCT device storage
Microgravity (in space travel)
Radiation (in space travel)

Logically, one might expect that vibration and unpredictable motion changes would influence POCT operator error in a transport setting. However, problems with testing reliability may be uncovered only after an extended period of field use. In one study nonanalytical POCT test failures were reported in a critical care transport setting over 6 years (4). They found 76 nonanalytical POCT test failures using the i-STAT® analyzer (i-STAT, East Windsor, NJ, USA) during 1146 patient tests, or ~7%. Reasons for these failures were determined to be cartridge failure (55%), operator error (42%), or analyzer failure requiring repair by the manufacturer (3%). Importantly, in all cases of these failures, results were not reported; the analyzer suppressed display of results. Repeat testing was done in all cases except the two analyzer failures requiring repair by the manufacturer. It was suggested that the operator errors could partially be attributed to the moving environment in which testing occurs.

It was suggested that regular maintenance, quality control, and assurance programs contributed to dependable operation (4). The issues of quality control, regular maintenance, proper training, and continuing education are likely to be important factors in maintaining the accuracy and reliability of POCT in a transport setting. To interpret test results from POCT appropriately, it is important for clinicians to have data regarding comparisons with central laboratory test methods and any differences in test values or reference ranges. One study described the benefits of a mobile POCT anticoagulation therapy management program (5); however, the variability of international normalized ratios (INRs) from these POCT systems has

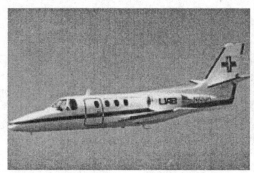
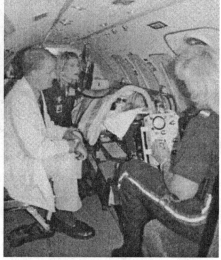

Figure 23-1   Critical care transport environment: The critical care transport environment often presents challenges of motion and limited space for POCT, as in this example of jet transport.

led to recommendations for better methods of quality control including the need for external quality control of these instruments (6).

POCT in space presents the additional problems of microgravity and radiation. The microgravity environment affects various physiological systems including the skeletal, muscular, and erythropoietic, as well as body fluid compartments. Microgravity also affects blood collection techniques and equipment designed to operate under normal gravity. One study investigated the utility of a commercial portable clinical blood analyzer on the space shuttle (7). The analyzer demonstrated good between-day precision in space, and control samples agreed well with ground-based measurements using control samples with the exception of sodium. Sodium was slightly decreased in flight but within Clinical Laboratory Improvement Amendments (CLIA) performance guidelines. These analyses may prove useful in providing important information regarding the health status of the crew during space flights. Obtaining transcutaneous measurements or substituting urine or saliva for blood specimens may minimize the intrusiveness of testing. In fact, transcutaneous glucose monitoring is commercially available at present (8). The application of nanotechnology to human fluid analysis may also become a routine aspect of future space travel. Validation of new technologies in the space medicine clinical research program and a transition to the routine application of those technologies will be an important challenge for future space flight.

In summary, technical factors present important challenges for POCT in a transport setting, as does their evaluation. Nevertheless, these challenges are beginning to be addressed. The impetus for overcoming them will be provided as benefits both in patient care and cost savings are realized.

Financial Factors

One of the most controversial aspects of POCT is the cost (9–12). In the intensive care unit, it may not be cost-effective to use POCT when a significantly less expensive central laboratory test is available. As previously mentioned in the transport setting, the issue is the cost of POCT versus no testing at all. Cost analysis of POCT in a critical care transport setting over a prolonged period of testing has been described (4). Of a total of 3500 cartridges purchased over 6 years, 1146 were used for patient testing, an average of 1.6 cartridges per case. The supply cost for a cartridge averaged about $5. For this low-volume testing environment, more than half of all cartridges were used for quality assurance testing or personnel training, or expired before use. Total capital costs were about $15,000, and no additional staff time was required. Costs averaged about $50 per case where POCT was used or about $8 per case if divided among all transports. Costs were allocated over all transports because the technology was available on all trips.

This study concluded that POCT represented a very small fraction of overall transport costs, a relatively small cost per case, and a potential for significant clinical benefit. One concern with POCT in critical care transport is the potential for excessive utilization because of the availability and ease of testing. A primary finding of this study was the low rate of utilization. Although POCT equipment was available for all transports for more than 6 years, testing was performed in only 17% of cases. Usage was higher in patients with high acuity than for patients with more stable conditions. The annual rate of use was relatively constant, and rampant overuse of laboratory testing in this environment clearly did not occur. Notably in this study, only one-quarter of all POCT was performed in the ambulance or jet during actual transport. This prior-to-transport portion of testing may affect overall transport costs by decreasing transport time and thereby reducing costs. In fact, one study supports the contention that patient blood gas POCT at the referring hospital reduces the time and costs of interfacility transport (13). Another scenario in which prior-to-transport testing may be useful is in an organ procurement organization/donor management setting where rapid bedside testing allowed more immediate clinical management decisions concerning deceased organ donors and permitted the organ placement calls to begin sooner (14).

Considering that the direct costs of virtually any medical complications can surpass the costs for POCT, there is the potential for cost savings. A number of reports conclude that POCT can improve patient care (2, 3, 7, 13, 15–18). However, the benefit part of the cost–benefit analysis is often difficult to measure in dollar terms and thus these savings can be difficult to quantify.

EVIDENCE FOR CLINICAL VALUE OF POCT IN MOBILE SETTINGS

A study of the impact of POCT on the care of 81 patients transported by helicopters serving as air ambulances was performed by the Mayo Clinic (3). In this study, POCT measurements of glucose, sodium, potassium, chloride, urea, and hematocrit were performed. Twenty of the patients (25%) received a treatment other than intravenous fluids that was related to POCT measurements. Sixteen patients received blood transfusions. Two patients were treated with insulin. One patient was treated for severe hypoglycemia. One patient was treated with an infusion of plasma and platelets.

A more extended 6-year study of the clinical value of POCT during the transport of patients by ambulance and aircraft was performed by the University of Alabama Critical Care Transport service (4). A total of 4276 cases were evaluated in which POCT with a test menu of glucose, sodium, potassium, chloride, ionized calcium, pH, bicarbonate, Po_2, Pco_2, and hematocrit was available during the transport. Each case had a team of a respiratory therapist, nurse, and physician conducting patient transport between healthcare facilities; the average duration of transports was 3 h. About 80% of the patients were critically ill, requiring ventilator or heart-assist pumps or were seriously ill, requiring admission to an intensive-care unit. POCT was performed during 706 of the cases. Although POCT was used in only about one-sixth of cases, POCT led to changes in patient therapy approximately 30% of the time that testing was performed. Therapeutic yields of POCT measurements are summarized in Table 23-3. (Therapeutic yield, expressed as a percentage, was considered to be the number of times that testing resulted in therapeutic changes divided by the total number of testing episodes.) Measurements of blood gases led to the most frequent therapeutic changes (therapeutic yield of 23%) such as adjustment of ventilator settings, intubation of patients, or other interventions affecting ventilation. When testing of electrolytes was performed, 16% of the time there were changes in therapy such as adjustment of intravenous fluids, starting or discontinuing potassium administration, and administration of bicarbonate or calcium. Measurement of hematocrit and glucose each led to changes in treatment about 5% of the time. Surprisingly, review of the sites where testing was performed found that 77% of the testing was performed at the hospital where the transport was initiated. This was considered to speed the evaluation and stabilization of patients, and it may have saved significant time and labor costs. However, it was an unexpected testing component, and it may have represented a convenience rather than a medical necessity considering that laboratory testing should have been available in those instances. Based on the volume of testing performed in this scenario the issue of pretransport testing should be addressed in future studies and should be considered as a separate component with different medical necessity.

Table 23-3 Treatment Changes Based on POCT Results[a]
Summary of results for 706 episodes of use of POCT during critical care transport.

Treatment change	Episodes
Blood gases: therapeutic yield 23%	
Adjust ventilator settings	102
Intubation	46
Adjust oxygen delivery, i.e., mask or nasal cannula	17
Administer surfactant	4
Administer albuterol	2
Electrolytes: therapeutic yield 16%	
Start or adjust intravenous fluids	44
Start or discontinue potassium	38
Administer bicarbonate	28
Administer calcium gluconate or calcium chloride	5
Hematocrit: therapeutic yield 5%	
Blood transfusion	33
Glucose: therapeutic yield 3%	
Administer or discontinue insulin	16
Administer dextrose	3

[a] Total cartridges used, 1146: 6+, 137; G3, 147; EG7+, 582; glucose, 280.
Data from (4).

The two preceding studies cited provide evidence that POCT can have a significant impact on the treatment of patients during extended transport of critically ill patients. Nevertheless, the studies do not go so far as to prove that POCT in this setting directly affects traditional measures of patient outcomes such as morbidity, mortality, or patient satisfaction (19). Occurrence of death and severe medical complications during transport are relatively rare events, and it may be difficult to conclude whether availability of POCT or other factors contribute to a change in outcomes. Therefore, a true outcome study examining the effects of POCT on traditional outcome measures is very difficult to perform. At present, there is no direct experimental evidence about whether the therapeutic changes resulting from POCT yield significant improvements in patient outcome. Instead we are left with more subjective measures of POCT on outcome. Review of individual cases identified a number of instances where POCT was subjectively considered to improve the patient's condition significantly (4). For 182 of the cases where POCT was performed, physicians caring for the patients were surveyed about the impact of POCT on patient care. The subjective assessment of the physicians was that POCT resulted in a moderate or substantial improvement in patient condition for 14% of the patients where testing was performed.

There are a wide variety of other mobile settings besides the care of critically ill or injured patients in ambulances where POCT potentially could have clinical value. Application of POCT by visiting nurses could assist in monitoring anticoagulant therapy. Use of a POCT device appeared to achieve just as effective adjustment of dosing of anticoagulation as did laboratory monitoring, and patients indicated greater satisfaction with community monitoring (5, 20). In a variety of mobile clinic settings, POCT might have a value similar to that of a typical physician office laboratory setting. Testing for drugs of abuse in a variety of settings outside the traditional healthcare settings may have value for forensic use or guidance of drug treatment programs, although interpretation of results can be challenging (21).

In summary, evaluation of the potential medical benefit of POCT in a mobile setting depends on consideration of access to medical facilities, the patient's clinical condition, and therapeutic capability. There are data indicating that POCT influences patient treatment but proof is lacking that patient outcomes are improved. At present, the decision to offer POCT in mobile settings is a matter of medical judgment.

As more sophisticated and even noninvasive POCT becomes available, this type of testing will undoubtedly increase in transport settings in the future.

REFERENCES

1. Johnson K, Pearce F, Westenskow D, Ogden LL, Farnsworth S, Peterson S, et al. Clinical evaluation of the life support for trauma and transport (LSTAT) platform. Crit Care 2002;6:439–46.
2. Burritt MF, Santrach PJ, Hankins DG, Herr D, Newton NC. Evaluation of the i-STAT® portable clinical analyzer for use in a helicopter. Scand J Clin Lab Invest 1996;56(Suppl 224):121–8.

3. Herr DM, Bewton NC, Santrach PJ, Hankins DG, Burritt MF. Airborne and rescue point-of-care testing. Am J Clin Pathol 1995;104:S54–S58.

4. Gruszecki AC, Hortin G, Lam J, Kahler D, Smith D, Vines J, et al. Utilization, reliability and clinical impact of point-of-care testing during critical care transport: six years of experience. Clin Chem 2003;49:1017–9.

5. Gill JM, Landis MK. Benefits of a mobile, point-of-care anticoagulation therapy management program. Jt Comm J Qual Improv 2002;28:625–30.

6. Poller L, Keown M, Chauhan N, Van Den Besselaar AM, Tripodi A, Shiach C, Jespersen J. ECCA Steering Group Members. European concerted action on anticoagulation. Correction of displayed international normalized ratio on two point-of-care test whole-blood prothrombin time monitors (CoaguChek Mini and TAS PT-NC) by independent international sensitivity index calibration Br J Haematol 2003;122:944–9.

7. Smith SM, Davis-Street JE, Fontenot TB, Lane HW. Assessment of a portable clinical blood analyzer during space flight. Clin Chem 1997;43:1056–65.

8. Chase HP, Roberts MD, Wightman C, Klingensmith G, Garg SK, Van Wyhe M, et al. Use of the GlucoWatch biographer in children with type 1 diabetes. Pediatrics 2003;111:790–4.

9. Price CP. Point-of-care testing. Br Med J 2001;322:1285–8.

10. Crook MA. Near patient testing and pathology in the new millennium. J Clin Pathol 2000;53:27–30.

11. Murphy MJ, Paterson JR. Point-of-care testing: no pain no gain [Editorial]. Q J Med 2001;94:571–3.

12. St-Louis P. Status of point of care testing: promise, realities, and possibilities. Clin Biochem 2000;33:427–40.

13. Macnab AJ, Grant G, Stevens K, Gagnon F, Noble R, Sun C. Cost:benefit of point of care blood gas analysis vs. laboratory measurement during stabilization prior to transport. Prehospital Disaster Medicine 2003;18:24–8.

14. Baier KA, Markham LE, Flaigle SP, Nelson PW, Shield CF, Muruve NA et al. Point-of-care testing in an organ procurement organization donor management setting. Clin Transplant 2003; 17(Suppl 9):48–51.

15. Davey AL, Macnab AJ, Green G. Changes in pCO_2 during air medical transport of children with closed head injuries. Air Med J 2001;20:27–30.

16. Randolph V, Kahler D, Howard C, Hortin G. Laboratories on the move: blood gas analysis. Lab Med 2000;31:45–8.

17. Kost GJ. Preventing medical errors in point-of-care testing; security, validation, safeguards, and connectivity. Arch Pathol Lab Med 2001;125:1307–15.

18. Price CP. Point-of-care testing impact on medical outcomes. Clinics Lab Med 2001;21:285–303.

19. Price CP. Medical and economic outcomes of point-of-care testing. Clin Chem Lab Med 2002;40:246–51.

20. Schiach CR, Campbell B, Poller L, Keown M, Chauhan N. Reliability of point-of-care prothrombin time testing in a community clinic: a randomized crossover comparison with hospital laboratory testing. Br J Haematol 2002;119:370–75.

21. George S, Braithwaite RA. Use of on-site testing for drugs of abuse. Clin Chem 2002;48:1639–46.

Chapter 24

Point-of-Care Testing in the Emergency Department

Richard P. Taylor

THE ARGUMENT FOR POINT-OF-CARE TESTING IN THE EMERGENCY DEPARTMENT

Point-of-Care Testing Is Intuitively Useful

If the function of point-of-care testing (POCT) is to produce timely information for patient diagnosis or to influence patient management decisions, then intuitively the emergency department (ED) should be an ideal setting for its implementation. This supposition has influenced the implementation of POCT in the ED, although the benefits have been difficult to establish objectively. It has been driven by ED physicians who argue that faster results provide additional information to support clinical decisions and allow more effective utilization of their time; ED physicians have long argued that laboratory turnaround times (TATs) are too slow for their needs (1), a view that appears to be supported by comprehensive surveys showing no improvement in TATs over a decade (2). Furthermore, a randomized controlled trial demonstrated that patient management decisions could be made significantly earlier if POCT was used for patients whose management was dependent on blood results (3). The diagnostics industry has developed tests for POCT use to fulfill the demand for faster results. Technological advances have resulted in the development of instruments that use whole blood specimens and can generate results in minutes, apparently simply and conveniently. The instruments are designed to eliminate the clerical and administrative tasks associated with sending specimens to the laboratory and to reduce the inconvenience of variable waiting times for results.

However, it can also be argued that POCT generates additional analytical costs, as well as instrument support and staff training requirements. It has a different set of data-recording and management processes that may be less robust than those in the laboratory (4). A randomized controlled study also found that POCT had no effect on the time patients spent in the ED, their length of stay in the hospital, admission rates, or mortality (3). Thus, what may be beneficial to the patient and to the working practices of ED staff in the patient's first few hours may provide no overall benefit and incur additional costs and duties for staff. So, what are the potential outcomes from the use of POCT in the ED? Is the use of POCT so well established that it is now part of the standard of care? Are there other tests that could be provided by POCT that would have a greater effect on emergency care?

Laboratory and ED Collaboration

Numerous studies have been performed to establish the nature and extent of benefits from POCT in the ED. What is clear is the complexity of the process of diagnosis and initiating treatment in the ED, and of referring patients to other specialties for further care if appropriate. POCT in the ED is just one part of this, and the time spent in the ED is just one part of what may be a complex patient journey. These complexities have contributed to the difficulty of carrying out studies to identify the benefits of POCT. The time required for other investigations such as radiology and electrocardiography and delays in availability of beds in referral departments influence a patient's length of stay in the ED.

As rapid production of test results is a key benefit of POCT, comparison of TAT with the local laboratory is an important factor. However, transport and specimen handling arrangements and the distance between the laboratory and the ED apparently vary so much between institutions that it is difficult to draw definitive conclusions from published studies. The definition of TAT itself has been a matter of debate. The way forward is for the laboratory to work in closer partnership with the ED so that all of those involved can gain a clearer understanding of how POCT influences patient care (5, 6). The role of ED physicians is to resuscitate, stabilize, and institute appropriate treatment for their acutely ill, unconscious, or traumatized patients. The available tests should be sufficient to facilitate this but do not necessarily have to provide a comprehensive diagnosis (7). The laboratory's role is to validate POCT assay accuracy and precision, ensure agreement with parallel laboratory methods, and ensure that quality assurance procedures are in place and that results are recorded appropriately. Laboratory staff should liaise closely with nursing and other clinical staff to implement training and education for effective POCT. Ideally the processes of POCT should be recorded electronically and integrated into the hospital information system. Most importantly, POCT tests must be integrated with central or satellite laboratory services.

The clinical laboratory has to respond to the demands of its users and should aim to support and adopt measures that will genuinely benefit patient outcomes, or contribute to cost or efficiency improvements within the hospital. The laboratory should work to improve its service to all users by addressing specimen transport and preanalytical automation, analyzer throughput, rapid reporting, and knowledge support. All of these factors influence the relative value of POCT and laboratory-based tests for the management of ED patients.

This chapter addresses the potential role of POCT in the management of the wide range of conditions patients present to the ED, discusses which tests are of value, reviews the literature, and suggests how further progress can be made to establish the role of POCT in the management of ED patients.

POTENTIAL APPLICATIONS FOR POCT

The Patient Case Mix Presenting at the ED

The first column of data in Table 24-1 gives the diagnostic categories for nonminor patient cases that present most commonly to the John Radcliffe Hospital ED as a percentage of all patients, whether or not they require laboratory tests. One-fourth of the patients present with chest pain, abdominal pain, or respiratory dysfunction, each requiring laboratory tests as part of the initial investigation. POCT or laboratory testing is performed for well over half of the nonminor admissions. Many may require other investigations, such as radiology, electrocardiography, and physiological measurements. Table 24-1 also gives diagnostic categories for patients in published studies (3, 8–10) from several EDs for whom laboratory tests were performed. These data exclude patients for whom no laboratory tests were done. Although there are some categorization differences, Table 24-1 again shows that the most common presentations are chest pain, abdominal pain, and respiratory illnesses. Their occurrence is similar between hospitals, and together these presentations constitute one-fourth to one-half of all patient cases tested. Trauma accounts for a further 5%. Other conditions such as collapse, overdose, nausea and vomiting, and gastrointestinal bleeding each account for approximately 5% to 10% of cases. Thus, POCT or rapid central laboratory tests have a role in the management of a wide range of ED patients.

ED physicians have to diagnose and treat patients with this very wide range of conditions, and as departments become busier they are under managerial pressure to become ever more

Table 24-1 Breakdown Analysis of Emergency Department Cases

Presenting symptom[a]	Oxford; % of all nonminor ED cases	Kendall (3): cases with POC tests	Kendall (3): cases with lab tests	Parvin (8): cases in control periods	Parvin (8): cases in experimental period	Sands (9): cases with POC tests	Tsai (10): cases with POC tests
Number of patients	1711	860	868	2918	1722	960	210
Psychiatric	11						
Chest pain	10	16	16	11	12	13	13
Abdominal pain	10	16	16	9	9	7	7
Musculoskeletal	9						
Wound	5						
Trauma		5	6	7	4	11	
SOB/respiratory	6	14	11	8	10	12	11
Nausea/vomiting				6	6	6	5
Hemorrhage						10	
Weakness/dizziness				5	5		9
Seizure				3	2	3	4
Cough/URI				2	3		
Diabetes						3	3
Syncope				1	2		
UTI symptoms				1	2		
Collapse		10	12				
Altered mental status						13	3
Overdose		6	7			3	
Gastrointestinal bleeding		5	3				
Unwell		8	8				
Bruise/superficial injury	7						
CNS, excluding stroke	5						
Fracture	4						
Other	33	19	20	38	34	26[b]	45
Unknown				9	11		

[a] CNS, central nervous system; SOB, shortness of breath; URI, upper respiratory infection; UTI, urinary tract infection.
[b] Some patients appear in multiple categories.

efficient. For many conditions, laboratory tests may speed decisions on treatment; in some cases laboratory tests may help to rule out one diagnosis and point to an alternative diagnosis. In some instances the test result may simply help to allay the concerns of the admitting physician in relation to a particular hypothesis (e.g., intake of toxic drugs). The appropriate tests should be available to facilitate this but do not necessarily have to provide a comprehensive diagnosis (7).

Diagnoses for Which Rapid Testing Has a Role in Patient Management

Table 24-2 gives an illustrative summary of conditions for which POCT is likely to improve diagnosis, initiation of treatment, or referral or discharge of patients presenting to the ED (11). POCT can be considered beneficial if the tests are acted on rapidly and appropriately. In almost all cases the necessary POCT systems are available. The devices provide results that help a physician make the decision to admit the patient, that influence early treatment, or that give an indication of the presence and severity of complications associated with the diagnosis. POCT may contribute to improved management of many other patient conditions as well, depending on local circumstances and the availability or development of suitable tests (11). Table 24-3 outlines some point-of-care (POC) tests that are likely to be of use in managing patients where knowledge of test results is required (11).

Tests Useful for Investigating a Wide Range of ED Patients

A group of core tests is useful for many conditions, but more than one test result is often necessary, requiring a number of different analyzers or readers. The grouping of tests has major practical implications, as discussed later. Many of the most widely useful tests give information on vital processes that can be abnormal in a range of different conditions. They provide important information for assessing lung ventilation and perfusion, the oxygen-carrying capacity of the blood, fluid and electrolyte balance, and blood pH. The clinical state of critically ill patients can change quickly, requiring rapid assessment to guide prompt treatment. The critical tests are outlined in the following sections.

Blood Gases and pH. Establishing and maintaining adequate tissue oxygenation and normal acid–base status are important aims of patient management in the ED. They are aided by measuring pH, Po_2, and Pco_2 in arterial blood. Additional parameters such as bicarbonate, base excess, and oxygen saturation are calculated by the instruments. A continuous measurement of oxygen saturation of hemoglobin in peripheral tissues can be obtained by pulse oximetry. This complements the intermittent measurement of blood gases. Pulse oximetry is not always reliable, for example, if tissue perfusion is inadequate or if the hemoglobin concentration is abnormal or hemoglobin variants are present. A continuous measurement of end-tidal CO_2 by capnography to complement the measurement of blood gases is recommended for ventilated patients.

Hemoglobin and Hematocrit. Adequate circulating plasma volume and red cell hemoglobin are necessary for tissue perfusion and transport of oxygen to the tissues. These require urgent assessment in a patient who is actively bleeding. Rapid availability of hemoglobin and hematocrit information alongside the clinical assessment is important for guiding treatment with fluids and blood.

Electrolytes. Maintenance of sodium and water balance and physiological concentrations of potassium and calcium is important for normal metabolism and organ function. In critically ill patients, homeostatic mechanisms may not function correctly and rapid deterioration can occur. Sodium, potassium, and calcium concentrations can be measured in whole blood to provide the information necessary for rapid corrective therapy. Sodium and water balance must be maintained and rapid changes avoided. Serious complications of fluid electrolyte imbalance are seizures and cerebral edema. Potassium concentrations may be deranged as a result of diuretic therapy. In diabetic ketoacidosis, potassium concentrations can be affected by losses from the body and by redistribution caused by acid–base changes or insulin therapy. Abnormal potassium concentrations can cause cardiac arrhythmias. Ionized calcium levels may fall after administration of large amounts of blood and high-volume fluid resuscitation, causing cardiac and neuromuscular dysfunction.

Lactate. Measurement of whole blood lactate can provide useful information on the adequacy of tissue perfusion and the presence of ischemia or hypoxia. It can be a prognostic marker for the success of treatment (12), especially in patients with severe sepsis and poor tissue oxygenation (13). It has been shown that a single blood lactate measurement can identify patients with a high likelihood of mortality (14). With appropriate and careful interpretation in the clinical context, blood lactate complements other information on oxygen delivery and

Table 24-2 Conditions for Which POCT May Improve Patient Treatment Time or Disposition

Chest pain
Congestive cardiac failure
Respiratory disorders, e.g., breathlessness
Metabolic or electrolyte disorders
Altered consciousness
Ectopic pregnancy
Conditions with associated hemorrhage, e.g., trauma, gastrointestinal bleeding
Some overdoses and poisonings, e.g., acetaminophen (paracetamol), salicylate, digoxin, carbon monoxide
Fever of unknown origin
Suspected hypoglycemia
Acute renal failure
Suspected deep-vein thrombosis or pulmonary embolism with low or moderate clinical risk
Pancreatitis
Generalized weakness
Tetany

Table 24-3 Tests Used for Management of ED Patients That Should Be Considered for POCT

Diagnosis	POC tests[a]	Supplementary tests
Suspected myocardial infarction	Myoglobin, CK-MB, TnI/TnT, FBC/CBC, glucose, Na$^+$, K$^+$, PT, aPTT	
Syncope	Na$^+$, K$^+$, glucose, urea/creatinine, FBC/CBC	
Congestive heart failure	BNP/NT-proBNP	
Cerebrovascular accident/ ischemic stroke	Glucose, FBC/CBC, PT, aPTT	
Delirium	Na$^+$, K$^+$, glucose, FBC/CBC, urea/creatinine, Ca^{2+}, urinalysis, arterial pH, P_{O_2}, P_{CO_2}, O$_2$ saturation	Ethanol/toxicology
Seizure	Glucose, Na$^+$, K$^+$, Ca^{2+}, anticonvulsants, Mg^{2+}, LFTs	
Diabetic ketoacidosis	Arterial pH, P_{O_2}, P_{CO_2}, O$_2$ saturation, Na$^+$, K$^+$, glucose, ketones	FBC/CBC, cultures
Abdominal pain	Amylase, glucose, FBC/CBC, urinalysis, LFTs	
Acute cholecystitis or ascending cholangitis	Amylase, FBC/CBC, LFTs	Blood cultures
Appendicitis	FBC/CBC, urinalysis	Urine cultures
Pancreatitis	Amylase, glucose, AST/ALT, urea, creatinine, FBC/CBC, P_{O_2}, T_{CO_2}, Ca^{2+}	Blood cultures
Vomiting	Na$^+$, K$^+$, Cl$^-$, T_{CO_2}, urea, creatinine, glucose, FBC/CBC	LFTs
Osteomyelitis	CRP, FBC/CBC	Tissue and blood cultures
Pediatric fever of unknown origin	FBC/CBC, urinalysis	Blood and urine cultures
Pneumonia	Arterial pH, P_{O_2}, P_{CO_2}, FBC/CBC, urea, creatinine, CRP	Blood cultures
Necrotising fasciitis	FBC/CBC, Na$^+$, K$^+$, urea/creatinine	Tissue and blood cultures
Pyelonephritis	Na$^+$, K$^+$, urea/creatinine, urinalysis, FBC/CBC	Blood and urine cultures
Sepsis	FBC/CBC, urinalysis, glucose, urea/creatinine, LFTs, PT, aPTT, D-dimer, LFTs	Blood cultures
Acute renal failure	Urea/creatinine, Na$^+$, K$^+$, Cl$^-$, T_{CO_2}, glucose, Ca^{2+}, FBC/CBC, urinalysis	Urine microscopy
Nephrolithiasis with renal colic	Urea/creatinine, FBC/CBC, urinalysis	Urine cultures
Ectopic pregnancy	Hemoglobin, hematocrit, urinary β-hCG	β-hCG, Type ± cross-match
Preeclampsia	AST/ALT, bilirubin, urea/creatinine, FBC/CBC, urinalysis, glucose, PT, aPTT, Mg^{2+}, urate	
Pulmonary embolus	Arterial pH, P_{O_2}, P_{CO_2}, O$_2$ saturation, D-dimer	
Acetaminophen (paracetamol) overdose	Acetaminophen, AST/ALT, PT, aPTT, urea/creatinine, glucose, Na$^+$, K$^+$, bilirubin	
Salicylate	Arterial pH, P_{O_2}, P_{CO_2}, Na$^+$, K$^+$, urea/creatinine, glucose	
Digoxin	Digoxin, urea/creatinine, Na$^+$, K$^+$	
Carbon monoxide poisoning	COHb, arterial pH, P_{O_2}, P_{CO_2}, lactate	
Major trauma	FBC/CBC, urinalysis, urea/creatinine	Type and cross-match

[a] ALT, alanine aminotransferase; AST, aspartate aminotransferase; aPTT, activated partial thromboplastin time; CRP, C-reactive protein; LFT, liver function test; PT, prothrombin time; PTT, partial thromboplastin time; T_{CO_2}, total carbon dioxide content. Other abbreviations as in text.

cardiac, respiratory, and hepatic function. In many seriously ill patients, the monitoring of lactate is likely to form part of the continuing assessment of the patient (15).

Urea and/or Creatinine. Measurement of the patient's renal function may be useful for deciding on appropriate fluid therapy.

Glucose. Severe or prolonged hypoglycemia can lead to neurological damage. It is part of the differential diagnosis and investigation of altered consciousness and seizures. Rapid measurement of blood glucose can establish the diagnosis and ensure immediate treatment. It is commonly a consequence of an imbalance in insulin or oral hypoglycemic therapy in diabetic patients. Confirmation of hyperglycemia in diabetic ke-

toacidosis or hyperosmolar nonketotic coma, together with assessment of fluid balance, acid–base status, electrolytes, ketones, and renal function, can establish the diagnosis and ensure that appropriate treatment is given. Glucose can be measured together with other analyses on blood gas analyzers or equivalent critical care analyzers. Glucose can easily be measured separately with test-strip and meter systems. Parallel measurement of blood ketones can assist in optimizing the amount of insulin administered (16).

Bleeding and Indices of Clotting. Measurement of the cellular components of blood [i.e., the full (or complete) blood count (FBC or CBC)] can be of use in some circumstances. An elevated white cell count can provide evidence of infection of various types, which may be a cause of conditions such as pneumonia, delirium, or abdominal pain, but knowledge of the white cell count may not influence initial management. Measurement of the hemoglobin or red cell components in blunt trauma or ectopic pregnancy can indicate if severe bleeding is occurring. Clotting disturbances may occur in sepsis, trauma, malignancy, pregnancy, or shock and complicate patient management. Rapid measurement of coagulation markers may speed treatment.

Urine Testing. Simple and rapid urine dipstick testing can give semiquantitative information on red blood cells, ketones, leukocyte esterase, nitrites, and β-human chorionic gonadotrophin (β-hCG). It is useful for investigating urinary tract infection, hematuria, renal colic, and ectopic pregnancy, or for confirming pregnancy (17, 18).

Investigation of Specific Diagnoses

The role that POCT in the ED can play is outlined in the following for some of the conditions listed in Tables 24-2 and 24-3. As stated earlier, the tests are always part of a broader clinical assessment, but can help to establish the diagnosis or diagnoses, as well as the severity and the presence of complicating factors (19).

Acute Coronary Syndromes and Heart Failure. Biochemical markers are valuable in the assessment of cardiac ischemia, myocardial infarction, and heart failure. The analytes of use for assessing cardiac dysfunction are myoglobin, creatine kinase-MB (CK-MB), cardiac troponin-I (TnI), and cardiac troponin-T (TnT). Myoglobin is the earliest marker of necrosis (20). CK-MB is also an early marker (21). The troponin markers rise later but have high sensitivity and specificity for cardiac necrosis (22). Congestive heart failure can be investigated with B-type natriuretic peptide (BNP) and N-terminal pro-BNP (NT-proBNP). They can be used for the differential diagnosis of dyspnea and heart failure and may provide additional information to troponin for risk stratification in acute coronary syndromes (23). Many studies have been performed to establish the value of the cardiac markers for diagnosis, risk stratification, prognosis, and rule-out, using both POCT and laboratory testing. BNP has been proposed as a useful POC test in the ED for the investigation of dyspnea (24). A detailed discussion of these tests is the subject of another chapter.

Diabetic Ketoacidosis. Acid–base, fluid, and electrolyte disturbances can be investigated with arterial whole blood specimens on blood gas analyzer–type instruments. Blood glucose can be measured on the same system or with dedicated glucose meters and test strips. Ketones, preferably β-hydroxybutyrate in blood, can be measured with a test strip and meter. The ketones reflect the degree of metabolic decompensation and may influence the insulin dose administered (16). Other tests are required to investigate possible precipitating factors, particularly infections. Specimens for blood cultures, urine/sputum microscopy and culture, and throat and wound swabs can be taken but are unlikely to influence the initial management of the metabolic abnormalities. A rapidly

available FBC or CBC could give an early indication of infection if the white cell count was elevated, although it rises in response to stress. A normal white cell count would indicate the need to search for other precipitating causes.

Abdominal Pain. Investigation of the causes of abdominal pain can be variously assisted by measurement of glucose, urea, and electrolytes to assess fluid and electrolyte status; FBC or CBC for blood loss or infection; and cardiac markers, amylase, and liver function tests to investigate the origin of the pain. Urinalysis with microscopy followed by urine culture is useful for urinary tract–related causes. In suspected acute pancreatitis, useful initial tests are amylase, arterial blood gases, glucose, FBC or CBC, urea and creatinine, calcium, and liver function tests. Coagulation tests are useful if complications are suspected (25).

Pulmonary Embolus. Pulmonary embolus (PE) is difficult to diagnose clinically. Useful initial investigations are arterial blood gas and oxygen saturation tests, electrocardiogram (ECG), and chest x-ray. Patients at low or intermediate risk of PE can usefully be tested with a rapid but laboratory-quality test for D-dimer, a degradation product of circulating cross-linked fibrin (26). In those patients who are not at high risk, a low D-dimer level rules out PE. Patients with an elevated D-dimer level require further investigation with ventilation-perfusion pulmonary scans or computerized tomography. These time-consuming and relatively expensive investigations can thereby be avoided in patients in whom D-dimer testing rules out PE.

Acute Renal Failure. Acute renal failure causes electrolye and acid–base disturbances. A potentially serious complication is severe hyperkalemia, causing cardiac arrhythmias which can be monitored by ECG. Hyperkalemia can be detected rapidly by POCT and appropriate treatment can be initiated. Other electrolyte and acid–base abnormalities can be investigated with the blood gas analyzer-type instruments used to measure potassium and, if necessary, stabilized prior to dialysis.

Complications of Early Pregnancy. Vaginal bleeding may occur in uterine pregnancy or in ectopic pregnancy. A urinary or blood β-hCG pregnancy test and hemoglobin or hematocrit reading to assess blood loss can be done rapidly by POCT. Resuscitation and referral must not be delayed by waiting for investigations. If the pregnancy test is positive, the patient should be blood-typed and cross-matched. An ultrasound scan is performed if there is clinical suspicion of ectopic pregnancy.

Trauma. A study evaluating the treatment of trauma patients using the central laboratory or a limited test repertoire on a POC microanalyzer showed that the POC repertoire of hemoglobin, hematocrit, electrolytes, glucose, calcium, and arterial blood gas measurement was sufficient for the evaluation of most trauma patients (27). In a prospective noninterventional study of the management of major trauma, hemoglobin, blood gas, lactate, and glucose testing were found on some occasions to possibly reduce morbidity or conserve resources, whereas electrolyte and urea testing did not (28).

Toxicology. The management of toxicology cases in the ED covers a wide range of possible agents. In some instances, the measurement of the substance is necessary to guide therapy. In others, the treatment is supportive, and accurate measurement of the substance is not an essential prerequisite. Practice guidelines for toxicology testing in the ED have been published recently (29). The expert committee proposed that the laboratory should be able to provide results on serum or plasma within 1 h for acetaminophen, lithium, salicylate, theophylline, valproate, carbamazepine, digoxin, phenobarbital, iron, transferrin, and ethanol. Urine tests for the commonly abused drugs cocaine, opiates, barbiturates, amphetamines, propoxyphene, phencyclidine, and tricyclic antidepressants should also be available, but they have lower urgency than serum assays, do not correlate well with clinical effects, and suffer from sensitivity and specificity problems. Tricyclic antidepressant results have significant specificity limitations and require careful interpretation alongside clinical information. The need for STAT qualitative urine assays was questioned by many participating ED physicians. A major conclusion was that improved assays are required for the commonly abused amphetamines, benzodiazepines, and opioids, and for tricyclic antidepressants. For possible drugs-of-abuse toxicity, the rapid immunoassays for testing urine concentrations cannot be relied on because of their inherent limitations of sensitivity and specificity (29). Many physicians are not aware of these limitations, particularly the problems with cross-reactivity (30). Treatment is supportive, and it is not essential to identify the substances at this point. Reliance on a rapid but unconfirmed result may lead to misdiagnosis and subsequent inappropriate treatment. However, the more reliable chromatographic methods currently available in laboratories can take much longer than is practicable for patient assessment in the ED, but they do provide definitive results to guide subsequent patient management (31).

Ethanol can conveniently be tested in breath, urine, or blood. Breath alcohol measurement is convenient and rapid but must be covered by the laboratory's quality assurance program. Knowledge of the patient's ethanol reading may assist in determining the cause of presenting signs and symptoms. A low ethanol reading may direct attention to other etiologies and diagnostic procedures. In cases of head injury with suspected alcohol ingestion, it is not safe to assume that ethanol accounts for altered consciousness, and the presence of ethanol should not lead to underinvestigation of the head injury. Rapid confirmation of methanol or ethylene glycol ingestion would be valuable information for initiating therapy, but there are no rapid methods available for ED use. Investigation by measurement of the osmolar gap is not very reliable, particularly in the presence of ethanol. An assessment of the metabolic state can be made with measurements of blood pH, gases, and lactate, which are all possible in the ED.

Knowledge of acetaminophen concentration is essential for making treatment decisions, but 4 h must elapse after ingestion before it is measured. There is a therapeutic window of several hours beyond this point. Therefore, more rapid acetaminophen measurement in the ED may add little to treatment decisions. Routine screening for acetaminophen has been proposed, but there are no outcome studies to demonstrate this provides medical benefit or is cost-effective. Salicylate overdose usually presents with characteristic symptoms, and a respiratory alkalosis or metabolic acidosis that can be investigated with a blood gas analyzer. The diagnosis can be confirmed by measurement of salicylate levels in blood, but the signs and symptoms may provide sufficient evidence to initiate treatment. This is directed at correcting the metabolic disturbances, ensuring adequate hydration, reducing salicylate absorption, and increasing its elimination. Prognosis is influenced by the metabolic effects rather than the measured salicylate concentration.

Iron overdose presents with nonspecific gastrointestinal and cardiac symptoms, but the history and clinical examination are important for identifying the cause. The laboratory should provide a rapid serum or plasma iron assay on a specimen taken before administration of a chelating agent, as it may interfere in colorimetric iron assays. An assessment of free iron can be made by measuring transferrin in the laboratory. In suspected digoxin toxicity, the ECG is recorded and the potassium and creatinine or urea concentrations measured. The potassium concentration should be monitored regularly. The digoxin concentration can be measured by immunoassay but is less urgent. In suspected lithium toxicity, the serum lithium concentration can be measured by ion-selective electrode (ISE) in the laboratory. Carbon monoxide poisoning can be investigated by measuring blood carboxyhemoglobin levels, but this does not correlate well with clinical features. Any resulting tissue hypoxia can be assessed with arterial blood gas measurements. In conscious patients, carbon monoxide can also be readily measured in expired air with a breath carbon monoxide meter.

Toxicological assays have a role to play in the management of patients in the ED, but in most cases acute management decisions are based on vital signs and mental status. Although POCT assays with improved performance may become available, the laboratory will continue to provide essential analytical support. Improvements in specimen transport and reporting are important and require attention to achieve the 1-h TATs demanded.

ANALYTICAL APPROACHES TO TESTS THAT MAY INFLUENCE PATIENT OUTCOMES OR IMPROVE ED THROUGHPUT

POCT Analyzers

Tests that are of value in the treatment of patients in the ED are listed in Table 24-4, grouped according to the type of instrument or test format in which they are usually used. Some of the tests are available in more than one format. For example, glucose is available as a channel on blood gas analyzers and as a test strip read on a dedicated handheld meter. The table is not exhaustive, and a detailed description can be found elsewhere (32). The available repertoire is changing rapidly, further increasing the options for POCT in the ED.

Table 24-4   Assay Presentation for Tests that May Influence Outcome or Speed ED Throughput[a]

1. Available as POC tests on sophisticated benchtop, portable, or handheld cartridge-based analyzers
   pH, Po_2, Pco_2, COHb
   O_2 saturation
   Cooximetry
   Hemoglobin, hematocrit, FBC/CBC
   Na^+, K^+, Cl^-, TCO_2 (bicarbonate), anion gap
   iCa^{2+}
   Glucose[b]
   Lactate
   Creatinine
   Bilirubin
   Urea
   iMg^{2+}
   White cell count
   D-dimer
   ACT
   Myoglobin, CK-MB, TnI, TnT
2. Available as POC tests in cartridge or strip format read with dedicated devices or by eye
   BNP, NT-proBNP
   Myoglobin, CK-MB, TnI, TnT
   PT, aPTT
   INR
   Blood ketones (β-hydroxybutyrate)
   Acetaminophen
   Breath, saliva, or blood ethanol
   Urine β-hCG
   Urinalysis [leukocyte esterase, nitrite, ketones, glucose, protein, albumin (as ratio to creatinine)]
   Drugs-of-abuse screening tests
   Digoxin
   CRP
3. Available in benchtop analyzers in a POCT format that requires operators to have laboratory competencies
   ALT, AST, ALP
   Amylase
4. Not readily available in POCT format but can be measured in the laboratory
   Salicylate
   Iron
   Lithium
   Fibrinogen
   Ethylene glycol, methanol
   Theophylline

[a] ALP, alkaline phosphotransferase; ALT, alanine aminotransferase; aPTT, activated partial thromboplastin time; AST, aspartate aminotransferase; CRP, complement-reactive protein; INR, international normalized ratio; PTT, partial thromboplastin time. Other abbreviations as in text.
[b] Glucose is commonly measured in the format of test strip and dedicated handheld device (category 2).

The first group comprises blood gas analyzers or cartridge-based systems. These analyzers give laboratory-quality results. They have comprehensive electronic data interfaces compliant with current standards. The results can be readily integrated into the hospital electronic patient record system. The test repertoires vary between suppliers, but the core tests for pH, blood gases, hemoglobin and hematocrit, glucose, and lactate are available on nearly all instruments. They are designed for easy introduction of the specimen, which is whole blood. Many instruments can measure additional tests by adding extra electrode modules or by using a different single-use multitest cartridge. This flexibility may enable the repertoire available in the ED to be changed without the obstacle of funding a completely new instrument with high capital costs.

The second category comprises POC tests in cartridge or strip format with a dedicated reading device that can objectively determine the result and transmit necessary data to the laboratory. These include the patient's test result and associated quality-control results, the user, and the date, time, and location. Some tests may also be read by eye. This is much less desirable because of the risk of human error in obtaining the result and documenting it. Many of the tests in this second category are immunoassays presented in POC format for rapid and easy use. As is the case with all immunoassays, cross-reactivity, sensitivity, and cutoff values must be established before the assays are introduced. The POCT assay performance may differ from that of the counterpart assay in the laboratory, and it is essential that the clinical significance of any differences between the assays are fully understood by ED and laboratory staff involved in interpreting results. The capital cost of the dedicated instruments is often relatively low, but depends on the range of features incorporated to simplify use and to manage the test-associated data.

Tests in the third and fourth categories require more complex instrumentation, requiring the user to have some degree of laboratory skills to carry out the POC test, or are more appropriately measured in the laboratory. POCT versions of some of these assays are likely to become available, and their role in improving patient care will require evaluation.

Selection of the POCT Repertoire

It is difficult to define a minimum set of tests that it is strictly necessary to have available in the ED. Several analytical systems with different procedures for use are likely to be required. This has implications for ED operator training, laboratory supervision, and maintenance. If adding more tests to the existing repertoire is being considered, the flexibility to change the repertoire afforded by many POCT systems means that in practice this may be possible without replacing the analyzer or reader. However, if a wider POCT repertoire involves the introduction of additional analytical platforms there will be significant cost and workforce implications for ED operator training, laboratory supervision, and maintenance costs (6, 33). These considerations must be evaluated locally at the planning stage.

Analytical Performance of POCT Analyzers

Ideally, the performance of a test should be good enough to meet the medical use to which it will be applied, irrespective of the type of assay or the setting where it is carried out. POCT methods are designed to produce rapid results using low volumes of specimen, commonly whole blood. The results produced by modern POCT systems are often operator independent after minimal training (34). However, the attainment of increased speed or convenience must not unduly affect the precision, bias, limit of detection, or measuring range of the test (35). The design characteristics of an assay required to make it suitable for a POCT setting may affect its performance relative to laboratory methods, emphasizing the need for careful assessment in the actual clinical setting (36, 37, 38). In general, the performance characteristics for bias and precision can be based on the known within-subject and between-subject variation for each analyte. If a test is to be used for repeated monitoring of an individual patient, the analytical variation should be small relative to the intraindividual variation. The widely accepted figure of an analytical variation of 50% of the intraindividual variation gives an added variability due to assay imprecision of ~10%. The contribution to the error resulting from other degrees of analytical variability can be predicted (39). Differences in bias between assays used jointly for sequential monitoring influence the ability to distinguish genuine changes in an analyte. A commonly accepted figure is one-quarter of the group biological variation (40). Generally applicable data for components of biological variation for a wide range of analytes are available (41), so that the effects of POCT and laboratory assay variability and bias on assay utility can be assessed. Other approaches for assessing assay performance are based on the recommendations of professional groups, regulatory bodies, or external quality assessment schemes, but they tend to have empirical or subjective components (35). For POC tests giving a positive/negative answer the decision point must be known, as it will determine the division of patients. If such a test is used as a first-line test to select for further testing in the laboratory, the implications for the number of further tests should be assessed.

It is important that the laboratory should address the analytical performance of complementary laboratory and POCT tests because they can influence the management of patients. Observed discrepancies between the POCT and laboratory methods can undermine clinicians' confidence in results and lead to additional testing, causing delays in treatment, wasted staff time, and additional costs.

MEASURING THE BENEFITS OF POCT IN THE ED

Physicians' Impressions and Opinions

ED physicians' perception that laboratory TATs are inadequate is long-standing and widespread. In Q-probe surveys of potassium and hemoglobin, TAT has not improved significantly over many years (2). Large hospitals had longer TATs than small hospitals. Specimen type had a significant effect, with results on serum 8 min slower than those on plasma, which were 22 min slower than for whole blood for potassium results. In a questionnaire, 61% of ED physicians thought that laboratory TAT delayed patient length of stay "always," "usually," or

"often," and more than 40% perceived that laboratory TAT delays similarly delayed treatment. The satisfaction rankings from ED physicians were lower than from other specialties. Pneumatic tube use is increasing, but TATs do not show a corresponding reduction. This clearly illustrates that specimen transport has to be actively managed across the hospital for optimum efficiency, particularly if components of the transport process are not directly managed by the laboratory. Satellite laboratories with relatively low throughput may induce delays when an influx of specimens saturates capacity, leading to queues (42). It is clear that laboratories should engage in schemes for continuous quality improvement in collaboration with ED staff and other hospital staff who can assist. It may be relevant that, more than other physicians, ED physicians tend to define TAT as ending when the result reaches the ED rather than the physician (2). This could have implications for the speed with which results are acted on when received in the ED. Appropriate use of electronic transmission can ensure the delivery of results to the optimum locations and individuals. However, as Kilpatrick and Holding (43) showed in an elegant study, even when electronic transmission of results to the ED is implemented, this is no guarantee that the ED physicians will access and act on the results. In their audit study they showed that more than 40% of results were never accessed after the introduction of electronic transmission.

Formal Outcome Studies of POCT in the ED

The Q-probe surveys give a picture that combines objective measures of TAT and subjective assessments of the value of POCT. Other studies have supported the clinicians' view that POCT is useful. Hutsko (44) used the i-STAT (i-STAT Corporation, East Windsor, NJ, USA) for testing patients with metabolic and electrolyte disorders, trauma, gastrointestinal bleeding, cardiac and respiratory disorders, and sepsis. Its use was at the physician's discretion, amounting to 5–10% of tests, with 90–95% sent to the central laboratory. The tests were thought to improve patient care, but no formal investigation was done. A number of studies have formally assessed the value of POCT in the ED, measuring apparent benefits in many different ways, often assessing TAT and the effect on clinical decisions or patient outcomes. Study designs have ranged from physician surveys of theoretical results through retrospective studies to prospective randomized controlled trials. It is instructive to review the studies that have been done to investigate the effects on TAT, clinical decision making, treatment outcomes, and the economic impact. It is also worth examining ways to perform further useful studies that will guide the implementation of POCT alongside traditional laboratory testing for the ED. Potential measures of outcome that have been used and could be applied to future studies are given in Table 24-5.

Effect on TAT

Tsai et al. (10) carried out a prospective observational study of patients presenting to the ED and found the test TAT with

Table 24-5   Measures of Outcome for Assessing the Value of POCT in the ED and the Institution

Clinical—within the ED
  Proportion of patients in whom POCT changed
    management in ED
  Proportion of Patients in whom POCT speeded time to
    initiation of treatment
Clinical—all episodes of care
  Length of stay in hospital
    Time to discharge from ED
    Time to transfer to another clinical unit
  Mortality
Clinical—ED and laboratory components
  Admission rates from ED
  Patient's total time in ED
  Therapeutic turnaround time (i.e., from test order to
    implementation of management decision or treatment)
    comprising phases a + b + c + e + f or a + d + e + f.
  Testing process phases:
    a. Test order to specimen collection
    b. Specimen collection to receipt in laboratory
    c. Specimen receipt in laboratory to result availability on
       ED
    d. Specimen collection to POCT result availability
    e. Result availability to management decision/treatment
    f. Management/treatment decision to implementation
Satisfaction
  Physician
  Patient
  Nurse
Economic
  Cost of POC tests
  Sum of POC plus laboratory test costs
  Sum of all laboratory and ED-related costs
  Total cost of hospital stay

POCT (8 min) was much faster than in the central laboratory (59 min). The physicians reported that POCT, independent of other rate-limiting steps, would have resulted in earlier therapeutic action in 19% of patients. Frankel et al. (27) found the TAT with POCT was 6 min compared to 64 min for the central laboratory. Sands et al. (9) carried out a prospective nonrandomized study comparing POCT with the central laboratory. Those treating the patients were provided only with the central laboratory results. POCT results for the range of analytes tested would have been available 31 to 44 min sooner than the laboratory results. The physicians thought that the POCT results would have led to earlier therapy in 9.5% of cases. However, decisions to discharge or admit were based on laboratory results for only 10.7% of patients, and none of the patient clinical outcomes would have been influenced by POC testing. Saxena and Wong (45) recognized that the process of testing is subject to delays at many stages, including the time taken by physicians to review the results. They suggested that continuous quality improvement programs should be implemented. A study by Fleisher and Schwartz (46) also illustrated the importance of ensuring that all stages of the specimen

transport are optimized. Mohammad et al. (47) improved the TAT of satellite laboratories. Kendall et al. (3), in a prospective randomized controlled trial of 1728 patients, confirmed that POCT markedly reduced TAT. Van Heyningen et al. (48) investigated a blood gas analyzer profile and Ng et al. (49), McCord et al. (50), and Altinier et al. (37) studied cardiac markers; all observed shorter TATs. This was perceived as improving the working efficiency of the ED.

Effect on Clinical Decision Making and Outcomes

Some of these studies and a number of others have been performed to investigate whether the faster TAT leads to improved clinical decision making or patient outcomes. Tsai et al. (10) and Sands et al. (9) used retrospective physician surveys. This study design is not very reliable, but they found that patient treatment would have been influenced in 19% and 9.5% of cases, respectively. The prospective randomized controlled trial of Kendall et al. (3) found that in the POCT arm of the trial, treatment of 14% of the 859 patients was influenced by POCT, and 7% of the 859 patients received time-critical changes in management. Decisions in the POCT arm were made 86 min earlier for urea, electrolytes, glucose, and hemoglobin and 21 min earlier for blood gases. These findings confirm the observations of the earlier studies.

However, the faster treatment does not readily translate into improved outcomes. Parvin et al. (8) performed a large prospective study with consecutive laboratory testing and POCT phases, measuring urea, electrolytes, and glucose. They found that the length of stay in the two phases was not significantly different (209 vs. 201 min, respectively). Van Heyningen et al. (48) reached the same conclusion. Similarly, Kendall et al. (3) found no differences between the laboratory and POC testing groups in the time spent in the ED (188 min for POCT vs. 193 min for laboratory testing). There were also no differences in hospital length of stay, admission rates, or mortality. They concluded that in their ED the rapid provision of test results was not a rate-determining step in transferring patients to other wards. The hospital length of stay was taken as a surrogate marker for patient morbidity in the heterogeneous ED population, implying that the earlier treatment did not influence patient recovery. They propose that significant benefits may be observed if specific patient subgroups are studied. A smaller randomized controlled trial by Murray et al. (51) found that the 93 patients randomized to POCT had a significantly shorter overall median ED length of stay of 208 min, compared to 262 min for the 87 patients whose specimens were tested in the laboratory. However, for the patients admitted to hospital, the length of stay in the ED was defined as the interval between triage and the time at which the admission decision was made by the consulting physician and did not take into account the additional factors influencing the management of patients. There was a significantly shorter length of stay for patients who were to be discharged home from the ED (185 min for POCT vs. 257 min for laboratory testing). This is an important finding, as they comprised 72% of the POCT group and 78% of the laboratory tested group. However, for the patients who were admitted there was no difference in median length of stay. The POCT test repertoire in this study was urea, creatinine, electrolytes, total CO_2, glucose, hematocrit, qualitative CK-MB, and myoglobin. The authors noted that with these tests the proportion of patients who could be tested with POC tests alone was quite small. In an assessment of accelerated critical treatment pathways for chest pain evaluation, Ng et al. (49) found that POCT for myoglobin, CK-MB, and TnI contributed to decreased CCU admissions and improved the appropriate discharge home of low-risk patients. Altinier et al. (37) found that POCT cardiac markers contributed to faster discharge of a small number of patients, which was thought to be a useful benefit. Di Serio et al. (52) found that POCT for cardiac markers improved the TAT and the triage process. Lee-Lewandrowski et al. (53) found that providing urine hCG, simple urinalysis by dipstick, and CK-MB and troponin results from a POCT satellite laboratory reduced the length of stay when the influence of these tests was combined.

Costs of Implementing POCT

Implementing POCT is likely to incur additional costs to the organization if the fixed costs associated with existing staffing and infrastructure for the central laboratory remain, as is likely (7). On the other hand, if POCT leads to outcome benefits such as faster discharge home, decreased length of stay, decreased morbidity, or increased patient throughput in the ED the additional testing costs are likely to be small in comparison to the benefits. The practice of departmental or "silo" budgeting, which only considers departmental costs in isolation and does not consider the whole process, complicates the assessment of overall financial benefits to the organization. The treatment and efficiency benefits may be apparent in the clinical units but the additional expenditure is incurred by the laboratory. Only an analysis of the entire process will reveal this clearly.

Several of the studies discussed above (10, 27, 36, 47, 48) and others (54, 55) have attempted to assess the relative cost of laboratory testing and POCT. It is apparent that organizational structures, laboratory services, and working practice differ markedly between institutions, such that conclusions on cost benefits are not readily transferable. Each hospital must carry out its own economic analysis to set alongside the clinical benefits (56). As discussed below, convincing evidence of financial benefit may be gained without a detailed knowledge of the costs, which is difficult to achieve (57–60). Patients admitted from the ED receive care in many units and specialties, which complicates the assessment of costs.

Performing Outcome Studies in the ED

Kendall et al. (3) suggested that the patient mix in their ED study is representative of that found in other hospitals. They propose that their findings, in conjunction with relatively small studies, can be used to interpret the consequences of implementing POCT in other hospitals where the provision of central laboratory testing is different from theirs. However, Murray et al. (51) noted the difficulty of controlling for the many factors that can influence patient management decisions in a complex organization. Asimos (28) commented on the difficulties of establishing the true effect of POCT on emergent diagnostic and therapeutic interventions. It is clear that the design of suitable studies to establish any benefits of POCT in our own institutions requires careful consideration. The application of techniques for performing outcome studies to healthcare has recently become more common, and general guidance is available (61, 62). The particular complexities of outcomes assessment for POCT have been recognized, and careful thought must be applied to study design. Rainey (63) presented some practical principles, listed in Table 24-6, in response to a well-designed outcome study of therapeutic TAT in a tertiary care teaching hospital (64). The assessment of institution-specific factors is especially important. The increasing use of practice guidelines and care paths should help to strengthen the link between results and interventions (65). Assessment of costs is difficult but a full analysis may not be necessary to reach useful conclusions. It may be possible to select a setting in which an intrinsic financial value is associated with other positive outcomes such as decreased length of stay (57). Practically useful information may be obtained from relatively small studies, and may require the active application of audit principles to the complex processes involved (58).

FUTURE DEVELOPMENTS

Developments in continuous monitoring in vivo for well-established analytes such as glucose or urea could bring laboratory tests to new levels of convenience and clinical utility. New analytes will require an assessment of whether the tests are really appropriate for ED use or for later care on other units. As an illustration, the protein S-100B shows potential as a rapid serum marker for cerebral injury and has possible applicability to the ED. A small study showed that the serum concentration of S-100B was related to outcome. The results were time dependent, with the best information obtained from early sampling (66). Several other studies have reached similar conclu-

Table 24-6   How to Perform Outcome Studies in ED

1. Carry out an observational study.
2. Carry out a prospective study.
3. Limit the study to a single well-defined procedure.
4. Use management protocols and clinical pathways to obtain standardized interventions.
5. Use outcome measures that can be quantified.
6. Use outcome measures with close temporal proximity to the testing event.
7. Use outcomes that may be surrogates for longer term outcomes.
8. Choose outcomes with an intrinsic financial value.
9. Identify institution-specific factors that may have affected the results.

From (63).

sions (67). These characteristics would be appropriate for a POCT application, but further work needs to be done to assess its role in decision making in the diagnosis and management of cerebral damage. The availability of a reliable laboratory assay (68) will help to elucidate its value, the optimum time for testing and the relative merit of using it at the point of care.

The development of new technologies will present further opportunities to assess the value of POCT in the ED. Analyzers with broader potential repertoires will enable POCT to be applied to more patients without the need for supplementary laboratory tests in the initial assessment and patient stabilization. The current drive to consolidation of laboratory instrumentation contrasts with the present proliferation of instruments and devices for POCT. Developments in device-readable autoidentification and instrument connectivity should improve the integration of POCT with the central laboratory service. Developments in ward ordering, pneumatic tube systems, and preanalytical automation in the laboratory will reduce laboratory TAT, at the least contributing to faster delivery of follow up tests that may influence patient disposition after initial treatment. Better knowledge management to support clinicians' use of results will increase their clinical value.

The laboratory must be closely involved with clinical colleagues in many specialties to ensure that new developments are introduced appropriately for cost effective improvements in patient care. Appropriate education and training of all those involved is necessary to derive the full benefits.

Acknowledgments

I am grateful to Dr. R. Pullinger and Dr. M. Darwent of the Emergency Department at the John Radcliffe Hospital, Oxford, for their invaluable advice in the preparation of this chapter.

REFERENCES

1. Valenstein P. Can we satisfy clinicians' demands for faster service? Should we try? Am J Clin Pathol 1989;91:705–6.
2. Steindel SJ, Howanitz. Physician satisfaction and emergency department laboratory test turnaround time. Arch Pathol Lab Med 2001;125:863–71.
3. Kendall J, Reeves B, Clancy M. Point of care testing: randomised controlled trial of clinical outcome. Br Med J 1998;316:1052–7.
4. Drenck N-E. Point of care testing in critical care medicine: the clinician's view. Clin Chim Acta 2001;307:3–7.
5. Murphy MJ, Paterson JR. Point-of-care testing: no pain, no gain. Q J Med 2001;94:571–3.
6. Jahn UR, Van Aken H. Near-patient testing—point-of-care or point of costs and convenience? Br J Anaesth 2003;90:425–7.
7. Kendall JM. The emergency department. In: Price CP, Hicks JM, eds. Point-of-care testing. Washington: AACC Press, 1999:337–58.
8. Parvin CA, Lo SF, Deuser SM, Weaver LG, Lewis LM, Scott MG. Impact of point-of-care testing on patients' length of stay in a large emergency department. Clin Chem 1996;42:711–7.
9. Sands VM, Auerbach PS, Birnbaum J, Green M. Evaluation of a portable blood analyzer in the emergency department. Acad Emerg Med 1995;2:172–8.
10. Tsai W, Nash DB, Seamonds B, Weir GJ. Point-of-care versus central laboratory testing: an economic analysis in an academic medical center. Clin Ther 1994;16:898–910.
11. Bourke SE, Kirk JD, Kost GJ. Point of-care testing in emergency medicine. In: Kost GJ, ed. Principles & practice of point-of-care testing. Philadelphia: Lippincott Williams &Wilkins, 2002:99–118.
12. Bakker J, Schieveld SSJ, Brinkert W. Using point-of-care lactate to predict patient outcomes. In: Kost GJ, ed. Principles & practice of point-of-care testing. Philadelphia: Lippincott Williams & Wilkins, 2002:567–76.
13. Pittard A. Does blood lactate measurement have a role in the management of the critically ill patient? Ann Clin Biochem 1999;36:401–7.
14. Stacpoole PW, Wright EC, Baumgartner TG, Bersin RM, Buchalter S, Curry SH et al. Natural history and course of acquired lactic acidosis in adults. DCA-Lactic Acidosis Study Group. Am J Med 1994;97:47–54.
15. Holloway PAH. Point of-care testing in intensive care. In: Kost GJ, ed. Principles & practice of point-of-care testing. Philadelphia: Lippincott Williams &Wilkins, 2002:133–56.
16. Wallace TM, Meston NM, Gardner SG, Matthews DR. The hospital and home use of a 30-second hand-held blood ketone meter: guidelines for clinical practice. Diabet Med 2001;18:640–5.
17. Jou WW, Powers RD. Utility of urinalysis as a guide to management of adults with suspected infection or hematuria. South Med J 1998;91:266–9.
18. O'Connor RE, Bibro CM, Pegg PJ, Bouzoukis JK. The comparative sensitivity and specificity of serum and urine HCG determinations in the ED. Am J Emerg Med 1993;11:434–6.
19. Wyatt JP, Illingworth RN, Clancy MJ, Munro P, Robertson CE, eds. Oxford handbook of accident and emergency medicine. Oxford: Oxford University Press, 1999:782pp.
20. De Lemos JA, Morrow DA, Gibson CM, Murphy SA, Sabatine MS, Rifai N, et al. The prognostic value of serum myoglobin in patients with non-ST-segment elevation acute coronary syndromes. Results from the TIMI 11B and TACTICS-TIMI 18 studies. J Am Coll Cardiol 2002;40:238–44.
21. Wu AH, Lane PL. Metaanalysis in clinical chemistry: validation of cardiac troponin T as a marker for ischemic heart diseases. Clin Chem 1995;41:1228–33.
22. Alpert JS, Thygesen K, Antman E, Bassand JP. Myocardial infarction redefined—a consensus document of the Joint European Society of Cardiology/American College of Cardiology Committee for the Redefinition of Myocardial Infarction. J Am Coll Cardiol 2000;36:959–69.
23. Cowie MR, Jourdain P, Maisel A, Dahlstrom U, Follath F, Isnard R, et al. Clinical applications of B-type natriuretic peptide (BNP) testing. Eur Heart J 2003;24:1710–8.
24. Mueller C, Scholer A, Laule-Kilian K, Martina B, Schindler C, Buser P, et al. Use of B-type natriuretic peptide in the evaluation and management of acute dyspnea. N Engl J Med 2004;350:647–54.
25. Nagurney JT, Brown DFM, Chang Y, Sane S, Wang AC, Weiner JB. Use of diagnostic testing in the emergency department for patients presenting with non-traumatic abdominal pain. J Emerg Med 2003;25:363–71.
26. Sadosty AT, Goyal DG, Boie ET, Chiu CK. Emergency department D-dimer testing. J Emerg Med 2001;21:423–9.
27. Frankel HL, Royzicki GS, Ochsner MG, McCabe JE, Harviel JD, Jeng JC, et al. Minimizing admission laboratory testing in trauma patients: use of a microanalyzer. J Trauma 1994;37:728–36.

28. Asimos AW, Gibbs MA, Marx JA, Jacobs DG, Erwin RJ, Norton HJ, et al. Value of point-of-care blood testing in emergent trauma management. J Trauma 2000;48:1101–8.

29. Wu AHB, McKay C, Broussard LA, Hoffman RS, Kwong TC, Moyer TP, et al. National Academy of Clinical Biochemistry laboratory medicine practice guidelines: recommendations for the use of laboratory tests to support poisoned patients who present to the emergency department. Clin Chem 2003;49:357–79.

30. Yang JM, Lewandrowski KB. Urine drugs of abuse testing at the point-of-care: clinical interpretation and programmatic considerations with specific reference to the Syva Rapid Test. Clin Chim Acta 2001;307:27–32.

31. George S, Braithwaite R. Use of on-site testing for drugs of abuse. Clin Chem 2002;48:1639–46.

32. Tang Z, Louie RF, Kost GJ. Principles and performance of point-of-care testing instruments. In: Kost GJ, ed. Principles & practice of point-of-care testing. Philadelphia: Lippincott Williams & Wilkins, 2002:67–92.

33. Fermann GJ, Suyama J. Point of care testing in the emergency department. J Emerg Med 2002;22:393–404.

34. Bingham D, Kendall J, Clancy M. The portable laboratory: an evaluation of the accuracy and reproducibility of i-STAT. Ann Clin Biochem 1999;36:66–71.

35. Fraser CG. Optimal analytical performance for point of care testing. Clin Chim Acta 2001;307:37–43.

36. Ng VL, Kraemer R, Hogan C, Eckman D, Siobal M. The rise and fall of i-STAT point-of-care blood gas testing in an acute care hospital. Am J Clin Pathol 2000;114:128–38.

37. Altinier S, Zaninotto M, Mion M, Carraro P, Rocco S, Tosato F, et al. Point-of-care testing of cardiac markers: results from an experience in an emergency department. Clin Chim Acta 2001;311:67–72.

38. Johi RR, Cross MH, Hansbro SD. Near-patient testing for coagulopathy after cardiac surgery. Br J Anaesth 2003;90:499–501.

39. Fraser CG, Hyltoft Petersen P, Libeer JC, Ricos C. Proposals for setting generally applicable quality goals solely based on biology. Ann Clin Biochem 1997;34:8–12.

40. Gowans EMS, Hyltoft Petersen P, Blaabjerg O, Horder M. Analytical goals for the acceptance of common reference intervals for laboratories throughout a geographical area. Scand J Clin Lab Invest 1988;48:757–64.

41. Sebastian-Gambaro MA, Liron-Hernandez FJ, Fuentes-Arderiu X. Intra- and inter-individual biological variability data bank. Eur J Clin Chem Clin Biochem 1997;35:845–52 [also available at www.westgard.com].

42. Steindel SJ, Novis DA. Using outlier events to monitor test turnaround time. Arch Pathol Lab Med 1999;123:607–14.

43. Kilpatrick ES, Holding S. Use of computer terminals on wards to access emergency test results; a retrospective audit. Br Med J 2001;322:1101–3.

44. Hutsko GM, Jones JB, Danielson L. Using point-of-care testing to speed patient care: one emergency department's experience. J Emerg Nurs 1995;21:408–12.

45. Saxena S, Wong ET. Does the emergency department need a dedicated stat laboratory? Am J Clin Pathol 1993;100:606–10.

46. Fleisher M, Schwartz M. Automated approaches to rapid-response testing. A comparative evaluation of point-of-care and centralized laboratory testing. Am J Clin Pathol 1995;104:S18–S25.

47. Mohammad AA, Summers H, Burchfield JA, Petersen JR, Bissell MG, Okorodudu AO. STAT turnaround time. Satellite and point-to-point testing. Lab Med 1996;27:684–8.

48. van Heyningen C, Watson ID, Morrice AE. Point-of-care testing outcomes in an emergency department [Letter]. Clin Chem 1999;45:437–8.

49. Ng SM, Krishnaswamy P, Morissey R, Clopton P, Fitzgerald R, Maisel AS. Ninety-minute accelerated critical pathway for chest pain evaluation. Am J Cardiol 2001;88:611–7.

50. McCord J, Nowak RM, McCullough PA, Foreback C, Borzak S, Tokarski G, et al. Ninety-minute exclusion of acute myocardial infarction by use of quantitative point-of-care testing of myoglobin and troponin I. Circulation 2001;104:1483–7.

51. Murray RP, Leroux M, Sabga E, Palatnick W, Ludwig L. Effect of point of care testing on length of stay in an adult emergency department. J Emerg Med 1999;17:811–4.

52. Di Serio F, Antonelli G, Trerotoli P, Tampoia M, Matarrese A, Pansini N. Appropriateness of point-of-care testing (POCT) in an emergency department. Clin Chim Acta 2003;333:185–9.

53. Lee-Lewandrowski E, Corboy D, Lewandrowski K, Sinclair J, McDermot S, Benzer TJ. Implementation of a point-of-care satellite laboratory in the emergency department of an academic medical center. Impact on test turnaround time and patient emergency department length of stay. Arch Pathol Lab Med 2003;127:456–60.

54. Tortella BJ, Lavery RF, Doran JV, Siegel JH. Precision, accuracy, and managed care implications of a hand-held whole blood analyzer in the prehospital setting. Am J Clin Pathol 1996;106:124–7.

55. Bailey TM, Topham TM, Wantz S, Grant M, Cox C, Jones D, et al. Laboratory process improvement through point-of-care testing. Jt Comm J Qual Improv 1997;23:362–80.

56. Kost GJ. Controlling economics, preventing errors, and optimizing outcomes in point-of-care testing. In: Kost GJ, ed. Principles & practice of point-of-care testing. Philadelphia: Lippincott Williams & Wilkins, 2002:577–600.

57. Scott MG. Faster is better—it's rarely that simple! Clin Chem 2000;46:441–2.

58. Nichols JH, Kickler TS, Dyer KL, Humbertson SK, Cooper PC, Maughan WL, et al. Clinical outcomes of point-of-care testing in the interventional radiology and invasive cardiology setting. Clin Chem 2000;46:543–50.

59. Statland BE, Brzys K. Evaluating STAT testing alternatives by calculating annual laboratory costs. Chest 1990;97:198S–203S.

60. De Cresce R, Phillips D, Howanitz P. Financial justification of alternate site testing. Arch Pathol Lab Med 1995;119:898–901.

61. Bruns DE. Laboratory-related outcomes in healthcare. Clin Chem 2001;47:1547–52.

62. Price CP. Point of care testing. Br Med J 2001;322:1285–8.

63. Rainey PM. Outcomes assessment for point-of-care testing. Clin Chem 1998;44:1595–6.

64. Kilgore ML, Steindel SJ, Smith JA. Evaluating stat testing options in an academic health center: therapeutic turnaround time and staff satisfaction. Clin Chem 1998;44:1597–1603.

65. Indrikovs AJ. The role of point-of-care testing in care paths. In: Kost GJ, ed. Principles & practice of point-of-care testing. Philadelphia: Lippincott Williams & Wilkins, 2002:543–53.

66. Jackson RG, Samra GS, Radcliffe J, Clark GH, Price CP. The early fall in levels of S-100 beta in traumatic brain injury. Clin Chem Lab Med 2000;38:1165–7.

67. Raabe A, Kopetsch O, Woszczyk A, Lang J, Gerlach R, Zimmermann M, Seifert V. Serum S-100B protein as a molecular marker in severe traumatic brain injury. Restor Neurol Neurosci 2003;21:159–69.

68. Biberthaler P, Mussack T, Kanz KG, Linsenmaier U, Pfeifer KJ, Mutschler W, et al. Identification of high-risk patients after minor craniocerebral trauma. Measurement of nerve tissue protein S100. Unfallchirurg 2004;107:197–202.

Chapter 25

Point-of-Care Testing in the Operating Room

Majed A. Refaai, George J. Despotis, Charles Eby, and Mitchell G. Scott

The increasing costs of healthcare have placed continued pressure to minimize cost, resulting in reductions in the number of inpatient hospital beds, more outpatient care, and decreased lengths of stay (1, 2).

Concurrently, technical advancements in point-of-care testing (POCT) during the last decade have increased the demand for POCT in settings where decreased length of stay and faster turnaround time are a focus. In addition to outpatient clinics, emergency departments, and intensive care units, operating rooms are increasingly recognizing the potential benefits of POCT. Decreasing test turnaround time is hypothesized to improve patient care and outcomes by leading to faster clinical and surgical decisions. Many of the outcomes in the operating room (OR) that are hypothesized to improve as a result of POCT, such as operating room time, hospital length of stay, and resource utilization, can be easily measured. Thus, the effects of POCT in the OR can potentially be readily assessed. Examples of measurable OR outcomes that will be discussed in detail in this chapter include blood products usage, blood loss, hospital length of stay, use of anesthesia, and use of frozen sections (3–5).

In most institutions the laboratory should play a role in POCT implementation decisions. These decisions should be guided by: (*i*) hypothesized improved outcome or service, (*ii*) how readily the outcome is measurable, and (*iii*) improved outcome vs. cost. Although reagents for POCT are invariably more expensive than those used in central laboratory testing, these costs may be negligible if some of the previously described outcomes can be realized in the OR as a result of POCT implementation (1, 2, 6).

The central laboratory should also play a role in the oversight and the management of POCT in the OR. All data, including calibrations and quality controls, should be reviewed on a timely basis by laboratory personnel in order to fulfill the requirements of regulatory and certifying bodies. Since POCT in the operating room is often performed by nonlaboratory staff, it is essential that the operator be well trained. Maintenance, calibrations, and quality control also have to be maintained, recorded, and reported by operating room personnel. Training and oversight of these functions usually falls upon the laboratory personnel (5, 7).

In 1966, POCT in the OR was first described by Hattersley using a locally invented whole-blood activated clotting time (ACT) test, which has become the routine test for heparin monitoring (8, 9). In 1975, Bull et al. (10) proposed a simplified heparin monitoring protocol using a POCT ACT method, and variations of this approach have been used ever since (10). Near-patient satellite laboratory testing for blood gases and pH for operating rooms followed in the early 1980s, and in the last 10 years the potential menu for POCT in the OR has expanded tremendously (11).

Here we will discuss the use of POCT in several specific OR settings and review the literature that assesses the impact of POCT on measurable outcomes.

CARDIOTHORACIC OPERATING ROOM

Approximately 500,000 coronary artery bypass graft (CABG) procedures are performed each year in the United States, and each patient receives an average of 4 U of blood (1). A unit of blood costs the patient approximately $250, so the average annual cost of transfusing blood products for cardiothoracic surgery approaches $500 million (2). In addition to these economic considerations, there are transfusion reactions and other risks related to blood transfusions that could be minimized if less blood were required during these procedures.

In general, patients undergoing cardiac surgery with cardiopulmonary bypass (CPB) are at increased risk for excessive perioperative blood loss and often require transfusion of blood products. The need for blood products can depend on patient-specific factors, the type of procedure, and the duration of being on the pump during CPB. Excessive activation of the hemostatic system, as a result of the extensive interaction of blood with nonendothelial surfaces, activation of the extrinsic pathway from surgical trauma, and retransfusion of pericardial blood during CPB surgery is considered one of the important factors leading to increased blood product usage (2). In addition, there is significant hemodilution related to crystalloid infusion via CPB and with cardioplegia. All of these can lead to bleeding complications and necessitate the use of blood products, particularly those that help overcome the effects of a subclinical disseminated intravascular coagulopathy (DIC) (12–16). Some of the coagulation disorders associated with CPB include both qualitative and quantitative platelet dysfunction, increased consumption of coagulation factors, and excess heparin or protamine in the systemic circulation. Historically, dosing of heparin and protamine, as well as administration of fresh frozen plasma and red blood cells, have been done empirically (16).

MANAGEMENT OF BLEEDING AFTER CARDIAC SURGERY

Because of these coagulation disorders and their potentially life-threatening nature, the use of a panel of rapidly performed screening tests such as the prothrombin time (PT), activated partial thromboplastin time (aPTT), thrombin time, platelet count (PLT), and fibrinogen concentration has been recommended to rapidly define the etiology of intraoperative disorders of hemostasis and to make decisions regarding implementation of therapy (17). Although central laboratory coagulation assays facilitate diagnosis and treatment of coagulation disorders after surgery, delays in obtaining results can limit their usefulness in the OR. Thus, it has been hypothesized that rapid POCT for coagulation will decrease the use of blood products used to maintain hemostasis. The utility of rapid determination of whole blood PT, aPTT, and PLT in the cardiothoracic operating room (CTOR) has been evaluated in a transfusion algorithm based on these POCT coagulation results (18).

In several studies, it was shown that the use of POCT in the intraoperative setting coupled with transfusion protocols can reduce the amount of postoperative bleeding and reduce blood product usage (19, 20). In one study, 66 patients undergoing CPB with microvascular bleeding were randomized to either standard therapy using central laboratory data and empirical decisions or to POCT. Whole blood PT, aPTT, and platelet count POCT was used in this study. The coagulopathy causing the microvascular bleeding was identified more rapidly when POCT was used, which allowed for the appropriate therapy to be initiated in a more timely manner. Consequently, the patients with POCT in the OR compared to the central laboratory group received less-fresh frozen plasma intraoperatively (0.4 U vs. 2.4 U; $P = 0.0006$), had less postoperative bleeding, and required fewer red cell and platelet transfusions

(1.9 U vs. 4.1 U; $P = 0.01$ and 1.6 U vs. 6.4 U; $P = 0.02$, respectively) (19).

Additional studies have shown that PT and aPTT coagulation measurements during CPB can identify patients at risk for excessive bleeding postsurgery (21–23). However, other studies have not supported these findings (24–30). The inability of these tests to identify patients at risk for increased bleeding may be in part related to the substantial variability that can be observed between various reagents or test methods (31).

A variety of POCT devices for PT and aPTT (Tables 25-1 and 25-2) testing are available. Most of these devices are small, portable, and utilize single-use cartridges, strips containing different thromboplastin reagents, or test tubes. Clot detection is accomplished by several methods, including cessation of capillary or pump-induced fluid movement, change in oscillation of paramagnetic particles, or alteration of fluorescence. Most devices use small amounts of fresh capillary, arterial, or venous whole blood as a sample, and some also allow the use of citrated blood specimens.

Platelet-Related Abnormalities

Platelet count alone cannot be used to identify individual patients at risk for excessive bleeding after cardiac surgery (24–30). Although a platelet count of less than $100,000/\mu L$ has been suggested and is often used empirically as a trigger for platelet transfusion, the most appropriate platelet concentration threshold for platelet transfusion is difficult to define for any single patient (18, 32–34). Depending on the functional state of the circulating platelets, the minimum platelet concentration for normal hemostasis varies from 50,000 to 200,000 per μL. Nevertheless, one can calculate the normal circulating platelet pool by using the platelet concentration, blood volume, and an estimate for splenic stores (e.g., $200,000/\mu L \times 5$ L $= 10 \times 10^{11} \times 120\% = 12 \times 10^{11}$ circulating platelets), and this may be helpful with empiric use of POCT platelet count measurements in the OR (35). The normal content of alloge-

Table 25-1 Prothrombin Time Point-of-Care Instruments

Instrument	Manufacturer	Sample type		Method of detection
		Fresh whole blood	Citrated whole blood/plasma	
CoaguChek S	Roche Diagnostics, Indianapolis, IN	Yes	No	Metal particles
CoaguChek Plus		Yes	No	Laser photometry
CoaguChek Pro DM		Yes	No	Laser photometry
GEM PCL	Instrumentation Laboratory, Lexington, MA	Yes	No	Optical
Hemochron Jr. Signature	International Technidyne, Edison, NJ	Yes	No	Optical
ProTime Microcoagulation System		Yes	No	Optical
Rapidpoint Coag	Bayer Diagnostics, Tarrytown, NY	Yes	Yes	Metal particles
Thrombolytic assessment system (TAS)		Yes	Yes	Metal particles

Table 25-2 Activated Partial Thromboplastin Time Point-of-Care Instruments

| Instrument | Manufacturer | Sample type | | Method of detection |
		Fresh whole blood	Citrated whole blood/plasma	
CoaguChek Plus	Roche Diagnostics, Indianapolis, IN	Yes	No	Laser photometry
CoaguChek Pro DM		Yes	No	Laser photometry
GEM PCL	Instrumentation Laboratory, Lexington, MA	Yes	No	Optical
Hemochron Jr. Signature	International Technidyne, Edison, NJ	Yes	No	Optical
Rapidpoint Coag	Bayer Diagnostics, Tarrytown, NY	Yes	Yes	Metal particles
Thrombolytic assessment system (TAS)		Yes	Yes	Metal particles

neic platelets (6 concentrated units or 1 apheresis unit) contains approximately 3.5×10^{11} platelets and generally increases the count by 30,000 to 60,000 per μL based on the variable dose of platelets administered and varying patient blood volumes.

Measuring platelet count during these procedures can be obtained by using small, compact, and automated instruments as point-of-care tests that can provide accurate CBC results using whole-blood specimens. These include the following: Coulter T540, MD 16, and A^cT8 (Coulter Electronics, Hialeah, FL, USA), Cell-Dyne 1400 and 1700 (Abbott, Abbott Park, IL, USA), K-800, K-1000 or SF-3000 (Sysmex Corporation, Long Grove, IL, USA), QBC (Becton Dickenson, Sparks, MD, USA), 9100 series (Biochem Immunosystems, Allentown, PA, USA), and the ICHOR (Array Medical, West Ridgewater, NJ, USA) (35). The T540 and MD 16 Coulter instruments, which provide precise and accurate cell counts and hemoglobin values, (36, 37) have been incorporated into treatment algorithms (6, 18).

Platelet Function

Several central laboratory–based platelet-function assays (e.g., aggregation, glass bead retention test, activation/receptor expression via flow cytometry) have been used to identify specific abnormalities of platelet function that were initially identified by abnormal bleeding time (38, 39). Several studies have verified a platelet function abnormality using aggregometry (22, 29, 38, 40–48), but these findings have not been universal (49). A relationship between excessive post-CPB bleeding and impaired platelet aggregation has been demonstrated in multiple studies (40, 45, 47). However, central laboratory-based platelet function studies are of limited clinical utility in the OR because they require substantial technical expertise, are expensive, and involve long turnaround times for both performance and interpretation. The bleeding time, which measures the interaction between platelets and the vessel wall, is the most commonly used screening test to evaluate in vivo platelet function (50). However, its results are arbitrarily elevated when platelet counts are <100,000/μL and can be influenced by a large number of diseases, physiological factors, test performance conditions, and therapeutic actions, which may or may

not reflect actual abnormalities in platelet function (51). In a recent review, preoperative bleeding time measurements were not shown to predict excessive blood loss or bleeding complications. However, bleeding time values may be useful in predicting postsurgical blood loss when performed in the postoperative interval (51). Prolonged bleeding time values have been documented in several studies after cardiac surgery (29, 43, 44, 49, 52–54).

Numerous tests have been developed to assess the response of platelets to a variety of platelet agonists within whole blood. One of these POCT systems (i.e., modified whole-blood aggregometer; Chrono-log, Havertown, PA, USA) that evaluates platelet function in a similar technique to platelet-rich plasma (PRP)-based turbidometric aggregometry was recently examined. Changes in its turbidometric measurements have been correlated to the blockage of GP IIb/IIIa receptor by abciximab (55). The Rapid Platelet Function Analyzer (RPFA; Accumetrics, San Diego, CA, USA) is based on the ability of platelets in whole blood to promptly agglutinate fibrinogen-coated beads when stimulated with an agonist peptide (56).

Other tests that use platelet agonists to evaluate platelet function include the PFA-100, ICHOR, and hemoSTATUS test systems. The PFA-100 Test (Dade Diagnostika, Germany) was developed as a point-of-care method to overcome the limitations of the standard bleeding time (57). Using either citrate-anticoagulated platelet-rich plasma or whole blood, the dual-channel Thrombostat 4000 (VDG-von der Goltz, Seeon, Germany) instrument provides an automated in vitro estimate of bleeding time (58). A comparison between the in vitro estimate of bleeding time at the end of surgery and blood loss in the first 24 h following surgery was demonstrated in 54 patients undergoing cardiac surgery and showed a significant ($P = 0.04$) but weak ($r^2 = 0.07$) relationship (58). The ICHOR system (Array Medical, West Ridgewater, NJ, USA) assists evaluation of platelet function by comparing platelet counts before and after in vitro addition of platelet agonists. The hemoSTATUS (Medtronic Blood Management, Parker, CO, USA) assay uses the kaolin-activated ACT to evaluate the effects of platelet activating factor (PAF) on acceleration of coagulation (22, 29, 59).

Anticoagulation for CPB

Activated Coagulation Time. The extracorporeal circuit of CPB requires high concentrations of heparin in order to prevent overt or subclinical clotting. Rapid reversal of the heparin at completion is necessary to minimize postoperative bleeding. Whole-blood ACT, first described by Hattersley (9) in 1966, has become the routine test for heparin monitoring. ACT is a whole-blood coagulation test method that is initiated by a contact activator such as celite (diamateous earth) or kaolin. It is similar to the aPTT and thus it will be prolonged in case of deficiency of one or more of the intrinsic factors (XII, XI, IX, VIII) and/or common pathway factors (X, V, II), and in the presence of heparin. It is different from aPTT, in that disorders of platelets will prolong results as the test is performed with whole blood. Fresh whole blood is added to an activator in a test tube or cartridge, and a timer records the time until a clot is formed; some assays can use citrated whole blood.

ACT is designed to monitor high-dose heparin therapy (in vivo heparin concentration of 1–6 U/mL) as used in CPB, vascular surgery, cardiac catheterization, and interventional radiology studies. In vitro studies have shown that the test is linearly responsive to heparin concentrations above 1 U/mL (1–7 U/mL). Although the degree of heparin response varies between patients, the linearity is fairly well maintained within each patient when blood from each individual anticoagulated patient is analyzed several times during the procedure (60, 61). Although ACT measurements linearly relate to heparin concentration, this relationship is dysfunctional with certain clinical scenarios, such as with platelet defects (e.g., IIb/IIIa inhibitors), CPB (e.g., ACT prolongation related to hypothermia, hemodilution), factor deficiency states (contact factors), or with anticardiolipin antibody or antiphospholipid antibody syndromes (62). Currently, many of the ACT-POC instruments (Table 25-3) have the ability to perform multiple coagulation tests in addition to ACT.

Heparin Concentration Methods. Determination of heparin concentrations in the patient's blood is an alternative approach for monitoring heparin therapy. Studies have shown variability of the heparin dose response, the variability in heparin half-life, and the lack of correlation between ACT and plasma heparin concentrations during CPB (10, 63–65). Studies have verified that after the initial heparin bolus during CPB, ACTs decline only gradually while heparin concentrations exhibit a rapid initial drop followed by a more gradual one. This is thought to be due to the effects of hemodilution and hypothermia on the ACT, which may, in part, cause a continued high ACT not reflective of actual heparin function (66, 67).

A comparison of heparin concentration measured by the Hepcon HMS to plasma antifactor Xa measured by a gold-standard antifactor Xa chromogenic substrate assay was studied in cardiac surgery patients (66, 68). An excellent correlation between the two assays was achieved, and a mean difference of 0.002 ± 0.53 U/mL. In contrast, another study (69) reported a greater difference between paired samples, particularly in samples obtained during CPB only. Only one-third of these data fell within their prearranged acceptance parameter of ± 0.7 U/mL, and the mean difference was 1.4 U/mL. Schluter et al. (70) performed similar comparisons at the heparin range of 0–1.6 U/mL. These studies showed good linearity over the tested range, excellent precision, and a slight underestimation of the actual heparin concentration. In general, heparin assay performance, in comparison to ACT, appears better at low concentrations (<1.5 U/mL), with more variability at higher concentrations.

Heparin and Protamine Dosing, Protocol, and Outcome. A POCT heparin monitoring protocol for CPB was developed by Bull et al. (10) in 1975 and has been modified several times since then. This protocol consists of (*i*) baseline

Table 25-3   Activated Coagulation Time Point-of-Care Instruments for High-Dose Heparin Therapy

Instrument	Manufacturer	Activator	Sample type	
			Fresh whole blood	Citrated whole blood/plasma
Actalyke	Helena Point of Care, Beaumont, TX	Celite or kaolin	Yes	No
HemoTec	Medtronic, Parker, CO	Kaolin	Yes	No
Hepcon HMS		Kaolin	Yes	No
CoaguChek Pro DM	Roche Diagnostics, Indianapolis, IN	Celite	Yes	No
GEM PCL	Instrumentation Laboratory, Lexington, MA	Celite	Yes	No
Hemochron Jr. Signature	International Technidyne, Edison, NJ	Kaolin with silica and phospholipids	Yes	No
Hemochron series (401, 801, 8000)		Celite or kaolin	Yes	No
Rapidpoint Coag	Bayer Diagnostics, Tarrytown, NY	Celite	Yes	Yes
Thrombolytic Assessment System (TAS)		Celite	Yes	Yes
i-STAT	i-STAT Corporation, East Windsor, NJ	Celite	Yes	No

ACT for bypass patients (reference interval <190 s), (*ii*) intravenous administration of a weight-based dose of heparin, (*iii*) goal of ACT >480 s, (*iv*) when bypass begins, extracorporeal circuit should contain an additional 5000 U of heparin to minimize the dilution factor of heparin, (*v*) ACT performed every 30–60 min during bypass, (*vi*) additional heparin given when ACT <480 s, (*vii*) protamine sulfate given (0.8–1.3 mg protamine/100 U of heparin administered) at completion of bypass, and (*viii*) goal of ACT returned to baseline, but (*ix*) if not, more protamine to be infused.

Although heparin dose response and clearance vary among patients, the ACT threshold of 480 s was set somewhat arbitrarily; in fact, a recent survey showed that most centers maintain ACT values of 400–480 s for CPB (62). The lack of clotting in the extracorporeal circuit was the only gold standard for adequacy of heparinization. Recently, the performances of new POCT monitoring protocols that determine the heparin dose response for each individual patient, the monitoring of heparin concentration during bypass, and more individualized determination of the postbypass protamine dose have been studied to determine whether simple POCT monitoring of individual dose-response heparin levels could improve outcomes during and after CPB. Both the Hepcon HMS (Medtronic Hemotec, Englewood, CO, USA) and Hemochron RxDx (International Technidyne, Edison, NJ, USA) systems have been evaluated in these situations.

The Hepcon HMS system is a multipurpose system that performs in vitro diagnostic procedures such as heparin assay test, heparin dose response, heparin-protamine titration to verify heparin concentration, and ACT to monitor anticoagulation functionality. After pipeting the blood into a single-use cartridge, which initiates test timing, a plunger in the cartridge is lifted and dropped through the sample/reagent mixture, where a fibrin web forms around a daisy located at the bottom of the plunger. The end point of the test is achieved by the clot formation, which blocks plunger movement and stops the timer in the instrument.

The Hemochron RxDx system also provides testing that can determine the appropriate doses of heparin and protamine during CPB. The heparin response test consists of two ACTs; one uses celite activator alone, while the other contains celite activator and 6 U of heparin. In order to achieve an ACT higher than 480 s (CPB application), the results of these two ACTs are compared in order to determine a heparin dose-response curve and compute the amount of heparin to be infused. The protamine response test also consists of two ACTs. One uses celite activator alone; the other contains celite activator and 40 μg of protamine sulfate. As above, the results of these two tests are required to determine a protamine dose-response curve and to calculate the dose of protamine to be administered in order to neutralize the circulating heparin.

Determining the heparin dose for each individual patient, using the RxDx system was hypothesized to improve patient outcomes by reducing blood loss and decreasing use of blood products. A POCT Hemochron RxDx monitoring protocol was compared to the standard monitoring approach by Jobes et al. (71). The RxDx protocol consisted of an initial dose of heparin

that was determined by a heparin response test, ongoing maintenance of a heparin concentration, and a protamine dose determined by the protamine response test. In addition, this protocol involved assessment of the adequacy of neutralization by adding an extra 10 mg of protamine each time heparin was detected. This process continued until no heparin was detectable. An ACT, thrombin time, and heparin-neutralized thrombin time were performed after the administration of the initial protamine dose. The RxDx group received more heparin and less protamine, but exhibited less 24-h chest tube drainage (671 ± 333 vs. 1298 ± 747 mL, $P = 0.01$) and was transfused less (9/22 vs. 18/24, $P = 0.02$).

Despotis et al. (6) compared a standard ACT monitoring protocol to one using Hepcon HMS to maintain patient-specific heparin levels in 254 patients undergoing CPB. The initial heparin dose in the study group was determined by the results of the heparin dose-response test. The optimal heparin concentration was determined by the dose-response test, and additional doses were given as needed to maintain a patient-specific heparin concentration. At the end of the bypass procedure, protamine doses were identified based on residual heparin concentration. Sufficiency of neutralization was assessed by ACT. Postoperative bleeding tendency was evaluated with POCT (PT, aPTT, and platelet count). Results showed that the study group received about 33% more heparin than the control group (612 ± 147 vs. 462 ± 114 U/kg); however, protamine doses postbypass were equal for both groups. Despite the increased heparin administration during bypass, the postbypass PT and aPTT were significantly lower in the study group. In comparison to the control group, the study group also received less platelets (1.7 ± 3.6 vs. 3.7 ± 6.7 U, $P = 0.003$), fresh frozen plasma (0.4 ± 1.3 vs. 1.4 ± 2.5 U, $P = 0.0001$), and cryoprecipitate units (0.0 ± 0.0 vs. 0.2 ± 1.2 U, $P = 0.04$) during the perioperative interval. The study group also had shorter operative times for closure (92 ± 32 vs. 102 ± 34 min, $P = 0.02$).

Taken together, these and other studies suggest that POCT in the CTOR can indeed decrease resource utilization and lead to improved measurable outcomes.

Role of Desmopressin. Desmopressin (DDAVP) is an arginine vasopressin analogue of antidiuretic hormone (ADH). A significant decrease in bleeding time values has been observed following the administration of DDAVP (72). DDAVP increases the plasma level of high- molecular-weight multimers of von Willebrand's factor, which are released by endothelial cells in response to secretion of PAF by monocytes (72–74). In an early randomized, prospective, double-blind study, a significant reduction in blood loss was achieved intraoperatively and in the early postoperative period when DDAVP (0.3 μg/kg IV infusion) was administered immediately after protamine (75). However, subsequent studies did not consistently confirm this prophylactic effect of DDAVP, as studies (76–79) with similar positive outcomes (36, 76–79) were slightly outnumbered by studies that showed no differences (80–85).

Recently, newer studies have revealed that certain subsets of patients may benefit from DDAVP, such as those requiring prolonged use of CPB, (75) those with excessive postoperative bleeding (e.g., >1180 mL/24 h) (86), patients on platelet-inhibiting drugs (36, 78, 87, 88), or patients at high risk for excessive bleeding as identified by tests of hemostatic function (89, 90).

One point-of-care test of hemostatic function that might predict a subset of patients that could benefit from DDAVP therapy is the thromboelastograph (TEG; see next section). Mongan et al. (89) studied the use of TEG testing for risk stratification of patients when evaluating post-CPB coagulation status. Hematocrit, platelet counts, PT, aPTT, and fibrinogen measurements were obtained in addition to TEG measurements after neutralization of heparin and discontinuation of bypass. Patients were randomly assigned to receive either normal saline (placebo) or 0.3 μg/kg of DDAVP. A post hoc analysis divided the patients into normal or abnormal TEG groups based on TEG maximum amplitude (MA) measurements. The mediastinal chest tube drainage in the placebo-treated, abnormal MA (>50 mm) patients was substantially greater when compared with normal (<50 mm) MA patients, indicating that TEG could identify patients at risk for excessive bleeding. Of interest, the blood loss was similar in both DDAVP-treated patients with abnormal TEG values and placebo-treated patients who had normal TEG values. These findings indicate that DDAVP can improve hemostasis in patients who have abnormal TEG and who are at risk for increased blood loss. DDAVP also seemed to be effective in reducing blood loss and blood component administration in the early postoperative period in patients at risk for increased blood loss (TEG:MA <50) (89).

In another recent trial, which utilized the hemoSTATUS test, 203 patients scheduled for elective cardiac surgical procedures were enrolled in this prospective, double-blind, placebo-controlled trial. This test compares clotting times in the presence of heparin and varying amounts of PAF (0–150 nmol/L) to determine a clot ratio. Clot ratios are mathematically determined by the following formula : 1 − (clotting time in PAF channel/clotting time in non-PAF channel). These clot ratios can be further characterized as a percentage of the maximal response, which is determined by the actual clot ratio obtained with 150 nmol/L PAF (channel 6) in normal volunteers [e.g., 0.5 (PAF = 150 nmol/L in channel 6)/0.3 (PAF = 12.5 nmol/L in channel 5)]. Thirty patients who required intraoperative management of microvascular bleeding with hemostatic blood products were excluded. Of the remaining 173 patients, 72 patients with normal clot ratio values were excluded, while the remaining 101 patients with abnormal clot ratio values (percent maximal <60 in channel 5) after administration of protamine were randomly assigned to either placebo (n = 51) or DDAVP (n = 50) treatment arms. Desmopressin-treated patients had a 50% reduction in red cells (1.1 vs. 2.2 U), 95% reduction in platelets (0.1 vs. 1.9 U), and 87% reduction in fresh frozen plasma (0.1 vs. 0.8 U) units transfused, with an overall 69% reduction in total donor exposures (1.6 vs 5.2 U) when compared to placebo patients. When compared to placebo-treated patients, patients who received Desmopressin also had a 39% (182 vs. 297 mL), 42% (299 vs. 513 mL), and 39% (624 vs. 1028 mL) reduction in blood loss in the first 4, 8, and 24 postoperative hours, respectively (91). These findings indicate that platelet function POCT systems may be useful in the identification of patients at risk for excessive bleeding and who may benefit from administration of pharmacologic agents (e.g., desmopressin) or in directing administration of hemostatic blood products.

POCT DURING LIVER TRANSPLANTATION

Orthotopic liver transplantation (OLT) is recognized as a potentially lifesaving therapy for eligible patients with end-stage liver disease. However, massive perioperative blood loss is still a prime concern. Liver hepatocytes synthesize fibrinogen and coagulation factors II, V, VII, IX, X, XI, and XII; coagulation inhibitors protein C, protein S, and antithrombin III (AT-III); and plasminogen. As a result, the concentrations of many of these hemostatic proteins are decreased in the setting of acute or chronic liver failure (92). Additional hemostatic defects, such as thrombocytopenia, acquired platelet dysfunction, and hyperfibrinolysis may also accompany advanced liver disease. The presence of these abnormalities in a patient undergoing a liver transplant may lead to excessive intraoperative bleeding (92). Additional humoral and metabolic factors, such as hemodilution, hypothermia, ionized hypocalcemia, and acidosis, may also contribute to hemostatic dysfunction. As a result, transfusion of multiple blood products frequently is required during OLT, and prompt assessment of hemostasis parameters may be beneficial in the selection of these blood components (92).

The thromboelastograph (TEG) is a point-of-care instrument that measures the viscoelastic properties of whole blood. First described by Hartert in 1948 (93), the TEG has primarily been used to assess coagulation abnormalities during OLT and CPB. The principle components of the TEG are a cylindrical cup and a pin. A whole-blood specimen (340–360 μL) (94, 95) is placed into the warmed cup; a pin is freely suspended in the cup by a torsion wire, and the cup then oscillates through a 4.45° angle (Figure 25-1). As clotting occurs in the cup, fibrin strands form between the walls of the cup and the pin, and the motion of the cup is transmitted to the pin. Increased or decreased torque over time, due to progressive fibrin formation or lysis, respectively, was directly transferred to a strip chart recording on older instruments and is now electronically transmitted to a computer screen (Figures 25-2 and 25-3). The clot's viscoelastic qualities are dependent on the interaction of fibrinogen and platelets, coagulation, and fibrinolytic proteins (94, 96).

Although originally validated with whole-blood specimens, TEG analysis can be performed on citrated and heparinized whole-blood specimens following recalcification and heparin neutralization steps, respectively (95, 97). Efforts to accelerate TEG analysis time include addition of intrinsic pathway (98) or extrinsic pathway (99) activators.

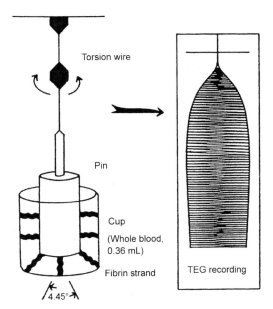

Figure 25-1 Thromboelastograph (TEG) instrument components (*left*), and normal TEG trace (*right*).

Multiple parameters (Figure 25-3) may be measured from the TEG tracing, either manually or with computer software. These parameters are: reaction time R, the interval between the start of the tracing to the onset of clot formation; clot formation time K, the time from clot formation to a fixed level of clot firmness; angle α, the slope from the initiation of clot formation point to the shoulder tangent of the tracing; maximum amplitude MA, the widest point of the tracing; and clot lysis Ly_{30}, the rate of decrease in amplitude 30 min after MA.

Several studies have compared TEG parameters to traditional laboratory coagulation tests. A positive correlation exists between the time R and the aPTT (27, 92). Tuman et al. (100) showed that celite activator shortened the time R in CPB patients consistent with accelerated activation of intrinsic pathway coagulation factors. Vig et al. (94) also showed a shorter time R with tissue factor activator. Spiess et al. (27) demon-

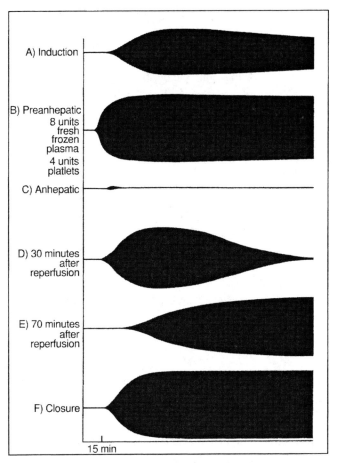

Figure 25-3 Thromboelastography tracings during different phases of orthotopic liver transplantation (OLT) operation: (*A*) prolonged time R and smaller α and MA (due to coagulopathy associated with chronic liver failure), (*B*) shortened R and increased α and MA values post–FFP transfusion, (*C*) worsening coagulopathy (prolonged R, decreased MA) and severe hyperfibrinolysis (decreased A_{60}/MA $\times$ 100) during the anhepatic phase, (*D*) improving coagulopathy (shortened R) with partial resolution of hyperfibrinolysis at the beginning of the reperfusion phase, (*E*) temporary relapse of coagulopathy (prolonged R, decreased MA) and resolving hyperfibrinolysis by the end of the reperfusion phase, and (*F*) near-normal TEG tracing at the end of the OLT procedure.

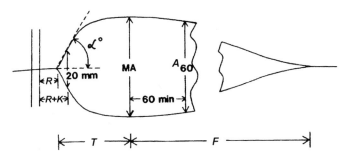

Figure 25-2 Variables and normal values measured by thromboelastography: reaction time R, 6–8 min; R + coagulation time K, 10–12 min; clot formation rate α, >50°; maximum amplitude MA, 50–70 mm; amplitude 60 min after MA, A_{60}; whole-blood clot lysis index A_{60}/MA $\times$ 100, >85%; and whole-blood clot lysis time F, >300 min.

strated similar correlations between aPTT and both time K and angle α in CPB patients. Multiple studies have shown a correlation between MA and platelet count, platelet function, and fibrinogen concentration (92, 100–103).

Changes in TEG parameters have been associated with different clinical conditions or in response to transfusion of specific blood components. Thrombocytopenia, platelet dysfunction, and hypofibrinogenemia decrease MA. While times R and K are prolonged in patients with coagulation factor deficiencies due to hemophilia or oral anticoagulation therapy, shortened times R and K plus increased angle α have been described in patients with hypercoagulable states (104, 105). Platelet transfusion increases both MA and angle α and, due to the presence of the coagulation factors in the plasma of the platelet product, decreases time R (104–106). Shorter time R and larger angle α were observed after transfusion of cryoprecipitate, which is rich in factor VIII and fibrinogen (92).

Only a few studies have compared clinical outcomes between patients in whom hemostatic function was monitored by TEG versus platelet counts, PT, aPTT, and fibrinogen during OLT or CPB. Based on their experience monitoring hemostatic function with the TEG during OLTs, Kang et al. (92) developed an empiric transfusion algorithm: fresh frozen plasma (FFP) when $R > 15$ min, platelet transfusion when MA <40 mm, and cryoprecipitate when α <45°. When compared to a historical control group using conventional coagulation tests to guide transfusion therapy, patients undergoing OLT who were monitored with the TEG-based algorithm received fewer transfusions of fresh frozen plasma and red blood cells, and more platelet and cryoprecipitate transfusions. While there was no significant difference in total blood products transfused, there was a significant reduction in the total volume of blood and crystalloid infused in the TEG monitored group (107). When Spiess et al. (27) compared postprotamine TEG monitoring in open-heart surgery patients to ACT and routine coagulation profile, TEG results more accurately predicted excessive postoperative hemorrhage. A prospective, randomized study comparing a different TEG-guided transfusion algorithm and an algorithm based on ACT, platelet count, PT, aPTT, and fibrinogen measurements during CPB found no difference between groups regarding intraoperative transfusion rates or postoperative mediastinal blood loss (99). Surprisingly, the TEG group received significantly less FFP ($P < 0.002$) and platelets ($P < 0.05$) postoperatively.

In summary, TEG provides a rapid assessment of multiple hemostatic abnormalities, including coagulation factors, fibrinolytic activity, and quantitative and qualitative platelet disorders. When used as a point-of-care device, TEG monitoring could potentially improve the management of hemostasis complications in patients undergoing OLT or CPB procedures by improving selection of replacement blood components and by appropriately administrating pharmacologic therapy. However, additional prospective studies are needed to determine whether TEG monitoring consistently leads to improvement of important clinical outcomes such as blood loss, transfusion exposure, and reexploration.

POCT IN PARATHYROIDECTOMY

The use of rapid intraoperative parathyroid hormone (PTH) measurements for patients undergoing parathyroidectomy is another example of POCT possibly leading to significant cost savings in the operating room (108). Primary hyperparathyroidism is the most common cause of hypercalcemia and has an estimated annual incidence of 1–2 per 1000 (109). Approximately 85% of the cases are caused by a solitary adenoma, with the remainder due to parathyroid hyperplasia and very rarely parathyroid carcinoma (109). In addition to clinical symptoms, the diagnosis of primary hyperparathyroidism requires elevated serum calcium values in the presence of inappropriately high

PTH values (109). In most cases, the recommended therapy is parathyroidectomy (109). Previous approaches to surgical treatment involved bilateral, open-neck exploration under general anesthesia with intraoperative frozen-section histopathologic examination of the parathyroid glands. Historically, patients stayed an average of 2–3 days in the hospital (110). Failure rates for this approach have been reported to exceed 10% in some institutions (111). Advances in surgical techniques have led to the use of concise parathyroidectomy, which is performed with smaller, less invasive incisions resulting in less postoperative complications (112). However, even these minimal approaches can require bilateral exploration, overnight hospital stays, and the use of general anesthesia (112). Furthermore, the failure of standard intraoperative frozen section diagnosis to agree with definitive histology in up to 10% of cases can impact intra- and postoperative management (113–115). Therefore, an improved means of assessing the intraoperative success of surgery was needed to improve upon the limitations of intraoperative frozen sections.

Recent implementation of two new technologies have greatly helped to simplify parathyroidectomy surgery and simultaneously decrease costs—preoperative Tc-99m sestamibi parathyroid imaging (108, 116–118) and a rapid point-of-care assay for intact PTH performed during the surgical procedure (119–122). Preoperative Tc-99m sestamibi parathyroid scanning can identify adenomatous or hyperactive glands in up to 90% of cases (108, 117, 118), thus reducing the need for routine bilateral neck exploration (110). However, this approach can miss a second diseased gland present in 2% to 5% of patients (118). Rapid intraoperative PTH assays have been hypothesized to circumvent this problem by serving as a "biological frozen section" (119, 123) to confirm the removal of all hyperfunctioning parathyroid tissue.

The 5-min half-life of intact parathyroid hormone allows it to serve as a practical intraoperative marker, and studies suggest that a 50% decrease in PTH values from the presurgical value following removal of the diseased gland(s) reliably predicts postoperative normocalcemia (119, 120, 122). Rapid immunoradiometric assay (IMRA) for PTH have been modified so that incubation times are now as short as 7 min, making them very attractive for POCT intraoperative utilization (119).

In a recent report, Ferrer et al. (124) measured PTH intraoperatively on 32 consecutive parathyroidectomy patients before the removal of abnormal parathyroid tissue and 10 min afterward. They used an immunochemiluminometric assay with a 7-min incubation time, and results were available in ≤15 min. A decrease in PTH value of more than 60% was confirmed in 30 patients (94%). A successful removal of a single adenoma was achieved in 26 of these 30 cases, while multiple hyperplastic glands were removed in the remaining 4 cases. In the two cases in which PTH failed to decrease below 60%, patients were diagnosed with parathyroid hyperplasia; however, following the removal of these hyperplastic glands, PTH dropped to more than 60% of the highest level.

In another study (125), the intact parathyroid hormone (iPTH) of 341 consecutive patients undergoing parathyroidectomy was measured by the quick parathyroid hormone assay (QPTH) intraoperatively. A drop in the iPTH levels of $\geq 50\%$ 10 min after gland excision was found to be significantly correlated ($329/341 = 96\%$) with the predicted postoperative calcium levels, while the operative outcome was incorrectly predicted in 12 patients (3.5%).

Sebag et al. (126) utilized an intraoperative parathyroid hormone assay (IOPTH) in a retrospective study that included two different groups of hyperparathyroidism patients who underwent a reoperation for persistent or recurrent sporadic primary hyperparathyroidism. IOPTH was not used in the first group ($n = 58$), but it was used in the second group ($n = 50$). A sufficient result was considered if a drop of at least 50% in the PTH values, from the highest value, was obtained within 10 min following the removal of the abnormal parathyroid tissue. In 36 patients out of 50 (72%; group 2), IOPTH results were reliable in predicting accurate outcomes. However, false-positive results were verified in five patients who had a drop of 50% or more in the PTH values with the presence of abnormal parathyroid tissues, as confirmed surgically. False-negative results were also determined in four different patients.

Several studies have hypothesized that the combination of sestamibi imaging and POCT rapid intraoperative PTH assays will lead to better clinical outcomes, decreased costs through less exposure to anesthesia, fewer frozen sections, and shorter hospital stays (127). In one study, laboratory and pathology costs, length of hospital stay, type of surgery (bilateral vs. unilateral neck dissection), and type of anesthesia was compared between 55 patients prior to implementation of a rapid intraoperative PTH to 49 patients following its implementation (128). The median drop in PTH values from baseline was 88% (range 33–99). Although the clinical outcome was similar for both groups, the use of the rapid PTH assay saved over $300 per patient in surgical pathology costs alone, and 37% of these patients did not stay overnight in the hospital (128). Thirty-seven patients required two intraoperative PTH determinations, seven required three, four required four, and one required five determinations. Compared to the retrospective control group, the group utilizing the intraoperative PTH assay had significantly fewer frozen sections (1.4 vs. 2.5, $P < 0.0001$), shorter hospital stays (17 discharged on day of surgery vs. none, $P < 0.0001$), greater use of local anesthesia (33% vs. 0%, $p < 0.001$), and more unilateral, rather than bilateral, neck explorations (35% vs. 0%, $P < 0.001$). These authors concluded that the combination of intraoperative Turbo PTH assay and preoperative Tc99m sestamibi scans can lead to significant decreases in laboratory and surgical pathology costs, hospital stay, and exposure to general anesthesia by facilitating the concise parathyroidectomy surgery.

A recent review of the literature in this field undertaken by Carter and Howanitz (129) showed that the utilization of intraoperative parathyroid hormone assays had significantly improved the parathyroidectomy procedure. Its unique ability to detect an occult residue of hyperfunctioning parathyroid tissue during parathyroid surgery, along with the preoperative imaging of parathyroid glands, enhanced the parathyroidectomy outcome. Thus, the use of this assay will avert the need for frozen section in most routine cases. It also facilitates minimally invasive parathyroidectomy for single parathyroid adenomas, which, in turn, improves cost-effectiveness and cosmetic outcome.

One of the remarkable outcomes of the rapid PTH assay has been the progress of surgery for primary hyperthyroidism from an approach using a bilateral neck exploration under general anesthesia to a minimally invasive approach. Since 85% to 90% of patients with primary hyperthyroidism have a single parathyroid adenoma, the use of preoperative sestamibi tomography along with intraoperative PTH assay will guide to a more directed surgery under a local or regional anesthesia (130). Thus, parathyroidectomy surgery has often become a 1-day procedure with less complication, a more successful rate, and a small incision.

CALCIUM POCT IN THE OPERATING ROOM

Due to the presence of citrate in transfused blood products, massive blood transfusion during surgery may contribute to the elevation of total calcium concentrations. Citrate binds ionized calcium (Ca^{2+}), which may drop dramatically in these situations, causing adverse outcomes. Since Ca^{2+} is essential for acute patient management, a rapid turnaround time testing approach is needed in order to achieve instant clinical/surgical decisions.

Severe ionized hypocalcemia may cause cardiac arrest, which can become refractory to resuscitation despite the substitution of Ca^{2+} to normal concentration. Clinically, ionized hypocalcemia is multifactorial and may result from hypomagnesemia, transient hypoparathyroidism, elevated circulating cytokines, vitamin D deficiency, resistance to PTH or vitamin D, calcium binding, chelation, or cellular redistribution and sequestration. When Ca^{2+} concentration drops to a level of 1.0 mmol/L (4.0 mg/dL) or less, neurological and cardiovascular disorders, including dysrhythmias and hypotension, emerge (11, 131). Cardiac arrest cases have been reported when the Ca^{2+} level reached values of 0.47 to 0.60 mmol/L (1.9 to 2.4 mg/dL). Depending on the change rate in the Ca^{2+} level and the patient's clinical condition, some values can be fatal (11, 131, 132). Therefore, a low Ca^{2+} level is an early predictor of mortality in critically ill surgical patients (133). On the other hand, significant clinical risks can also arise if calcium treatment is given when not indicated (11). Thus, frequent monitoring of Ca^{2+} is essential in the OR setting.

The goals of POCT systems optimization for Ca^{2+} monitoring in the OR are : (*i*) to establish a feedback system with rapid process cycle time, (*ii*) to provide adequate physiologic information for fast diagnosis and therapy, and (*iii*) to detect abnormalities in other important contextual analytes, such as potassium, that may change unexpectedly during surgical and transplant procedures.

Therefore, utilizing direct whole-blood analysis of Ca^{2+} levels by POCT in operating rooms, which accomplishes a turnaround time of ~5 min, was claimed to improve surgical outcomes, but these were not specified (11).

Other POCT, such as monitoring blood glucose, blood gases, electrolytes, and hemoglobin and hematocrit, can be utilized in the OR setting and provide a useful aid in physicians' clinical and surgical decisions. Although these point-of-care tests are commonly used in surgical settings, there is a paucity of outcome studies that examine whether their use improves any measurable outcomes. Nevertheless, such testing is routinely performed under the premise that faster is better, and it is up to the laboratories to make sure all operators are trained, quality assurance is maintained, and regulatory and compliance issues are followed. Because these types of POCT are so common in many ORs today, it is unlikely that we will see true outcome studies where the control arm would require removal of POCT.

CONCLUSIONS

Utilizing POCT in the OR setting provides valuable advantages, clinically by setting up the appropriate decisions and economically by reducing the operation time and LOS. The fast and early detection of any undesirable values may and will change the clinical and surgical decisions, which, as a result, will prevent many complications and reduce the morbidity and mortality rates. In addition to the better clinical outcome, the assessment of POCT in the OR has added a significant improvement on the cost effectiveness, as shown by reducing the LOS for parathyroidectomy patients and minimizing blood products transfusions in both CTOR and OLT. Other common point-of-care tests in the OR have not been evaluated as rigorously, but oversight of all POCT by the central laboratory will ensure that POCT is performed well and meets all regulatory requirements.

REFERENCES

1. Conn RB, Snyder JW. Changes in the American health care system: crisis in the clinical laboratory. Clin Chim Acta 1997; 267:33–49.
2. Kricka LJ, Parsons D, Coolen RB. Healthcare in the United States and the practice of laboratory medicine. Clin Chim Acta 1997;267:5–32.
3. Hicks JM, Haeckel R, Price CP, Lewandrowski K, Wu AH. Recommendations and opinions for the use of point-of-care testing for hospitals and primary care: summary of a 1999 symposium. Clin Chim Acta 2001;303:1–17.
4. Rainey PM. Outcomes assessment for point-of-care testing. Clin Chem 1998;44:1595–6.
5. Scott MG. Faster is better—it's rarely that simple! Clin Chem 2000;46:441–2.
6. Despotis GJ, Joist JH, Hogue CW, Alsoufiev A, Kater K, Goodnough LT, et al. The impact of heparin concentration and activated clotting time monitoring on blood conservation: a prospective, randomized evaluation in patients undergoing cardiac operations. J Thorac Cardiovasc Surg 1995;110:46–54.
7. Greendyke RM. Cost analysis. Bedside blood glucose testing. Am J Clin Pathol 1992;97:106–7.
8. Hackel DB, Wagner GS. Acute circumferential subendocardial infarction. Clin Cardiol 1992;15:373–6.
9. Hattersley PG. Activated coagulation time of whole blood. JAMA 1966;196:436–40.
10. Bull BS, Korpman RA, Huse WM, Briggs BD. Heparin therapy during extracorporeal circulation. I. Problems inherent in existing heparin protocols J Thorac Cardiovasc Surg 1975;69:674–84.
11. Kost GJ, Jammal MA, Ward RE, Safwat AM. Monitoring of ionized calcium during human hepatic transplantation. Critical values and their relevance to cardiac and hemodynamic. Am J Clin Pathol 1986;86:61–70.
12. Kalter RD, Saul CM, Wetstein L, Soriano C, Reiss RF. Cardiopulmonary bypass. Associated hemostatic abnormalities. J Thorac Cardiovasc Surg 1979;77:427–35.
13. Heimark RL, Kurachi K, Fujikawa K, Davie EW. Surface activation of blood coagulation, fibrinolysis and kinin formation. Nature 1980;286:456–60.
14. Boisclair MD, Lane DA, Philippou H, Esnouf MP, Sheikh S, Hunt B, et al. Mechanisms of thrombin generation during surgery and cardiopulmonary bypass. Blood 1993;82:3350–7.
15. de Haan J, Boonstra PW, Monnink SH, Ebels T, van Oeveren W. Retransfusion of suctioned blood during cardiopulmonary bypass impairs hemostasis. Ann Thorac Surg 1995;59:901–7.
16. Goodnough LT, Johnston MF, Toy PT. The variability of transfusion practice in coronary artery bypass surgery. Transfusion Medicine Academic Award Group. JAMA 1991;265:86–90.
17. Fleisher M, Schwartz MK. Automated approaches to rapid-response testing. A comparative evaluation of point-of-care and centralized laboratory testing. Am J Clin Pathol 1995;104:S18–25.
18. Despotis GJ, Santoro SA, Spitznagel E, Kater KM, Cox JL, Barnes P, et al. Prospective evaluation and clinical utility of on-site monitoring of coagulation in patients undergoing cardiac operation. J Thorac Cardiovasc Surg 1994;107:271–9.
19. Metz S, Keats AS. Low activated coagulation time during cardiopulmonary bypass does not increase postoperative bleeding. Ann Thorac Surg 1990;49:440–4.
20. Hooper TL, Conroy J, McArdle B, Dell A, Watson B, Pearson DT, et al. The use of the Hemochron in assessment of heparin reversal after cardiopulmonary bypass perfusion. 1988;3:295–300.
21. Dorman BH, Spinale FG, Bailey MK, Kratz JM, Roy RC. Identification of patients at risk for excessive blood loss during coronary artery bypass surgery: thromboelastography versus coagulation screen. Anesth Analg 1993;76:694–700.
22. Ereth MH, Nuttall GA, Klindworth JT, MacVeigh I, Santrach PJ, Orszulak TA, et al. Does the platelet-activated clotting test (HemoSTATUS) predict blood loss and platelet dysfunction associated with cardiopulmonary bypass? Anesth Analg 1997; 85:259–64.
23. Nuttall GA, Oliver WC, Ereth MH, Santrach PJ. Coagulation tests predict bleeding after cardiopulmonary bypass. J Cardiothorac Vasc Anesth 1997;11:815–23.
24. Gravlee GP, Arora S, Lavender SW, Mills SA, Hudspeth AS, Cordell AR, et al. Predictive value of blood clotting tests in cardiac surgical patients. Ann Thorac Surg 1994;58:216–21.
25. Essell JH, Martin TJ, Salinas J, Thompson JM, Smith VC. Comparison of thromboelastography to bleeding time and standard coagulation tests in patients after cardiopulmonary bypass. J Cardiothorac Vasc Anesth 1993;7:410–5.

26. Fassin W, Himpe D, Alexander JP, Borms S, Theunissen W, Muylaert P, et al. Predictive value of coagulation testing in cardiopulmonary bypass surgery. Acta Anaesthesiol Belg 1991; 42:191–8.

27. Spiess BD, Tuman KJ, McCarthy RJ, DeLaria GA, Schillo R, Ivankovich AD. Thromboelastography as an indicator of post-cardiopulmonary bypass coagulopathies. J Clin Monit 1987;3: 25–30.

28. Gelb AB, Roth RI, Levin J, London MJ, Noall RA, Hauck WW, et al. Changes in blood coagulation during and following cardiopulmonary bypass: lack of correlation with clinical bleeding. Am J Clin Pathol 1996;106:87–99.

29. Despotis GJ, Levine V, Filos KS, Santoro SA, Joist JH, Spitznagel E, et al. Evaluation of a new, point-of-care test that measures PAF-mediated acceleration of coagulation in cardiac surgical patients. Anesthesiology 1996;85:1311–23.

30. Despotis GJ, Levine V, Goodnough LT. The relationship between leukocyte count and patient risk for excessive blood loss after cardiac surgery. Crit Care Med 1996;30:120–5.

31. Murray D, Pennell B, Olson J. Variability of prothrombin time and activated partial thromboplastin time in the diagnosis of increased surgical bleeding. Transfusion 1999;39:56–62.

32. Goodnough LT, Johnston MF, Ramsey G, Sayers MH, Eisenstadt RS, Anderson KC, et al. Guidelines for transfusion support in patients undergoing coronary artery bypass grafting. Transfusion Practices Committee of the American Association of Blood Banks. Ann Thorac Surg 1990;50:675–83.

33. Paone G, Spencer T, Silverman NA. Blood conservation in coronary artery surgery. Surgery 1994;116:672–7.

34. Spiess BD, Gillies BS, Chandler W, Verrier E. Changes in transfusion therapy and reexploration rate after institution of a blood management program in cardiac surgical patients. J Cardiothorac Vasc Anesth 1995;9:168–73.

35. Despotis GJ, Saleem R, Bigham M, Barnes P. Clinical evaluation of a new, point-of-care hemocytometer. Crit Care Med 2000;28:1185–90.

36. Dilthey G, Dietrich W, Spannagl M, Richter JA. Influence of desmopressin acetate on homologous blood requirements in cardiac surgical patients pretreated with aspirin. J Cardiothorac Vasc Anesth 1993;7:425–30.

37. Despotis GJ, Alsoufiev A, Hogue CW, Zoys TN, Goodnough LT, Santoro SA, et al. Comparison of CBC results from a new, on-site hemocytometer to a laboratory-based hemocytometer. Crit Care Med 1996;24:1163–7.

38. Zilla P, Fasol R, Groscurth P, Klepetko W, Reichenspurner H, Wolner E. Blood platelets in cardiopulmonary bypass operations. Recovery occurs after initial stimulation, rather than continual activation. J Thorac Cardiovasc Surg 1989;97:379–88.

39. Despotis GJ, Joist JH, Hogue CW, Alsoufiev A, Joiner-Maier D, Santoro SA, et al. More effective suppression of hemostatic system activation in patients undergoing cardiac surgery by heparin dosing based on heparin blood concentrations rather than ACT. Thromb Haemostas 1996;76:902–8.

40. Holloway DS, Summaria L, Sandesara J, Vagher JP, Alexander JC, Caprini JA. Decreased platelet number and function and increased fibrinolysis contribute to postoperative bleeding in cardiopulmonary bypass patients. Thromb Haemost 1988;59: 62–7.

41. Zimmerman JL, Dellinger RP. Initial evaluation of a new intra-arterial blood gas system in humans. Crit Care Med 1993;21: 495–500.

42. Harker LA. Bleeding after cardiopulmonary bypass. N Engl J Med 1986;314:1446–8.

43. Bick RL. Alterations of hemostasis associated with malignancy: etiology, pathophysiology, diagnosis and management. Sem Thromb Hemost 1978;5:1–26.

44. Edmunds LH, Jr., Ellison N, Colman RW, Niewiarowski S, Rao AK, Addonizio VP, Jr., et al. Platelet function during cardiac operation: comparison of membrane and bubble oxygenators. J Thorac Cardiovasc Surg 1982;83:805–12.

45. Ferraris VA, Ferraris SP, Singh A, Fuhr W, Koppel D, McKenna D, et al. The platelet thrombin receptor and postoperative bleeding. Ann Thorac Surg 1998;65:352–8.

46. Ray MJ, Hawson GA, Just SJ, McLachlan G, O'Brien M. Relationship of platelet aggregation to bleeding after cardiopulmonary bypass. Ann Thorac Surg 1994;57:981–6.

47. Soslau G, Horrow J, Brodsky I. Effect of tranexamic acid on platelet ADP during extracorporeal circulation. Am J Hematol 1991;38:113–9.

48. Rinder CS, Bohnert J, Rinder HM, Mitchell J, Ault K, Hillman R. Platelet activation and aggregation during cardiopulmonary bypass. Anesthesiology 1991;75:388–93.

49. Kestin AS, Valeri CR, Khuri SF, Loscalzo J, Ellis PA, MacGregor H, et al. The platelet function defect of cardiopulmonary bypass. Blood 1993;82:107–17.

50. Harker LA, Slichter SJ. The bleeding time as a screening test for evaluation of platelet function. N Engl J Med 1972;287:155–9.

51. Rodgers RP, Levin J. A critical reappraisal of the bleeding time. Semin Thromb Hemost 1990;16:1–20.

52. Khuri SF, Wolfe JA, Josa M, Axford TC, Szymanski I, Assousa S, et al. Hematologic changes during and after cardiopulmonary bypass and their relationship to the bleeding time and nonsurgical blood loss. J Thorac Cardiovasc Surg 1992;104:94–107.

53. Mammen EF, Koets MH, Washington BC, Wolk LW, Brown JM, Burdick M, et al. Hemostasis changes during cardiopulmonary bypass surgery. Sem Thromb Hemost 1985;11:281–92.

54. Addonizio VP, Jr., Fisher CA, Kappa JR, Ellison N. Prevention of heparin-induced thrombocytopenia during open heart surgery with iloprost (ZK36374). Surgery 1987;102:796–807.

55. Mascelli MA, Worley S, Veriabo NJ, Lance ET, Mack S, Schaible T, et al. Rapid assessment of platelet function with a modified whole-blood aggregometer in percutaneous transluminal coronary angioplasty patients receiving anti-GP IIb/IIIa therapy. Circulation 1997;96:3860–6.

56. Coller BS, Lang D, Scudder LE. Rapid and simple platelet function assay to assess glycoprotein IIb/IIIa receptor blockade. Circulation 1997;95:860–6.

57. Uchiyama S, Stropp JQ, Claypool DA, Didisheim P, Dewanjee MK. Filter bleeding time: a new in vitro test of hemostasis. I. Evaluation in normal and thrombocytopenic subjects Thromb Res 1983;31:99–115.

58. Kratzer MA, Born GV. Simulation of primary haemostasis in vitro. Haemostasis 1985;15:357–62.

59. Klindworth JT, MacVeigh I, and Ereth MH. The platelet activated clotting test (PACT) predicts platelet dysfunction associated with cardiopulmonary bypass (CPB) [Abstract]. Anesth Analg 1996;82:99–100.

60. Mulry CC, Le Veen RF, Sobel M, Lampe PJ, Burke DR. Assessment of heparin anticoagulation during peripheral angioplasty. J Vasc Interv Radiol 1991;2:133–9.

61. Dougherty KG, Gaos CM, Bush HS, Leachman DR, Ferguson JJ. Activated clotting times and activated partial thromboplastin

times in patients undergoing coronary angioplasty who receive bolus doses of heparin. Cathet Cardiovasc Diagn 1992;26: 260–3.

62. Despotis GJ, Gravlee GP, Filos KS, Levy JH. Anticoagulation monitoring during cardiac surgery: a review of current and emerging techniques. Anesthesiology 1999;91:1122–51.

63. Murray DJ, Brosnahan WJ, Pennell B, Kapalanski D, Weiler JM, Olson J. Heparin detection by the activated coagulation time: a comparison of the sensitivity of coagulation tests and heparin assays. J Cardiothroac Vasc Anesth 1997;11:24–8.

64. Bull BS, Huse WM, Brauer FS, Korpman RA. Heparin therapy during extracorporeal circulation. II. The use of a dose-response curve to individualize heparin and protamine dosage. J Thorac Cardiovasc Surg 1975;69:685–9.

65. Esposito RA, Culliford AT, Colvin SB, Thomas SJ, Lackner H, Spencer FC. The role of the activated clotting time in heparin administration and neutralization for cardiopulmonary bypass. J Thorac Cardiovasc Surg 1983;85:174–85.

66. Despotis GJ, Summerfield AL, Joist JH, Goodnough LT, Santoro SA, Spitznagel E, et al. Comparison of activated coagulation time and whole blood heparin measurements with laboratory plasma anti-Xa heparin concentration in patients having cardiac operations. J Thorac Cardiovasc Surg 1994;108:1076–82.

67. Huyzen RJ, van Oeveren W, Wei F, Stellingwerf P, Boonstra PW, Gu YJ. In vitro effect of hemodilution on activated clotting time and. Ann Thorac Surg 1996;62:533–7.

68. Despotis GJ, Joist JH, Goodnough LT, Santoro SA, Spitznagel E. Whole blood heparin concentration measurements by automated protamine titration agree with plasma anti-Xa measurements. J Thorac Cardiovasc Surg 1996;170:611–3.

69. Hardy JF, Belisle S, Robitaille D, Perrault J, Roy M, Gragnon L. Measurement of heparin concentration in whole blood with the hepcon/HMS device does not agree with laboratory determination of plasma heparin concentration using a chromogenic substrate for activated factor X. J Thorac Cardiovasc Surg 1996;112:154–61.

70. Schlueter AJ, Pennell BJ, Olson JD. Evaluation of a new protamine titration method to assay heparin in whole blood and plasma. Am J Clin Pathol 1997;107:511–20.

71. Jobes DR, Schaffer GW, Aitken GL. Increased accuracy and precision of heparin and protamine dosing reduces blood loss and transfusion in patients undergoing primary cardiac operations. J Thorac Cardiovasc Surg 1995;110:36–45.

72. Beck KH, Bleckmann U, Mohr P, Kretschmer V. DDAVP's shortening of the bleeding time seems due to plasma von Willebrand factor. Semin Thromb Hemost 1995;21:40–3.

73. Mannucci PM, Aberg M, Nilsson IM, Robertson B. Mechanism of plasminogen activator and factor VIII increase after vasoactive drugs. Br J Haematol 1975;30:81–93.

74. Hashemi S, Palmer DS, Aye MT, Ganz PR. Platelet-activating factor secreted by DDAVP-treated monocytes mediates von Willebrand factor release from endothelial cells. J Cell Physiol 1993;154:496–505.

75. Salzman EW, Weinstein MJ, Weintraub RM, Ware JA, Thurer RL, Robertson, et al. Treatment with desmopressin acetate to reduce blood loss after cardiac surgery. A double-blind randomized trial. N Engl J Med 1986;314:1402–6.

76. Salzman EW, Weinstein MJ, Reilly D, Ware JA. Adventures in hemostasis. Desmopressin in cardiac surgery [Review]. Arch Surg 1993;128:212–7.

77. Sheridan DP, Card RT, Pinilla JC, Harding SM, Thomson DJ, Gauthier L, Drotar D. Use of desmopressin acetate to reduce blood transfusion requirements during cardiac surgery in patients with acetylsalicylic acid-induced platelet dysfunction. Can J Surg 1994;37:33–6.

78. Gratz I, Koehler J, Olsen D, Afshar M, DeCastro N, Spagna PM, et al. The effect of desmopressin acetate on postoperative hemorrhage in patients receiving aspirin therapy before coronary artery bypass operations. J Thorac Cardiovasc Surg 1992;104:1417–22.

79. Fremes SE, Wong BI, Lee E, Mai R, Christakis GT, McLean RF, et al. Metaanalysis of prophylactic drug treatment in the prevention of postoperative bleeding. Ann Thorac Surg 1994;58:1580–8.

80. Hackmann T, Gascoyne RD, Naiman SC, Growe GH, Burchill LD, Jamieson WR, et al. A trial of desmopressin (1-desamino-8-D-arginine vasopressin) to reduce blood loss in uncomplicated cardiac surgery. N Engl J Med 1989;321:1437–43.

81. Lazenby WD, Russo I, Zadeh BJ, Zelano JA, Ko W, Lynch CC, et al. Treatment with desmopressin acetate in routine coronary artery bypass surgery to improve postoperative hemostasis. Circulation 1990;82:IV413–9.

82. Ansell J, Klassen V, Lew R, Ball S, Weinstein M, VanderSalm T, et al. Does desmopressin acetate prophylaxis reduce blood loss after valvular heart operations? A randomized, double-blind study. J Thorac Cardiovasc Surg 1992;104:117–23.

83. Casas JI, Zuazu-Jausoro I, Mateo J, Oliver A, Litvan H, Muniz-Diaz E, et al. Aprotinin versus desmopressin for patients undergoing operations with cardiopulmonary bypass. A double-blind placebo-controlled study. J Thorac Cardiovasc Surg 1995;110:1107–17.

84. Temeck BK, Bachenheimer LC, Katz NM, Coughlin SS, Wallace RB. Desmopressin acetate in cardiac surgery: a double-blind, randomized study. South Med J 1994;87:611–5.

85. de Prost D, Barbier-Boehm G, Hazebroucq J, Ibrahim H, Bielsky MC, Hvass U, et al. Desmopressin has no beneficial effect on excessive postoperative bleeding or blood product requirements associated with cardiopulmonary bypass. Thromb Haemost 1992;68:106–10.

86. Cattaneo M, Harris AS, Stromber U, Mannucci PM. The effect of desmopressin on reducing blood loss in cardiac surgery: a meta-analysis of double-blind, placebo-controlled trials. Thromb Hemostas 1995;74:1064–70.

87. Sheridan DP, Card RT, Pinilla JC, Harding SM, Thomson DJ, Gauthier L, et al. Use of desmopressin acetate to reduce blood transfusion requirements during cardiac surgery in patients with acetylsalicylic-acid-induced platelet dysfunction. Can J Surg 1994;37:33–6.

88. Laupacis A, Fergusson D. Drugs to minimize perioperative blood loss in cardiac surgery: meta-analyses using perioperative blood transfusion as the outcome. The International Study of Peri-operative Transfusion (ISPOT) Investigators. Anesth Analg 1997;85:1258–67.

89. Mongan PD, Hosking MP. The role of desmopressin acetate in patients undergoing coronary artery bypass surgery. A controlled clinical trial with thromboelastographic risk stratification. Anesthesiology 1992;77:38–46.

90. Czer LS, Bateman TM, Gray RJ, Raymond M, Stewart ME, Lee S, et al. Treatment of severe platelet dysfunction and hemorrhage after cardiopulmonary bypass: reduction in blood product usage with desmopressin. J Am Coll Cardiol 1987;9:1139–47.

91. Despotis GJ, Levine V, Saleem R, Spitznagel E, Joist JH. Use of point-of-care test in identification of patients who can benefit from desmopressin during cardiac surgery: a randomised controlled trial. Lancet 1999;354:106–10.

92. Kang YG, Martin DJ, Marquez J, Lewis JH, Bontempo FA, Shaw BW, Jr., et al. Intraoperative changes in blood coagulation and thrombelastographic monitoring in liver transplantation. Anesth Analg 1985;64:888–96.

93. Hartert H. Blutgerinnung studien mit der thromelastographie, einen neuen untersuchingsverfahren. Klin Wochenschr 1948;26:577–83.

94. Vig S, Chitolie A, Bevan DH, Halliday A, Dormandy J. Thromboelastography: a reliable test? Blood Coagul Fibrinolysis 2001;12:555–61.

95. Camenzind V, Bombeli T, Seifert B, Jamnicki M, Popovic D, Pasch T, Spahn DR. Citrate storage affects Thrombelastograph analysis. Anesthesiology 2000;92:1242–9.

96. Salooja N, Perry DJ. Thrombelastography. Blood Coagul Fibrinolysis 2001;12:327–37.

97. Bowbrick VA, Mikhailidis DP, Stansby G. The use of citrated whole blood in thromboelastography. Anesth Analg 2000;90:1086–8.

98. Yamakage M, Tsujiguchi N, Kohro S, Tsuchida H, Namiki A. The usefulness of celite-activated thromboelastography for evaluation of fibrinolysis. Can J Anaesth 1998;45:993–6.

99. Shore-Lesserson L, Manspeizer HE, DePerio M, Francis S, Vela-Cantos F, Ergin MA. Thromboelastography-guided transfusion algorithm reduces transfusions in complex cardiac surgery. Anesth Analg 1999;88:312–9.

100. Tuman KJ, McCarthy RJ, Patel RV, Patel RB, Ivankovich AD. Comparison of thromboelastography and platelet agregometry. Anesthesiology 1991;75:A433.

101. Gottumukkala VN, Sharma SK, Philip J. Assessing platelet and fibrinogen contribution to clot strength using modified thromboelastography in pregnant women. Anesth Analg 1999;89:1453–5.

102. Kettner SC, Panzer OP, Kozek SA, Seibt FA, Stoiser B, Kofler J, et al. Use of abciximab-modified thrombelastography in patients undergoing cardiac surgery. Anesth Analg 1999;89:580–4.

103. Oshita K, Az-ma T, Osawa Y, Yuge O. Quantitative measurement of thromboclastography as a function of. Anesth Analg 1999;89:296–9.

104. Clayton DG, Miro AM, Kramer DJ, Rodman N, Wearden S. Quantification of thrombelastographic changes after blood component transfusion in patients with liver disease in the intensive care unit. Anesth Analg 1995;81:272–8.

105. Tuman KJ, Spiess BD, McCarthy RJ, Ivankovich AD. Effects of progressive blood loss on coagulation as measured by thromboelastography. Anesth Analg 1987;66:856–63.

106. Toy PT, Strauss RG, Stehling LC, Sears R, Price TH, Rossi EC, et al. Predeposited autologous blood for elective surgery. A national multicenter study. N Engl J Med 1987;316:517–20.

107. Plevak D, Divertie G, Carton E, Bowie EJ, Rettke S, Taswell H, et al. Blood product transfusion therapy after liver transplantation. Transplant Proc 1993;25:1838.

108. Hindie E, Melliere D, Perlemuter L, Jeanguillaume C, Galle P. Primary hyperparathyroidism: higher success rate of first surgery after preoperative Tc-99m sestamibi-I-123 subtraction scanning. Radiology 1997;204:221–8.

109. Batelle Medical Technology Assessment and Policy Research. The economic and clinical efficiency of point-of-care testing for critically ill patients. Med Laboratory Observer 1996;27:12–6.

110. Carty SE, Worsey J, Virji MA, Brown ML, Watson CG. Concise parathyroidectomy: the impact of preoperative SPECT 99mTc sestamibi scanning and intraoperative quick parathormone assay. Surgery 1997;122:1107–14.

111. Curren DJ. Industry struggles with tight labor market. In: Crisis in the clinical laboratory. Clin Chem Acta 1997;267:33–49.

112. Lowney JK, Weber B, Johnson S, Doherty GM. Minimal incision parathyroidectomy: cure, cosmesis, and cost. World J Surg 2000;24:1442–5.

113. Levin KE, Clark OH. The reasons for failure in parathyroid operations. Arch Surg 1989;124:911–4.

114. Prey MU, Vitale T, Martin SA. Guidelines for practical utilization of intraoperative frozen sections. Arch Surg 1989;124:331–5.

115. Cusumano RJ, Mahadevia P, Silver CE. Intraoperative histologic evaluation in exploration of the parathyroid glands. Surg Gynecol Obstet 1989;169:506–10.

116. Malhotra A, Silver CE, Deshpande V, Freeman LM. Preoperative parathyroid localization with sestamibi. Am J Surg 1996;172:637–40.

117. Bergman JA, Pallant R. Thallium/technetium subtraction scanning for primary hyperparathyroidism: scan sensitivity and effect on operative time. Ear Nose Throat J 1998;77:404–7.

118. Purcell GP, Dirbas FM, Jeffrey RB, Lane MJ, Desser T, McDougall IR, Weigel RJ. Parathyroid localization with high-resolution ultrasound and technetium Tc 99m sestamibi. Arch Surg 1999;134:824–8.

119. Nussbaum SR, Thompson AR, Hutcheson KA, Gaz RD, Wang CA. Intraoperative measurement of parathyroid hormone in the surgical management of hyperparathyroidism. Surgery 1988;104:1121–7.

120. Irvin GL, III, Dembrow VD, Prudhomme DL. Clinical usefulness of an intraoperative "quick parathyroid hormone" assay. Surgery 1993;114:1019–22.

121. Michelangeli VP, Heyma P, Colman PG, Ebeling PR. Evaluation of a new, rapid and automated immunochemiluminometric assay for the measurement of serum intact parathyroid hormone. Ann Clin Biochem 1997;34:97–103.

122. Sokoll LJ, Drew H, Udelsman R. Intraoperative parathyroid hormone analysis: a study of 200 consecutive cases. Clin Chem 2000;46:1662–8.

123. Irvin GL, III, Carneiro DM. Management changes in primary hyperparathyroidism. JAMA 2000;284:934–6.

124. Ferrer Ramirez MJ, Lopez GA, Oliver Oliver MJ, Canos L, I, Lopez MR. Value of the intraoperative determination of parathyroid hormone (PTH) in hyperparathyroidism surgery. Acta Otorrinolaringol Esp 2003;54:273–6.

125. Carneiro DM, Solorzano CC, Nader MC, Ramirez M, Irvin GL, III. Comparison of intraoperative iPTH assay (QPTH) criteria in guiding parathyroidectomy: which criterion is the most accurate? Surgery 2003;134:973–9.

126. Sebag F, Shen W, Brunaud L, Kebebew E, Duh QY, Clark OH. Intraoperative parathyroid hormone assay and parathyroid reoperations. Surgery 2003;134:1049–55.

127. Chen H, Sokoll LJ, Udelsman R. Outpatient minimally invasive parathyroidectomy: a combination of sestamibi-SPECT local-

ization, cervical block anesthesia, and intraoperative parathyroid hormone assay. Surgery 1999;126:1016–21.

128. Johnson LR, Doherty G, Lairmore T, Moley JF, Brunt LM, Koenig J, et al. Evaluation of the performance and clinical impact of a rapid intraoperative parathyroid hormone assay in conjunction with preoperative imaging and concise parathyroidectomy. Clin Chem 2001;47:919–25.

129. Carter AB, Howanitz PJ. Intraoperative testing for parathyroid hormone: a comprehensive review of the use of the assay and the relevant literature. Arch Pathol Lab Med 2003;127: 1424–42.

130. Udelsman R, Donovan PI, Sokoll LJ. One hundred consecutive minimally invasive parathyroid explorations. Ann Surg 2000; 232:331–9.

131. Drop LJ. Ionized calcium, the heart, and hemodynamic function. Anesth Analg 1985;64:432–51.

132. Urban P, Scheidegger D, Buchmann B, Barth D. Cardiac arrest and blood ionized calcium levels. Ann Intern Med 1988;109: 110–3.

133. Burchard KW, Gann DS, Colliton J, Forster J. Ionized calcium, parathormone, and mortality in critically ill surgical patients. Ann Surg 1990;212:543–9.

Chapter **26**

Point-of-Care Testing in the Intensive Care Unit

Peter Gosling, Paul A. H. Holloway, and Anne Sutcliffe

The birth of the intensive care unit (ICU) can be traced to the Danish poliomyelitis epidemic in 1953, which highlighted the lifesaving benefit of prolonged ventilation for the treatment of respiratory failure. This led to the rapid development of mechanical ventilators and the appointment of specialized staff to care for ventilated patients. Since then, intensive care medicine has become increasingly sophisticated, and today support is provided for most major organ systems. The role of the ICU is to provide organ support, allowing the patient to recover from the initial injury or insult. It is the monitoring of organ function, and providing a form of "surrogate homeostasis," that determines the requirements for point-of-care testing (POCT).

Mechanical ventilation requires rapid assessment of the oxygen and acid-base status of the patient, and coincided with the development of the first integrated clinical blood-gas measuring system (1). Although blood gas was initially a laboratory-based measurement, growth in hospital size increased the distance of the ICU from the laboratory, introducing specimen transport delays, making POCT attractive. By the late 1970s, ICUs had bedside blood-gas analytical systems that were used by nursing and medical staff. The continuing development in sensor technology and the ability to measure other analytes on a syringe sample of heparinized whole blood soon led to the addition of sodium, potassium, chloride, and ionized calcium. Microprocessor-controlled derivative spectroscopy of whole-blood hemolysates made it possible to estimate hemoglobin fractions and thereby measure not only total hemoglobin but also oxygen saturation, and hence derive the oxygen-carrying capacity of the blood. Further advances in sensor design have provided glucose, lactate, urea, and in some instruments ionized magnesium, all of which can be measured with less than 1 mL of fresh heparinized blood.

The increase in sophistication of instrumentation and range of available analyses, coupled with increasing user-friendliness toward nonlaboratory staff, has resulted in an enormous expansion in POCT in ICUs. In all modern ICUs, POCT has become an indispensable aid to clinical management. The rapid technological advancements in POCT have the potential to bring genomics, pharmacogenomics, proteomics, and metabonomics to the bedside within the next decade.

This chapter discusses the requirements for ICU analytical services from a clinical perspective, reviews the ways in which POCT may be most effectively used, and discusses some analytes that show promise for future application as point-of-care tests in the ICU of the future. These include early markers of bacterial and nonbacterial sepsis, assessment of microvascular patency, and genomic characterization of individual patient response to acute inflammatory insults.

CLINICAL QUESTIONS IN THE ICU

Who Needs Intensive Care?

The most common reason patients require intensive care is respiratory failure, necessitating one-to-one nursing and, frequently, endotracheal intubation and mechanical ventilation. Other common reasons for ICU admission are severe acid-base disorders due, for example, to diabetic ketoacidosis, cardiopulmonary arrest, or poisoning. Many hospitals in the United Kingdom have an ICU outreach team that is asked to assess patients who may require ICU care. POCT has an important role in the rapid assessment of patients on the ward or in the emergency department who may require intensive care. An important factor in deciding if such patients require ICU care is their blood-gas and acid-base status, and results are usually required within 5–10 min of a member of the ICU team being called to see the patient. POCT is the only practical way in which these results can be obtained within this time frame.

Is the Blood Carrying Enough Oxygen?

Patients reaching the ICU are by definition at risk of losing or have lost their normal homeostatic mechanisms, which are essential for cellular function. The most important cellular requirement is an adequate oxygen supply to the cells. Interruption of the oxygen supply will cause brain damage within 2–3 min and death within 10 min. The mechanisms leading to respiratory failure are numerous and complex but can be summarized from a clinical perspective (Table 26-1).

Both respiratory muscle failure and inadequate gas exchange are treated by mechanical ventilation. Only by estimation of oxygen saturation of hemoglobin and arterial blood-gas measurement can the adequacy of ventilation be assessed.

Mechanical ventilation is also used to manipulate arterial blood-gas tensions in head injury patients with raised intracranial pressure. Adequate oxygenation of the injured brain is essential, and maintenance of the arterial carbon dioxide tension at the lower end of normal helps to reduce the volume of intracranial contents and thus reduces intracranial pressure.

Table 26-1 Summary of Some Common Causes of Respiratory Failure

1. The airway must be patent.
   Causes of obstruction include:
   Tongue falling backward in unconscious patients
   Inhalation of a foreign body
   Swelling caused by accidental injury, allergy, or inhalation of hot smoke
   Surgery blocking the airway
   With the exception of foreign bodies, which must be removed, other forms of airway inadequacy are treated by endotracheal intubation.
2. The respiratory muscles must be functioning adequately.
   Inadequate muscle function may be due to:
   Infections such as poliomyelitis
   Autoimmune neurological dysfunction such as Guillain-Barre syndrome
   Injury to the chest wall or spinal cord
3. The lung tissue must be capable of gas exchange.
   Gas exchange may be compromised by:
   Collapsed alveoli due to trauma
   Alveoli obliterated by blood following injury, infected sputum, or edema fluid.

Both the primary disease process and the sedative and paralyzing drugs used to facilitate mechanical ventilation compromise the patient's homeostatic processes, which maintain normal oxygenation and carbon dioxide removal.

Except for patients with profound derangement, the adequacy of blood oxygenation and carbon dioxide removal is impossible to assess accurately using clinical features such as skin color, perfusion, and heart rate. In a single-observer blind study of pulse oximetry in patients undergoing surgery and postoperative care, the incidence of mild hypoxia (Hb saturation 86% to 90%) were 53% and 55%, respectively, and severe hypoxia (Hb saturation <81%) were 20% and 13%, respectively. When pulse oximetry data were made available in real time, extreme hypoxia (Hb saturation <76%) was avoided completely in the operating room and recovery room. Several changes were associated with the availability of pulse oximetry data, including high flow rates of supplemental oxygen, oxygen therapy on discharge to the ward, and increased use of naxolone. Compared with a control group, there was a 19-fold increase in diagnosed hypoxemia in patients from whom pulse oximetry data were available (2).

Care must be exercised in interpreting pulse oximetry data, since the accuracy of pulse oximetry deteriorates as hypoxemia worsens. Confirmation of arterial blood oyxhemoglobin saturation by cooximetry is essential when precise determination of arterial oyxhemoglobin is critical (3). Nevertheless, these results suggest that continuous monitoring of blood oxygenation by pulse oximetry and confirmatory blood-gas measurements are mandatory for patients undergoing general anesthesia and for patients in the ICU. Only in this way will sudden deterioration in oxygenation be detected.

Is Oxygen Delivery Optimal?

Estimating the hemoglobin oxygen saturation with pulse oximetry or by measurement of the arterial PaO_2 does not, however, indicate whether enough oxygen is reaching the tissues. Oxygen delivery depends not only on the oxygen content of the blood but also the adequacy of blood flow to the tissues. The oxygen content of blood can be calculated from the measured values of total hemoglobin and oxyhemoglobin. The flow rate to the tissues depends on the adequacy of vascular filling and myocardial contractility. The adequacy of flow can be inferred by invasive measurement of the cardiac output, pulmonary capillary occlusion pressure, and systemic vascular resistance using a pulmonary artery flotation catheter (PAFC). PAFCs have blood sampling ports that permit the oxygen content of mixed venous blood to be estimated. Subtraction of the mixed venous oxygen content from the arterial oxygen content gives an indication of global oxygen extraction by the tissues. A similar calculation using the oxygen content of blood, sampled from a catheter placed in the jugular bulb, allows an assessment to be made of the adequacy of cerebral oxygenation, but as of yet it is not possible to perform similar measurements for other individual organs.

Transesophageal doppler probes are less invasive and directly measure the blood flow generated by the heart. In contrast to the PAFC and jugular bulb catheter, blood samples cannot be obtained for measurement of oxygen flux.

Assessment of the global adequacy of tissue oxygenation can also be made by measurement of the acid-base status, since anaerobic metabolism will be associated with a nonrespiratory acidosis. However, in patients suspected of having hypovolemic shock, a low-standard bicarbonate and increased anion gap (AG) cannot be assumed to indicate lactic acidosis (4). Measurement of blood lactate can be helpful in differentiating between a nonrespiratory acidosis due to other causes [e.g., ketosis (high AG) or hyperchloremia (normal AG)] and tissue hypoxia. Nevertheless, interpretation of blood lactate values requires some care. An increased blood lactate value may reflect not only tissue hypoxia, but also failure of hepatic lactate metabolism (Cori cycle) due to liver disease, poisoning, or ischemia. Recent studies suggest that mitochondrial failure in severe sepsis may also cause lactic acidosis despite adequate delivery of oxygen to the tissues (5, 6). Conversely, in a hypovolemic patient with intense adrenergic vasoconstriction, the arterial blood lactate may underreport the severity of tissue hypoxia because of arteriovenous shunting. Under these circumstances, the blood lactate concentration may rise when the circulation is restored due to a washout of ischemic tissue. This understanding of the limitations of interpreting raised blood lactate concentrations is important, as inappropriate resuscitation treatment can be hazardous. Despite these limitations, successful resuscitation of a patient suffering hypovolemic shock, for example, will be associated with serial blood lactate concentrations falling from high values to normal within 4–6 h. This gives some indication of the requisite turnaround time required for the measurement to be used for clinical guidance, and the reason for its increasing use in monitoring ICU patients as part of a panel of measurements on modern POCT blood-gas analyzers. It is important to recognize that infusions of lactate—for example, with lactate-buffered hemofiltration replacement fluid—can lead to significant but transient elevations in levels of blood lactate (5–6 mmol/L). There are some data suggesting that lactate intolerance may be harmful, and in these circumstances alternative buffers are recommended (7).

Another approach to assess oxygen delivery is to measure the gastric mucosal pCO_2 using a gastric tonometer filled with saline, bicarbonate solution, or air, which is allowed to equilibrate with the CO_2 tension in the lumen of the stomach. By measuring the tonometer pCO_2 and using the derived bicarbonate from a simultaneous arterial blood-gas measurement, it is possible to calculate the intramucosal pH, known as the pHi. During periods of gut hypoperfusion, the pHi can drop dramatically as the gut becomes ischemic, and this technique is used as an additional marker of tissue perfusion and oxygenation (8–10). Although this technique is performed at the bedside, the tonometer takes a long time to equilibrate, and thus the method cannot be used to detect rapid changes in physiological status.

An alternative methodology for assessing regional rather than systemic ischemia is the application of microdialysis. This method requires the placement of a microdialysis probe adjacent to the site at risk (e.g., a skin flap or surgical anastomosis) and serial analysis of dialyzed interstitial fluid for metabolites lactate and pyruvate. The lactate–pyruvate ratio is an indicator of the redox state of the adjacent tissues, and several studies have shown the potential of this method to anticipate destructive tissue ischemia. This technique has yet to reach widespread use and awaits the support from further research evidence (11).

How Can Oxygenation Be Improved?

Mechanical ventilation allows the oxygen content of the inspired gas to vary from 21% (room air) to 100% (pure oxygen). Comparison of the PaO_2 and the fractional inspired oxygen tension (FiO_2) gives an indication of how well the blood supply to the lungs is matched to their ventilation. At its simplest, the efficiency of the lungs can be described by dividing PaO_2 by FiO_2. In a normal person, this is about 430 (90 mmHg/0.2) while for a patient with lung failure, the value might be 113 (90 mmHg/0.8).[a] Poor gas exchange may be due to failure to ventilate all the alveoli (e.g., as a result of pulmonary edema), or failure of the blood supply to the lungs (because of heart failure), or hypovolemia. The positive intrathoracic pressure required for mechanical ventilation can itself cause lung injury, including pneumothorax and increased risk of chest infection. Different ventilator techniques are now employed to reduce the risk of "barotrauma," associated with mechanical ventilation (12). Removal of interstitial edema by fluid restriction and careful use of diuretics may also help to increase the number of alveoli that are ventilated. Physiotherapy will also assist by removing lung secretions that mechanically obstruct the airways within the lung. Blood flow to the lungs can

[a] Using pO_2 in kPa, these values are 57 and 15 respectively.

be increased by correction of hypovolemia, optimizing cardiac output through manipulation of the cardiac filling pressures and pharmacological adjustment in the patient's vascular tone with inotropes. Selective pulmonary vasodilatation, by adding nitric oxide (NO) to the inspired gas, is now used to improve lung blood flow without producing an undesirable fall in systemic blood pressure. However, nitric oxide administration has yet to be shown to improve outcome and must be carefully controlled, since in concentrations >25 ppm there is a risk of toxicity due to formation of toxic peroxynitrite free radicals (13). One feature of toxicity is the formation of methemoglobin, which can be monitored by oximetry in the ICU, and this is now an essential parameter for POCT in units that use NO therapy.

For a critically ill patient, it may be necessary to make frequent adjustments to several aspects of the treatment regime to optimize tissue oxygenation. Ideally, only one or two changes are made at a time so that the effects of changing each component of therapy can be clearly identified. Consequently, frequent measurements of PaO_2, hemoglobin, oxyhemoglobin, and oxygen content are essential for appropriate management of mechanically ventilated patients. For example, changes in ventilator settings would be expected to influence parameters of oxygenation within 5–10 min. Clearly, the results must be available within this time frame or the patient's clinical condition may require another change in treatment before the effect of previous changes are known. In the absence of exceptionally rapid specimen transport to the laboratory, POCT is the only way of providing these results.

What Is the Patient's Acid-Base Status?

Simultaneous measurement of arterial carbon dioxide and hydrogen ion concentration (pH) gives an indication of how well the lungs are removing carbon dioxide and the effect this is having on the net balance of acid production and removal. For example, in a patient with poor gas exchange and carbon dioxide retention for 24 h or more, the initial excess of hydrogen ions due to formation of carbonic acid is normally corrected by renal synthesis (recycling) of additional bicarbonate. Patients with nonrespiratory acidosis due, for example, to diabetic ketoacidosis will tend to hyperventilate, thereby lowering their pCO_2 and restoring their extracellular fluid (ECF) hydrogen ion concentration to normal. The effectiveness of this compensation can be assessed by measurement of arterial H^+ (pH) and pCO_2. Acid-base status can change extremely rapidly in the critically ill patient. For example, a patient suffering a cardiopulmonary arrest will develop a mixed respiratory and nonrespiratory acidosis within 2 min. Assuming resuscitation is effective and cardiac and lung function are restored, the patient's acidosis will generally clear within 30–60 min. Failure of acidosis to resolve within this period indicates further complications, and the patient may require inotropic support, bicarbonate infusion, and alteration in the mode of ventilation. The calculated parameter of base excess (or deficit) is used as a way of assessing the degree of nonrespiratory or metabolic acid-base disturbance. This parameter, if abnormal, does not give an indication of the cause of the metabolic disturbance, but it is common to rely on this (e.g., base deficit in a metabolic acidosis) as a barometer of change. Current concepts of acid-base include not only the traditional buffer base Henderson-Hasselbach equation but also the electroneutrality concept described by Stewart (14).

In all aqueous systems, the balance of anions and cations must retain electrical neutrality. There are only three major independent determinants that control acid-base balance: pCO_2, weak acids (albumin and phosphate), and the strong ion difference (SID). In practice, the SID describes the mathematical difference between plasma Na^+, K^+, Ca^+, and Mg^+ (strong cations) and Cl^- and $lactate^-$ (strong anions) and is normally between 38 and 42 mmol/L (38 and 42 mEq/L). If one of these ions increases in concentration (e.g., Cl^-), then the SID will be reduced. To retain electrical neutrality, more hydrogen ions dissociate from water and the hydrogen ion concentration increases, the pH falls, and the patient becomes acidotic. However, the change in hydrogen ion concentration is in the nanomolar range and is insufficient to maintain electrical neutrality when the chloride rises by millimoles; thus, the plasma proteins play the major role in restoring electrical neutrality. The reverse happens in patients with a chloride deficit, such as might arise with loss of nasogastric aspirate from the upper gastrointestinal tract. This leads to a decrease in the chloride–sodium ratio, an increase in the SID, and thus a decrease in water dissociation and a fall in hydrogen ion activity (hypochloremic alkalosis). Thus assessment of chloride, and in particular the chloride–sodium ratio, becomes of real value in determining the acid-base disturbance and assessing treatment in critically ill patients (14). Assessment of SID can be used as a quantitative guideline for chloride (NaCl or KCl) replacement. The full implications of this concept await studies to demonstrate an influence on patient outcome, but there is no doubt that chloride is now considered an essential contributor to acid-base assessment in the ICU and needs to be available from POCT. This is another example illustrating how POCT is essential for guiding treatment in the ICU.

Diagnosis and treatment of metabolic acidosis must include an assessment of unmeasured anions. Although lactate is usually available on POCT blood gas analyzers, unmeasured anions include phosphate, sulphate, and hippurate in renal failure, and ketones in starvation and diabetic ketoacidosis, as well as other anions after poisoning (e.g., methanol). Careful inspection of the anion gap may suggest a significant contribution from these unmeasured anions. For example, starvation ketoacidosis is frequently a significant problem in ICU patients, yet can easily be missed or ignored. Point-of-care analysis of blood ketones (ideally hydroxybutyrate) should be considered a high priority in the assessment of a metabolic acidosis.

What Is the Patient's Extracellular Potassium Concentration?

Acute hypokalemia causes muscle weakness, and when severe carries a risk of cardiac arrhythmia. Hypokalemia may develop gradually, due, for example, to increased urinary losses asso-

ciated with diuretic administration or excessive gastrointestinal losses. However, in the mechanically ventilated ICU patient, hypokalemia can occur within 1 h or so. For example, in patients with chronic CO_2 retention, there is a compensatory rise in ECF bicarbonate produced by the kidneys, which tends to offset the respiratory acidosis, bringing the H^+ (pH) back to normal. Under these circumstances a sudden fall in pCO_2 (e.g., due to commencement of mechanical ventilation or an abrupt change in ventilator settings) will rapidly remove CO_2 and precipitate an acute alkalosis due to the residual high circulating bicarbonate concentration. The acute alkalosis produces a shift of potassium ions into the cells, lowering the patient's extracellular potassium concentration. This process may be further influenced by endocrine changes (e.g., both glucocorticoid and mineralocorticoid) and by pharmacological interventions (e.g., low-dose hydrocortisone and thiazide diuretics). Abnormalities in renal tubular function such as renal tubular acidosis are recognized complications in critically ill patients (e.g., drug induced, as a complication of diabetic ketoacidosis, or from acute tubular necrosis), and the possibility of such conditions should caution the intensivist to evaluate urine electrolytes, pH, and anion gap. Although these are difficult to evaluate at the point of care, the delays from remote analysis are one of the reasons why these tests are often neglected. Access to rapid urine analysis at the point of care would enhance electrolyte and acid-base assessment and would seem a high priority for development. Serum potassium concentrations can fall from 4.0 to 2.5 mmol/L within 2 h in extreme cases, and this is a well-recognized cause of cardiac arrhythmia and cardiac arrest.

Hyperkalemia is also common in ICU patients, both due to movement of potassium from within the cells in exchange for hydrogen ions during acidosis and because of reduced renal excretion of potassium due to renal impairment. Severe hyperkalemia carries a risk of cardiac arrhythmia and cardiac arrest. Administration of insulin and glucose, either as part of intensive control of blood glucose (see later) or for correction of acidosis, will drive potassium back into the cells and may result in a rapid fall in extracellular potassium. Renal replacement therapies such as hemofiltration also correct acidosis and will remove extracellular potassium. Thus, sudden changes in extracellular potassium concentrations are not uncommon in ICU patients and require regular monitoring of blood potassium, and in some circumstances results need to be available within in a few minutes. Figure 26-1 provides an example of how rapidly oxygenation, acid-base, potassium, and ionized calcium can change in a critically ill postoperative patient and how POCT data influence patient management.

Are the Patient's Ionized Calcium and Magnesium Optimal?

In addition to the extracellular potassium concentration, neuromuscular function is also influenced by the extracellular ionized calcium activity. Both may affect the ease with which a patient can be weaned from mechanical ventilation. Hypocalcemia is associated with hyperexcitability of neuromuscular

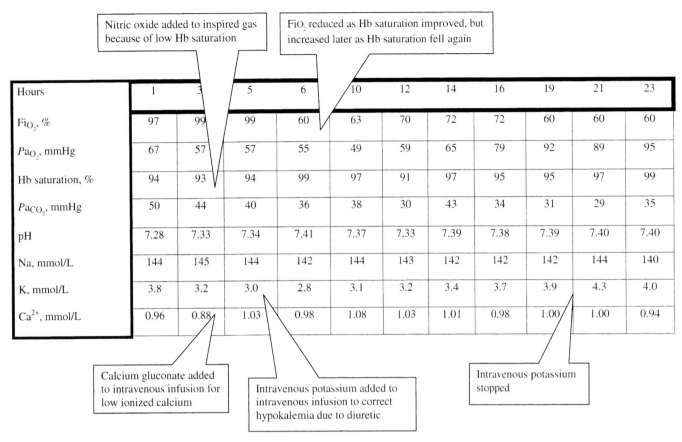

Nitric oxide added to inspired gas because of low Hb saturation

FiO_2 reduced as Hb saturation improved, but increased later as Hb saturation fell again

Hours	1	3	5	6	10	12	14	16	19	21	23
FiO_2, %	97	99	99	60	63	70	72	72	60	60	60
PaO_2, mmHg	67	57	57	55	49	59	65	79	92	89	95
Hb saturation, %	94	93	94	99	97	91	97	95	95	97	99
$PaCO_2$, mmHg	50	44	40	36	38	30	43	34	31	29	35
pH	7.28	7.33	7.34	7.41	7.37	7.33	7.39	7.38	7.39	7.40	7.40
Na, mmol/L	144	145	144	142	144	143	142	142	142	144	140
K, mmol/L	3.8	3.2	3.0	2.8	3.1	3.2	3.4	3.7	3.9	4.3	4.0
Ca^{2+}, mmol/L	0.96	0.88	1.03	0.98	1.08	1.03	1.01	0.98	1.00	1.00	0.94

Calcium gluconate added to intravenous infusion for low ionized calcium

Intravenous potassium added to intravenous infusion to correct hypokalemia due to diuretic

Intravenous potassium stopped

Figure 26-1 POCT data for a patient admitted to the ICU after gastroduodenectomy for a large arterial bleed. The patient had pulmonary edema and raised central venous pressure. A diuretic was given to help mobilize fluid in the lungs, inspired nitric oxide was given to produce pulmonary vasodilatation, and potassium and calcium were given based on POCT results.

junctions, while hypercalcemia depresses neuromuscular function. Low plasma ionized calcium concentration may occur in patients who have been transfused with large volumes of blood, since calcium is bound to citrate, used as an anticoagulant in stored blood. This may be particularly marked in the anhepatic phase of liver transplantation, when citrate metabolism is impaired. Laboratory measurement of total calcium is a poor measure of ionized calcium, since about 50% of calcium is either complexed with other anions or bound to protein (chiefly albumin), and "calcium correction for albumin" is at best semiquantitative (15). For this reason, ionized calcium methodologies have been developed, and ionized calcium sensors are frequently included in the repertoire of POCT equipment.

Over the past 10 years, interest has centered on magnesium in critically ill patients (16). In a study of patients undergoing cardiopulmonary bypass, plasma ionized magnesium was significantly reduced 24 h after the operation, with no change in total magnesium (17). Manifestations of magnesium deficiency include hypokalemia, hypocalcemia, neuromuscular hyperexcitability, respiratory muscle weakness, and intractable cardiac arrhythmias. A possible link has been made between respiratory distress syndrome of the premature infant, sudden infant death syndrome, and mag-

nesium deficiency. The proposed mechanism involves acute magnesium deficiency leading to platelet aggregation, microvascular congestion, hemorrhage, and edema affecting the lungs in particular (18).

Other studies have revealed a high incidence of abnormal serum and erythrocyte magnesium abnormalities in the critically ill, with hypermagnesemia being associated with increased mortality (19). As with calcium, about 50% of circulating magnesium is protein bound; thus, total magnesium measurements may be misleading in patients with hypoalbuminemia–an extremely common finding in ICU patients (20). There is no convincing evidence, however, to suggest that ionized magnesium measurement offers an advantage to serum total magnesium, and thus daily central laboratory serum magnesium assays are still most common in ICU practice in the United Kingdom, and most units have developed protocols to initiate magnesium replacement regimes.

Are the Patient's Capillaries Leaking?

Any inflammatory stimulus (e.g., surgery, sepsis, acute pancreatitis, trauma, burn injury, or ischemia and reperfusion) produces an increase in systemic capillary permeability (21). Systemic capillary permeability can be monitored by measurement of low-level urinary albumin excretion (microalbuminuria), because the renal concentrating mechanism amplifies changes in glomerular permeability (22). In a variety of clinical conditions such as major surgery, trauma, bacterial meningitis, and acute pancreatitis, microalbuminuria has been found to be predictive of later complications, particularly pulmonary dysfunction and organ failures. In general ICU admissions, microalbuminuria has been found to be a predictor of sepsis and multiple organ failure (23–25).

Microalbuminuria appears to be predictive of later complications because increased vascular permeability is associated with severe stimulation of the inflammatory pathways. Unopposed acute inflammation is central to the pathogenesis of multiple organ failure (26), and an increase in systemic capillary permeability, known as clinical capillary leak syndrome, is a very early feature of this process (27). Therefore, hourly bedside measurement of microalbuminuria, corrected for the urine flow rate, provides a way of monitoring the early postinsult inflammatory process and identifies patients who are at particular risk of later organ failure (28). Figure 26-2 illustrates how increased capillary permeability assessed by microalbuminuria predicts mortality on the ICU within 4–6 h of ICU admission (29).

Knowledge of the duration and extent of capillary leak in the critically ill not only predicts complications, but also allows intravenous fluid administration to be tailored to the individual patient. Patients in the ICU who develop pulmonary edema, acute respiratory distress syndrome, and multiple organ failure are characterized by a positive fluid balance of many liters. The fluid accumulation is in the interstitial space and is caused by increased capillary permeability, which allows protein and water to escape from the vascular compartment. Every gram of albumin moving into the interstitial space is accompanied by 18 g of water.

Interstitial edema in the lungs prevents effective gas exchange, and in other organs compromises blood flow by increasing the pressure within the microvascular capillary bed, and increasing the distance between capillaries and cells, across which oxygen and other substrates must diffuse. In order to minimize interstitial edema, intravenous resuscitation fluids are now being used that are better retained within the vascular compartment at times of increased capillary leak. The use of human albumin solutions for volume expansion of the critically ill has been criticized because of an association with increased mortality (30), which has been attributed to its failure to be retained in the circulation. Larger-molecular-weight synthetic colloids, such as hydroxyethyl starches (mean molecular weight = 200,000 Da), are better retained in the circulation during periods of capillary leak. There is evidence that their administration in surgical patients produces less splanchnic ischemia compared with albumin solutions (31) and gelatine (32), and better lung function (33).

It has also been shown that hydroxyethyl starch resuscitation of trauma victims improves pulmonary gas exchange and reduces trauma capillary leak to less than half, compared with resuscitation with low-molecular-weight colloids (34, 35). Point-of-care assessment of vascular permeability by urine albumin measurement should make it possible to control capillary leak with synthetic colloids such as hydroxyethyl starches. Studies are yet to be done to show whether this approach will reduce complications such as acute respiratory distress syndrome and organ failure in the ICU population. Since the average cost per day of an ICU bed in the United Kingdom is ~$3000 (£1500), reducing the time patients spend in ICU by improved fluid management would make a major saving.

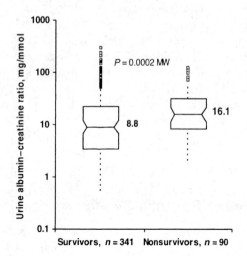

Median ACR within 15 min of ICU admission

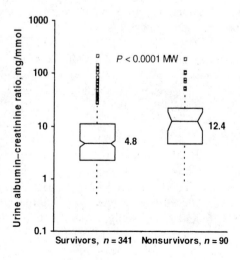

Median ACR 4–6 h post–ICU admission

Figure 26-2 Median (95% CI) urine albumin:creatinine ratio within 15 min of ICU admission and after 4–6 h for 431 patients, compared with ICU mortality. [Data from Gosling et al. (29).]

What Is the Patient's Colloidal Oncotic Pressure?

In the past, serum albumin concentrations have been used as a crude estimation of plasma colloidal oncotic pressure, and albumin was sometimes given in an attempt to raise oncotic pressure and reduce edema in ICU patients. The increasing use of synthetic colloids, rather than human blood products (e.g., human albumin solution or plasma protein fraction) for more effective volume expansion, frequently results in very low patient serum concentrations of albumin and total protein. Because the effective plasma life of different synthetic colloids varies, depending both on the product's structure and its variable distribution in individual patients, it is impossible to estimate whether a patient's colloidal oncotic pressure is sufficient to prevent worsening of interstitial edema. Conversely, there is concern that excessive administration of colloids could have damaging effects on vulnerable cell membranes such as renal glomerulus and tubule (36). For this reason, plasma colloidal oncotic pressure measurement may become increasingly in demand. A bedside measurement would be ideal (although not essential, provided there is a prompt laboratory service) because the oncotic pressure is likely to change dramatically in critically ill patients who have lost large volumes of blood due to hemorrhage, and proteins and water into their interstitial space due to capillary leakage.

What Is the Patient's Blood Volume, and Is Circulation Adequate?

Most modern blood-gas equipment has the ability to provide an accurate hemoglobin measurement. However, measured hematocrit or hemoglobin is a poor indicator of anemia in critically ill patients. This is because acute blood loss is accompanied by vasoconstriction, especially in the splanchnic circulation, resulting in maintenance of normal hemoglobin concentrations despite a contracted vascular volume. In addition, increased capillary permeability associated with the acute inflammatory response, which is invariably present in such patients, allows leakage of protein and water into the interstitial space, causing a relative concentration of red blood cells in the vascular compartment. Although medical and nursing staff experienced in caring for the critically ill are generally aware of this phenomenon, and interpret hemoglobin results with caution until it is judged that the patient's blood volume has been restored to normal with fluid, this can be extremely difficult to assess (37). For these reasons efforts have been made to develop practical bedside methods of estimating blood volume. Dilution studies using erythrocytes labeled with ^{51}Cr have been the most widely used method of determining circulating blood volume, but such techniques are cumbersome, involve radioisotopes, and cannot be easily repeated in the same patient. Other approaches have included injection of indocyanine green (38), addition of carbon monoxide to the inhaled gas and estimation of carboxyhemoglobin (39), and injection of fluorescent-labeled large-molecular-weight col-

loids (40). To date, there is no commercially available technique that can be used for bedside blood-volume estimation. Consequently, it is likely that occult anemia is often present in ICU patients.

Intricately linked to the assessment of circulating volume is that of hydration status, and for this, regular monitoring of serum sodium is essential. Regardless of the mechanisms involved, hypernatremia has been shown in several studies and audits to be associated with increased morbidity and mortality, and outcome would appear to be influenced by the degree of correction of either admission or subsequent development of hypernatremia. Although the clinician is more readily aware of the risks of hyponatremia and fluid overload, identifying the cause and then correction of hypernatremia are often complex conundrums that take up a disproportionate percentage of the ward round discussions at the bedside. For these to be meaningful and effective, regular serum, and ideally urine, sodium measurements at the point of care are essential and complement the other parameters of circulating volume and cardiac function.

Is the Patient's Coagulation under Control?

Abnormalities of blood coagulation are common in critically ill patients. They may be due to dilution following resuscitation and major transfusion, liver failure, and the inability to synthesize coagulation proteins or disseminated intravascular coagulation—the hematological manifestation of multiple organ failure. Abnormalities of clotting can also occur after some surgical procedures that require anticoagulation. Cardiopulmonary bypass, percutaneous revascularization for acute myocardial infarction, and coiling of intracerebral aneurysms are examples of such procedures. Furthermore, in the ICU, continuous venovenous hemofiltration for the treatment of acute renal failure requires carefully controlled anticoagulation. It is important that coagulation is checked regularly to ensure that either reversal is complete or that the degree of anticoagulation is appropriate. Many procedures performed in the ICU are undertaken percutaneously and are effectively blind when compared to surgical procedures where any bleeding blood vessel can be seen and dealt with. Consequently, it is important that coagulation is within the normal range so that if a vessel is inadvertently punctured, bleeding stops rapidly by natural means. Such ICU procedures include the placement of large-bore intravascular cannulae for dialysis or cardiovascular monitoring and percutaneous tracheostomy. As with other ICU techniques, it is often important to perform these techniques without undue delay. Therefore, the portable bedside equipment now available for the measurement of prothrombin time, activated partial thromboplastin time, thrombin time, and heparin-neutralization time could be immensely useful. However, comparison with laboratory-based methods gives mixed results (41), although activated partial thromboplastin time can be measured at the bedside (42), and is perhaps the most valuable measure because heparin anticoagulation is frequently used in ICUs because of its easy reversibility.

Thromboelastography is a well-established method for dynamic assessment of the coagulation process. Although it is more commonly used during cardiac surgery, as the technology improves it is also emerging as part of the point-of-care repertoire in the ICU. It remains to be demonstrated whether this will supplant existing central laboratory–based methods. Recombinant activated protein C has emerged as one of the only intervention therapies to date that can improve the outcome from severe sepsis, but the studies that demonstrated the benefit did not suggest that monitoring levels are of value either before or during therapy.

Is the Patient's Blood Glucose under Control?

The critically ill patient's ability to maintain blood glucose concentrations within the limits defined for normal subjects is often impaired. Moderate hyperglycemia is frequently found following an acute inflammatory stimulus (e.g., surgery, myocardial infarction, sepsis, trauma, or burns) and is attributed to release of glycocorticoids and catecholamines, which stimulate gluconeogenesis. Hyperglycemia can worsen a hyperosmotic state such as uremia and may predispose a patient to infection.

A more serious risk in critically ill patients is hypoglycemia, which if untreated can cause brain damage and death. In a healthy fasting subject, the glycogen reserves in the liver and muscle will provide glucose (glucose 6 phosphate in muscle) for about 24 h, after which the glucose supply is derived from gluconeogensis. In contrast, a critically ill patient who is hypercatabolic will use up the glycogen stores within a few hours and risk becoming hypoglycemic if gluconeogenic pathways cannot meet the increased glucose demand. This is particularly true in neonates.

Concerns about risks from hypoglycemia, combined with the lack of information to suggest an "ideal" blood glucose level in critical illness and concerns about the accuracy of glucose stick tests caution against aggressive control of blood glucose. In 2001, a large randomized controlled study that compared conventional glucose control (8–11.0 mmol/L) with intensive control (4–5.5 mmol/L) was stopped following an interim assessment when it was demonstrated that there was significantly lower mortality in the intensive treatment group (43). This study, which did not demonstrate an increased risk from hypoglycemia in the intensive treatment group, had an immediate global effect on the management of blood glucose in ICU patients, and the intensive control target values were widely accepted. There is not a clear understanding of the mechanism for the influence on mortality, but it seems likely that the major influence comes from the insulin treatment and the complex metabolic and endocrine effects that it induces rather than from the normalization of blood glucose per se. For this regime to be effective and safe, accurate measurements of blood glucose must be a high priority for point-of-care analysis, and these are usually now provided by a blood-gas analyzer with integral metabolite electrodes. As intravenous infusions of dextrose and insulin can produce rapid alterations in blood glucose, normoglycemia in the critically ill patient can only be maintained by frequent monitoring, with results being rapidly available.

POTENTIAL ANALYTES FOR FUTURE ICU POCT

Markers of Sepsis

The term *sepsis* in ICU patients generally refers to patient response to a severe inflammatory stimulus, which can be caused by insults such as trauma, surgery, ischemia reperfusion injury, or bacterial infection. The clinical features include pyrexia, confusion, or loss of consciousness, with hypotension, tachycardia, and vasodilatation with either a rapid fall or rapid increase in white cell count outside the reference range. This combination of symptoms has been defined as the systemic inflammatory response syndrome (SIRS), and carries an increased risk of organ failure and death (26). Although the clinical features are fairly consistent, the initiating cause of inflammation may not be obvious. Studies of ICU patients with SIRS have failed to identify an infective organism in about 40% of cases, which has supported the concept that many cases of SIRS are due to noninfective inflammatory processes. There is an alternative view, which is that most patients with SIRS are suffering from an infection, but that laboratory investigations have failed to identify an infective organism. However, in order to treat patients effectively, it is important to differentiate between infective and noninfective causes of SIRS. For this reason, there has been a search for more sensitive and specific markers of bacterial sepsis. There follows a brief overview of markers of sepsis and an attempt to evaluate their potential use as point-of-care analyses.

Procalcitonin

Procalcitonin is a 14-kDa protein encoded by the Calc-1 gene along with calcitonin and katacalcin, which is elevated in patients with sepsis and severe infections. In a study of 123 consecutive ICU patients with SIRS, Bell et al. (44) found that procalcitoinin was 10 times higher in those with positive blood cultures, together with C-reactive protein (CRP) was more sensitive than either test alone, and differentiated between patients who died in the hospital or survived. In a comparison of procalcitonin with interleukin (IL)-2 and IL-8 in 33 patients with sepsis or septic shock, all three markers increased in parallel with illness severity. However procalcitonin exhibited the greatest sensitivity (85%) and specificity (91%) in differentiating patients with SIRS from those with sepsis. The authors suggested that daily determination of procalcitonin may be helpful in the follow-up of critically ill patients (45). In 116 neonates and children up to 12 years old with sepsis, Enguix et al. (46) compared procalcitonin with CRP and serum amyloid A on admission or when a bacterial sepsis was suspected. In critically ill neonates, procalcitonin, CRP, and amyloid A all had similar diagnostic efficiency as markers of sepsis, but procalcitonin concentration >8.1 ng/mL identified all children with bacterial sepsis. In 101 consecutive patients admitted to a medical ICU, serum procalcitonin concentration was a more sensitive and specific marker of sepsis, compared with serum CRP, IL-6, and lactate levels (47). Finally, a follow-up of 405 trauma patients suggested that procalcitonin is a sensitive predictor of posttrauma complications such as severe sepsis and organ failure (48).

These studies suggest that procalcitonin is a more specific marker for bacterial sepsis than serum CRP or proinflammatory cytokines such as IL-2, IL-6, or tumor necrosis factor. However, this alone does not justify its provision as a point-of-care test unless the rapid turnaround time can be shown to be of benefit. Bacterial sepsis evolves over hours rather than minutes; thus, provided blood specimens can be delivered promptly to the local laboratory, a same-day procalcitonin service would seem to be adequate. However, other factors may influence the need for a point-of-care procalcitonin provision. For example, in remote regions, the local laboratory might be unable to provide a procalcitonin service, and a result would be helpful in making the decision whether to transfer a patient to a specialist ICU.

POCT for Identification of Infectious Agents in the ICU

Another area of molecular and metabolic medicine in development is rapid PCR rule-out diagnosis of bacterial and other infections. These are good systems that could be used at point of care, and are capable of providing this service for a wide range of pathogens, producing sensitive data to diagnose or rule out the pathogens selected within 6 h, as compared to several days from existing culture techniques. The systems are currently being evaluated, with an emphasis on cost-benefit being of paramount importance as costs are still high for this technology. Functional genomics, pharmacogenomics, proteomics, and metabolomics are expected to reveal new insights into systems biology and, in particular, highlight variations in host response that could help segment treatment targets and characterize patients early in their admission to the ICU. If these technologies are to enhance clinical assessment and management in the ICU they will need to be provided with rapid turnaround (within minutes if possible) and would be expected to be provided at, or near, the point of care by dedicated personnel.

REASONS WHY POCT IS APPROPRIATE IN THE ICU

The obvious advantage of POCT in an ICU setting is that the result is immediately available and therapeutic decisions can be made more rapidly. In identifying which measurements are appropriate for point-of-care provision in the ICU, it is important to consider the questions that the investigation is being used to help answer. For example, suppose the questions were:

- Is there evidence of worsening sepsis?
- Is there significant change in liver or renal function?

If it is assumed that there is a conventional laboratory service that can provide results within 2–3 h, then laboratory-based measurements of, for example, differential leukocyte count, serum CRP, liver enzymes, and serum creatinine would normally be adequate to help answer these questions. This is because these parameters will not generally change so rapidly that more than daily measurement is required.

However, there may be operational reasons why these investigations might be requested urgently. For example, a patient with little clinical history may have just been admitted to the ICU after suffering a collapse. Therefore, baseline measurements are required to aid or exclude a diagnosis. In general, such requests form a small proportion of the laboratory workload coming from the ICU and do not warrant provision of a full hematology and biochemistry service next to the patient. In contrast, some questions require rapid responses:

- Is oxygen delivery and utilization adequate?
- What is the acid-base and potassium status?
- Is the patient hypovolemic?
- Is the patient's glucose level optimal?
- Are the patient's capillaries leaky?

Delay in treating hypoxia, hypovolemia, acidemia, hypo- or hyperkalemia, hypo- or hyperglycemia, or pulmonary edema risks death or an unnecessary worsening of the patient's condition and a longer stay in the ICU.

There is another aspect of caring for critically ill patients that demands point-of-care availability of key parameters. In the paralyzed and sedated patient, homeostatic systems may be compromised due to disease or be overridden by mechanical ventilation, renal replacement therapy, or drugs. It is only by repeated measurement of key parameters that the adequacy of delivery of cellular substrates (oxygen, glucose, water, sodium, potassium, etc.) can be assessed. Thus, in concept, the point-of-care measuring system becomes a surrogate component of the patient's own homeostatic mechanisms. From this it follows that because of our very imperfect ability to artificially maintain the "milieu interior," as described by Claude Bernard, the earliest possible warning is required of deviation from set levels of oxygenation, glycemic control, and acid-base control, etc. This is because the cause of the homeostatic derangement may not be obvious from clinical signs and is only suspected when laboratory measurements fall outside the normal range. Interpretation of the results may suggest a cause and lead to manipulation of ventilator settings, fluid input, and inotrope dosage, etc. The correctness of the chosen approach can only be assessed if the effect of these manipulations can be immediately seen by point-of-care measurement.

ORGANIZATION AND MANAGEMENT OF POCT IN THE ICU

Who Does the Analysis and Where?

A number of studies have demonstrated that near-patient blood-gas and electrolyte analysis in the ICU can be carried out by nonlaboratory staff, with results comparable to those obtained by laboratory technicians (49, 50). In a survey of critical care nurses in the United States, POCT was carried out exclusively by nursing staff in 35% of units, laboratory technicians and critical care nurses in 32.5%, and other personnel in 25% (51). Of the nurses doing analyses, 95.5% performed blood glucose measurement, 18.7% arterial blood gases, 4.5% electrolytes, and 4.5% hematology profiles. Of particular interest was that although the majority of nurses felt that emergency (stat) laboratory tests were not reported promptly enough, thereby necessitating bedside testing, they would prefer laboratory personnel to do the testing, freeing them for other patient care responsibilities. Thus, while the clinical need for selected analytes, such as blood gases, to be available within 5 min of blood collection is clear, where and by whom the analysis should be done is less obvious. This may be a cultural problem. In a recent UK study of 82 ICUs, the most common point-of-care investigation was blood glucose followed by blood gases and urine analysis (52) (Figure 26-3).

The same study showed that in the United Kingdom, the majority of POCT in the ICU was performed by nursing staff (Figure 26-4). In the United Kingdom, ICU nurses routinely perform blood glucose and electrolyte estimations, as well as arterial blood-gas analysis. They regard this as part of their role and in some centers audit their work to ensure that it is appropriate for optimal patient care.

The concept of the ICU stat laboratory was first described nearly 30 years ago, and a report from 1981 describes provision of data on blood gases; hematocrit, hemoglobin, and hemoglobin fractions; lactate; electrolytes; osmolality; colloidal oncotic pressure; and plasma protein content within 11 min of receipt of an arterial or mixed venous blood sample (53). However, by the early 1990s, the influence of whole-blood POCT instruments was such that, with the important exception

of colloidal oncotic pressure, all the above analytes were available using bedside equipment from 0.2 mL of blood within 2–5 min (54, 55). It is worth emphasizing that this time the interval includes transport, analysis, and reporting. In his guidelines for POCT, Gerald Kost (56) points out that "rapid response testing should be available continuously during critical emergencies (such as cardiac arrest)" and that whole blood analysis is essential whether the analysis is done next to the patient or in the laboratory, since centrifugation introduces an unacceptable delay, and results must be available within 5 min or less. This turnaround time would be hard to match in many hospitals even with a rapid specimen transport system, a centralized emergency laboratory facility, and computerized reporting. Furthermore, the costs of staffing a 24-h-per-day dedicated emergency laboratory make POCT systems economically attractive.

However, this view has been challenged by at least one group that compared turnaround time for blood-gas analysis from a satellite laboratory within a neonatal intensive care unit and a central laboratory linked by a pneumatic tube system and computerized reporting (57). The mean turnaround time for the results from the satellite laboratory was 4.5 min compared to 6 min from the central laboratory. The authors concluded that, since the cost for the result from the satellite laboratory was considerably higher that that for the central laboratory, the cost savings outweighed the minor difference in turnaround time. No comparison was made with the cost if analyses were performed by nonlaboratory staff, (e.g., nurses) using equipment in the ICU.

Critical care nurses closely monitor patients, observing and, where computerized data handling is not in place, manually recording physiological data, such as pulse rate, blood and

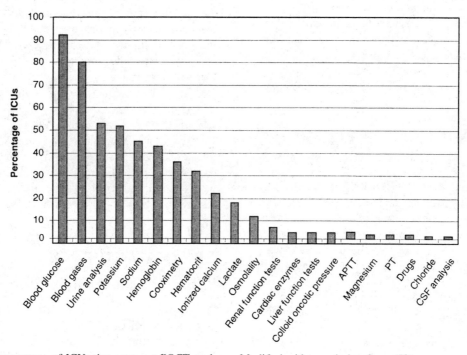

Figure 26-3 The percentage of ICUs that carry out POCT analyses. Modified with permission from (52).

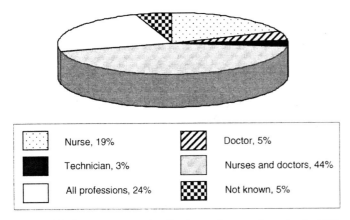

Nurse, 19%   Doctor, 5%

Technician, 3%   Nurses and doctors, 44%

All professions, 24%   Not known, 5%

Figure 26-4 The range of staff who perform analyses in the ICU. Modified with permission from (52).

central venous pressure, and temperature, derived from in vivo sensors. In the authors' view, their role in bedside laboratory monitoring is crucial because the results of analyses can be an important part of nursing management protocols for the patient. This is particularly true in cardiac ICUs, where potassium replacement is a common requirement, and in many general ICUs, where nurses undertake protocol-guided weaning from ventilators.

Choice of Equipment

There are obvious advantages in a close liaison between the intensive care unit and the local laboratory in the choice, purchase, and maintenance of near-patient testing equipment. Unification to a single design and manufacturer for ICU blood-gas and related equipment makes training of both clinical users and laboratory staff simpler. This results in fewer problems associated with misuse by nursing and clinical staff. In addition, laboratory staff have only to learn how to maintain and troubleshoot a single type of instrument, which allows greater flexibility when rostering staff for these duties. Finally, purchase of a common system should result in savings when purchasing consumables and maintenance contracts.

Quality Assessment

Quality assessment can be classified as *internal* or *external*. Internal quality assessment describes the analysis of a material for which there is a prescribed range of acceptable values; it is used to ensure that the instrument is working satisfactorily for clinical purposes. External quality assessment describes the analysis of a material whose assigned value is withheld from the analyst; test performance is reviewed retrospectively when the scheme organizers circulate units with their results and the mean performance of the other scheme participants. In a recent survey of 82 UK ICUs using blood-gas and related equipment, 25% of units did not perform any form of internal quality control, and 64% did not participate in any external quality assessment scheme (52). These findings highlight the need for basic quality assessment procedures.

Maintenance and Troubleshooting

Although the maintenance requirements of modern ICU POCT equipment are decreasing, regular maintenance is still essential. It is also essential that there are arrangements for a prompt response for dealing with instrument failures, which can range from simple blockages due to blood clots to major hardware problems. The maintenance can be broadly classified into two categories: that needed for day-to-day operation (e.g., emptying of waste containers, changing printer paper rolls, and replenishment of reagents) and more extensive maintenance such as deproteinization and sample-path cleaning. In the UK survey of 82 ICUs already referred to, the equipment was maintained by the local clinical biochemistry department in 47%, and in the remainder by a variety of groups, including ICU consultants (21%), ICU technicians or operating department assistants (19%), and biomedical engineers (6%) (52). There are advantages to having the local laboratory provide maintenance:

- Laboratory staff will be familiar with the sensor technologies employed in the instrument.
- Laboratory staff will understand the clinical significance of the results produced and be able to make value judgments of the requisite analytical performance required for clinical use.
- Internal and external quality assessment is most conveniently organized through the local laboratory.
- Results from the equipment can be made comparable with those produced by the local laboratory (e.g., Na, K, Hb).
- The laboratory is in an ideal position to arrange emergency, hospitalwide backup arrangements when equipment fails, for example, transferring specimens to a nearby ICU with similar equipment or installing a portable blood-gas analyzer as a temporary measure.
- Modern systems are now being networked both within and between hospital sites, allowing centralized monitoring of individual instruments from a laboratory-based workstation. An outline of the possible arrangements is given in Figure 26-5. In this way, sensor performance can be continuously monitored and advance warning can be given of an imminent failure, allowing measures to be taken to correct the problem. This may be either from the remote workstation (e.g., initiating additional calibration or wash cycles) or through a visit from laboratory staff. If an analytical channel is likely to give dangerously erroneous results, it can also be shut down from the remote site. In addition, patient and calibration data stored from a large number of instruments can be accessed centrally.

Data Security and Storage

In the United Kingdom, laboratory accreditation requires that patient results are securely stored. By extension, these should include POCT results. It is commonplace for a blood-gas analysis printout to be lost by a doctor under the pressure of a clinical emergency, and unless the results are written in the patient notes, there will be no written record either that the analysis was per-

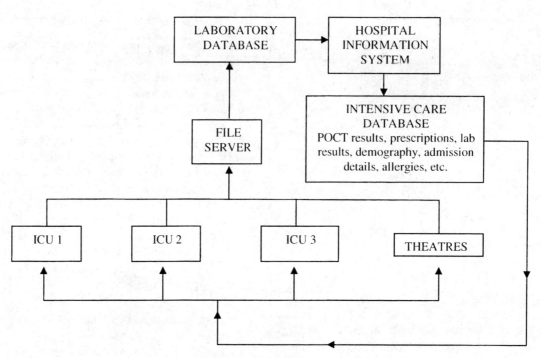

Figure 26-5 Outline of a network for monitoring POCT systems and storing POCT patient results via the hospital information system. Using radio-linked handheld monitors, POCT and laboratory results can be brought to the patient's bed, together with prescribing information, clinical summaries, information on allergies, and other important data. The system can utilize an existing hospital computer network, since the amount of traffic involved in monitoring POCT equipment and transmitting POCT patient results is small. By using the same network, patient POCT data can be included in the ICU database and made available.

formed or of the results. In an increasingly litigious society, steps must be taken to put in place some form of data storage for point-of-care results. Most instruments have the ability to store patient demographics, results, and user identity, together with calibration and quality-control information. In the authors' experience, the major hurdle is reliable inputting of the patient's name and registration number. In hospitals that produce machine-readable (barcoded) patient identity labels, this information can be scanned in, but when this information is not available, or not available in this form, reliance is placed on the user to key some form of unique patient ID data into the instrument. The user is often unwilling to input this information, since it is apparently unnecessary when treating an acutely ill patient. However, when users are reminded of coroners' cases, or hospital inquiries into suspected negligence, the need for reliable recording of patient results is generally viewed sympathetically. In the authors' experience, where POCT results are filed on the ICU database, nursing staff are happy to enter the patient's hospital number and name while waiting the 40 s or so for the analysis to be completed.

BENEFITS AND DISADVANTAGES OF POCT IN THE ICU

Since arterial blood-gas samples are stable for at best 30 min even when cooled in ice, rapid transportation to the point of measurement is essential, together with speedy return of results to the ICU. There have been different approaches to meet these requirements. In addition to the provision of POCT equipment

on the ICU, these include rapid specimen transport to the laboratory via pneumatic tubes and the development of a satellite laboratory dedicated to the ICU, which have already been discussed (Table 26-2).

A rapid transport system has the advantage of allowing centralization of blood-gas and related equipment, avoiding the need for duplication of systems across the hospital's high-dependence units. Other advantages include the avoidance of having to train nursing and clinical staff to use the equipment and a reduced risk of instrument failure due to misuse. Disadvantages include the absolute requirement of a rapid transport system from the ICU to the laboratory and rapid processing by the laboratory, which includes patient data entry into the laboratory or hospital database, and analysis and communication of results to the ICU. In the authors' experience, this approach cannot match the turnaround time of POCT on the ICU.

In the United Kingdom, nurses generally carry out analyses on blood drawn from arterial lines, and the point has been made that this is a drain on nursing time that might be better directed to patient care. However, a major component of the nurses' role in caring for ICU patients is monitoring their condition, and the time taken for blood analysis within the unit is probably less than that required for preparing and packing a blood sample in ice, completing a pathology test request form, and arranging suitable transport to the laboratory. At least one published nursing view is in favor of POCT in the critically ill: "[POCT] will reduce unnecessary testing, provide timely mea-

Table 26-2 Advantages and Disadvantages of POCT in the ICU

Advantages

Results available within 2–4 min, facilitating rapid clinical decision making

Reduced risk of transcription errors of telephoned results or results taken from a hospital computer database

Parameters such as pH/H$^+$ blood gases, potassium, or lactate are unstable, and immediate measurement will give more accurate results compared to those from a specimen transported to the laboratory

Reduced risk of infection, due, for example, to breakage or leakage in a mailing tube, since the specimen never leaves the ICU

Results can be instantly combined with physiological measurements, drug therapy, laboratory results, etc., on the ICU patient database, giving a more complete picture of the patient's condition

Disadvantages

Duplication of equipment, hence increased capital and running costs

Erosion of nursing time, which could be dedicated to patient care

Drain on laboratory staff, maintaining and troubleshooting equipment

Risk of instrument failure due to misuse

Nursing and clinical staff training required before using equipment

Risk of overtesting because results are easily available—needs appropriate protocols and/or training and/or understanding of the appropriateness of measurement

surements of critical values and avoid unnecessary and catastrophic mistakes" (58).

A further disadvantage of POCT in the ICU is the risk of basing clinical decisions on erroneous results. However, the most important factor influencing the quality of results for blood-gas and related analytes is the quality of the blood sample and the effects of delayed analysis. The authors' view is that nursing and medical staff are equally able to interpret and recognize erroneous POCT results that do not fit the patient's clinical picture as they are to recognize a misplaced pulmonary artery flotation catheter or a faulty pulse oximeter.

Near-patient testing is moving toward online patient monitoring. Thus, in addition to the now commonplace continuous monitoring of pulse, blood pressure, central venous pressure, respiratory rate, pulse oximetry, ECG, and core–peripheral temperature, indwelling sensors providing pH, pO_2, and pCO_2 are now being developed. This allows all data to be presented simultaneously, giving an overall picture of the patient's condition. For example, i-STAT™ (i-STAT Corporation, East Windsor, NJ, USA) bedside measurement of Na, K, Cl, blood urea nitrogen, ionized Ca, pH, pCO_2, pO_2, and hematocrit can be integrated into the patient monitoring data system together with physiological and ventilator data (59).

ECONOMIC ANALYSIS OF POCT IN THE ICU

The cost of healthcare continues to rise, and laboratory services are a significant component of this increase. The increasing reliance on laboratory results in diagnosis and patient management reflects a technological revolution both in automation, allowing larger numbers of analyses to be provided more rapidly, and in the development of more clinically useful investigations. Laboratory test costs are now under scrutiny together with other ICU costs such as radiography, blood products, and drugs, and significant cost reductions have been claimed (60). Winkelman and Wybenga (57) compared an ICU satellite laboratory with a centralized laboratory served by a pneumatic tube for the provision of blood-gas analyses. Despite the longer turnaround time, the authors concluded that this was acceptable in a cost–benefit analysis, and that a centralized laboratory service was more cost-effective. However, a more recent study in a neonatal intensive care unit indicated an overall significant saving by POCT (61). Worldwide, there are clearly differences in practice for the provision of critical results for ICU patients, and published comparisons have centered on satellite and centralized laboratories in the United States (62). Simple qualitative analysis suggests that provision of POCT instrumentation in the ICU, which is used by nursing and medical staff, is cheaper than the same equipment being operated 24 h per day in a satellite laboratory because of the staff costs incurred by the latter. This view is supported by the findings of Frankel et al. (63), who compared the costs of initial laboratory investigations for 200 consecutive admissions to a level 1 trauma center. They found that not only were the mean turnaround times for results from the POCT system and the laboratory 6 and 64 min, respectively; the POCT system represented a cost savings of $166 per analysis. When a centralized 24-h laboratory service is already in place and several ICUs are being served, then savings over POCT might be made. However, a rapid specimen transport system would be a prerequisite, and laboratory staffing would need to be at levels that could provide instantaneous sample processing 24 h per day. Even under optimal circumstances, the turnaround time could not match POCT in the ICU.

However, in attempting an economic analysis of POCT compared with a centralized laboratory service for ICU patient care, the authors were impressed by the lack of published studies, despite this need being highlighted in 1990 (64). There are few, if any, cost analyses of true POCT in the ICU versus a centralized laboratory-based service. Cost reductions in laboratory services have been achieved by more critical analysis of which individual results are required for ICU patient care, rather than carrying out a battery of tests that includes the analyte of interest (65, 66). These measures have been directed toward centralized laboratory services, but a similar problem seems to be occurring with POCT. Modern instruments now provide an increasing number of analytes, all of which are measured and reported even when, for example, only blood-gas results are required. A cost–benefit analysis, which needs to be done for POCT in the ICU, is a review of the provision of analytes such as lactate, urea, and ionized calcium, which are measured with every blood-gas specimen. While on occasion rapid availability of these results is valuable, they do not need to accompany every pO_2 measurement. In summary, a comprehensive cost–benefit analysis of POCT in comparison with either a satellite laboratory service or a centralized service has not been done, but a centralized laboratory service for the ICU cannot provide a comparable turnaround time with POCT. Savings in avoiding duplication of POCT equipment by centralization are offset by the costs of providing a level of staffing that will give instant 24-h-per-day analytical response, together with a high-capacity rapid specimen transport system.

CONCLUSION

The advances in user-friendly POCT equipment have widened the analytical repertoire, which in combination with the discovery of new biomarkers for predicting disease severity and the response to therapy has the potential to expand POCT in the intensive care area far beyond measurement of acid-base, blood gases, electrolytes, and metabolites. Although there are still no comprehensive cost–benefit studies of POCT in intensive care, its essential role in the care of the critically ill is now irrefutable. From a clinical perspective, not only are the choice, installation, and monitoring of POCT equipment in the ICU best done in collaboration with the local pathology service, it is crucial not to lose regular clinical liaison between the laboratory staff and front-line staff in the ICU. Care of the critically ill remains a team effort, of which an essential component is an informed and responsive pathology service.

REFERENCES

1. Siggaard-Andersen O. Blood acid-base alignment nomograms. Scales for pH, pCO_2, base excess of whole blood of different haemoglobin concentrations, plasma bicarbonate and plasma total CO_2. Scan J Clin Lab Invest 1963;27:239–45.
2. Miller JT. Anesthesia related hypoxemia. The effect of pulse oximetry monitoring on perimoperative events and postoperative complications. Dan Med Bull 1994;41:489–500.
3. Thrush D, Hodges MR. Accuracy of pulse oximetry during hypoxemia. South Med J 1994;87:518–21.
4. Mikulaschek A, Henry SM, Donovan R, Scalea TM. Serum lactate is not predicted by anion gap or base excess after trauma resuscitation. J Trauma 1996;40:218–23.
5. Fink MP. Cytopathic hypoxia. Mitochondrial dysfunction as a mechanism contributing to organ dysfunction in sepsis. Crit Care Clin 2001;17:219–37.
6. Cairns CB, Moore FA, Haenel JB, Gallea BL, Ortner JP, Rose SJ, Moore EE. Evidence for early supply independent mitochondrial dysfunction in patients developing multiple organ failure after trauma. J Trauma 1997;42:532–6.
7. Holloway P, Benham S, St John A. The value of blood lactate measurements in ICU: an evaluation of the role in the management of patients on haemofiltration. Clin Chim Acta 2001;307:9–13.
8. Fiddian-Green RG. Splanchnic ischaemia and multiple organ failure in the critically ill. Ann R Coll Surg Engl 1988;70:128–34.
9. Solverman HJ. Gastric tonometry: an index of splanchnic oxygenation? Crit Cai Med 1991;19:1223–4.
10. Kavarana MN, Frumento RJ, Hirsch AL, Oz MC, Lee DC, Bennett-Guerrero E. Gastric hypercarbia and adverse outcome after cardiac surgery. Intensive Care Med 2003;29:742–8.
11. Binnert C, Tappy L. Microdialysis in the intensive care unit: a novel tool for clinical investigation or monitoring? Curr Opin Clin Nutr Metab Care 2002;5:185–8.
12. Malarkkan N, Snook NJ, Lumb AB. New aspects of ventilation in acute lung injury. Anaesthesia 2003;58:647–67.
13. Greene JH, Klinger JR. The efficacy of inhaled nitric oxide in the treatment of acute respiratory distress syndrome. An evidence-based medicine approach. Crit Care Clin 1998;14:387–409.
14. Story DA, Morimatsu H, Bellomo R. Strong ions, weak acids and base excess: a simplified Fencl-Stewart approach to clinical acid-base disorders. Br J Anaesth 2004;92:54–60.
15. Pain RW, Rowland KM, Phillips PJ, Duncan B McL. Current "corrected" calcium challenged. BMJ 1975;4:617–9.
16. Dacey MJ. Hypomagnesemic disorders. Crit Care Clin 2001;17: 155–73.
17. Brookes CI, Fry CH. Ionised magnesium and calcium in plasma from healthy volunteers and patients undergoing cardiopulmonary bypass. Br Heart J 1993;69:404–8.
18. Caddell JL. Hypothesis: possible links between the respiratory distress syndrome of the premature neonate, the sudden infant death syndrome, and magnesium deficiency shock. Magnes Res 1993;6:25–32.
19. Guerin C, Cousin C, Mignot F, Manchon M, Fournier G. Serum and erythrocyte magnesium in critically ill patients. Intensive Care Med 1996;22:724–7.
20. Kulpmann WR, Rossler J, Brunkhorst R, Schuler A. Ionised and total magnesium serum concentrations in renal and hepatic diseases. Eur J Clin Chem Clin Biochem 1996;34:257–64.
21. Fleck A, Raines G, Hawker F, Trotter J, Wallace PI, Ledingham IM, et al. Increased vascular permeability: a major cause of hypoalbuminaemia in disease and injury. Lancet 1985;1:781–4.
22. Gosling P. Microalbuminuria: a marker of systemic disease. Br J Hosp Med 1995;54:285–90.
23. MacKinnon KL, Molnar Z, Watson ID, Shearer E, Lowe D. Use of microalbuminuria as an indicator for the development of sepsis and multiple organ failure. Br J Anaesth 1997:678P.
24. Gosling P, Brudney S, McGrath L, Riseboro S, Manji M. Mortality prediction at admission to intensive care: a comparison of microalbuminuria with acute physiology scores after 24 hours. Crit Care Med 2003;31:98–103.
25. Thorevska N, Sabahi R, Upadya A, Manthous C, Amoateng-Adjepong Y. Microalbuminuria in critically ill medical patients: prevalence, predictors, and prognostic significance. Crit Care Med 2003;31:1075–81.
26. Davies MG, Hagen PO. Systemic inflammatory response syndrome. Br J Surg 1997;64:920–35.
27. Zikria BA, Bascom JU. Mechanisms of multiple organ failure. In: Zikria BA, Oz MO, Carlson RW, eds. Reperfusion injuries and clinical capillary leak syndrome. Armonk, NY: Futura, 1994: 443–92.
28. Gosling P. Prevention of post-traumatic clinical capillary leak syndrome. Trauma 1999;1:91–103.
29. Gosling P, Czyz J, Manji M. Bedside measurement of microalbuminuria in 431 patients admitted to ICU predicts mortality and

organ function. Proceedings of the Association of Clinical Biochemists National Meeting, 2004.

30. Cochrane Injuries Group Albumin Reviewers. Human albumin administration in the critically ill: systematic review of controlled trials Why albumin may not work. BMJ 1998;317:235–40.

31. Boldt J, Heesen M, Muller M, Pabsdorf M, Hempelmann G. The effects of albumin versus hydroxyethyl starch solution on cardiorespiratory and circulatory variables in critically ill patients. Anesth Analg 1996;83:254–61.

32. Rittoo D, Gosling P, Bonnici C, Burnley S, Millns P, Simms MH, et al. Splanchnic oxygenation in patients undergoing abdominal aortic aneurysm repair and volume expansion with eloHAES. Cardiovasc Surg 2002;10:128–33.

33. Rittoo D, Gosling P, Burnley S, Bonnici C, Millns P, Simms MH, et al. Randomized study comparing the effects of hydroxyethyl starch solution with Gelofusine on pulmonary function in patients undergoing abdominal aortic aneurysm surgery. Br J Anaesth 2004;92:61–6.

34. J Allison KP, Gosling P, Jones S, Pallister I, Porter KM. Randomized trial of hydroxyethyl starch versus gelatine for trauma resuscitation. Trauma 1999;47:1114–21.

35. Dieterich HJ. Recent developments in European colloid solutions. J Trauma 2003;54(Suppl 5):S26–30.

36. Schortgen F, Lacherade JC, Bruneel F, Cattaneo I, Hemery F, Lemaire F, Brochard L. Effects of hydroxyethylstarch and gelatin on renal function in severe sepsis: a multicentre randomised study. Lancet 2001;357:911–6.

37. Hudson I, Cooke A, Holland B, Houston A, Jones JG, Turner T, et al. Red cell volume and cardiac output in anaemic preterm infants. Arch Dis Child 1990;65:672–5.

38. Busse MW, Zisowsky S, Henschen S, Panning B, Reilmann L. Determination of circulating blood volume by measurement of indocyanine green dye in hemolysate: a preliminary study. Life Sci 1990;46:647–52.

39. Fogh-Anderson N, Thomsen JK, Foldager N, Siggaard-Anderson O. pH effect on the COHb absorption spectrum: importance for calibration of the OSM3 and measurement of circulating hemoglobin and blood volume. Scan J Clin Lab Invest Suppl 1990; 203:247–52.

40. Massey EJ, de Souza P, Findlay G, Smithies M, Shah S, Spark P, et al. Clinically practical blood volume assessment with fluorescein labeled HES. Transfusion 2004,44:151–7.

41. Reich DL, Yanakakis MJ, Vela-Cantos FP, DePerio M, Jacobs E. Comparison of bedside coagulation monitoring tests with standard laboratory tests in patients after cardiac surgery Anaesth Analg 1993;77:673–9.

42. Blumenthal RS, Carter AJ, Resar JR, Coombs V, Gloth ST, Dalal J, et al. Comparison of bedside and hospital laboratory coagulation studies during and after coronary intervention. Cathet Cardiovasc Diagn 1995;35:9–17.

43. Finney SJ, Zekveld C, Elia A, Evans TW. Glucose control and mortality in critically ill patients. JAMA 2003;290:2041–7.

44. Bell K, Wattie M, Byth K, Silvestrini R, Clark P, Stachowski E, et al. Procalcitonin: a marker of bacteraemia in SIRS. Anaesth Intensive Care 2003;31:629–36.

45. Balcl C, Sungurtekin H, Gurses E, Sungurtekin U, Kaptanoglu B. Usefulness of procalcitonin for diagnosis of sepsis in the intensive care unit. Crit Care 2003;7:85–90.

46. Enguix A, Rey C, Concha A, Medina A, Coto D, Dieguez MA. Comparison of procalcitonin with C-reactive protein and serum amyloid for the early diagnosis of bacterial sepsis in critically ill neonates and children. Intensive Care Med 2001;27:211–5.

47. Muller B, Becker KL, Schachinger H, Rickenbacher PR, Huber PR, Zimmerli W, et al. Calcitonin precursors are reliable markers of sepsis in a medical intensive care unit. Crit Care Med 2000; 28:977–83.

48. Wanner GA, Keel M, Steckholzer U, Beier W, Stocker R, Ertel W. Relationship between procalcitonin plasma levels and severity of injury, sepsis, organ failure, and mortality in injured patients. Crit Care Med 2000;28:950–7.

49. Zaloga GP, Dudas L, Roberts P, Bortenschlager L, Black K, Prielipp R. Near-patient blood gas and electrolyte analyses are accurate when performed by non-laboratory-trained individuals. J Clin Monit 1993;9:341–6.

50. Bishop MS, Hussain I, Aldred M, Kost GJ. Multisite point-of-care potassium testing for patient-focused care. Arch Pathol Lab Med 1994;118:797–800.

51. Lamb LS, Parrish RS, Goran SF, Biel MH. Current nursing practice of point-of-care laboratory diagnostic testing in critical care units. Am J Crit Care 1995;4:429–34.

52. Cox DJA, Naidoo R. The intensive care laboratory—a report of current UK practice and recommendations for the implementation of required minimum standards. Care of the Critically Ill 1995; 11:98–103.

53. Weil MH, Michaels S, Puri VK, Carlson RW. The stat laboratory: facilitating blood gas and biochemical measurements for the critically ill and injured. Am J Clin Pathol 1981;76:34–42.

54. Shirley TL. Critical care profiling for informed treatment of severely ill patients. Am J Clin Path 1995;104:S79–87.

55. Kost GJ. New whole blood analysers and their impact on cardiac and critical care. Crit Rev Clin Lab Sci 1993;30:153–202.

56. Kost GJ. Guidelines for point-of-care testing. Am J Clin Path 1995;104:S111–27.

57. Winkelman JW, Wybenga DR. Quantification of medical and operational factors determining central versus satellite laboratory testing of blood gases. Am J Clin Pathol 1994;102:7–10.

58. Bayne CG. Point of care testing: testing the system? Nurs Manage 1997;28:34–6.

59. Shabot MM. The HP CareVue clinical information system. Int J Clin Monit Comput 1997;14:177–84.

60. Barie PS, Hydo LJ. Learning not to know: results of a program for ancillary cost reduction in surgical critical care. J Trauma 1996; 41:714–20.

61. Am Alves-Dunkerson JA, Hilsenrath PE, Cress GA, Widness JA. Cost analysis of a neonatal point-of-care monitor J Clin Pathol 2002;117:809–18.

62. Castro HJ, Oropello JM, Halpern N. Point-of-care testing in the intensive care unit. The intensive care physician's perspective. Am J Clin Path 1995;104:S95–9.

63. Frankel HL, Rozycki GS, Ochsner MG, McCabe JE, Harviel JD, Jeng JC, et al. Minimising admission laboratory testing in trauma patients: use of a microanalyzer. J Trauma 1994;37: 728–36.

64. Zaloga GP. Evaluation of bedside testing for the critical care unit. Chest 1990;97:85S–90.

65. Kirton OC, Civetta JM, Hudson-Civetta J. Cost effectiveness in the intensive care unit. Surg Clin North Am 1996;76:175–200.

66. Novich M, Gillis L, Tauber AI. The laboratory test justified. An effective means to reduce routine laboratory testing. Am J Clin Pathol 1985;84:756–9.

Chapter 27

Point-of-Care Testing in the Home via Telehealth

Craig A. Lehmann

Most diagnostic vendors have added point-of-care testing (POCT) technology to their portfolio of services. For most laboratorians, POCT has become just another segment of clinical laboratory services. One of the primary concerns associated with POCT has been cost. Typically, POCT is far more expensive (when considered as cost per test) than tests performed in the clinical laboratory. Up until now, these added costs have been ignored, primarily because many practitioners feel that the improved turnaround time of test results improves overall patient care and, for now, it looks as though hospital in-house POCT will continue to grow. While this holds true for most hospital laboratories, it should be noted that some laboratories have been able to decrease the use of POCT by improving the central laboratory's efficiency.

The economics of performing POCT in one's home will be far less controversial because costs associated with specimen collection and transportation issues are high. In addition, there are many specimen variables associated with home collection. For example, there are times when a home healthcare provider cannot drop off a specimen for analysis until the end of the workday. This leaves the specimen idle in a holding box for a few hours, with the possibility that it will deteriorate and produce incorrect test results. Typically, such scenarios require a return visit from the home healthcare provider to obtain a new specimen. The additional costs associated with the return visit places increased costs on home health agencies at a time when the US government is cutting back on reimbursement. This situation is also being experienced elsewhere in the world.

Home healthcare is one of the fastest growing markets in the United States and encompasses more than 7000 agencies (1). There are a number of reasons behind this growth, and economics is at the top of the list.

Recently, the home health industry has engaged in vital sign technology that enables the home patient the opportunity to perform a number of vital sign measurements (e.g., blood pressure monitoring) and POCT at home and send the results to their healthcare provider via a phone or cable line. This accessibility gives the patient the ability to manage their ailment from the privacy of their own home, decreases unnecessary visits to physician offices and emergency departments, and lessens extended hospitalizations.

This chapter will discuss population trends, economics, and the influences of telehealth technology in the home healthcare market place.

POPULATION TRENDS/HEALTHCARE COSTS

One of the major challenges facing our nation today is providing healthcare to our ever-growing aging population. Not only will there be more individuals reaching the age of 65, but they will be living longer. Along with longevity comes chronic ailments such as arthritis, diabetes, and heart disease, all of which infringe on one's independence. This scenario has challenged the US government's Centers for Medicare and Medicaid Services (CMS) not only to find a solution for providing healthcare for the elderly, but to do so economically. Many now believe that a combination of home health and telehealth could be the answer. Because of this and other factors, the home health industry has become an important link in providing economical healthcare. Presently, home healthcare services cover the spectrum of individuals who require medical or nursing care, social work, and/or assistance with daily therapeutic treatment or activities. The primary providers of these services have been nurses; physical, occupational, respiratory, infusion and speech therapists; and home health aids. In 1998 this workforce totaled 671,600 with the highest percentage consisting of nurses (registered nurses, 129,304; licensed practical nurses, 40,849) and home health aids (146,989). From 1990 to 1997 Medicare home health spending went from $3.3 billion to $18 billion. This growth was considered one of the primary reasons for the passing of the Balanced Budget Act in 1997, which was the precursor to the prospective payment system (PPS) passed in October 2000. As with diagnostic-related groups this system encourages the economic and efficient delivery of healthcare. CMS developed and implemented the Outcome and Assessment Information Set (OASIS) to ensure the quality of the industry. The 2003 Medicare Payment Advisory Commission report to Congress confirmed that there has been no decline in quality over the years (1, 2).

Providing healthcare for the elderly is not a problem unique to the United States, and many other industrialized nations are faced with growing numbers of aging individuals

(3). For example, China has the largest elderly population (in 1990, >63 million individuals over 65 years of age), and the elderly populations of Canada and Japan will more than double over the next 25–30 years. This increase will result in an international healthcare crisis.

The US population has continued to increase at a rate of ~10% per year since 1984, and projections are that it could reach 0.5 billion by the year 2050. As of 2000, the population of individuals 65 years of age or older was 35 million. Many predict that by 2030, the geriatric (65 years or older) population will be more than 69 million and by 2050 will rise to 80 million. Already, these individuals (baby boomers) are demanding appropriate healthcare from their government (e.g., prescription drugs) and will make it an issue for many of their political representatives. The US government, through Medicare/Medicaid and Veterans Affairs, is responsible for a very large portion of healthcare expenditures (>43%). As life expectancy continues to grow (life expectancy in 2010 is predicted to be 74.5 for males and 81.3 for females) so will the government's health costs. Many of the diseases associated with the geriatric population are chronic in nature and will require long-term care. As of today, the leading causes of death in the geriatric population are heart disease, cancer, cerebrovascular disease, chronic obstructive pulmonary disease, pneumonia, and influenza, all of which have a significant effect on healthcare costs. In 2002, healthcare spending increased by 9.3%, the largest increase in 11 years. Health spending has reached a total of $1.55 trillion, accounting for 15% of the nation's economy. The average amount spent for each US citizen came to $5440 per year. Even though 43 million Americans are uninsured, the United States spends more money per capita on healthcare than any other country. This is at a time when everyone is trying to reduce healthcare costs. For example, over the past few years healthcare payers have attempted to decrease utilization of healthcare by increasing copayments. On the average, for every $100 spent on healthcare, consumers pay $14 out of pocket (4).

The economic pressures placed on hospitals by the government (e.g., diagnostic-related groups) and managed care have encouraged hospitals to find ways to remain economically sound. One of the strategies was to shorten patient length of stay. As a result, many patients will require some form of home healthcare. The National Association for Home Care estimated that 7.4 million Americans received home health services in 1997, and there are projections that as many as 11 million additional Americans could use home care services. Many believe that more than three quarters of the elderly with severe disabilities are not receiving any form of professional home health services. One possible solution that may help alleviate this problem is telehealth.

TELEHEALTH TECHNOLOGY

The recent advances made in telehealth technology have enabled many healthcare providers to treat, evaluate, and educate patients from remote locations (e.g., the individual's home). As a result, costs have decreased, transmission has improved, and a variety of measurement capabilities have been added. The industry reached $13.8 billion in 1998 and has been on the increase ever since. As seen in Figure 27-1, some of this technology can measure a variety of vital signs and enable POCT, as well as record and disseminate the information to a variety of healthcare providers. The opportunity to measure pulse, blood pressure, temperature, weight, and blood oxygen percent saturation, along with the ability to listen to cardiac and lung sounds make the technology very attractive to the home health industry. Some of the POCT devices in Figure 27-1 also have the ability to send data. Even if the POCT technology is not interfaced, the patient can still enter the results manually and have them sent to their own web address. All the data is secured with advanced encryption technology and complies with all HIPAA standards (Figure 27-2). Once the data is sent to the patient's web address, healthcare providers can access the files by using a password. For example, if a nurse enters the system and pulls up a patient's records, the system presents the records in an actionable format. If a patient's vital signs or POCT results are out of the normal range, the file is placed on top of the list and is coded red, indicating that immediate attention is needed. Results that are slightly out of range but do not pose an immediate threat to the patient are coded yellow. All acceptable ranges are coded green, indicating that the results fall within the normal range. Another feature of the software is that the practitioner can access trend graphs (Figure 27-3), which enable quick recognition of subtle changes. The software also allows one to set up schedules for medication adherence, vital sign and POCT measurements, appointments (e.g., physician's office) and ask questions or provide instruction. The Viterion 500®, shown in Figure 27-1, has the capability to take digitized pictures (e.g., for wound documentation) as well as provide two-way, real-time video conferencing between patient and practitioner.

HOME HEALTHCARE

As previously stated, home healthcare is one of the nation's most rapidly growing healthcare industries. As of 2003, there were more than 7000 home healthcare providers. In 2001, home health spending reached nearly $45 billion. In the early 1990s, home health was one of the fastest growing industries. In fact, from 1990 to 1997 Medicare spending for these services increased 45%, reaching $18 billion. Because of this, in 1997 the government passed the Balanced Budget Act to curtail these runaway costs. Under this legislation, reimbursement declined from $18 billion to $8.3 billion in 1999, and as of 2002 was $10 billion. In October 2000 a prospective payment system (PPS) was implemented. The PPS applied caps to the existing system and reimbursed based on costs. This system is based on 60 days of episodes of care. Following PPS, CMS has developed and mandated standardized assessment that monitors the quality of home care, now referred to as the Outcome and Assessment Information Set (OASIS). A 2003

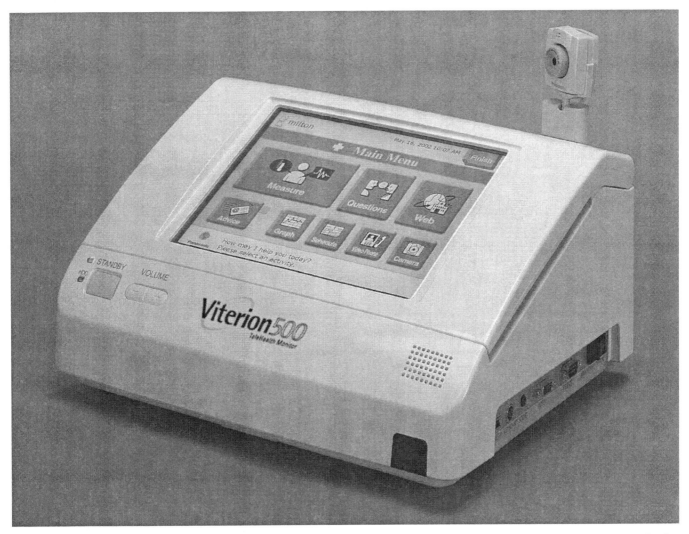

Figure 27-1. Viterion 500, produced by Viterion Telehealthcare, a Bayer-Panasonic company. Reprinted with permission from Viterion Telehealthcare LLC, Tarrytown, NY; info@viterion.com.

report by the Medicare Payment Advisory Commission demonstrated that there has been a decline in home visits and costs per visit under PPS, but there has been no decline in quality (1, 2).

The largest group of patients requesting and receiving home healthcare services are those who have diseases of the circulatory system (33.5%), many of whom receive healthcare services from skilled nursing (registered nurse). Some of the other dominant diagnostic-related groups receiving home healthcare are major joint and limb reattachment, heart failure, cerebrovascular, simple pneumonia and pleurisy, diabetes, arthritis, and pulmonary disease. The mean numbers of visits for the top ten ICD-9-CM Codes range from a low of 29.3 visits to a high of 58 visits (1, 2).

The caregiver group that supplies services to these patients is a combination of professionals and paraprofessionals. The two dominant caregivers are registered nurses [129,304 full-time equivalents (FTEs)] and home healthcare aides (326,633 FTEs). Other home healthcare providers are licensed practical nurses, physical therapists, occupational therapists, speech pathologists, and social workers. All together, according to the US Department of Labor, Bureau of Labor Statistics, National Industry-Occupational Employment Matrix (excludes hospital-based and public agencies), in 1998 there were a total of 671,600 FTEs providing services. The average number of home care visits per 8-h day for the group is 4.4, resulting in the social worker having the least number of visits (3 visits/8-h day) and the physical therapist having the most visits (6 visits/8-h day). The median reimbursement for home healthcare providers ranges from $15.00 for the home health aide to $45.46 for the social worker. In comparison to hospital charges ($2753/day) and skilled nursing facilities ($421/day) home healthcare is far more cost-effective ($100/visit) (1).

Although the benefits of home healthcare seem obvious, that is not the consensus of most individuals. At one time, the delivery of healthcare for physicians included home healthcare. However, that is no longer true, as healthcare has been cen-

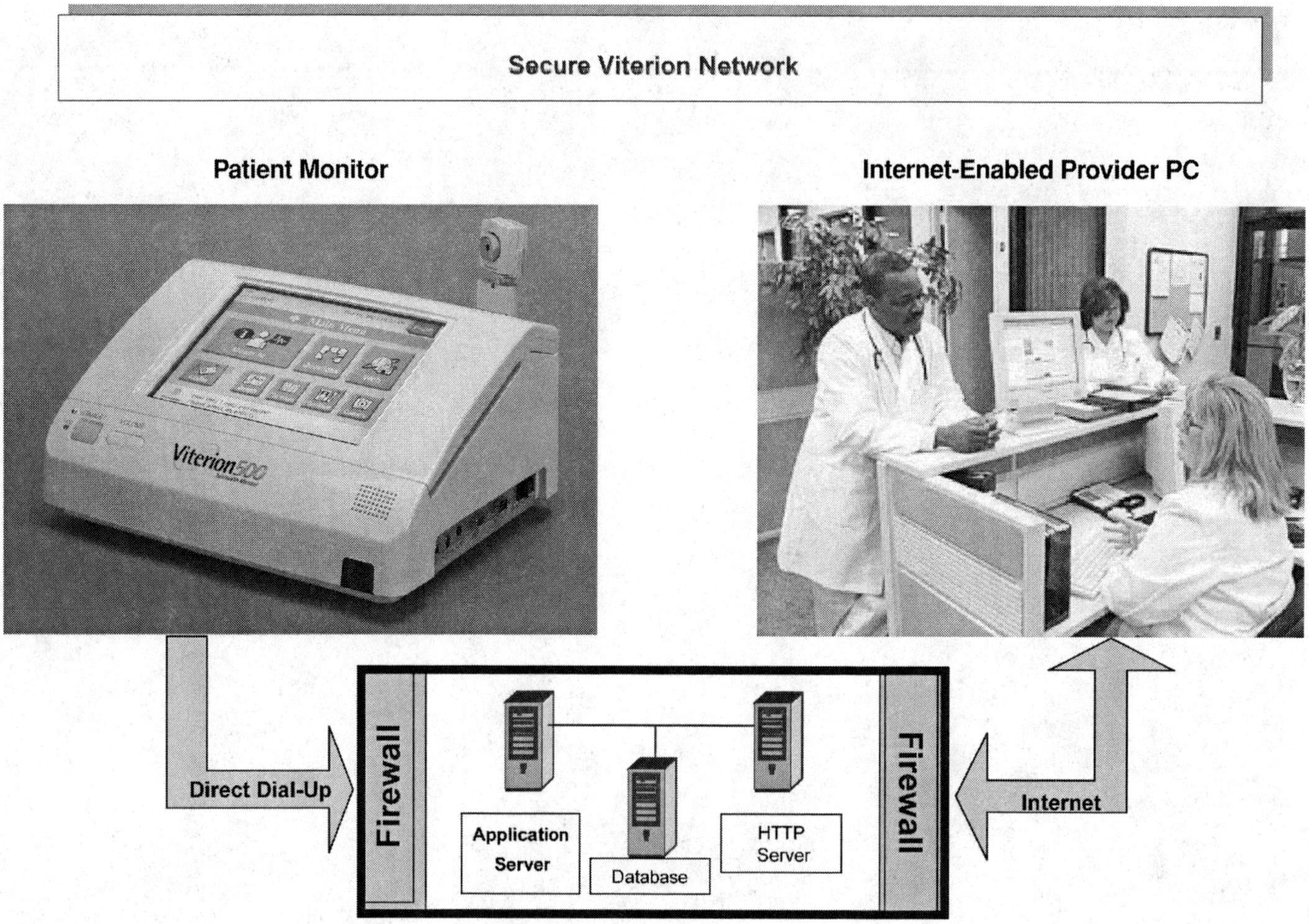

Secure Viterion Network

Patient Monitor   **Internet-Enabled Provider PC**

Figure 27-2. Viterion's web-based patient repository.

tralized in the hospital for many years. Physicians see their office and the hospital as the primary sites for the delivery of healthcare and are not convinced that they should once again include the home. As hospitals take on more and more home healthcare responsibility, the development of more universal standards will occur, thus standardizing healthcare practices. The ever-growing abundance and variety (primary care physicians, physician assistants, and nurse practitioners) of primary care providers will encourage such individuals to pursue new environments in which to practice (e.g., home visits). Hospitals, agencies, and government will encourage these healthcare providers to enter the home healthcare market, especially if outcomes can be improved. The curriculum for many of these healthcare providers now includes a course in clinical laboratory sciences, and within the course content there is generally a section on POCT. In addition, physician assistants and nurse practitioners have prescription rights, thereby negating the need to contact a physician for medication or changes. Because of the knowledge base and prescription privileges of these individuals, it behooves the healthcare industry to take a closer look at their possible role. As the market for healthcare practitioners becomes more competitive, salary levels will surely decrease. This could encourage the use of primary care physicians, physician assistants, and nurse practitioners as primary

home healthcare providers. Because of the competitiveness of the market, home visits might not only be available to the homebound patient. It is possible that in the future, home visits could be available to many in the general public.

CONGESTIVE HEART FAILURE AND DIABETES IN THE HOME HEALTHCARE ENVIRONMENT

Congestive Heart Failure

There are almost 5 million Americans with congestive heart failure (CHF) and 500,000 new cases are added each year. CHF accounts for 875,000 hospitalizations, and for the elderly (65 years or older) it is the most common hospitalization diagnosis. In 1993, CHF patients accounted for more than 2.9 million physician office visits and 65,000 home care visits. The costs for CHF in 1993 were estimated to be almost $18 billion. The numbers of patients with CHF will continue to grow over the years, primarily because of the predicted growth of the elderly population and new medical procedures such as coronary bypass and cardiac stents. These medical procedures will afford many cardiac patients the opportunity to live much longer with their disease, increasing their opportunity to de-

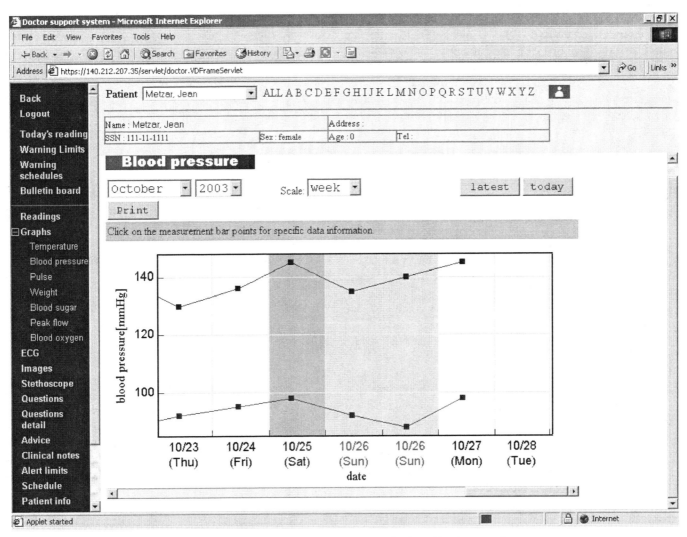

Figure 27-3. Viterion system provides trend graphs of the patient's test results (e.g., blood pressure).

velop CHF (5). As with other chronic diseases, appropriate management improves both quality and longevity of life. Telehealth for CHF patients can offer not only independence, but the ability to perform some sophisticated clinical and diagnostic measurements such as oxygen saturation, heart and lung sounds, and electrocardiograms.

A pilot study recently evaluated the impact of providing some CHF patients with telehealth technology in their home in the hope of reducing readmissions to the hospital via the emergency department (6). Twenty patients were randomly separated into control and study groups. The control group had no changes in their nursing visits and continued to phone in their weight. The study group was given a 1-h training session on how to use the Viterion 500®. Each patient was instructed to contact their nurse with any concerns about their vital signs. The study group measured blood pressure, weight, and blood oxygen saturation. In addition, they were instructed to use the stethoscope to record their heart or lung sounds if they experienced any problems associated with breathing or felt any cardiac variations. The electronic stethoscope takes a 3-min

recording and places it in the patient's database. A practitioner can access this recording at any time for review. Over the 6-month study period, 2 patients or 20% of the control group were rehospitalized via the emergency department, while none of the study group either visited the emergency department or were rehospitalized.

Diabetes

Diabetes is a worldwide disease that affects about 125 million individuals. Diabetes affects more than 16 million individuals in the United States and costs more than $100 billion annually. The direct medical costs associated with diabetes are $44.1 billion (7). Healthcare utilization by diabetes patients is substantial; they have 96.1 million outpatient medical encounters, 26.9 million visits to physicians' offices, and 16.4 million visits to ambulatory care settings. Diabetes patients visit their physicians an average of 15.5 times a year, compared to 4.9 for the general population (8). A recent study demonstrated that, of diabetic patients who had been hospitalized, 30% had two or more stays that contributed to 55% of total hospitalizations and 54% of total hospital costs. The study also revealed that costs are 3 times as high for patients with multiple stays as they are for those with a single stay ($23,119 vs. $8508) and that chronic complications are more prevalent among adults (9, 10). All of this documents the high cost of the diabetes patient and the need to better manage this chronic condition whose incidence continues to rise.

Many diabetes patients monitor their condition using POCT in their home. Capillary blood glucose measurements performed in the home can help patients manage their diabetes. There are a variety of glucometers available on the market, at an average cost of $75. These systems provide accurate glucose measurements via the measurement of color produced on a glucose oxidase strip. Each glucose assay strip costs about $0.75 (7). One of the problems with individuals managing their own condition is compliance. Early studies of individuals using telehealth vs. the telephone demonstrate better compliance for those using telehealth (11, 12).

Over 1.4 million patients have Type 1 diabetes, while another 14.5 million or more have Type 2. Recently Medicare has added Type 2 to its reimbursement menu. There are also estimates that there are an additional 6 million individuals with undiagnosed Type 2 diabetes mellitus. The prevalence of Type 2 diabetes will continue to grow due to the growth of the aging population. Complications related to diabetes will also increase. Heart disease is the leading cause of diabetes-related deaths. Adults with diabetes are 2–4 times more likely to die of heart disease or stroke than other adults. In addition, more than 73% of diabetes patients have high blood pressure. Diabetes is the leading cause of blindness and is a major contributor to dental disease. One of the most common single causes of end-stage renal disease (ESRD) is diabetes. In 2000, the cost associated with treating diabetes-related ESRD was greater than $4 billion (7, 13).

The earliest clinical sign of ESRD is the presence of microalbuminuria. Continual and/or increasing microalbuminuria is a strong indication of ESRD. Diabetic patients (Type 1 and 2) with increased and/or continual microalbuminuria have a 20-fold risk of developing ESRD (3, 14, 15). The Ad Hoc Committee of the Council on Diabetes Mellitus of the National Kidney Foundation has recommended the measurement of the urinary albumin:creatinine ratio as the screening test for albuminuria. POCT for urinary albumin:creatinine ratio is available. The home healthcare provider or the patient can perform a simple dipstick method in the home. Early detection could lead to treatment that would prevent or delay ESRD.

Diabetes is a lifelong disease and is the sixth leading cause of death among the US population. Because Type 2 diabetes is more prevalent in the geriatric population, which is increasing in size as well as living longer, it would make economic sense to manage the healthcare of these individuals with telehealth technology. The patient can record each glucose test result into the database through a wireless glucometer. Each time the patient performs the assay, the data is placed in their file with the date and time of assay. Either the patient or a practitioner can review the data at any time. The data can also be plotted out in graph form so results can be compared over time. All other POCT results (e.g., albumin:creatinine ratio) can be manually entered and plotted out. Self-testing results such as triglycerides and total cholesterol, entered over time, will provide early detection of cardiovascular disease. Such diagnostic tests, along with documented clinical vital signs (e.g., blood pressure) can provide the visiting nurse, as well as the patient, with a more complete picture of the patient's physical condition.

The crippling effects of CHF and diabetes in the elderly population demonstrate how these individuals can have a major effect on healthcare economics and utilization. Better management and early detection of secondary disorders is necessary if cost containment is to be achieved. As demonstrated in the pilot study, the use of vital sign technology can reduce healthcare utilization, which ultimately will result in reduced healthcare costs.

SELF-TESTING

Many feel that there is a market for diagnostic testing offered directly to the consumer. In addition to getting results within a few minutes, self-testing by the consumer offers privacy and convenience direct from the home. The menu for self-testing is growing, with one website (http://www.home-healthtesting. com) showing almost two dozen diagnostic tests for consumers. They range from a simple cholesterol test to more sophisticated tests for Alzheimer's disease, drugs in hair and urine, and prostate cancer. Many of the more sophisticated tests are not offered as self-tests because they require sending off samples for analysis. The reasons for testing are as diverse as the menu of tests offered and include the opportunity for individuals to manage their ailments (e.g., self-testing glucose), monitor their health by ensuring they are eating properly (e.g., antioxidants), and test themselves or a family member for substance abuse (e.g., alcohol and drugs). Self-testing can also be provided by a healthcare provider when the patient is reluctant to perform the test, the method is more complicated, or the value is more critical (e.g., prothrombin time).

Of all of the self-tests offered, the only ones that seem to have significant sales are glucose, ovulation, and pregnancy kits. Testing oneself in the home for glucose levels is not new, and based on the number of diabetics, it is understandable that the demand is high. Ovulation and pregnancy kits are popular for a number of reasons. Ovulation kits detect a woman's most fertile days during the monthly cycle and the method is relatively simple. For a saliva-based fertility monitor, a woman's saliva is placed on a minimicroscope first thing in the morning. When the saliva has dried, one looks into the microscope, and if fern-like patterns exist, ovulation is occurring. The theory is that when a woman is fertile her saliva contains a high level of salts, which form a fern-like pattern as the saliva dries (16). With home pregnancy tests, women have the opportunity to be the first to know whether or not they are pregnant instead of having to wait for the physician to call, and these tests are easy to use and are fairly accurate.

The reluctance of consumers to purchase some of the other self-testing kits on the market might be due to the type of sample required (e.g., blood from a fingerstick) and/or the lack of knowledge about the relevance of the test. Another problem with self-testing kits is the number of variables associated with these assays. The importance of quality control, proper specimen collection (e.g., hemolyzing), and pre-testing preparation (e.g., fasting for triglycerides) are not always known by individuals. Because of these variables, many individuals might end up in a physician's office for additional testing due to erroneous results, which in turn may result in increased healthcare costs.

For these reasons and others, the healthcare industry must assess who really should be performing POCT and how to better educate the user. This does not suggest that home patients should not monitor their condition or test for specific complications. It merely suggests that there be a strong educational component associated with this task. Diabetic patients are a good example. Those that have been educated and continually perform self-testing are reasonably proficient at performing the test and are knowledgeable about quality control. Healthcare workers performing POCT can include a wide spectrum of healthcare providers, ranging from home healthcare aides to primary care providers. Diagnostic technology available for POCT is simple and accurate and provides quality assurance. The abundance of glucose monitoring devices for both patients and healthcare providers is a good example. Other technologies offer POCT coagulation testing. A coagulation analyzer designed for the home healthcare market has met with mixed reviews in the United States, but many patients are using the system in Germany. Even though the analyzer is in the Clinical Laboratory Improvement Amendments (CLIA) waived category, it requires a training course, is dispensed via a physician, and has not been widely accepted by individuals and/or agencies. There could be many reasons for this: Physicians may be reluctant to put this responsibility on their patients even though there has been good success for those who have implemented this POCT, or it could be that the patients are reluctant. Whatever the reason, it demonstrates that home POCT is still a complex arena and is not easily definable. Whether in the hands of the patient or a healthcare provider, the ability to produce accurate POCT results with quality assurance is going to play a major role in the delivery of home healthcare.

EFFECTS OF TELEHEALTH ON SELF-TESTING QUALITY ASSURANCE

Home healthcare agencies are seeing the need to provide more diagnostic and therapeutic services for their patients as the severity, complications, and/or comorbidity of the patients' conditions increase.

Vital sign measurements are not new for the homebound patient. Blood pressure, weight, and pulse rates have a long history in this market. However, as pressures increase to release individuals from hospitals sooner, the quantity of homebound patients and the severity of their conditions have increased. Telehealth technology has provided both the patient and the home healthcare provider an opportunity to standardize and record these vital sign measurements. Every time a patient performs a vital sign measurement, it is recorded on the patient's web-based record. Each measurement can be reviewed and compared to previous measurements. The technology used is standardized, and educational programs are implemented at the time the technology is placed in the home. In addition, instructions and consultations can be accessed via the technology.

At the same time, POCT diagnostic technology has improved. Over the past few years, POCT has also made some major strides in ease of use and quality control and now affords individuals with minimum training the opportunity to perform select tests. As previously stated, among the highest percentages of home healthcare patients are those with circulatory problems. Many of these patients are at risk for thromboembolic events. Individuals who are undergoing long-term Coumadin (warfarin) treatment are at risk of clotting (underdose) or abnormal bleeding (overdose) and therefore require frequent prothrombin time (PT) or international normalized ratio (INR) monitoring. The 1999 data reveal that more than 20 million individuals were taking warfarin. Testing of these patients is generally performed in a hospital or commercial laboratory. There is POCT for PT/INR on the market, and some individuals/agencies do use them, particularly in European countries. INRs performed at home by the patient or the healthcare provider lead to better control of anticoagulation and fewer bleeding episodes due to the frequency of measurements (17). In the United States, most home care practitioners either send the patient to the hospital to have a specimen drawn or draw a specimen from the patient at home and have their INR tests performed by a hospital or commercial laboratory. Either scenario results in delays of diagnostic results. If, for any reason, the results are abnormal, the nurse must first contact the physician and then return to the patient's home to correct the dosage. The transportation and storage of such samples are also variables because they can render the sample unacceptable by the laboratory or produce spurious results. This outcome also requires that the healthcare provider return to the patient's home to collect another specimen. Either of these scenarios leads to increased return visits to the patient's home, thereby increasing costs. The ability to perform the test via POCT and send it by way of telehealth technology to the patient's web-based record has many advantages. Once again the ability to compare current results to previous recordings as well as plot results over time provides a visual picture of the patient's results. If the test is abnormal, the physician and/or the laboratorian can be alerted and questioned as to the appropriate response.

The same argument that is being made about POCT in the hospital can be applied to the home healthcare market: Is the increased cost of doing the test by the bedside providing a better outcome? As demonstrated by this scenario, there is a major difference between the hospital patient and the home healthcare patient in that the distance between the laboratory and the patient can be extensive. This alone has a major impact on turnaround time and costs. The time spent traveling to a site to drop off the specimen as well as the time it takes to actually receive test results can hinder patient care. If the laboratory results are abnormal they may require additional visits, thus increasing overall costs.

ADVANCES IN INFORMATION TECHNOLOGY: TELEHEALTH PROVIDES AN INTERNET DATABASE

Information is going to be a key ingredient in providing healthcare in the home. It plays an important role in effectively delivering, monitoring, and assessing an individual's health. The efficient delivery of healthcare across a region will require the movement of information. All sites delivering healthcare (including the home) will require the availability of information and connectivity to the electronic patient record. The legacy systems presently being used are not structured to facilitate the data sharing necessary in a patient care–focused system. In addition, they are not using effective productivity tools essential for clinician-driven information technology.

The ability to support integrated models with multiple facilities has placed a variety of constraints on present information systems. The integrated models of tomorrow will demand flexibility and functional scalability. The ability to access and disseminate information across such a system has been hindered by aging platforms and architectures that utilize dated technology. In addition to the movement of information, the integrated systems will require security. As information moves from the physician's office to the home and from the home to the laboratory information system and/or hospital information system, there will be a need to restrict access. As healthcare systems move more toward decentralization and ambulatory care, the need for interactive technology will be imperative. The ability of the home healthcare provider or patient to download POCT and vital sign results to both the physician and hospital laboratory information system will help in making the appropriate decision (e.g., change in medication) at the time of the next home visit. As mentioned before, the Viterion 500 system automatically downloads all data to the patient's web-based file, which can then be accessed by any healthcare provider in the system who has the appropriate access authority. This allows the home health practitioner to monitor the patient in the home as well as review the data prior to the next meeting. This also affords the physician the opportunity to review all the patient's vital signs and POCT reports before the next office visit, thereby expediting the visit. The next step in improving the care provided during the home health visit should be to provide the practitioner with the ability to download previous laboratory data on the patient (e.g., Δ check) when at the patient's home. It is just a matter of time before the information can go in both directions, allowing practitioners in the home to access data from the hospital laboratory, physician office visits, hospital stays, etc. The connectivity of information will eventually allow one to perform outcome studies and monitor trends. This will provide the opportunity to evaluate impacts of strategies and/or protocols such as POCT in home healthcare, monitor specific case mixes with home healthcare visits with and without POCT, document return visits based on testing on or off site, and build a database on home POCT screening programs. These are just a few of the cost management analysis opportunities that could be available.

The role of the laboratory will depend very much on the creativity of laboratory information system vendors. As pointed out by Cooper, "The future of the laboratory information system and its role in diagnostic services will be dependent on its ability to keep up with the advances of information technology (18)."

CONCLUSION

Home healthcare is one of the fastest-growing segments in healthcare. Telehealth technology is becoming wireless and very interactive. More and more practitioners are making the virtual home visit in place of the traditional one-on-one visit. It appears that both practitioners and home patients are embracing the technology. Each new generation of telehealth technology has a broader vital sign menu and enhanced software. The telehealth system utilizes wireless glucometers that automatically release data to the patient's web-based record. The data demonstrate increased patient compliance when recording their vital signs and/or performing POC tests (from approximately 30% to >90%), which is a primary goal of patient management. As telehealth grows, the costs will decline. This, along with information technology connectivity, will surely guarantee its place in healthcare.

Long hospital stays and extensive utilization of medical specialists are commodities that today's healthcare system can no longer afford. The alternatives to such costly encounters involve maximizing the services of a full spectrum of healthcare providers such as primary care physicians, physician assistants, nurse practitioners, subacute healthcare centers, and home healthcare personnel. To ensure that cost reduction strategies are sound, cost-effective, and in the best interest of the patient, managed care and governmental agencies must step back and look at the bigger picture. They need to give patients continuity of healthcare from the hospital to the home and take a long-term view rather than focusing on immediate savings. Programs for homebound patients that include diagnostic testing, monitoring, and screening can save a considerable amount of money (short- and long-term) if implemented correctly and among appropriate populations. For example, home health programs utilize respiratory care professionals for clinical treatments as a cost-saving measure (e.g., setting up technology and patient education). If telehealth afforded home healthcare providers the opportunity to perform POCT for blood gases and electrolytes, as well as other diagnostic tests such as INRs and renal function tests, it would ultimately reduce the number of return visits to the hospital and/or emergency departments and/or the use of more sophisticated technology (e.g., renal dialysis).

It is clear that to compete in this new environment, healthcare systems will have to focus on the continuity of care and the costs associated with treatment, monitoring, and quality of life. It appears that home healthcare will play an integral part in meeting these criteria. The more technology advances, and the simpler and less invasive diagnostic tests become, the more attractive they will be.

The laboratory's role in telehealth POCT, as with hospital POCT, will most likely be consultative. However, this will happen only if laboratory information systems can keep up with technological advances in information systems.

REFERENCES

1. Centers for Medicare and Medicaid Services, Health and Human Services. http://www.cms.hhs.gov/marketupdate (accessed September 22, 2003).
2. National Association for Home Care. http://www.nahc.org/consumer/hcstats.html (accessed September 29, 2003).
3. Miller SM. Diabetes: get a clearer picture. MLO Med Lab Obs 2003;35:10–22.
4. Pear R. Spending on healthcare increased sharply in 2001. New York Times January 9, 2004:8.
5. National Heart, Lung and Blood Institute, National Institutes of Health. http:www.nhlbi.nih.gov (accessed December 12, 2003).
6. Lehmann C, Lopatin W, Gaur P, Miyazaki J, Lesch J, Mitzner I. Impact of technology on home bound congestive heart failure patients. J Telemed Telecare 2002;8:253–4.
7. Masharani U. Diabetes mellitus & hypoglycemia. In: Tierney, LM Jr, McPhee SJ, Papadakis MA, eds. Current medical diagnosis & treatment. 43rd ed. New York: McGraw-Hill, 2004; 1146–90.
8. Centers for Disease Control. http://www.cdc.gov (accessed December 12, 2003).
9. Jiang HJ, Stryer D. Multiple hospitalizations for patients with diabetes. Diabetes Care 2003;26:1421–6.
10. Horgan P, Dall T, Nikolov P. Economic costs of diabetes in the US in 2002. Diabetes Care 2003;26:917–32.
11. Mebra MR, Uber P, Chomsky DB, Oren R. Emergence of electronic home monitoring in chronic heart failure: rationale, feasibility, and easy results with the HomMed Sentry-Observer System. Congest Heart Fail 2000;6:137–9.
12. Peddicord H. Extending disease management: a home monitoring system for vital signs. Am Clin Lab 2000;19:22.
13. Centers for Disease Control. http://www.cdc.gov/diabetes activated (accessed November 3, 2003).
14. American Diabetes Association. Clinical practice recommendations. Diabetes Care 2003;26:1–148.
15. Sacks DB, Bruns DE, Goldstein DE, Maclaren NK, McDonald JM, Parrott M. Guidelines and recommendations for laboratory analysis in the diagnosis and management of diabetes mellitus. Clin Chem 2002;48:1140–2.
16. Guida M, Barbato M, Bruno P, Lauro G, Lampariello C. Salivary ferning and the menstrual cycle of women. Clin Exp Obstet Gynecol 1993;20:48–54.
17. Lehmann CA. The future of home testing—implications for traditional laboratories. Clin Chim Acta 2002;323:31–6.
18. Cooper SD. The role of the laboratory information system in clinical diagnostic technology. In: Ward-Cook KM, Lehmann CA, Schoeff LE, Williams RH, eds. Clinical diagnostic technology: the total testing process, vol. 1. Washington, DC: AACC Press, 2003.

Chapter 28

Point-of-Care Testing in Primary Care

Christopher P. Price and Andrew St John

For many decades, primary care has been seen as the major medical interface between the public and the healthcare system—hence the term "primary care." It has, for many years, comprised a number of healthcare professionals including doctors, midwifes, health visitors, and more recently, practice nurses. Today it comprises an even wider range of professionals, including a number of allied health personnel. Traditionally they have provided a repertoire of care that embraces both health promotion as well as management of disease and ways of dealing with illness. In his book, *From Cradle to Grave; Fifty Years of the NHS*, Geoffrey Rivett (1) describes the history of the National Health Service (NHS) in the United Kingdom from its inception in 1948 to the modern day. He describes a period from 1958 to 1967 as a "renaissance of general practice and the hospitals"— general practice being effectively what we call primary care today. There was a "General Practitioner's Charter" in 1965 that included "increasing recruitment, undergraduate education oriented toward practice and good postgraduate education, a maximum number of patients on a list, incentives for skills and experience, pay to reflect workload, reasonable working hours, and a worthwhile, effective, and satisfying career with clinical freedom in a personal family doctor service." Twenty years later, the work of Cochrane on the quality and effectiveness of healthcare began to attract attention, and there was discussion of structure, process, and outcome, and the role of primary care at the center of a "planned health service" was envisaged. The effect of this was a dramatic increase in work for all healthcare professionals and an escalating cost of care. At the same time, an explosion of technological innovation helped contribute to soaring costs. As might be expected, the increasing costs led to further reviews, and fresh plans, while the trends in increasing work and demands on the service continued unabated. In the meantime, the patient was also becoming more demanding and beginning to choose alternative routes to obtain care, including seeking immediate attention for minor ailments from the emergency services as well as from the general practitioner. At the present time the United Kingdom's NHS is undergoing a further reorganization that is attempting to address many of the issues and pressures that are arising today.

There is no doubt that similar changes have been occurring in healthcare systems throughout the world, exhibiting many of the same trends and pressures, as well as seeking solutions in a similar manner. In addition, many of the trends seen in the healthcare systems are also evident in laboratory services, with technological innovation and demand leapfrogging each other

as the reason for increased costs. Technology to enable testing at the point of care has added to this evolution in a way that challenges many of the policy decisions that have been made and are being made today, especially in the thinking around patient-centered care and a health service led by primary care. These themes are being expounded around the world and are already being practiced to some degree in various countries. In this context it is interesting to speculate on the potential of point-of-care testing (POCT) to resolve some of the problems seen in the delivery of care today, and various examples are quoted in the chapters of this book.

In the first edition of this book (1999), Richard Hobbs (2) drew attention to a number of pressures that constantly beset the primary care physician, including:

- An intolerance of late diagnosis
- An increasing requirement to filter access to specialist care, especially in managed care systems such as the NHS in the United Kingdom or health maintenance organizations (HMOs) in the United States
- The earlier discharge of patients from hospital
- Demands to manage the surveillance of long-term disease

Many of these observations illustrate the changes occurring in primary care today across the world.

Hobbs et al. (3) undertook a systematic review of POCT in primary care and found little evidence to support the use of POCT in this setting. They found very few papers that addressed the issue of the clinical need for which the test result might be required, with most of the papers being concerned with the technical performance of the POCT devices described. This chapter reviews the evidence on the application of POCT in the primary care setting in the context of the way in which today's primary care is evolving.

MODERN PRIMARY CARE

More than 90% of patient contacts within a health system such as the NHS occur in primary care (4). Classically, the role of the primary care physician is seen as a gatekeeper to secondary care. Approximately 65% of the patients seen in primary care are suffering from minor and/or self-limiting conditions, while about 20% have a chronic disease and/or a permanent disability; the remaining 15% have a major or life-threatening condition (5). Approximately 400 referrals per year are made to secondary care by a primary care physician, but only 5% of primary care consultations lead to a referral (5). Against the background of these simple statistics, it is clear why the use of telephone advisory services [e.g., NHS Direct in the United Kingdom (6) and Health Direct in Australia (7)] have arisen. A recent systematic review of the quality of clinical care in primary care in the United Kingdom, Australia, and New Zealand showed that most of the care for common and chronic conditions was provided in the primary care sector (8). Using outcome measures based on access, clinical effectiveness, interpersonal effectiveness, equity, and efficiency, the authors found that acceptable quality standards were not attained. The study showed that guidelines were not always being followed, a conclusion that was also drawn by another study that looked at the use of guidelines in primary care (9). It must be stressed, however, that the quality of some of the studies reported was quite poor, and both of the authors recommended that further studies were required before robust conclusions could be drawn.

There is a considerable literature on the consultation process in primary and secondary care, and, despite its complexity, it is worth briefly looking at some of the conclusions. Engstrom et al. (10) attempted to compare the effectiveness of primary and specialist care to try to determine whether primary care was effective, by undertaking a systematic review of the literature. They found limitations in many studies but concluded that increased accessibility to physicians working in primary care contributed to better health outcomes and lower costs in the healthcare system. They also noted that there were few studies that investigated the best way in which to organize primary care. Harrington et al. (11) undertook a systematic review on improving patient communication with doctors. They reviewed the literature on intervention studies designed to increase patient participation in medical consultations. Half of the interventions resulted in increased patient participation; however, of the 10 written interventions, only 2 reported a significant increase in patient questions. Patient satisfaction was the most commonly measured outcome, but few significant improvements were found. However, there were significant improvements in perceptions of control over health, preferences for an active role in healthcare, recall of information, adherence to recommendations, attendance, and clinical outcomes. Wilson and Childs (12) reviewed the literature on the relationship between the consultation length, process, and outcomes in the primary care setting, using objectively measured process or health outcomes. The authors concluded that, although the average consultation length may be a marker of other doctor attributes, the evidence suggests that patients seeking help from a doctor who spends more time with them are more likely to have a consultation that includes important elements of care. Overall, the literature does suggest that more time spent with a patient is beneficial to the outcome. Thiru et al. (13) performed a systematic review of the scope and quality of the electronic patient record in primary care. They found a total of 52 papers that met their inclusion criteria, of which 48 were concerned with diagnostic data. Interestingly, the authors

found that prescribing data held in the record was generally of better quality than the diagnostic data. The authors also stressed the value of electronic capture of data, and the fact that this often does not occur may explain the poorer showing of the diagnostic information in the review.

Some of the issues highlighted in the literature discussed earlier have contributed to a broadening of the role of other healthcare professionals to become the first point of contact for the patient with the health service. This is best exemplified in the expansion of the role of the nurse (14, 15), and more recently that of the community pharmacist (16), developments that have been established for several years in the United States but only more recently have gained momentum in the United Kingdom (see Chapter 35). Horrocks et al. (17) undertook a systematic review of the literature to determine whether nurse practitioners could provide an equivalent level of care to doctors. They found 34 studies meeting the inclusion criteria for the review. The studies showed that patient satisfaction was improved with nurse care, but there was no difference in health status outcome. Interestingly, nurses were found to undertake significantly more investigations and had longer consultations than doctors. The quality of care provided by nurses was considered to be at least as good as that provided by doctors. Several of the studies highlighted the role of the nurse practitioner in providing care to patients requesting same-day appointments predominantly for acute minor illness, working in a team supported by doctors. The review also included more recent papers describing the specialist nurse practitioner's role in caring for patients with chronic diseases (e.g., diabetes, hypertension, asthma, and heart failure). There were a number of limitations to the review, including exactly what was meant by the term *nurse practitioner*, as well as the level of training given to such a person. There were also significant variations in the data that were recorded and the outcome measures used. It was concluded, however, that further research was warranted on the role of the nurse practitioner.

It is interesting to review the observations made in the studies above in the context of the way in which the delivery of primary care may be developing, together with the potential role that POCT might have in supporting and complementing the change in practice. Some of the changes in practice of primary care that may affect health outcomes, including incorporation of POCT, are listed in Table 28-1.

THE POTENTIAL USE OF POCT IN PRIMARY CARE

Conventionally, an in vitro diagnostic test can be used (a) in screening for the presence or absence of a disease, (b) in making a diagnosis, (c) in optimizing and monitoring treatment, and (d) in assessing prognosis. To fulfill these roles, the diagnostic test must meet defined analytical and clinical performance criteria. The role of any test will initially have been established with an analytical system in a clinical laboratory; if the efficacy of the test has not been established in this way, it is unlikely that it will prove to be effective when using the

Table 28-1   Some of the Trends in Primary Care Services and Their Relation to the Introduction of POCT

First attendance with symptoms
Testing undertaken prior to consultation by patient
Testing undertaken prior to consultation by pharmacist
Testing undertaken prior to consultation by practice nurse
Testing undertaken by primary care physician
Patient asked to attend local laboratory for testing after consultation

Chronic disease management
Use of specialist miniclinic, e.g., diabetes, anticoagulation
Use of specialist nurse practitioner for routine consultation
Specialty trained primary care physician
Patient attends a week early for phlebotomy, testing by laboratory
Testing performed at health center
Testing and consultation performed in community pharmacy setting
Testing performed during consultation
Patient self-management and telemedicine consultation

Testing at-risk populations
As part of routine service undertaken by practice nurse with regular recall
Increased range of at risk testing services
Well-person clinic at health center
Well-person clinic at community pharmacy
Self-testing with aid of Internet advice

Statements in italics represent situation closest to current practice in many institutions.

POCT modality. Having said that, as stated elsewhere in this book, the essence of the value of POCT lies in the quick delivery of the result after the test has been ordered.

The key to the use of POCT in any setting, including primary care, is that the test result enables a decision to be made, and some action to be initiated at the time of the consultation. The decisions that POCT enables can be considered under the following broad headings:

- Acute diagnosis rule-out and disease exclusion
- Acute diagnosis rule-in and treatment
- Contribution to differential diagnosis
- Referral to secondary care rule-in
- Therapy effectiveness monitoring
- Chronic disease management
- Opportunistic screening of at-risk individuals
- Screening for disease

Hobbs (2) pointed to the fact that any POCT device that is going to be effective in the primary care environment must be unobtrusive in terms of its effect on the consultation period. This is potentially one of the most challenging aspects of the use of POCT in primary care because of the short consultation periods that pertain for most patients. Gutierres and Welty (18) made the point in their review of POCT that those studies that incorporated POCT with a change in the way patient care was delivered showed a significant improvement in patient out-

comes. They made the further point that although the cost of providing the testing was higher than that of using a central laboratory, the increased cost was offset by the improvement in patient outcomes and the reduction in utilization of healthcare resources. Nichols et al. (19), among others, found in a secondary care environment that a change in practice was required to deliver the expected benefit from POCT.

The publication of the new General Medical Services contract for primary care physicians in the United Kingdom incorporates a number of quality indicators that give an indication of the way in which primary care practice is envisaged as developing (20). These are listed in Table 28-2 and include a number of indices related to in vitro diagnostic tests. These applications span screening but are associated primarily with chronic disease management.

The point was made earlier that the ideal POCT device is one that does not interrupt the patient consultation, and in many cases this is an extremely difficult requirement to meet. Thus, at the present time it is most likely that there will need to be some reorganization of the patient flow through the primary care center, certainly in relation to unplanned visits by new patients. In the case of a regular patient, such as a diabetic person on a schedule of quarterly or half yearly review, it is possible to consider the organization of miniclinics, bringing together all of the expertise required for that group of patient consultations. Currently the testing component of such visits may be accommodated by asking the patient to attend for

Table 28-2   Quality Indicators Including Laboratory Indices in the New General Medical Services Contract for UK Primary Care Physicians as They Could Pertain to POCT[a]

Cardiovascular disease—secondary prevention
Cholesterol measurement over the past 15 months
Cholesterol concentration < 5.0 mmol/L (193 mg/dL)

Stroke or transient ischemic attacks
Cholesterol measurement over the past 15 months
Cholesterol concentration < 5.0 mmol/L (193 mg/dL)

Diabetes mellitus
HbA1c measurement over the past 15 months
HbA1c level < 7.4%
Serum creatinine measurement over the past 15 months
Urine microalbumin over the past 15 months
Cholesterol measurement over the past 15 months
Cholesterol concentration < 5.0 mmol/L (193 mg/dL)

Hypothyroidism
Thyroid function tests over the past 15 months

Mental health
For patients on lithium, a measurement over the past 15 months
For patients on lithium, a measurement level withiin the therapeutic range
For patients on lithium, a measurement of serum creatinine and thyroid function tests over the past 15 months

[a] Indicators are generally written in terms of the proportion of patients with a record of measurement within the past x months or the proportion of patients with values within a certain range.

phlebotomy a week ahead of the consultation, but this may not be convenient for the patient. This is where the community pharmacist may have a role in the future. It has been suggested that in another clinical setting, a patient describing symptoms of a urinary tract infection may be asked to take a fresh urine sample to the pharmacist or the health center nurse for testing prior to an appointment with the primary care physician. There is no doubt that these scenarios will be explored in the future as physicians and patients alike seek to improve the efficiency, effectiveness, and general user acceptability of the consultation process. Whatever process is chosen, quality control of its elements will be expected and required.

TECHNOLOGY, ORGANIZATION, AND MANAGEMENT OF POCT IN PRIMARY CARE

The early chapters in this book describe the principles underpinning the design of the POCT devices available today. The two key features to point out in relation to the application of POCT in primary care are (a) the operator-friendly design of the modern systems and (b) the repertoire of assays that are available. It must be recognized, however, that at the present time it would be necessary for any health center engaging in the full application of POCT to maintain a fairly extensive portfolio of equipment, with the ensuing costs associated with operator training, maintenance, and quality control.

Although regulations will determine how POCT is organized and managed in some countries, the guidance given in the earlier chapters on equipment procurement and implementation, training and certification of operators, quality control, and quality assurance are perhaps more apposite in the primary care setting, where there is less familiarity with analytical equipment. Reference has been made on several occasions to the need to maintain strong links between remote testing sites and the local clinical laboratory, which can provide expertise in staff training, evaluation of new equipment, and quality control. In addition, they can provide a valuable troubleshooting resource if problems occur, as well as a backup analytical service if things go wrong.

Because patients are frequently managed with a combination of POCT and central laboratory testing, it is important to ensure good concordance of results between the POCT site and the central laboratory, to minimize the need for repeat testing when the patient moves from one setting to the other. In addition, good concordance of data will increase the confidence of the primary care physician in the results produced by the POCT system. Hobbs et al. (21), in evaluating the performance of a number of POCT devices for measuring prothrombin time (PT) in a primary care setting, stressed the importance of good liaison with the local laboratory. Murray et al. (22) demonstrated, again with PT testing, that it is possible to run an external quality assurance program in primary care. One approach is to involve the local laboratory as the organizer, as this makes the expertise immediately available for consultation on the interpretation of findings.

EARLY GENERAL STUDIES ON POCT IN PRIMARY CARE

A number of studies have investigated in broad terms the use of POCT in primary care. One of the first was a before-and-after study conducted by Rink et al. (23) that involved a range of tests delivered by a laboratory service and by POCT. The tests chosen were for plasma urea and electrolytes, cholesterol, uric acid, and γ-glutamyl transferase, together with simple urinalysis and urine chlamydia testing. The main findings were that there was an increase in the recording of risk factors for heart disease together with more cholesterol testing when using POCT, and that the simple urinalysis could have led to a reduction in the number of samples being sent to the laboratory for culture and sensitivity in cases of suspected urinary tract infection. The economic analysis was limited to comparing the cost of testing, while a questionnaire to the primary care physicians indicated that they were unlikely to continue using POCT, possibly owing to the difficulty of fitting it into the routine of the practice.

In another study reported by Gillam et al. (24) the effects of providing results on full blood count, platelet count, urea and electrolytes, liver function tests, cholesterol, glucose, and creatine kinase by POCT were assessed. The authors found an increase in the testing workload together with an increase in testing costs. They found that the image of the health center was enhanced and that 87% of the patients preferred to have their tests performed by POCT. There was no further assessment on the longer-term effects of this modality of testing.

These studies are examples of the early forays into POCT and can really only be considered as exploratory studies of the overall concept and approach to POCT. They lacked the focus on the clinical challenges experienced by the primary care physicians, which may be reflected in the choice of analytes that were studied. The repertoire of tests may have reflected the most common tests ordered, as well as mirroring the type of POCT systems available at the time. The studies were too small to assess another feature of test orders by general practitioners, namely the huge variability seen in the number of orders made by individual practitioners (25)

It is interesting therefore to study the range of problems faced by the primary care physician. Wijk et al. (26) studied the ordering behavior of a group of 44 general practices in the Netherlands as part of a wider study on compliance with decision support for ordering blood tests. They found the highest proportion of tests was ordered for an indication of "vague symptoms" (30.1%). This was followed by more specific questions relating to risk factors for hypertension (9.1%), screening for hypercholesterolemia (8.6%), and so on. Wijk et al. (26) found that >80% of the work was related to 12 indications. The data are summarized in Table 28-3 and compared with an audit of the tests requested by a group of general practitioners in the United Kingdom, performed by Myers (5).

The study by Wijk et al. (26) is interesting because it looked at the compliance with guidelines on requesting laboratory investigations. The guidelines were based on a review of

Table 28-3 Comparison of the Main Symptoms of Primary Care Center[a] Patients Referred for Testing and the Main Tests Ordered by Another Center[b]

Center 1[a]		Center 2[b]	
Symptom	Percentage of total tests ordered	Test	Orders per year
Vague complaints	30.1	Full blood count	1100
Hypertension, assessing risk	9.1	Urea and electrolytes	620
Hypercholesterolemia, screening	8.6	Erythrocyte sedimentation rate/viscometry	450
Anemia, diagnosis	4.7	Liver function tests	360
Allergic rhinitis, diagnosis	4.4	Thyroid function tests	350
Hyperthyroidism, diagnosis	4.3	Cholesterol/lipids	350
Hypercholesterolemia, monitoring	3.7	Midstream urine culture	320
Rheumatoid arthritis, diagnosis	3.6	Blood glucose	270
Infectious mononucleosis, diagnosis	3.5	Blood group	150
Prostate cancer, diagnosis	3.2	Uric acid	130
Iron-deficiency anemia, diagnosis	2.9	HbA1c	120
Diabetes mellitus, monitoring	2.1	Lutenizing hormone/follicle-stimulating hormone	110
		Rubella *Treponema pallidum* hemagglutination assay titer	100

[a] Data from (26).
[b] Data from (5).

the literature, current medical practice, and a consensus among the group developing the guidelines (27, 28). The authors reported that the most common cause of noncompliance was the addition of new tests (e.g., triglycerides and HDL cholesterol in the case of a patient being screened for hypercholesterolemia). They concluded that this was most probably due to physicians applying new information on medical practice.

Takemura et al. (29) performed a large panel of 30 tests in 540 new symptomatic patients presenting to a primary care center, albeit it was probably a hospital outpatient clinic setting. They evaluated the utility of the panel in terms of the ability of the information gained from the results to contribute to the physician's diagnosis or decision making relating to a "tentative initial diagnosis" obtained from a history and physical examination alone. The investigators found 398 situations in which the results influenced the diagnosis or decision making and uncovered 261 occult diseases. Analysis of the data showed that 1592 test results contributed to this yield of information. The cost per effective test that contributed to diagnosis or decision making varied from less than $1 for a cholesterol measurement to just over $50 for a chest x-ray film. The authors suggested that it would be possible to refine the panel of tests to improve further the cost-effectiveness, the use of a large panel of tests not proving to be cost-effective (30). It is worth noting that the 540 patients were seen over a period of 6 years, which suggests that use of the test panel was not widespread. An earlier report on the same population indicated that the most common diseases detected were hypercholesterolemia and liver disease (31).

The overall impression is that there is a wide disparity of views concerning what tests are of real value in the primary care setting. Applying an evidence-based approach to this question prompts the observation that there needs to be a greater definition of the clinical questions that the primary care

physician is asking in order to ensure that the correct tests are made available at the point of care (32). Only then will it be possible to perform the requisite outcomes studies to ascertain whether POCT is valuable in the primary care setting. It is therefore interesting to note that the Australian government is embarking on a randomized controlled trial of POCT for certain analytes in a range of primary care centers across the country; the majority of the analytes are concerned with chronic disease management (33).

The remaining section of this chapter reviews some of the studies that have been undertaken in the primary care setting and addresses specific clinical situations.

SPECIFIC APPLICATIONS OF POCT IN PRIMARY CARE

Acute Presentations

Identification of Infectious Diseases. The study by Rink et al. (23) involved a pre-test–post-test study design; they assessed the potential benefits of urinalysis in primary care as part of a larger study. These investigators found a potential for reduction in the number of urine samples sent to the laboratory for testing when a urinary tract infection was suspected, using leukocyte esterase and nitrite tests to rule out the likelihood of urinary tract infection. The latter has been the topic of many studies, including that of Ditchburn et al. (34), who found that a dipstick test for leukocyte esterase and nitrite gave a 92% negative predictive value for urinary tract infection. Winkens et al. (35), however, reported a multicenter trial with only a 56% negative predictive value. The difference between the two studies is likely to be due to the influence of inter-operator variability in the latter study. This emphasizes the importance of reliable manufacture and storage of devices together with good operator training and continuing education. In addition, there may be a reduction in inter-operator variability as more of the test strips are read with the aid of an instrument (36). McNulty et al. (37) found that the use of the microbiology laboratory and the test positivity rate varied considerably. They used qualitative methods to determine how primary care physicians made decisions about the care of patients, taking into account the wide variation in frequency with which practitioners used the laboratory. Frequent users of the laboratory with low positivity did not use POCT, while those with high positivity used POCT to rule out the possibility of urinary tract infection, sending only the positive specimens to the laboratory for antibiotic susceptibility testing. Infrequent users of the laboratory did not use POCT, appearing to prescribe antibiotics even for minimal symptoms. The authors concluded that clear guidelines were required on the management of urinary tract infections, which set out the roles of POCT and the laboratory, and that these should form the basis for the education of primary care staff.

The role of C-reactive protein as a general marker of infection and inflammation has been suggested from time to time. Hobbs et al. (38) evaluated a POCT device for use in primary care on an "intent to investigate" basis, comparing results with a laboratory analyzer method. Over a 3-month period 181 tests were performed, with 81% used to establish a diagnosis and the remainder for disease monitoring. The agreement with the laboratory method was good, with a positive predictive value of 59% and 99% for positive and negative results, respectively. The investigators noted that the assay could be performed during the consultation period and concluded that the device was reliable for use in primary care. Seamark et al. (39) also found that C-reactive protein could be measured reliably in primary care.

Dahler-Eriksen et al. (40) investigated the effect of POCT for C-reactive protein on clinical, operational, and economic outcomes in primary care. They found that the use of the erythrocyte sedimentation rate decreased during the study, as did the number of specimens sent to the laboratory. The number of follow-up telephone calls to patients was reduced, but there was no change in the rate of prescribing of antibiotics. In patients with very high C-reactive protein levels, however, therapy was instituted earlier, compared with care when no POCT was available. The POCT service was thought to be cost effective mainly because of the reduction in use of the laboratory services. This follows other studies that have found the use of POCT for C-reactive protein to be useful in primary care (41, 42). Takemura et al. (43) looked at the effect of immediate availability of C-reactive protein and leukocyte counts on antimicrobial prescribing habits—albeit in an outpatient clinic setting. They found a significant reduction in the use of antibiotics in the POCT group ($P < 0.001$).

Several studies have investigated the use of POCT for influenza in children using either throat or nasal swabs (44) or with nasopharyngeal aspirates (45). Harnden et al. (45) performed a study in primary care using a POCT device (Quick-Vue, Quidel, San Diego, CA, USA) involving 157 children

with a cough and fever thought to be "more than a simple cold." Influenza was detected by the laboratory in 61 of the children, while the POCT device was positive in 27 of the 61, giving a sensitivity of 44% (95% CI = 32–58%) and a specificity of 97% (95% CI = 91–99%). The likelihood ratio for a positive test result was 14.2 (4.5–44.7) and for a negative result 0.58 (0.46–0.72). Rodriguez et al. (44) studied 116 children and compared four systems: (i) QuickVue Influenza Test (Quidel, Quidel Corporation, San Diego, CA, USA), (ii) Flu OIA (Biostar, Thermo Electron Corporation, Louisville, CO, USA), (iii) Z Stat Flu (ZymeTx, ZymeTx, Oklahoma City, OK, USA) and (iv) Directigen Flu A (Becton Dickinson, BD Diagnostic Systems, Sparks, MD, USA). The sensitivities of the four tests ranged from 72% to 95%, with the Z Stat differing markedly from the other three ($P = 0.001$). The specificities of all four tests were similar (76–86%). The positive predictive value of the four tests ranged from 80% to 86%. The negative predictive value of all four tests ranged from 75% to 94%, although the Z Stat Flu had a lower negative predictive value than the other three tests (75%; $P = 0.001$). The differences in the sensitivities in the two studies for the QuickVue system are probably due to the use of different reference methods; Harnden et al. (45) used a molecular technique on an aspirate, whereas Rodriguez et al. (44) used a culture technique on a swab. Harnden et al. (45) concluded that the QuickVue could be used to rule in but not to rule out influenza in children, and may improve the quality of care in children in primary care. Pregliasco et al. (46), however, studied 928 children over two separate years and found the sensitivities of the QuickVue system to be 36.5% and 54.5% for the two years, compared with culture in both years and a molecular technique in the second year. They concluded that the test was not good enough for surveillance and immediate management of children presenting with influenza-like symptoms.

Several POCT devices for the detection of group A streptococci are described in the literature. In an early evaluation of the Testpack Strep A (Abbott Laboratories, Abbott Park, IL, USA), Burke et al. (47) studied 250 patients with sore throat and found that the sensitivity of the test was 63% and the specificity 91.7% compared with 74% and 58% for clinical assessment alone. The investigators also found that the test results rarely led to previous prescribing decisions [in only 34 (13%) of episodes] being altered. Carey et al. (48), although using a different reference procedure for confirmation of infection, found a sensitivity of 79.4% and a specificity of 93.3%. These authors concluded that maximum cost-effectiveness was achieved, with respect to short-term costs and benefits, by diagnosing and treating solely on the basis of the POCT result. If positive complications were taken into account, then screening with POCT and confirmation of the positive results by the laboratory was recommended. Nerbrand et al. (49) evaluated the QuickVue In-Line One-Step Strep A test against a conventional culture method and found a sensitivity of 73.9% and a specificity of 86.8%. Kawakami et al. (50) also evaluated the Quidel assay and found it to be more sensitive than the Abbott Testpack assay; when compared with culture of 100 throat swabs they found a sensitivity of 94.4% and a specificity of 100%. They concluded, as did the previous investigators, that POCT is likely to play only a peripheral role in the diagnosis of Group A streptococci infection and its treatment.

The detection of *Helicobacter pylori* infection in patients presenting with dyspepsia using POCT has been reported in a number of studies. Jones et al. (51), using a POCT device, found that almost all of the patients that tested positive were treated with eradication therapy without any further intervention. However, Asante et al. (52) did not consider that such tests had the required accuracy compared with laboratory tests, a view also expressed by Duggan et al. (53) following an evaluation in primary care of a POCT antigen assay system. A systematic review (54) concluded that the sensitivity of a blood test varied between 77% and 92%, with specificity varying between 56% and 69%. In a more recent randomized controlled trial, however, Delaney et al. (55) found that use of POCT with open-access endoscopy for those patients with positive results did not lead to any improvement in clinical outcomes, and was more expensive, although more patients with peptic ulcer were diagnosed (7.4% vs. 2.1%, $P = 0.011$). It has been suggested that the urea breath test is the gold-standard technique for detection of *H. pylori* infection, and Opekun et al. (56) found that it was practical to use this technique in primary care and the results produced were reliable.

Chlamydia infection is associated with a number of serious complications, including ectopic pregnancy, pelvic inflammatory disease, and infertility—all of which may initially present in primary care. Hopwood et al. (57) assessed a POCT system (Clearview Chlamydia MF, Unipath, Bedford, UK) using endocervical swabs from women attending a pregnancy advisory service clinic. A total of 27 positive results were obtained, with 24 confirmed by the reference molecular technique, while 32 women tested positive by the molecular technique. The investigators concluded that POCT did not offer the required sensitivity, but it might be appropriate for optimal management in some cases where a quick result was needed (e.g., in the situation in which there was a risk that the patient may not return to receive the result, and any treatment offered). The case of screening for chlamydia infection is discussed later.

Cardiovascular Disease.   Mant et al. (58) recently reported on a systematic review and modeling of acute and chronic chest pain presenting in primary care. They report that there are no clinical features in isolation that rule in or rule out acute coronary syndromes, while the ST elevation was the most useful feature of the electrocardiogram (ECG) for identifying myocardial infarction (likelihood ratio 13.1), with a normal ECG ruling out a myocardial infarction (likelihood ratio 0.14). The observation was also made that POCT for troponins was cost-effective for triage of patients with suspected acute coronary syndrome. At present there are few data to substantiate this claim as far as studies in the primary care setting are concerned.

It has also been suggested that the measurement of the natriuretic peptides (BNP) may be of value in the screening of populations at risk of developing heart failure (59). The measurement may also be used for differential diagnosis of patients with dyspnea, fatigue, or peripheral edema—although this has not been rigorously tested in the primary care setting.

Chronic Disease Management

A number of studies have addressed the trend of chronic disease management in the primary care setting. Those that involve the use of POCT are discussed briefly in the following section.

Diabetes Mellitus.   A number of studies have investigated the benefits of diabetes care in the primary care setting. Griffin (60) undertook a systematic review and metaanalysis of the studies up to 1998, which attracted some criticism in relation to the robustness of the conclusions (61). When analyzing the data based on the use of the surrogate marker HbA1c, he found lower weighted mean differences consistent with a benefit associated with diabetes care in the primary care setting. When analyzing the morbidity and mortality indices, however, he could find no benefit. He concluded that unstructured follow-up was associated with poorer outcomes and that computerized recall systems could help patient management and this could lead to care that was equal to, or better, than that provided in the outpatient clinic. Renders et al. (62, 63) undertook a systematic review of trials evaluating interventions in the management of diabetes in primary care that confirmed the points made by Griffin (60). Hansen et al. (64) looked at the effect of encouraging regular follow-up of diabetic individuals over a 6-year period. They found that the indices of glycemic control initially improved but then fell in the later stages of the study. They concluded that active intervention on a continuing basis was essential to good diabetes management. Nocon et al. (65) described such an approach in a city in the United Kingdom. Williams et al. (66) studied the care of diabetes in the primary care setting in the United Kingdom and found that there was a considerable variation in the facilities available for specialist diabetes care. One example of active intervention is the use of a computerized database to monitor the processes and outcomes of diabetes care. Gegick et al. (67) demonstrated the use of such a system and showed improvements in HbA1c and lipid indices.

Few of the studies outlined earlier have included any mention of the role of POCT, and it is assumed that the primary care physician depends in most instances on the use of the individual patient's record of his or her blood glucose measurements, perhaps with the aid of stored data from the meter's memory. Furthermore, HbA1c results are requested at the time of the consultation, and the results are fed back to the patient at a later date. Alternative approaches are to ask the patient to attend a phlebotomy clinic the week before or to send a sample in to the laboratory using a specialized collection device (68). Data from secondary care studies show that the HbA1c result provided at the time of the clinic visit results in a significant fall in the HbA1c, presumably as a result of a more informed consultation with the physician or specialist nurse (69, 70). Miller et al. (71) demonstrated improved outcomes when using POCT for HbA1c in a rural primary care clinic. They showed greater intensification of therapy when the HbA1c reading was >7.0% at the baseline (51% compared to 32% of patients when no HbA1c result was available at the time of the clinic visit). The HbA1c result fell in the intervention group (8.4% to 8.1%, $P = 0.04$). Clearly it is best if the use of the POCT system (ideally), or at a minimum, the availability of the result, can be coordinated with the consultation process.

To date there does not appear to be any literature on the use of POCT systems for serum cholesterol, creatinine, and urine albumin excretion in the primary care diabetes setting, but it would seem reasonable to assume that, on the grounds of patient and diabetes specialist efficiency, it would be helpful to have all the results to hand so that decisions and counseling can be exercised promptly.

Anticoagulation Status. Anticoagulant management is based primarily on the measurement of prothrombin time (PT) as a surrogate marker of immediate coagulation status. The measurement is dogged by a number of issues surrounding the standardization of the PT assay, primarily as a result of the variation in the sensitivities of the reagents (see Chapter 41). To overcome this, the concept of an international normalized ratio (INR) was developed, and this has helped to reduce the interassay variability, which was originally a major problem for POCT systems. This is illustrated by the work of the European Concerted Action on Anticoagulation and one of the reports on the use of the INR with two POCT devices (72). Poller et al. (73) found that despite the use of the INR there was still significant variability at individual testing centers, which demonstrated the need for close links with the laboratory, and for participation in external quality assurance programs. Hobbs et al. (21) also found a similar experience when comparing performance between a number of laboratory and primary care centers. Poller et al. (73) also reported on experience with a quality assessment program. Shiach et al. (74) compared experience with POCT in primary care and laboratory testing in a crossover study design. The proportion of patients within the target range was 60.9% and 63.4% in two periods using POCT and 59.3% and 64.3% using a laboratory coagulometer for management. Patient questionnaires showed greater satisfaction with the community-based POCT monitoring program.

The importance of training of operators, whether healthcare professionals or patients, has been examined in a number of studies [e.g., Morsdorf et al. (75)], while Sawicki showed the value of a structured teaching and self-management program (76). Murray et al. (22) described experience with external quality assessment procedures in primary care in which patients were asked to analyze samples at home and under supervision in the health center. Health professionals also participated in the program. There was no significant difference in the median results on the quality assessment samples obtained by the patients and those obtained by professionals. In three instances patients obtained results that were outside of the consensus limits (results > 15% from the median INR) on

more than one occasion. The precision of the patient results in the program showed coefficients of variation ranging from 22.3% to as low as 5.4%. As the authors pointed out, there is a need to determine how this performance relates to clinical outcomes (e.g., time within normal INR range). Gill and Landis (77) described a mobile anticoagulation monitoring service where a nurse specialist traveled to a number of primary care centers. Education and testing were performed together with advice on changes in therapy. Over the period of the study (1 year) there was significant improvement in the percentage of in-range INRs (from 40.75% to 58.5%, $P < 0.001$).

In a series of papers Fitzmaurice et al. (78–80) described and then evaluated the use of a computerized decision support tool for anticoagulation management. They showed a significant improvement in INR control from 23% to 86% ($P < 0.001$) (78). When patients were randomly assigned to use the support tool or continue with conventional care, there was also a significant improvement in INR values ($P < 0.001$). The times between recall were extended using the support tool, and patient satisfaction was increased. The number of adverse outcomes was comparable between the support tool and conventional care groups. When a further randomized controlled trial of the computerized decision tool was undertaken (79), the investigators found that nurse-led anticoagulation clinics could be implemented in novice primary care settings with outcomes that were at least as good as those of hospital clinic-based care. They then went on to show that this approach was generally applicable to a wider community of practices outside of the research setting (80). Fitzmaurice et al. (81) also showed that patient self-management is equally as good as primary care management of oral anticoagulation. McCahon et al. (82) then reported on a larger multicenter study involving 49 general practices; they showed that the model of care for self-management could be extended beyond the unique environment of the earlier work, thereby overcoming earlier criticisms of selection bias and applicability to the UK health service. Poller et al. (83) and Manotti et al. (84) also evaluated the use of computerized decision support tools for monitoring anticoagulation treatment, and both showed that computer-aided management is at least as good as hospital-based specialist care.

All of these studies stress the basic tenets of good POCT, namely to ensure proper training of all operators, participation in quality control, and external quality assurance, as well as maintaining good links with the local laboratory professionals.

Hyperlipidemia. Several studies have evaluated the performance of POCT devices for cholesterol measurement (2). Although there have been no formal studies of POCT for cholesterol in the health center setting, a number of studies have investigated the role of the community pharmacist in providing POCT and advice on the results obtained. Thus Till et al. (85) demonstrated how a pharmacist took responsibility for ordering the tests and for advice on treatment changes. They showed a significant fall in low-density cholesterol levels compared with the clinical specialist management protocol (usual care) (18.5% vs. 6.5%, $P = 0.049$). The extent of the reduction was also directly associated with the number of pharmacy visits, compared with usual care. Mahtabjafari et al. (86) described their experience with POCT as part of a cholesterol education program that found, based on risk factor assessment and cholesterol measurement, that 50% of the attendees required intervention. Peterson et al. (87) undertook a randomized controlled study of a pharmacist home visit program that included POCT for cholesterol, as well as lifestyle guidance and assessment of compliance with therapy. There was a significant fall in the serum cholesterol over the 6 months of the study ($P < 0.005$), whereas there was no change in the control group who received standard medical care ($P = 0.26$). Nola et al. (88) reported on a study with a randomized pre-test–post-test control group design for screening individuals for hypercholesterolemia and entering them in a pharmacist-led lipid-lowering program. They found that 32% of the patients in the test group achieved their treatment goal, compared with only 13% in the control group. They also found that the patients' knowledge of hyperlipidemia increased significantly. Bluml et al. (89) reported on a study of 397 patients who were given lipid-lowering therapy and monitored in a community pharmacy setting. They found that a very high proportion of patients maintained their compliance, while 62.5% of the patients achieved their treatment goals over the period of the study.

Hypertension. Clearly the management of hypertension occurs to a large extent in the primary care sector. The role of POCT in this setting, however, is not clear. The technology to assess microalbuminuria by means of the albumin:creatinine ratio is now available, enabling the use of a spot urine test to screen the at-risk population (90). To date no studies have investigated the use of POCT with this group of patients.

Screening At-Risk Populations

There are a number of situations in which regular monitoring to enable the early identification of disease has been proposed and/or studied.

Chlamydia Infection. Pimenta et al. (91) investigated the feasibility of screening for genital chlamydia infection in a primary and secondary healthcare setting. They found the uptake was high in the two centers studied (67% and 84%), and that the relatively noninvasive use of a urine sample made it more acceptable. The same group had previously found that the POCT system based on immunoassay did not have the required sensitivity, so a molecular technique was used to establish a trial program. They found that the prevalence in women 16 to 24 years of age was ~9% in primary care, with a wider range in different locations (3.4–17.6%) (92). Earlier studies showed the cost-effectiveness of screening and treatment for chlamydia infection (93); thus, the option of using a more sensitive POCT technology might improve accessibility and ease of follow-up, especially in the primary care setting.

Diabetes Mellitus. There is increasing discussion over the merits of screening for type 2 diabetes as the prevalence of the disease continues to rise. Hirtzlin et al. (94) described a screening program in France, based on a fingerstick glucose measurement, and in so doing they identified some of the

problems associated with such a program. Pettitt et al. (95) described a school-based screening program for diabetes using Hba1c measurement on a fingerstick sample. Hoerger et al. (96) analyzed the cost-effectiveness of screening for type 2 diabetes and concluded that it was viable only if targeted at those people at risk, e.g., those with hypertension, and in those older than 55 years of age. Some community pharmacists are already offering blood glucose measurements as a screening test.

Hypercholesterolemia. Kanstrup et al. (97) showed, in a randomized prospective population-based study conducted over a period of 5 years, that the serum cholesterol levels were significantly lower in the intervention group compared with the control group, and that the decrease were most pronounced in those patients at greatest cardiovascular risk. This study used a laboratory for the biochemical measurements, but there is no reason why this cannot be undertaken using POCT.

Proteinuria. Guthrie and Lott (98), based on a study of urinalysis in a family practice, argued the case for regular dipstick monitoring for proteinuria in patients with diabetes and hypertension. Kissmeyer et al. (99), in an audit of case notes in 12 primary care practices, found a high prevalence of renal insufficiency in hypertensive and diabetic patients, using either plasma creatinine or proteinuria assessment, and advocated regular testing for proteinuria in this patient group in the primary care setting. The NKF-K/DOQI Clinical Guidelines (100) advocate testing for proteinuria in the at-risk population.

Craig et al. (101) undertook a feasibility study of whether mass screening for proteinuria would be worthwhile in the detection of early kidney disease using systematic review and meta-analysis methods. They found that in Australia about 1500 individuals developed ESRD each year, of whom two-thirds were >50 years of age (approximately 200 patients per million population per year). They found proteinuria to confer a 15-fold increased risk for ESRD, while the use of angiotensin-converting enzyme inhibitors (ACEIs) could reduce the risk of ESRD by about 30% over a 2- to 3-year period. The authors argued that with opportunistic at-risk testing, confirmation with a 24-h urine collection, and commencement of ACEIs in appropriate individuals, 20,000 individuals >50 years of age would need to be tested to prevent 1 case of ESRD, 100 people would be treated with drugs, and 1000 people would need the confirmatory urine test—of which 700 results would be false positives. It was concluded that this approach would save health resources, although some important unanswered questions remained, and a trial would be required to prove the model. Issues such as the effect of drug therapy on those people who tested positive remained unanswered, as did the effect of the testing on the individuals. The authors also felt that the use of a protein:creatinine or albumin:creatinine ratio test would improve the results of the study.

Boulware et al. (102) undertook a cost-effectiveness analysis using Markov decision analytical modeling to compare a strategy of annual screening with no screening (usual care) for proteinuria at 50 years of age, followed by treatment with an ACEI or an angiotensin II receptor blocker. They found that for individuals with neither hypertension nor diabetes, the cost-effectiveness ratio for screening versus no screening (usual care) was unfavorable. However, selective testing of such individuals beginning at 60 years of age yielded a more favorable ratio. For patients with hypertension, the ratio was highly favorable (~\$282,000 vs. \$53,000 vs. \$19,000 per quality adjusted life year, respectively, which equated to an improvement from 0.0022 to 0.03 quality-adjusted life years per person). The authors concluded that broad testing for early detection of urine protein in order to slow progression of chronic kidney disease and decrease mortality was not cost-effective unless selectively directed toward high-risk groups (older adults and patients with hypertension) or conducted at an infrequent interval of 10 years.

Garg et al. (103) studied the prevalence of albuminuria and renal insufficiency (as judged by serum creatinine) in the population covered by the Third National Health and Nutrition Examination Survey (NHANES III). They found that it would be necessary to test three individuals with diabetes, seven nondiabetic hypertensive individuals, or six individuals >60 years of age to identify one case of albuminuria. They also noted that about a third of the individuals with a reduced glomerular filtration rate (calculated at <30 mL $\cdot$ min^{-1} $\cdot$ 1.73 m^{-2}) showed no albuminuria. More than 8.0% of the study population had microalbuminuria, and 1.0% had macroalbuminuria.

It was anticipated in all of these studies that the testing would be undertaken using POCT systems with confirmation by the laboratory.

CONCLUSIONS

There is now a considerable body of literature that indicates the potential use of POCT in the primary care setting, although the literature is often of poor quality. There is clear evidence from other studies that there is a need for such testing in order to improve outcomes. Some of the observations made to date are speculative, but they indicate where changes may occur in the way that diagnostic testing is delivered. In addition, there is a strong body of opinion among policymakers and health planners that more care should be provided in the primary care setting. Against this background it is important to ensure that proper outcomes studies are performed to demonstrate the situations in which POCT could be of real value; many pointers are given in the literature cited in this chapter. Delaney et al. (104) have discussed the standards that are required for the evaluation of POCT in the primary care arena.

It will remain important to identify the decision that will be made on receipt of the POCT result, and the action that will then be taken. It will also be important to be open to the need to change practices in order to reap the full benefit. This is probably the most crucial issue in relation to the beneficial implementation of POCT.

REFERENCES

1. Rivett G. From cradle to grave; fifty years of the NHS. London: King's Fund Publishing, 1997;506.

2. Hobbs FDR. Point-of-care testing in primary care. In: Price CP, Hicks JM, eds. Point-of-care testing. Washington, DC: AACC Press, 1999,289–317.

3. Hobbs FD, Delaney BC, Fitzmaurice DA, Wilson S, Hyde CJ, Thorpe GH, et al. A review of near patient testing in primary care. Health Technol Assess 1997;1:1–230.

4. Wilson S, Delaney BC, Roalfe A, Roberts L, Redman V, Wearn AM, Hobbs FD. Randomised controlled trials in primary care: case study. Br Med J 2000;321:24–7.

5. Myers P. Primary care. In: Hooper J, McGreanor G, Marshall W, Myers P, eds. Primary care and laboratory medicine. London: ACB Venture, 1996:1–15.

6. NHS Direct Self-Help Guide. http://www.nhsdirect.nhs.uk/Self-Help/index.asp (accessed June 1, 2004).

7. Turner VF, Bentley PJ, Hodgson SA, Collard PJ, Drimatis R, Rabune C, Wilson AJ. Telephone triage in Western Australia. Med J Aust 2002;176:100–3.

8. Seddon ME, Marshall MN, Campbell SM, Roland MO. Systematic review of studies of quality of clinical care in general practice in the UK, Australia and New Zealand. Qual Health Care 2001;10:152–8.

9. Worrall G, Chaulk P, Freake D. The effects of clinical practice guidelines on patient outcomes in primary care: a systematic review. CMAJ 1997;156:1705–12.

10. Engstrom S, Foldevi M, Borgquist L. Is general practice effective? A systematic literature review. Scand J Prim Health Care 2001;19:131–44.

11. Harrington J, Noble LM. Newman SP. Improving patients' communication with doctors: a systematic review of intervention studies. Patient Educ Couns 2004;52:7–16.

12. Wilson A, Childs S. The relationship between consultation length, process and outcomes in general practice: a systematic review. Br J Gen Pract 2002;52:1012–20.

13. Thiru K, Hassey A, Sullivan F. Systematic review of scope and quality of electronic patient record data in primary care. Br Med J 2003;326:1070.

14. Sox HC Jr. Quality of patient care by nurse practitioners and physician's assistants: a ten-year perspective. Ann Intern Med 1979;91:459–68.

15. Department of Health. Making a difference: strengthening the nursing, midwifery and health visitor contribution to health and health care. London: Department of Health, 1999.

16. Murdock A. The consultant pharmacist and pharmacist technician in primary care. In: Lissauer R and Kendall L, eds. New practitioners in the future health service. London: IPPR, 2002: 13–20.

17. Horrocks S, Anderson E. Salisbury C. Systematic review of whether nurse practitioners working in primary care can provide equivalent care to doctors. Br Med J 2002;324:819–23.

18. Gutierres SL, Welty TE. Point-of-care testing: an introduction. Ann Pharmacother 2004;38:119–25.

19. Nichols JH, Kickler TS, Dyer KL, Humbertson SK, Cooper PC, Maughan WL, Oechsle DG. Clinical outcomes of point-of-care testing in the interventional radiology and invasive cardiology setting. Clin Chem 2000;46:543–50.

20. British Medical Association. Quality and outcomes framework guidance. Investing in general practice. The new General Medical Services contract. Annex A: Quality indicators—summary of points. http://www.bma.org.uk/ap.nsf/Content/NewGMS-Contract/\$file/gpcontractannexa.pdf. (accessed June 1, 2004).

21. Hobbs FD, Fitzmaurice DA, Murray ET, Holder R, Rose PE, Roper R. Is the international normalised ratio (INR) reliable? A trial of comparative measurements in hospital laboratory and primary care settings. J Clin Pathol 1999;52:494–7.

22. Murray ET, Kitchen DP, Kitchen S, Jennings I, Woods TA, Preston FE, Fitzmaurice DA. Patient self-management of oral anticoagulation and external quality assessment procedures. Br J Haematol 2003;122:825–8.

23. Rink E, Hilton S, Szczepura A, Fletcher J, Sibbald B, Davies C, et al. Impact of introducing near patient testing for standard investigations in general practice. Br Med J 1993;307:775–8.

24. Gillam S, Freedman D, Naughton B, Ridgwell P, Singer P. An evaluation of near patient testing in general practice. J Eval Clin Pract 1998;4:165–9.

25. Boyde AM, Earl R, Fardell S, Yeo N, Burrin JM, Price CP. Lessons for the laboratory from a general practitioner survey. J Clin Pathol 1997;50:283–7.

26. van Wijk MA, van der Lei J, Mosseveld M, Bohnen AM, van Bemmel JH. Compliance of general practitioners with a guideline-based decision support system for ordering blood tests. Clin Chem 2002;48:55–60.

27. van Wijk MA, van der Lei J, Mosseveld M, Bohnen AM, van Bemmel JH. Assessment of decision support for blood test ordering in primary care. A randomized trial. Ann Intern Med 2001;134:274–81.

28. van Wijk MA, Bohnen AM, van der Lei J. Analysis of the practice guidelines of the Dutch College of General Practitioners with respect to the use of blood tests. J Am Med Inform Assoc 1999;6:322–31.

29. Takemura Y, Ishida H, Inoue Y, Beck JR. Yield and cost of individual common diagnostic tests in new primary care outpatients in Japan. Clin Chem 2002;48:42–54.

30. Takemura Y, Ishida H, Inoue Y, Beck JR. Common diagnostic test panels for clinical evaluation of new primary care outpatients in Japan: a cost-effectiveness evaluation. Clin Chem 1999;45:1752–61.

31. Takemura Y, Ishida H, Inoue Y, Kobayashi H, Beck JR. Opportunistic discovery of occult disease by use of test panels in new, symptomatic primary care outpatients: yield and cost of case finding. Clin Chem 2000;46:1091–8.

32. Price CP, Christenson RH, eds. Evidence-based laboratory medicine. From principles to outcomes. Washington, DC: AACC Press, 2003:1–279.

33. Point-of-care testing trial general information and updates. http://www.health.gov.au/pathology/poctt/info.htm (accessed June 1, 2004).

34. Ditchburn RK, Ditchburn JS. A study of microscopical and chemical tests for the rapid diagnosis of urinary tract infections in general practice. Br J Gen Pract 1990;40:406–8.

35. Winkens RAG, Leffers P, Trienekens TAM, Stobberingh EE. The validity of urine examination for urinary tract infections in daily practice. Fam Pract 1995;12:290–3.

36. Pugia MJ, Lott JA, Luke KE, Shihabi ZK, Wians FH Jr, Phillips L. Comparison of instrument-read dipsticks for albumin and creatinine in urine with visual results and quantitative methods. J Clin Lab Anal 1998;12:280–4.

37. McNulty C, Freeman E, Nichols T, Kalima P. Laboratory diagnosis of urinary symptoms in primary care—a qualitative study. Commun Dis Publ Health 2003;6:44–50.

38. Hobbs FD, Kenkre JE, Carter YH, Thorpe GH, Holder RL. Reliability and feasibility of a near patient test for C-reactive protein in primary care. Br J Gen Pract 1996;46:395–400.

39. Seamark DA, Backhouse SN, Powell R. Field-testing and validation in a primary care setting of a point-of-care test for C-reactive protein. Ann Clin Biochem 2003;40:178–80.

40. Dahler-Eriksen BS, Lauritzen T, Lassen JF, Lund ED, Brandslund I. Near-patient test for C-reactive protein in general practice: assessment of clinical, organizational, and economic outcomes. Clin Chem 1999;45:478–85.

41. Hjortdahl P, Landaas S, Urdal P, Steinbakk M, Fuglerud P, Nygaard B. C-reactive protein: a new rapid assay for managing infectious disease in primary health care. Scand J Prim Health Care 1991;9:3–10.

42. Gulich MS, Matschiner A, Gluck R, Zeitler HP. Improving diagnostic accuracy of bacterial pharyngitis by near patient measurement of C-reactive protein (CRP) Br J Gen Pract 1999;49:119–21.

43. Takemura Y, Kakoi H, Ishida H, Kure H, Tatsuguchi-Harada Y, Sugawara M, et al. Immediate availability of C-reactive protein and leukocyte count data influenced physicians' decisions to prescribe antimicrobial drugs for new outpatients with acute infections. Clin Chem 2004;50:241–4.

44. Rodriguez WJ, Schwartz RH, Thorne MM. Evaluation of diagnostic tests for influenza in a pediatric practice. Pediatr Infect Dis J 2002;21:193–6.

45. Harnden A, Brueggemann A, Shepperd S, White J, Hayward AC, Zambon M, et al. Near patient testing for influenza in children in primary care: comparison with laboratory test. Br Med J 2003;326:480.

46. Pregliasco F, Puzelli S, Mensi C, Anselmi G, Marinello R, Tanzi ML, et al. Influenza virological surveillance in children: the use of the QuickVue rapid diagnostic test. J Med Virol 2004;73:269–73.

47. Burke P, Bain J, Lowes A, Athersuch R. Rational decisions in managing sore throat: evaluation of a rapid test. Br Med J (Clin Res Ed), 1988;296:1646–9.

48. Carey RD, Tilyard MW, Morris RW. Evaluation of a rapid diagnostic test for group A beta-haemolytic streptococcus in general practice. N Z Med J 1991;104:401–3.

49. Nerbrand C, Jasir A, Schalen C. Are current rapid detection tests for Group A Streptococci sensitive enough? Evaluation of 2 commercial kits. Scand J Infect Dis 2002;34:797–9.

50. Kawakami S, Ono Y, Yanagawa Y, Miyazawa Y. Basic and clinical evaluation of the new rapid diagnostic kit for detecting group A streptococci with the immunochromatographical method. Rinsho Biseibutshu Jinsoku Shindan Kenkyukai Shi 2003;14:9–16.

51. Jones R, Phillips I, Felix G, Tait C. An evaluation of near-patient testing for *Helicobacter pylori* in general practice. Aliment Pharmacol Ther 1997;11:101–5.

52. Asante MA, Mendall MA, Finlayson C, Ballam L, Northfield T. Screening dyspeptic patients for *Helicobacter pylori* prior to endoscopy: laboratory or near-patient testing? Eur J Gastroenterol Hepatol 1998;10:843–6.

53. Duggan AE, Elliott C, Logan RF. Testing for *Helicobacter pylori* infection: validation and diagnostic yield of a near patient test in primary care. Br Med J 1999;319:1236–9.

54. Roberts AP, Childs SM, Rubin G, de Wit NJ. Tests for *Helicobacter pylori*: a critical appraisal from primary care. Fam Pract 2000;17:S12–20.

55. Delaney BC, Wilson S, Roalfe A, Roberts L, Redman V, Wearn A, Hobbs FD. Randomised controlled trial of *Helicobacter pylori* testing and endoscopy for dyspepsia in primary care. Br Med J 2001;322:898–901.

56. Opekun AR, Abdalla N, Sutton FM, Hammoud F, Kuo GM, Torres E, et al. Urea breath testing and analysis in the primary care office. J Fam Pract 2002;51:1030–2.

57. Hopwood J, Mallinson H, Gleave T. Evaluation of near patient testing for *Chlamydia trachomatis* in a pregnancy termination service. J Fam Plann Reprod Health Care 2001;27:127–30.

58. Mant J, McManus RJ, Oakes RA, Delaney BC, Barton PM, Deeks JJ, et al. Systematic review and modelling of the investigation of acute and chronic chest pain presenting in primary care. Health Technol Assess 2004;8(3):1–158.

59. Cowie MR, Jourdain P, Maisel A, Dahlstrom U, Follath F, Isnard R, et al. Clinical applications of B-type natriuretic peptide (BNP) testing. Eur Heart J 2003;24:1710–8.

60. Griffin S. Diabetes care in general practice: meta-analysis of randomised controlled trials. Br Med J 1998;317:390–6.

61. Greenhalgh T. Commentary: meta-analysis is a blunt and potentially misleading instrument for analysing models of delivery of care. Br Med J 1998;317:395–6.

62. Renders CM, Valk GD, Griffin SJ, Wagner EH, Eijk Van JT, Assendelft WJ. Interventions to improve the management of diabetes in primary care, outpatient, and community settings: a systematic review. Diabetes Care 2001;24:1821–33.

63. Renders CM, Valk GD, Griffin S, Wagner EH, Eijk JT, Assendelft WJ. Interventions to improve the management of diabetes mellitus in primary care, outpatient and community settings. Cochrane Database Syst Rev 2001;(1):CD001481.

64. Hansen LJ, Olivarius Nde F, Siersma V, Beck-Nielsen H, Pedersen PA. Encouraging structured personalised diabetes care in general practice. A 6-year follow-up study of process and patient outcomes in newly diagnosed patients. Scand J Prim Health Care 2003;21:89–95.

65. Nocon A, Rhodes PJ, Wright JP, Eastham J, Williams DR, Harrison SR, Young RJ. Specialist general practitioners and diabetes clinics in primary care: a qualitative and descriptive evaluation. Diabet Med 2004;21:32–8.

66. Williams DR, Baxter HS, Airey CM, Ali S, Turner B. Diabetes UK funded surveys of the structural provision of primary care diabetes services in the UK. Diabet Med 2002;19(Suppl 4):21–6.

67. Gegick CG, Altheimer MD, Kissling GE. Benefits of computerized outcome analysis in diabetes management. Endocr Pract 2000;6:253–9.

68. Holman RR, Jelfs R, Causier PM, Moore JC, Turner RC. Glycosylated haemoglobin measurement on blood samples taken by patients: an additional aid to assessing diabetic control. Diabet Med 1987;4:71–3.

69. Cagliero E, Levina E, Nathan D. Immediate feedback of HbA1c levels improves glycemic control in type 1 and insulin-treated type 2 diabetic patients. Diabetes Care 1999;22:1785–9.

70. Grieve R, Beech R, Vincent J, Mazurkiewicz J. Near patient testing in diabetes clinics: appraising the costs and outcomes. Health Technol Assess 1999;3:1–74.

71. Miller CD, Barnes CS, Phillips LS, Ziemer DC, Gallina DL, Cook CB, et al. Rapid A1c availability improves clinical decision-making in an urban primary care clinic. Diabetes Care 2003;26:1158–63.

72. Poller L, Keown M, Chauhan N, Van Den Besselaar AM, Tripodi A, Shiach C, Jespersen J, ECCA Steering Group Members. European concerted action on anticoagulation. Correction of displayed international normalized ratio on two point-of-care test whole-blood prothrombin time monitors (CoaguChek Mini and TAS PT-NC) by independent international sensitivity index calibration. Br J Haematol 2003;122:944–9.

73. Poller L, Keown M, Chauhan N, van den Besselaar AM, Tripodi A, Shiach C, Jespersen J. European concerted action on anticoagulation. Quality assessment of the CoaguChek Mini and TAS PT-NC point-of-care whole-blood prothrombin time monitors. Clin Chem 2004;50:537–44.

74. Shiach CR, Campbell B, Poller L, Keown M, Chauhan N. Reliability of point-of-care prothrombin time testing in a community clinic: a randomized crossover comparison with hospital laboratory testing. Br J Haematol 2002;119:370–5.

75. Morsdorf S, Erdlenbruch W, Taborski U, Schenk JF, Erdlenbruch K, Novotny-Reichert G, et al. Training of patients for self-management of oral anticoagulant therapy: standards, patient suitability, and clinical aspects. Semin Thromb Hemost 1999;25:109–15.

76. Sawicki PT. A structured teaching and self-management program for patients receiving oral anticoagulation: a randomized controlled trial. Working Group for the Study of Patient Self-Management of Oral Anticoagulation. JAMA 1999;281:145–50.

77. Gill JM, Landis MK. Benefits of a mobile, point-of-care anticoagulation therapy management program. Jt Comm J Qual Improv 2002;28:625–30.

78. Fitzmaurice DA, Hobbs FD, Murray ET, Bradley CP, Holder R. Evaluation of computerized decision support for oral anticoagulation management based in primary care. Br J Gen Pract 1996;46:533–5.

79. Fitzmaurice DA, Hobbs FD, Murray ET, Holder RL, Allan TF, Rose PE. Oral anticoagulation management in primary care with the use of computerized decision support and near-patient testing: a randomized, controlled trial. Arch Intern Med 2000;160:2343–8.

80. Fitzmaurice DA, Murray ET, Gee KM, Allan TF. Does the Birmingham model of oral anticoagulation management in primary care work outside trial conditions? Br J Gen Pract 2001;51:828–9.

81. Fitzmaurice DA, Murray ET, Gee KM, Allan TF, Hobbs FD. A randomised controlled trial of patient self management of oral anticoagulation treatment compared with primary care management. J Clin Pathol 2002;55:845–9.

82. McCahon D, Fitzmaurice DA, Murray ET, Fuller CJ, Hobbs RF, Allan TF, Raftery JP. SMART: self-management of anticoagulation, a randomised trial [ISRCTN19313375]. BMC Fam Pract 2003;4:11.

83. Poller L, Shiach CR, MacCallum PK, Johansen AM, Munster AM, et al. Multicentre randomised study of computerised anticoagulant dosage. European concerted action on anticoagulation. Lancet 1998;352:1505–9.

84. Manotti C, Moia M, Palareti G, Pengo V, Ria L, Dettori AG. Effect of computer-aided management on the quality of treatment in anticoagulated patients: a prospective, randomized, multicenter trial of APROAT (Automated Program for Oral Anticoagulant Treatment). Haematologica 2001;86:1060–70.

85. Till LT, Voris JC, Horst JB. Assessment of clinical pharmacist management of lipid-lowering therapy in a primary care setting. J Manag Care Pharm 2003;9:269–73.

86. Mahtabjafari M, Masih M, Emerson AE. The value of pharmacist involvement in a point-of-care service, walk-in lipid screening program. Pharmacotherapy 2001;21:1403–6.

87. Peterson GM, Fitzmaurice KD, Naunton M, Vial JH, Stewart K, Krum H. Impact of pharmacist-conducted home visits on the outcomes of lipid-lowering drug therapy. J Clin Pharm Ther 2004;29:23–30.

88. Nola KM, Gourley DR, Portner TS, Gourley GK, Solomon DK, Elam M, Regal B. Clinical and humanistic outcomes of a lipid management programme in the community pharmacy setting. J Am Pharm Assoc 2000;40:166–73.

89. Bluml BM, McKenney JM, Cziraky MJ. Pharmaceutical care services and results in project ImPACT: hyperlipidemia. J Am Pharm Assoc 2000;40:57–65.

90. Claudi T, Cooper JG. Comparison of urinary albumin excretion rate in overnight urine and albumin creatinine ratio in spot urine in diabetic patients in general practice. Scand J Prim Health Care 2001;19:247–8.

91. Pimenta JM, Catchpole M, Rogers PA, Hopwood J, Randall S, Mallinson H, et al. Opportunistic screening for genital chlamydial infection. II: prevalence among healthcare attenders, outcome, and evaluation of positive cases. Sex Transm Infect 2003;79:22–7.

92. Pimenta JM, Catchpole M, Rogers PA, Perkins E, Jackson N, Carlisle C, et al. Opportunistic screening for genital chlamydial infection. I: acceptability of urine testing in primary and secondary healthcare settings. Sex Transm Infect 2003;79:16–21.

93. Howell MR, Quinn TC, Brathwaite W, Gaydos CA. Screening women for Chlamydia trachomatis in family planning clinics: the cost-effectiveness of DNA amplification assays. Sex Transm Dis 1998;25:108–17.

94. Hirtzlin I, Fagot-Campagna A, Girard-Le Gallo I, Vallier N, Poutignat N, Weill A, Le Laidier S. Screening for diabetes in France: data from the 2000–2001 Cohort of the national medical insurance system. Rev Epidemiol Sante Publique 2003;52:119–26.

95. Pettitt DJ, Giammattei J, Wollitzer AO, Jovanovic L. Glycohemoglobin (A1C) distribution in school children: results from a school-based screening program. Diabetes Res Clin Pract 2004;65:45–9.

96. Hoerger TJ, Harris R, Hicks KA, Donahue K, Sorensen S, Engelgau M. Screening for type 2 diabetes mellitus: a cost-effectiveness analysis. Ann Intern Med 2004;140:689–99.

97. Kanstrup H, Refsgaard J, Engberg M, Lassen JF, Larsen ML, Lauritzen T. Cholesterol reduction following health screening in general practice. Scand J Prim Health Care 2002;20:219–23.

98. Guthrie RM, Lott JA. Screening for proteinuria in patients with hypertension or diabetes mellitus. J Fam Pract 1993;37:253–6.

99. Kissmeyer L, Kong C, Cohen J, Unwin RJ, Woolfson RG, Neild GH. Community nephrology: audit of screening for renal insufficiency in a high risk population. Nephrol Dial Transplant 1999;14:2150–5.

100. National Kidney Foundation. K/DOQI clinical practice guidelines for chronic kidney disease: evaluation, classification and stratification. Am J Kidney Dis 2002;39(Suppl 1):S1–S266.

101. Craig JC, Barratt A, Cumming R, Irwig L, Salkeld G. Feasibility study of the early detection and treatment of renal disease by mass screening. Intern Med J 2002;32:6–14.

102. Boulware LE, Jaar BG, Tarver-Carr ME, Brancati FL, Powe NR. Screening for proteinuria in US adults: a cost-effectiveness analysis. JAMA 2003;290:3101–14.

103. Garg AX, Kiberd BA, Clark WF, Haynes RB, Clase CM. Albuminuria and renal insufficiency prevalence guides population screening: results from the NHANES III. Kidney Int 2002;61:2165–75.

104. Delaney B, Wilson S, Fitzmaurice D, Hyde C, Hobbs R. Near-patient tests in primary care: setting the standards for evaluation. J Health Serv Res Policy 2000;5:37–41.

Chapter **29**

Point-of-Care Testing in the Indigenous Rural Environment—The Australian Experience

Mark D. S. Shephard

The characteristics of rural health and the issues driving the delivery of healthcare services to the rural environment are very different from those of metropolitan centers. Geographical isolation and its effect on access to health services is the defining element of rural health (1). In addition, the differing social, lifestyle, and environmental determinants of health in the rural population, including a greater degree of cultural diversity; lack of employment opportunities; lower income levels; and poorer access to housing, education, and transport, significantly influence the mode of healthcare delivery, health status, and patterns of disease (2). Overall, the rural sector experiences higher mortality rates and poorer health status than metropolitan regions, a trend that becomes more apparent with increasing remoteness (3). Prevalence rates for both acute and chronic conditions and communicable and noncommunicable diseases are generally higher in rural than in metropolitan environments, and greatest in remote regions (4).

The challenge of reducing the health differential between rural and metropolitan environments lies with the development of inventive solutions to specific local health problems (1). The astute and practical application of point-of-care testing (POCT) can unquestionably be one of those inventive solutions in the broader context of improving rural healthcare delivery—in both the acute and chronic clinical context.

POINT-OF-CARE TESTING IN THE RURAL HEALTH ENVIRONMENT

A recent review of the role and value of POCT in general practice in Australia concluded that rural and remote health practices in particular could be major beneficiaries from the adoption of POCT (5).

There are a number of clinical conditions for which POCT represents a practical and viable option for the rural health practitioner. For acute trauma and/or emergency surgery where retrieval may be necessary, POCT for tests such as potassium and blood gases are of particular clinical relevance. Point-of-care (POC) measurement of cardiac markers such as the troponins, heart fatty acid binding protein, and ischemic modified albumin can provide important information in the differential diagnosis of chest pain and subsequent early initiation of thrombolytic treatment. Timely POC international normalized ratio (INR) monitoring is important in preventing thrombosis and avoiding excessive bleeding during surgical procedures. INR is also of use in monitoring of Coumadin® (warfarin) therapy.

There are several examples of innovative and effective rural hospital-based POCT models for some of these acute care tests being used in Australia. Queensland Health Pathology Service has developed an integrated state-wide network of approximately 50 rural and remote hospital sites that are all using the i-STAT® analyzer (i-STAT, East Windsor, NJ, USA) for onsite measurement of electrolytes and blood gases. All patient results and quality control data are captured following analysis and sent to a central data station, located at the Prince Charles Hospital in Brisbane, via a network downloader. Results with correct patient data entry are then forwarded to the hospital's laboratory information system (6).

In South Australia, the *iCARnet* group (Integrated Cardiac Assessment Regional Network) was established in 2001 to support rural general practitioners in the delivery of up-to-date evidence-based management of patients presenting with chest pain, or other symptoms suggestive of acute coronary syndrome. The network provides POC Troponin T testing using a cardiac reader (Roche Diagnostics, Mannheim, Germany), evidence-based triage, risk stratification and management guidelines, and 24-h on-call cardiologists (7).

In addition, many POC tests for the management and/or risk assessment of patients with chronic illnesses are being used in the rural environment. Hemoglobin A1c (HbA1c), glucose, and urine microalbumin or albumin:creatinine ratio (ACR) are key tests for the management of patients with diabetes that can be performed at the point of care (8, 9). Urine ACR is also a particularly useful test in the detection of early renal disease (8), and blood urea and creatinine can be monitored for the management of established renal disease. Blood lipids can be conveniently measured by POC technology as part of heart disease risk assessment and management (10), while urine ACR has also been shown to predict cardiovascular risk (11, 12). Whole blood hemoglobin can be measured at the point of care for assessment of anemia status, which may be of significant clinical benefit because anemia is very prevalent in rural tropical environments, particularly among indigenous women and young children (13, 14). There are now many POC tests for tumor makers such as prostate-specific antigen (PSA) and carcinoembryonic antigen. Working POCT models for some of these chronic disease tests are described later.

INDIGENOUS RURAL HEALTH ENVIRONMENT IN AUSTRALIA

Nowhere is the health differential between rural and metropolitan environments more profound than for indigenous peoples living in rural and remote regions. Regardless of which health indicator is used, the health status of Aboriginal people in Australia is worse than that of non-Aboriginal people (15, 16). The chronic diseases—diabetes, renal disease, and cardiovascular disease—typify the health disadvantage of Aboriginal people and collectively pose one of the most significant health issues for contemporary Australian Aboriginal society. For example, Aboriginal people suffer between 12 and 17 times more deaths attributable to non–insulin-dependent diabetes (NIDDM) than nonindigenous Australians. Overall prevalence rates of diabetes are generally within the range of 10% to 30%, and at least two to four times that of the non-Aboriginal population (16, 17). In some communities, nearly half of the entire adult indigenous population has diabetes.

During the 1990s there was a rapid escalation in the number of Aboriginal Australians with end-stage renal disease. Recent age- and sex-adjusted figures indicate Aboriginal people have ~9 times greater risk of developing end-stage renal disease than all other Australians. In some parts of Australia, notably the Tiwi Islands, rates of renal disease are among the highest in the world (18–21). In the Northern Territory, Aboriginal people comprise just over 20% of the population, but represent 95% of people on hemodialysis (22). Cardiovascular disease is the leading cause of mortality in Aboriginal Australians, with mortality rates attributable to coronary heart disease and stroke being twice those of non-Aboriginal Australians (23, 24). Of particular concern are the high death rates from coronary heart disease among young and middle-aged Aboriginal people, with death rates for people 25 to 44 years of age being more than 10 times those of other Australians (23). The extremely high rates of chronic disease among indigenous Australians are caused by a multitude of interrelated factors such as dispossession from their land, destruction of traditional culture and values, exposure to infectious diseases, poor environmental living conditions, and the effects of alcohol and Western diets that are high in fat and sugar.

These appalling statistics on chronic disease are not unique to Australian Aboriginal communities and are mirrored in many other indigenous populations living in rural parts of the world (25). For the Australian indigenous rural community, there is clearly an urgent clinical need to provide effective services for the monitoring of diabetes control to prevent the long-term complications of this debilitating condition. There is also a need to stem the tide of end-stage renal disease by developing community-controlled risk assessment programs for the early detection of this disease. Given that heart disease is the major cause of Aboriginal mortality, the need to characterize cardiovascular risk profiles, particularly among young Aboriginal people, is also of immediate concern. POCT can have a significant role in fulfilling each of these needs, but in this environment implementation and sustainability of POCT faces major challenges.

AUSTRALIAN ABORIGINAL MEDICAL SERVICE

Aboriginal medical services in Australia are either managed and controlled by local Aboriginal people with funding by the Commonwealth or state governments, or they are controlled and funded by state or territory governments. Aboriginal Community Controlled Health Services (ACCHSs) now represent the principal vehicle for delivering primary healthcare to Aboriginal and Torres Strait Islander peoples. There are more than 125 ACCHSs throughout Australia, more than 90% of which are located in rural and remote areas. A peak body called the National Aboriginal Community Controlled Health Organisation (NACCHO) represents the interests and affairs of ACCHSs nationally.

ACCHSs vary considerably in size, infrastructure, resources, and the number of Aboriginal people they service. Many are located several hundred, up to a thousand kilometers, from the nearest hospital or laboratory service. Staffing levels also vary widely, but most services generally have a medical doctor, a clinic nurse, and one or more Aboriginal health workers. The Aboriginal health worker is an Aboriginal person who lives and works in the local community and who has attained a primary healthcare qualification. The health worker provides the pivotal communication link between the community and non-Aboriginal professional staff at the health service.

POTENTIAL BENEFITS AND CHALLENGES OF POCT IN THE INDIGENOUS RURAL ENVIRONMENT

The most significant barrier to effective clinical services in rural and remote Aboriginal communities is limited access to pathology laboratories. As stated above, Aboriginal health services may be several hundred, even thousands, of kilometers from the nearest pathology service, and it may take up to several days for blood samples to reach that service, particularly if air transport is limited or unavailable. The return of results to the community and then to the individual patient incurs further delays. Conventional means of delivery of pathology services are time consuming and of less relevance to the patient, while clinical management is delayed. POCT services overcome these problems of "disadvantage by distance" and do not incur the additional costs associated with transport of pathology samples. Furthermore, distance, in either a temporal or geographical context, can also be associated with poor compliance, e.g., with reattendance at clinics, follow-up of results, and treatment changes. The benefits of POCT in relation to improved compliance have been demonstrated for diabetes and anticoagulation therapy in other communities (see Chapters 31 and 41).

POCT has other advantages specific to the Aboriginal healthcare setting. Through appropriate training, Aboriginal health workers can perform POCT, thereby empowering them to take greater responsibility for the health of their own community members. Immediate availability of results provides a more convenient and timely service for the patient. It also means that the Aboriginal patient does not have to come back for a follow-up visit, which may often be very difficult to organize in the Aboriginal community setting because other social and cultural priorities sometimes take precedence over health matters. By conducting the tests onsite, ownership and control of health information remains with the community, a factor crucial to the acceptance and success of indigenous health programs worldwide.

The challenges faced in providing an effective POCT service in the indigenous rural environment are considerable. Many rural Aboriginal medical services experience difficult working conditions such as dust, excessive heat and/or humidity, power fluctuations, and inadequate lighting and refrigerator space. High rates of staff turnover are a constant problem in many services, making health programs (including POCT services) difficult to sustain. This applies not only to administrative and clinical staff where health service priorities may change with new appointments, but also at the Aboriginal health worker level—the person generally responsible for daily operation and maintenance of POCT. POCT services need to be robust in the face of such change and, as described later, the ongoing delivery of education, training, and support services is critical for sustainability.

Specifically in relation to education and training, there is a real challenge for the non-Aboriginal health professional to translate complex scientific, medical, or laboratory concepts into culturally appropriate images that can be readily understood by an Aboriginal health worker team. This translation is even more important given that the transfer of information in Aboriginal culture is based on the spoken word and visual images. Highly visual laminated posters with simple step-by-step instructions showing how to perform POCT and how to conduct quality assurance testing procedures that consolidate detailed information into a practical, workable format have proven useful in our hands.

EFFECTIVE AND SUSTAINABLE POCT MODELS IN THE INDIGENOUS RURAL ENVIRONMENT

Three health models utilizing POCT for chronic disease prevention and management, which have proven successful in the rural Australian Aboriginal environment, are now described. They are the Umoona Kidney Project, the national Quality Assurance for Aboriginal Medical Services (QAAMS) Program for POC HbA1c testing, and the Point-of-Care in Aboriginal Hands Program (26). Each model is based on four fundamental elements: continuing education, training, quality management, and ongoing support for POCT. It is important to reemphasize that these models function outside the comfort zone of the hospital base, with the Aboriginal community and their associated health service driving the model (not the lab-

oratory). The POCT challenge has been to develop quality-assured, robust, sustainable, and clinically effective models for the community setting. Each model is discussed in turn under common themes of background, chronic disease focus, POCT instrumentation and markers used, principal activities and results, evaluation, sustainability, and transferability.

Umoona Kidney Project

The Umoona Kidney Project was a partnership between the Umoona Aboriginal community at Coober Pedy in South Australia's far north (850 km from Adelaide) and the Renal Units at Flinders Medical Centre and Women's and Children's Hospital, Adelaide, South Australia (27–31). The program involved a number of people and health professional groups. From the Umoona community, the board, the director, the clinical nurse, four Aboriginal health workers, and community members participated in the program. From the Flinders' and Women's and Children's Hospital teams, there were two nephrologists, two scientists, and one nutritionist from each site together with a medical student who worked under a National Health and Medical Research Council (NHMRC) Training Scholarship.

The primary focus of the Umoona Kidney Project was a voluntary (or opportunistic) renal disease risk assessment program for the >400 adults and children in the community. There was also a voluntary clinical management program for adults identified as being at risk for renal disease.

The DCA 2000 (Bayer Diagnostics, Tarrytown, NY, USA) was the cornerstone of both the renal risk assessment program and the clinical management arm. The device measures urine albumin:creatinine ratio (ACR) on 40 μL of a first morning urine, as a marker for early renal disease or microalbuminuria. Prior to the commencement of the program, the Adelaide team spent 6 months of groundwork speaking to the community, holding information forums, showing the POCT technology and discussing the ACR test, and educating and training the Aboriginal health worker team in the use of the technology and quality management practices. This groundwork unquestionably contributed to the successful use of the DCA 2000 and the program overall. In addition to the ACR test, risk assessment also involved the measurement of blood pressure, blood glucose, body mass index, and dipstick urinalysis, while a full medical examination and history was taken for each person.

The overall risk factor profile of the 158 adults assessed (which represented ~65% of the adults in the community) showed 42% of the people had high blood pressure, 24% had diabetes, and there was a large pool of incipient renal disease, with 19% of adults having persistent microalbuminuria and 9% macroalbuminuria. A significant association was observed between blood pressure, blood glucose, and body mass index and the progression of albuminuria (as measured by the DCA 2000). A strong association was also found between albuminuria and an increasing number of coexisting risk factors, with only 20% of people having a normal urine ACR in the presence of three or more risk factors (27).

In relation to clinical management, 35 people were identified as being at risk for renal disease. All were either overtly hypertensive, hypertensive with other risk factors, or diabetic with microalbuminuria. Each was voluntarily offered the opportunity to take the ACE inhibitor medication Coversyl (Perindopril, Servier Laboratories, Australia) to reduce blood pressure and stabilize renal function. They were monitored according to a management protocol set by the Flinders' renal specialists, who conducted a total of 231 onsite clinical consultations with the patients on medication from 1998 to 2000. A sustained and statistically significant drop in blood pressure to normal levels was observed, as well as a stabilization of renal function, with mean ACR of the group (monitored using the DCA 2000) falling from 17 to 12 mg/mmol (150 to 106 mg/g) ($P = 0.09$, paired t-test). Across this 2-year period, there was no change in the group potassium, urea, creatinine, or glomerular filtration rate (Table 29-1).

Across 2 years of continuous field testing ($n = 46$) the DCA 2000 exhibited a precision base (CV%) of 6.9% and 3.6% for urine albumin (for Bayer quality control samples with concentrations of 36 and 208 mg/L, respectively), 3.2% and 4.1% for creatinine [9 and 36 mmol/L (1018 and 4072 mg/L)] and 6.7% and 5.3% for urine ACR [ratios of 4.1 and 5.8 mg/mmol (36.2 and 51.3 mg/g)] (29). These are well within precision goals of 10%, 6%, and 12% for urine albumin, creatinine, and ACR that are derived from biological variation and other international consensus data on performance criteria (8, 32).

Members of the Umoona community evaluated the program internally through a survey conducted by community elders, supported by the NHMRC medical student. By all criteria, the community expressed a high level of satisfaction with the program and the use of POCT technology, with a greater than 90% satisfaction rating recorded for all questions. Education and training initiatives for ACR POCT began in earnest in September 1999. Over the next 15 months Umoona's Aboriginal health workers took an increasingly greater responsibility for performing onsite blood pressure measurements and

urine ACR testing on the DCA 2000. In December 2000, the program was handed over to the Umoona Community as a self-sustaining activity fully integrated into the health service infrastructure. Both the South Australian Government's Department of Human Services Renal and Urology Services Implementation Plan 2000–2011 and the Statewide Iga Warta Aboriginal Renal Disease Summit, 1999 endorsed the Umoona model for expansion to other Aboriginal communities in rural and remote South Australia.

One of the most pleasing aspects of the Umoona Kidney Project was that POCT became a focal point for raising community awareness about renal disease. Through the trust and respect gained from the renal program, a number of other community activities (for both adults and children) around related health issues and health promotion were conducted. These included developing a nutrition training program for Umoona's Aboriginal health workers at their request (28), staging a poster competition for the children at the local area school about healthy foods, and holding education days at the school about kidney health and the importance of good nutrition (sponsored by the Australian Kidney Foundation). A bush tucker trip was also conducted with the Umoona community elders for the school children, where the children were taught how to dig for witchetty grubs, collect other bush foods, and cook kangaroo.

National QAAMS Program for Point-of-Care HbA1c Testing

The QAAMS Program arose from a recommendation of the Australian National Diabetes Strategy in 1998 (33), commenced as a pilot program in June 1999, and is now fully integrated into mainstream Aboriginal healthcare in Australia (34, 35). Since its inception, the program has been a collaborative partnership between a number of groups including the Office for Aboriginal and Torres Strait Islander Health and the Diagnostics and Technology Branch within the Australian Government's Department of Health and Ageing, NACCHO,

Table 29-1   Reduction in Renal and Cardiovascular Risk Two Years after Commencing Coversyl

Marker	Measure/matrix	Units	Pre-Coversyl baseline, mean ± SEM	Post-Coversyl 2 years, mean ± SEM	P-value[a]
Blood pressure					
Standing	Systolic	mmHg	151 ± 3	137 ± 3	<0.0001
	Diastolic	mmHg	92 ± 2	84 ± 2	<0.0001
Lying	Systolic	mmHg	147 ± 3	131 ± 3	<0.0001
	Diastolic	mmHg	94 ± 2	84 ± 2	<0.0001
Albumin:creatinine ratio (ACR)	Urine	mg/mmol	16.5 ± 3.9	12.0 ± 2.8	NS
Potassium	Plasma	mmol/L	4.0 ± 0.1	4.0 ± 0.1	NS
Urea	Plasma	mmol/L	4.9 ± 0.3	5.1 ± 0.3	NS
Creatinine	Plasma	mmol/L	0.081 ± 0.003	0.077 ± 0.003	NS
Glomerular filtration rate (GFR)[b]		mL/min	110 ± 5	118 ± 8	0.019

[a] Values of $P < 0.05$ are significant; NS, not significant.
[b] Calculated GFR from (44).

the Royal College of Pathologists of Australasia (RCPA)'s Quality Assurance Programs, and the Community Point-of-Care Services unit within the Flinders University Rural Clinical School.

The chronic disease focus of the QAAMS program is the management of Aboriginal people with established diabetes. More than 2300 patients are involved in the program, which is being conducted at 50 commonwealth-, state-, and territory-funded Aboriginal medical services around Australia. These sites encompass every state and territory in Australia, with more than 90% located in rural or remote areas (Figure 29-1). The DCA 2000 was selected for use in this program following the recommendation of the National Diabetes Strategy (33) and all HbA1c tests are performed by Aboriginal health workers. An educational resource package was prepared for each site, which included a laminated A3-size book, video, and supporting posters for specific aspects of the program. Initial training was provided for Aboriginal health workers from every participating site. Health workers were given instruction on how to perform the HbA1c test on the DCA 2000 and on the principles and practice of quality control and quality assurance.

With 50 POCT devices in the field, it was critical that a formal surveillance mechanism was implemented to monitor the performance of results generated by these instruments. Therefore a quality assurance program was developed collaboratively by the Community Point-of-Care Services unit at Flinders University and the RCPA Quality Assurance Programs. The breadth of quality assurance programs available to central laboratories is well known but, to the author's knowledge, the QAAMS program is the first POCT program of this type to be developed for indigenous people anywhere in the world.

The QAAMS program is modeled on the laboratory quality assurance program system used by the RCPA. Each

QAAMS participant is provided with an annual kit of quality assurance samples for testing (with two samples to be tested per month), a single-page result sheet, and a monthly summary report with a graphical result format similar to, but more simplified than, that provided for laboratories. Each site has its own code number to ensure confidentiality of results. The government charter in establishing this program has been to provide education, training, and quality management support services and not to collect or analyze patient data. This remains the property of the participating services, under NACCHO's direction.

At the time of writing, nine 6-month testing cycles have now been completed over the past 4.5 years from July 1999 to December 2003. Some of the key performance indicators are as follows. Participation rate has averaged 86% (range 73% to 93%) across all nine testing cycles, with almost 4000 quality assurance results returned during this time. The percentage of results considered acceptable has averaged 83% (range 81% to 86%), using limits for acceptable performance that are the same as those for the laboratory-based glycohemoglobin program conducted by the RCPA (5%). The median precision (CV%) achieved by the DCA 2000 analyzers across nine cycles has averaged 3.8%, with the precision base consistently improving across time and a CV% of 3.2% being recorded in the most recent testing cycle (Table 29-2).

As mentioned, the RCPA runs a parallel glycohemoglobin program for laboratories in Australasia. Seventy-five laboratory DCA 2000 users are registered in this program, which uses an identical quality assurance material to that of QAAMS. Across the past six testing cycles, the precision base achieved by Aboriginal medical services in the QAAMS program has been equivalent to that achieved by the laboratories (Table 29-2). This reflects the intensive ongoing commitment to continuing education, training, and support for the participating services that the QAAMS program provides.

The importance of precise HbA1c results for serial monitoring of diabetes control is now well recognized following studies such as the Diabetes Control and Complications Trial and the UK Prospective Diabetes Study clinical trials (36, 37). The desirable precision goal (CV%) for HbA1c analysis now recommended by most professional groups is 3% or less (8, 38, 39). In the QAAMS program, the precision base of DCA 2000 is now approaching the 3% goal. In a practical sense, for rural and remote communities where geographical isolation is common and laboratory access is limited, the DCA 2000 analyzer clearly provides a reliable, robust, and timely means of obtaining HbA1c analyses.

In March 2001 NACCHO conducted an independent evaluation of the first 18 months of the QAAMS program (40). The executive summary of this report stated that the use of the DCA 2000 represented a major opportunity to provide better care for and management of Aboriginal clients with diabetes within the community setting, while the ability of POCT to generate rapid results served as a catalyst to enhance patient self-management. The summary also concluded that the DCA 2000's simplicity of use led to high levels of acceptance by Aboriginal

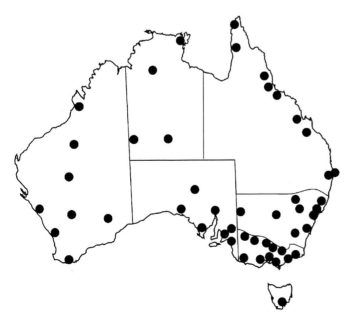

Figure 29-1 Map showing general location of QAAMS participants in 2003.

Table 29-2   Comparative Precision Base Over Last Six Testing Cycles[a]
Aboriginal community-controlled health services (ACCHS) versus laboratories using the Bayer DCA 2000

		Cycle period					
Program	Type of service	Jan–June 2001	July–Dec 2001	Jan–June 2002	July–Dec 2002	Jan–June 2003	July–Dec 2003
QAAMS	ACCHS	3.7	4.1	3.9	3.4	3.8	3.2
Glycohemoglobin	Laboratory	3.4	4.1	3.7	3.5	3.6	3.0

[a] Values are CV%, calculated by dividing the SD by the midpoint of the service's range of concentrations, expressed as a percentage. The SD is the error of the estimate $Sy \cdot x$ and represents the mean SD across the range of concentrations analyzed.

health workers nationally, with nearly two-thirds of services expressing the view that it had raised the self-esteem of their health workers. Importantly, the sense of community control was enhanced as a result of diabetes management becoming more focused within Aboriginal medical services.

In December 2000 the Australian Government's Health Minister announced that a Medicare rebate could be claimed for HbA1c testing performed by the DCA 2000 analyzer in Aboriginal Community Controlled Health Services under a separate item number established specifically for the QAAMS program. The rebate, which has ensured a sustainable funding mechanism for the program, is conditional on several factors including continuing participation in and sound analytical performance for quality assurance testing in the QAAMS program.

To enhance the sustainability of the program further, an annual workshop for participants has been held since 2001. These workshops have now become a key feature of the QAAMS calendar. The meetings are very interactive, with significant opportunities for retraining and networking. All participants now undergo competency assessment and certification (in both practical and theoretical elements of the program) at the workshop. In 2003, the island of Tonga from the Western Pacific region was recruited as the program's first international participant. Considerable interest remains from other Western Pacific islands and Canada. The QAAMS model is transferable to other types of POCT. In January 2003 a new QAAMS program commenced for the measurement of urine ACR on the DCA 2000. There are 30 ACCHSs enrolled in the program and ACR testing will be used to monitor microalbuminuria in Aboriginal patients with diabetes.

Point-of-Care in Aboriginal Hands Program

The Point-of-Care in Aboriginal Hands program commenced in mid-2001 (41). It is a partnership between the Community Point-of-Care Services unit at the Flinders University Rural Clinical School and four rural and remote Aboriginal health services at Port Lincoln, the Riverland, and Meningie, rural towns and regions in South Australia, varying from 200 to 650 km from metropolitan Adelaide, and at Kalgoorlie in Western Australia, a rural mining town almost 500 km from metropolitan Perth. Meningie is a small rural community, with one health worker and two doctors servicing the community. The

Port Lincoln Aboriginal Health Service and the Riverland Regional Health Service are well-resourced rural health centers, servicing larger population bases. The Bega Garnbirringu Aboriginal health service at Kalgoorlie is by far the largest health center, servicing Aboriginal people from the entire Goldfields region of outback Western Australia and having a very large health worker team and strong clinical and infrastructure support.

Education, training, and quality management of POCT again underpin the program and the local Aboriginal health worker is responsible for the day-to-day operation of the POC technology. The Point-of-Care in Aboriginal Hands program differs from the other models described in several fundamental ways. First, it has a greater local community focus with local medical officers and/or medical directors undertaking all clinical management at each health service, as opposed to the renal specialists associated with the previously described Umoona program. Second, the Point-of-Care in Aboriginal Hands program has a broader chronic disease focus that looks at the early detection and management of diabetes, renal disease, and cardiovascular disease collectively rather than having a single disease focus; for example, renal for the Umoona project or diabetes for the QAAMS HbA1c program. Finally, there is wider use of POCT. Aboriginal Health Workers are trained in how to use the Bayer DCA 2000 for both HbA1c and urine ACR testing and the Cholestech LDX lipid analyzer (Cholestech, Hayward, CA, USA), which provides a full lipid profile and a glucose measurement on a fingerprick of blood in 5 min (42).

The principal activities are education and training for the entire local health professional team and a voluntary (opportunistic) chronic disease risk assessment service for community members at each site with a concomitant chronic disease management arm. Although most of the point-of-care risk assessments are conducted in the clinic setting, the opportunity is taken whenever possible to conduct field-testing outside the clinic. For example, testing has been carried out at such diverse locations as a local ecotourism center, a local adult education college, and in a tin shed at the Port Lincoln Aboriginal Women's Centre (an event that was also linked with a nutrition health promotion activity). In the Riverland, a bus has been purchased and renovated to provide a mobile POCT service throughout the Riverland region (with risk assessment also linked to an eye examination for people with diabetes through a separate program). These examples highlight the flexibility and versatility of POCT in the community setting.

More than 600 chronic disease risk assessments have been performed by POCT across all four participating sites. A number of common trends relating to chronic disease risk between participating communities have been identified. Diabetes is extremely prevalent (ranging from 15% to 26% in the general community). Again, there is a large incipient pool of renal disease, with rates of microalbuminuria ranging from 19% to 26% in the general community. Elevated lipids are very common (35% to 44%), particularly in males and the younger age group (where increased lipids were found in 24% to 28% of people assessed). Obesity is extremely prevalent in females (ranging from 47% to 59%). An example of the risk assessment profile found in one community is shown in Figure 29-2.

For clinical management, flow charts for POCT processes have been developed in collaboration with each community, based on best practice evidence and input of the local clinicians. The frequency of follow-up testing is determined by diabetes, blood pressure, microalbumin, and lipid status. A well-defined niche for the use of POCT in chronic disease management has been identified, namely integration of POCT with the Australian government's Chronic Disease Self Management Care Plan initiative (43). At Port Lincoln, for example, a subset of 29 patients in the Point-of-Care in Aboriginal Hands program were entered into the Chronic Disease Self-Management Care Plan program during 2002. Their HbA1c (as performed by POCT on the DCA 2000) was measured at baseline and at 12 months. The mean HbA1c of the group improved from 7.8% at baseline to 7.4% after a year (43).

A number of case studies have also been identified across the program that clearly demonstrate the benefits of POCT in the early detection and diagnosis of chronic disease, more expedient initiation of treatment, improved clinical effectiveness, and greater patient satisfaction and motivation. Two case examples are described in the following.

The first case describes a 57-year-old man with NIDDM, obesity, and ischemic heart disease. He had been "lost to the health system" in the community for more than 2 years until he re-presented at clinic in December 2001. His POC results on presentation were: HbA1c, 10.5%; blood glucose, 11.6 mmol/L (209 mg/dL); urine ACR, 2.8 mg/mmol (24.8 mg/g); blood pressure, 150/90 mmHg; and weight, 124 kg (273 lb). Insulin was resumed immediately to treat his poor glycemic control. During the next year, regular HbA1c tests were performed using POCT, and the patient's HbA1c fell to 9.7% (February 2002), 8.8% (August 2002), and 8.4% (December 2002). Across this period, he received ongoing dietary, podiatry, and retinopathy review. He commented that regular POCT has helped motivate him to achieve improved diabetes control. He has also initiated lifestyle changes including taking bush trips every second day and consuming more bush foods and fish.

The second case describes a 32-year-old male student from a very remote Aboriginal community who was visiting "town" to attend a training course. He presented at the local health service complaining of headaches after drinking heavily the previous night. His POCT results were: HbA1c, 10.6%; blood glucose, 19.0 mmol/L (342 mg/dL); urine ACR 22.7, mg/mmol (200 mg/g); cholesterol, 12.0 mmol/L (463 mg/dL); nonfasting triglyceride >7.3 mmol/L (>650 mg/dL) (the upper measuring limit of the Cholestech LDX analyzer), and blood pressure, 156/115 mmHg. The patient's blood sample was also left standing on the bench, allowing the red blood cells to settle and reveal plasma that was strawberry milk in color. Opportunistic POCT led to the patient being identified as diabetic with poor glycemic control, microalbuminuria, and severe hyperlipidemia (as well as hypertension). Treatment was initiated immediately and the patient returned home and is now managed by the visiting Royal Flying Doctor Air Service. Visualization of the milky plasma also led to valuable education for the health worker team about heart disease and raised community awareness about blood fats, as this sample was photo-

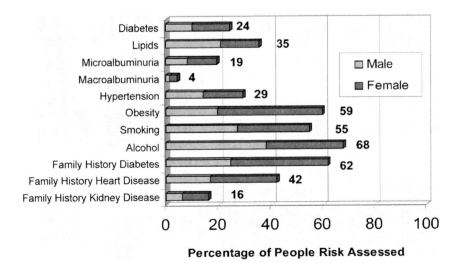

Percentage of People Risk Assessed

Figure 29-2 Chronic disease risk assessment profile in one community in the Point-of-Care in Aboriginal Hands program.

Table 29-3 Median Precision of QAAMS HbA1c and Urine ACR Testing by Four Sites in the Point-of-Care in Aboriginal Hands Program[a]

Site	HbA1c		Urine ACR	
	Median precision	Precision goal	Median precision	Precision goal
1	3.2	3	4.3	12
2	3.1	—	5.1	—
3	3.1	—	NA[b]	—
4	2.9	—	5.0	—

[a] Values are CV%.
[b] Data unavailable.

graphed and is now used as a teaching aid at community health promotion functions.

For quality management purposes, all sites are now enrolled in both national QAAMS programs for HbA1c and urine ACR. In addition, they conduct onsite internal quality control testing, the results of which are immediately faxed to and managed by the Flinders' Community Point-of-Care Services unit. There is also monthly communication between the unit and each participating site around a quality management checklist. Table 29-3 details the analytical performance achieved by each site for QAAMS testing in the most recent cycle. These results again clearly demonstrate that POCT can be carried out to a high level of analytical competency by Aboriginal health workers, provided they are supported by a quality management framework comprising ongoing education, training, and participation in structured quality management programs.

The Point-of-Care in Aboriginal Hands program has been well accepted by the participating Aboriginal communities, Aboriginal health workers, and supporting clinical staff. The program has worked effectively in four different rural communities, each with different levels of staff resources, infrastructure support, and clinical agendas.

REFERENCES

1. Wakerman J, Humphreys JS. Rural health: why it matters. Med J Aust 2002;176:457–8.
2. Australian Institute of Health and Welfare (AIHW). It's different in the bush—a comparison of general practice activity in metropolitan and rural areas of Australia, 1998–2000. Canberra: AIHW, 2001. (AIHW Catalogue No. GEP-6).
3. Australian Institute of Health and Welfare (AIHW). Health in rural and remote Australia. Canberra: AIHW, 2001;14. (AIHW Catalogue No. PHE-6).
4. Simmons D, Hsu-Hage B. Determinants of health, disease and disability: differences between country and city. In: Wilkinson D, Blue I, eds. The new rural health. Melbourne: Oxford University Press, 2002:79–93.
5. Guilbert R, Schattner P, Sikaris K, Churilov L, Leibowitz R, Matthews M. Review of the role and value of near patient testing in general practice. Report to the Pathology Section, Diagnostic and Technology Branch, Commonwealth Department of Health and Aged Care. 2001. http://www.health.gov.au/haf/docs/nptfinalrpt.htm.
6. Cole D, Kelly R, Taylor L, Dimeski G. POCT—connecting to the LIS and defeating the tyranny of distance. Clin Biochem Rev 2002;23:85.
7. Tirimacco R, Tideman P. Introduction of bedside troponin T testing protocols within an integrated cardiac assessment regional network (iCARnet). Clin Biochem Rev 2002;23:88.
8. Sacks DB, Bruns DE, Goldstein DE, MacLaren NK, McDonald JM, Parrott M. Guidelines and recommendations for laboratory analysis in the diagnosis and management of diabetes mellitus. Clin Chem 2002;48:436–72.
9. Diabetes Australia and The Royal Australian College of General Practitioners. Diabetes management in general practice. Diabetes Australia Publication NP 1020, 2002.
10. National Heart Foundation of Australia and Cardiac Society of Australia and New Zealand. Lipid management guidelines— 2001. Med J Aust 2001;175:S57–85.
11. Gerstein HC, Mann JF, Yi Q, Zinman B, Dinneen SF, Hoogwerf B, et al. Albuminuria and risk of cardiovascular events, death, and heart failure in diabetic and nondiabetic individuals. JAMA 2001; 286:421–6.
12. Bakris GL. Microalbuminuria: What is it? Why is it important? What should be done about it? J Clin Hyper 2001;3:99–102.
13. Hopkins RM, Gracey MS, Hobbs RP, Spargo RM, Yates M, Thompson RC. The prevalence of hookworm infection, iron deficiency and anaemia in an Aboriginal community in northwest Australia. Med J Aust 1997;168:241–4.
14. Couzos S, Murray R. Aboriginal primary health care. An evidence-based approach. Melbourne: Oxford University Press, 1999:51–3.
15. Miller P, Torzillo P. Health, an indigenous right: a review of Aboriginal health in Australia. Aust J Med Sci 1996;17:3–12.
16. Anderson I, Thomson N. Health of indigenous Australians: a rural perspective. In: Wilkinson D, Blue I, eds. The new rural health. Melbourne: Oxford University Press, 2002:110–25.
17. International Diabetes Institute. Review of the epidemiology, aetiology, pathogenesis and preventability of diabetes in Aboriginal and Torres Strait Islander populations. Canberra: Office for Aboriginal and Torres Strait Islander Health Services, Commonwealth Department of Health and Family Services, 1998 (Publication No. 2335).
18. Thomas MAB. Kidney disease in Australian Aboriginals: time for decisive action. Med J Aust 1998;168:532–3.
19. Spencer JL, Silva DT, Snelling P, Hoy WE. An epidemic of renal failure among Australian Aboriginals. Med J Aust 1998;168: 537–41.
20. Hoy W. Renal disease and the environment: lessons from Aboriginal Australia. Nephrology 2001;6:19–24.
21. Hoy WE, Baker PR, Kelly AM, Wang Z. Reducing premature death and renal failure in Aboriginal Australians. Med J Aust 2000;172:473–8.
22. Hoy W. Renal disease in Australian Aborigines. Nephrol Dial Transplant 2000;15:1293–7.
23. Thomson N, Winter J, Pumphrey M. Review of cardiovascular disease among Aboriginal and Torres Strait Islander populations. 1999. Australian Indigenous Health InfoNet. http://www.health-infonet.ecu.edu.au.
24. National Centre for Monitoring Cardiovascular Disease. Heart, stroke and vascular diseases: Australian facts 1999. Canberra:

Australian Institute of Health and Welfare and Heart Foundation of Australia, 1999.

25. Thomas M. Pugsley D. Renal disease in indigenous populations. Proceedings from the satellite meeting of the X1Vth International Congress of Nephrology. Nephrol 1998;4(Suppl):S1–124.

26. Shephard M. Point-of-care testing in the Aboriginal community. Aust J Med Sci 2003;24:10–6.

27. Shephard MDS, Allen GG, Barratt LJ, Paizis K, Brown M, Barbara JAJ, et al. Albuminuria in a remote South Australian Aboriginal community: results of a community-based screening program for renal disease. Rural and Remote Health 2003;3(Online). http://rrh.deakin.edu.au (February 8, 2003).

28. Zeunert S, Cerro N, Boesch L, Duff M, Shephard MDS, Jureidini KF, Braun J. Nutrition project in a remote Australian Aboriginal community. J Ren Nutr 2002;12:102–6.

29. Shephard MDS, Allen GG. Screening for renal disease in a remote Aboriginal community using the Bayer DCA 2000. Aust J Med Sci 2001;22:164–70.

30. Shephard MDS, Brown M, Hudson M, Riessen C, Braun J. The Umoona Kidney Project. Abor Island Hlth Work J 2000;24:12–5.

31. Shephard MDS. The Umoona Kidney Project—case study of effective Aboriginal health care. Sth Aust Med Rev 2000; 13:16–9.

32. Ricos C, Alvarez V, Cava F, Garcia-Lario JV, Hernandez A, Jiminez CV et al. Current databases on biological variation: pros, cons and progress. Scand J Clin Lab Inves 1999;59:491–500.

33. Colagiuri S, Colagiuri R, Ward J. National Diabetes Strategy and Implementation Plan. Canberra: Diabetes Australia, 1998.

34. Shephard MDS, Gill JP. Results of an innovative education, training and quality assurance program for point-of-care HbA1c testing using the Bayer DCA 2000 in Australian Aboriginal community controlled health services. Clin Biochem Rev 2003; 24:123–30.

35. Shephard MDS, Mundraby K. Assisting diabetes management through point-of-care HbA1c testing—the 'QAAMS' program for Aboriginal health workers. Abor Island Hlth Work J 2003; 27:12–8.

36. Diabetes Control and Complications Trial Research Group. The effect of intensive treatment of diabetes on the development and progression of long-term complications in insulin-dependent diabetes mellitus. N Engl J Med 1993;329:977–86.

37. UK Prospective Diabetes Study (UKPDS) Group. Intensive blood-glucose control with sulphonylureas or insulin compared with conventional treatment and risk of complications in patients with type 2 diabetes (UKPDS 33). Lancet 1998;352:837–53.

38. Coleman PG, Goodall GI, Garcia Webb P, Williams PF, Dunlop ME. Glycohaemoglobin: a crucial measurement in modern diabetes management. Progress towards standardisation and improved precision of measurement. Med J Aust 1997;167: 95–8.

39. Goodall I. The need for standardisation of glycohaemoglobin measurement. International standardisation 1996 IFCC/AACC proposals. In: Coulston L, ed. Diabetes, glycation and complications. The clinical biochemist monograph. Perth: Australian Association of Clinical Biochemists, 1996:87–96.

40. Brice G, Daley L, Bellis-Smith N. From 'major threat' to 'major opportunity'? Pilot project to assess the use of on-site haemoglobin A1c testing for managing persons with diabetes (using the Bayer DCA 2000 analyser) in Australian Aboriginal community controlled health services: June 1999 to August 2000. National Aboriginal Community Controlled Health Organisation, 2001.

41. Jones R, Mazzachi B, Shephard M. Point-of-care in Aboriginal hands. Abor Island Hlth Work J 2002;26:13–6.

42. Shephard MDS, Tallis G. Assessment of the point-of-care Cholestech Lipid Analyser for lipid screening in Aboriginal communities. Aust J Med Sci 2002;23:4–10.

43. Ah Kit J, Prideaux C, Harvey PW, Collins J, Battersby M, Mills PD et al. Chronic disease self management in Aboriginal communities: towards a sustainable program of care in rural communities. Aust J Prim Hlth 2003;9:168–76.

44. Cockcroft DW, Gault MH. Prediction of creatinine clearance from serum creatinine. Nephron 1976;16:31–41.

Chapter 30

Point-of-Care Testing in Sports Medicine

Marvin M. Adner and Terry Shirey

For decades athletes have been evaluated at the site of sports activity. They are monitored on the playing fields of organized team sports and in sporting activities involving small groups participating in areas remote from traditional medical facilities, such as high-altitude climbs, wilderness expeditions, and endurance events. Often the problem is the diagnosis and management of an athlete who has collapsed. Evaluation of the patient by obtaining a history and performing a physical examination often provides sufficient evidence to diagnose dehydration, heat stroke, hypothermia, and transient syncope. In recent years, point-of-care testing (POCT) has facilitated the early diagnosis and treatment of two causes of exercise-associated collapse, both of which are associated with high morbidity and mortality: (1) exercise-induced hyponatremia due to overhydration occurring primarily in endurance events such as triathalons, marathons, and ultramarathons and (2) cardiac disorders presenting as arrhythmias, cardiac arrest, and myocardial ischemia.

EXERCISE-ASSOCIATED HYPONATREMIA SECONDARY TO OVERHYDRATION

In 1972, Frank Shorter won the gold medal in the Olympic marathon. This was the beginning of the running boom. Completion of the historic Boston Marathon became for many the ultimate athletic achievement. In 1976, 2000 runners started in Hopkinton, Massachusetts. The temperature at the starting line was 100 °F, and there were no medical facilities along the route. Little fluid was available at the finish line. Upon completion of the race, runners were offered the traditional beef stew, and medical care was provided by a small team of medical physicians and podiatrists. Several of the participants belonging to the American Medical Joggers Association (AMJA) recognized the inadequacy of the medical coverage for the race. AMJA sponsored an organized medical team for the 1978 Boston Marathon. In preparing a medical care plan, the medical leadership reviewed information presented in the symposium published by the New York Academy of Sciences in 1977 on the medical aspects of marathon running. Authorities in the field provided information on body temperature regulation, fluid balance, sweating, heat stroke, and hypothermia. The major medical problem was sweat loss resulting in relative dehydration. Electrolyte abnormalities, such as hypokalemia and hyponatremia, were not perceived as a problem due to renal compensation that maintained electrolyte balance

(1). The subject index from the symposium did not contain the term *hyponatremia*.

Sparked by the challenge of running a 26-mile race, athletes began to participate in longer endurance events, including 100-mile ultramarathons and triathalons. These events resulted in more serious metabolic dysfunction with profound fluid volume and electrolyte depletion. These conditions caused significant morbidity but rarely resulted in death. Most notable was the development of severe hyponatremia. The pathophysiology was considered to be the loss of hypotonic sweat over many hours and its replacement by water, producing dilutional hyponatremia.

In 1987, the first report of hyponatremia in a marathon participant was published (2). The finishing time of the stricken runner was 5½ h, a relatively slow time for a marathon, but approximating finishing times observed in some ultraendurance events. In 1987, a symposium titled Medical Coverage of Endurance Athletic Events included presentations by medical directors of ultraendurance events, such as the Western States 100, the Iron Man Canada Triathalon in western Canada, and the Iron Man Triathalon in Hawaii (3). Medical directors of these events described biochemical measurements at the point of care that provided critical data to establish a diagnosis in disabled runners. At the same symposium, presentations by medical directors of 26-mile marathons did not describe use of POCT because there was a belief that these metabolic disorders did not occur in races with finishing times of usually <4 h. The greatest risks for participants were considered to be heat stroke and sudden death from cardiac disease, both of which were rare occurrences.

Heat stroke is generally not experienced by participants in the Boston Marathon, which is run in April when the temperatures are normally in the 50–60 °F range. To be a participant, athletes, who were predominantly male, had to have completed a marathon within the previous year with qualifying times ranging from 3 to 3½ h. About 5% of the participants in the Boston Marathon entered the finish-line medical tent for care (4). One-third of the runners' problems were due to minor musculoskeletal disorders. Frequently, runners developed mild hyper- and hypothermia. A number of runners became mildly volume depleted. Intravenous fluids were administered to those runners who could not tolerate oral fluids. Based on the recommendations of exercise physiologists at the Natick Army Laboratory (Natick, MA), the intravenous replacement fluid was "half normal" saline and 5% glucose, used to replace sweat loss and depleted carbohydrate stores.

From 1987 until later in the 1990s, there were isolated reports of hyponatremia in marathon runners. In the 1999 Boston Marathon, two young women who had completed the marathon developed seizures at home many hours after they had completed the race. They were hospitalized and diagnosed with hyponatremia. One of these women, who had been in the medical tent complaining of nausea and malaise, was treated with 2 L of hypotonic saline. She felt no better upon release, went home, and continued to drink water. These women were inexperienced, first-time marathoners, with finishing times of ~6 h.

The recognition of life-threatening hyponatremia was the stimulus for POCT at the Boston Marathon. No longer could ill patients be treated with intravenous fluids for perceived dehydration without ruling out hyponatremia. It was necessary to make an early diagnosis of hyponatremia at the 2000 Boston Marathon. In a planning meeting several months before the 2000 race, a recently published paper describing the presence of hyponatremia, cerebral edema, and noncardiac pulmonary edema occurring in seven marathon runners was reviewed (5). In this study, diagnoses were made at the time of hospitalization, not in the medical tent.

The Boston Marathon medical care team performed point-of-care biochemical monitoring at the 2000 Boston Marathon. In collaboration with Nova Biomedical Corporation (Waltham, MA), the team relied on three of Nova's Ultra M instruments, which measured blood pH, hematocrit, sodium, potassium, chloride, ionized calcium, magnesium, glucose, lactate, and blood urea nitrogen (BUN) levels of venous blood samples. Analysis turnaround time for each runner's sample was ~160 s, minimizing the time of delay for appropriate intervention.

Pre- and post-race blood specimens were drawn from 34 runner volunteers. In addition, 86 runners were triaged to the intensive care section of the medical tent for evaluation of abnormal signs and symptoms, including altered mental status, inability to walk, dyspnea, chest pain, vomiting, hypotension, and hypothermia. No life-threatening biochemical abnormalities, including hyponatremia, were found. However, clinically significant hyponatremia did develop in some runners who had collapsed along the race route or become ill after completing the race, but who had not sought medical attention (6).

Based on reports of hyponatremia occurring in runners of numerous marathons throughout the world, there was an increased understanding of the pathogenesis of the metabolic disorder. Overhydration was the principal cause for the dilutional hyponatremia. Increased salt loss through sweating was contributory, but not usually a major factor. The excess fluid intake was most likely to occur in runners with finishing times >4½ h who were of small stature and female gender. The use of nonsteroidal antiinflammatory agents increased the risk of developing hyponatremia (7).

In the 2002 Boston Marathon, POCT was to be performed on all runners who were candidates for intravenous fluid, regardless of their finishing time, and in those individuals finishing after 4 h whose clinical presentation matched the risk profile. A total of 80 runners underwent POCT. Three runners had sodium levels of 130–134 mmol/L (130–134 mEq/L). A female runner with a sodium level of 125 mmol/L (125 mEq/L) developed a grand mal seizure and was taken to the hospital, where she recovered without incident. Eighteen runners had sodium levels >145 mmol/L (>145 mEq/L). Five and a half hours into the race, a female runner who collapsed at mile 22 was brought from the course to a major Boston teaching hospital. She was determined to have profound hyponatremia with a sodium level of 113 mmol/L (113 mEq/L). Despite aggressive therapy, she died from complications related to cerebral edema due to hyponatremia secondary to overhydration. The death of a young healthy woman in the world's oldest and most prestigious marathon shocked the running community.

In preparation for the 2003 Boston Marathon, there was a focus on prevention of exercise-induced hyponatremia. A pamphlet describing the pathogenesis of hyponatremia, with measures to prevent overhydration during and after the race, was sent to all marathon participants. This information was reviewed with the 1000 charity runners. These individuals, many of whom were women, did not have to meet a qualifying time to gain entrance to the race. They qualified by participating in fund-raising for charities in a combined program with the Boston Athletic Association. Many of these participants fit the high-risk profile for hyponatremia. In the 2003 race, 154 runners were tested. Four women runners had sodium levels of 125–130 mmol/L (125–130 mEq/L), one of whom required triage to the hospital. The three other runners were treated in the tent with fluid restriction and sodium repletion. Fifty-three runners were hypernatremic, with sodium levels >145 mmol/L (>145 mEq/L).

POCT allows for early diagnosis of hyponatremia in runners brought to the medical tent at the finish line. Most runners do not require hospitalization. Those runners with severe hyponatremia can be transported from the medical tent to one of the major teaching hospitals located only a few minutes away by ambulance.

The Boston Marathon is a point-to-point race. It now has about 20,000 participants who run through crowded suburban and urban areas. POCT along the route is not currently feasible. However, in loop marathons, POCT can be performed at a single medical station providing care for runners both along the route and at the finish line. POCT should not be the standard of care for all marathons. In smaller races, in which the anticipated number developing this relatively uncommon disorder is low, runners can be transported to a local hospital emergency department. As marathon participants develop a greater understanding of proper hydration, it is likely that the number of runners who develop hyponatremia will decrease. However, POCT of Boston Marathon runners is currently necessary to establish an early diagnosis and appropriate treatment for life-threatening hyponatremia.

EXERCISE-ASSOCIATED MORBIDITY AND MORTALITY DUE TO CARDIAC DISORDERS

Sudden death occurring in children and young adults during vigorous exercise is primarily due to congenital abnormalities such as hypertrophic cardiomyopathy and coronary artery anomalies (8). The primary focus in preventing these deaths is preparticipation screening. POCT has little value in improving the prognosis in these disorders.

Habitual physical activity decreases the development of coronary artery disease and decreases the cardiac mortality in exercise-based cardiac rehabilitation programs (9). Underlying coronary artery disease is the major cause of exercise-related deaths in adults and occurs primarily in individuals who are inactive and with multiple cardiac risk factors (10). There have been two deaths due to coronary artery disease in 108 years of the running of the Boston Marathon. In 1973, a runner developed myocardial infarction during the race, was hospitalized, and died of complications of his cardiac disease 1 month later (11). In the 100th running of the Boston Marathon, in 1996, an elderly runner with known coronary artery disease collapsed at the finish line immediately after completing the race. The cardiac monitor revealed he was asystolic. Resuscitative measures failed to revive him.

The use of portable electrocardiographic (ECG/EKG) monitors and defibrillators to assess athletes with exercise-associated collapse enhances the capability of early diagnosis and treatment of cardiac disorders such as a cardiac arrhythmia, cardiac arrest, and myocardial infarction. However, patients with myocardial infarction may have no chest pain and have no specific ECG/EKG changes or no ECG/EKG changes at all. The diagnosis of myocardial infarction often depends on changes in cardiobiochemical markers, including troponin and creatine kinase (CK) isoenzymes, especially the MB isoenzyme, which is found predominantly in heart muscle. A study of CK-MB levels in trained marathoners measured after completing a race revealed total CK and percentage of MB isoenzymes in asymptomatic runners comparable to levels found in patients with myocardial infarction (12). Because of the non-specificity of the CK MB fraction in runners the measurement of this isoenzyme is of little value in making an early diagnosis of myocardial injury in athletes. A measurement of troponin1 is a much better marker because it is specific for cardiac injury (13). Point-of-care measurement of troponin1 in an emergency department accelerated the evaluation of patients presenting with chest pain (14). Evidence of a troponin leak in myocardial infarction occurs within 3–12 h of the injury. Therefore, the probability of finding evidence of myocardial damage in an athlete who collapses in an event of <3 h is small, but in endurance events lasting >3 h, troponins may have considerable value.

Blood lactate levels have been demonstrated to be useful in establishing a diagnosis of acute myocardial infarction within 3 h of symptom development (15). Sixteen of a group of 28 patients with acute myocardial infarction (MI) were seen in this time period, and all but one had elevated lactate levels [defined by the authors as >1.5 mmol/L (>13.5 mg/dL)] at the time of presentation. Elevated lactate levels were seen in a subset of runners who underwent biochemical monitoring at the Boston Marathon (6). However, clinical correlation was not performed. The elevation of lactate in a runner may well be a product of anaerobic metabolism. Therefore, using elevation of lactate levels to establish a diagnosis of acute MI in a collapsed runner is unlikely to be useful because of a low specificity, a situation comparable to measuring CK MB to rule out myocardial ischemia in collapsed runners. However, in the acute MI study there was a negative predictive value of blood lactate of 98%. Therefore, a normal lactate may be useful in ruling out acute MI in runners presenting with exercise-associated collapse.

LACTATE AS A MEASURE OF ATHLETIC PERFORMANCE

Lactate concentrations are typically increased in runner-patients entering the medical tent at the finish line of the Boston Marathon. While the reference range for lactate is 0.5–2.2 mmol/L (4.5–19.8 mg/dL), average lactate values for Boston Marathon runner-patients were 4.3 and 4.5 mmol/L (38.7 and 40.5 mg/dL), respectively, for the 2002 and 2003 marathon events. Values ranged from 1.9 to 13.4 mmol/L (17.1–120.6 mg/dL) in 2002 and from 0.9 to 13.1 mmol/L (8.1–117.9 mg/dL) in 2003. Is there any clinical significance to the higher lactate values? Elevated lactate values in critical care medicine (e.g., heart attack, hemorrhage, stroke, surgery, head injury) generally mean that tissues are not getting adequate oxygen. The magnitude of resulting tissue damage appears to depend on the tissues affected and the amount of oxygen debt that develops in these tissues. Oxygen deprivation of many tissues (e.g., brain, heart, kidney) correlates strongly with morbidity and mortality. Consequently, elevated lactate in many critical care settings demands its rapid discovery, an explanation for the oxygen deprivation, and rapid therapy to correct it.

In athletes, however, lactate is usually produced by skeletal muscle operating anaerobically. At a certain level of exercise, the rate of lactate generation begins to exceed that of lactate removal. This is the lactate threshold (LT). Elevated lactate levels, therefore, suggest that the LT has been exceeded. Elite athletes, such as cyclists, runners, and cross-country skiers, can sustain work levels substantially above their LTs for up to 1 h (16).

Several factors may contribute to the lactate elevations seen in runners. Intensity (speed at which exercise occurs), duration, muscle fiber composition, and the condition of the athlete are the most obvious. Even higher ambient temperature and humidity may increase lactate levels during exercise (17). Intense workloads may lead to rapid increases in lactate over relatively short periods of time. Peak lactate levels following brief sprints in one study were as follows: 8.1 mmol/L (7.3 mg/dL), 15 s; 11.2 mmol/L (100.8 mg/dL), 30 s; and 14.7 mmol/L (132.3 mg/dL), 45 s (18). Repeated bouts of exercise with brief rests between bouts led to lactate values as high as 32 mmol/L (288 mg/dL) (19).

Energy for exercise comes from adenosine triphosphate and creatine phosphate for the first 10 s, from glycogen going to lactate for the first minute of anaerobic exercise, from glycogen to CO_2 for the first hour of aerobic exercise, and from fatty acids to CO_2 for aerobic exercise exceeding 1 h. Fat metabolism does not produce lactate (16). The average lactate values immediately following the 2002 and 2003 Boston Marathon in runner-patients, and controls, nonpatient runners, were in line with the threefold increase in values typically seen in prolonged exercise (20). The lactate seen in most of these runners apparently comes from a degree of anaerobic metabolism of residual or newly synthesized glycogen, or glucose obtained over the course of the marathon, which are available for metabolism in the latter portion of the race.

With anaerobic metabolism comes the breakdown of ATP, resulting in the release of protons (acidity). An accumulation of protons results in the inhibition of local muscle contraction and pain resulting from the effects of the protons (lactate?) on nerve endings. Blame those heavy legs on the protons. Fatigue at prolonged sub-LT intensities includes carbohydrate depletion and dehydration (16). The magnitude of the difference in lactate concentrations among the runners may, in part, reflect differences in their tolerance for pain and fatigue and their individual desire to finish with a good personal time.

Conditioning can increase the intensity and duration of exercise before LT is reached. Adaptations such as increasing mitochondrial number and size, increasing capillary density, improving fatty acid oxidation capacity, and increasing myoglobin levels make this possible. Conditioning is highly specific to the exercise task. A conditioned cyclist may substantially increase the distance he or she can pedal in a given period of time before reaching his or her LT, but still become quickly fatigued when running a marathon (using different muscles) without appropriate conditioning or preparatory distance running (16). One approach used for conditioning athletes is to build their training regimens based on reaching a lactate value of 4 mmol/L (36 mg/dL) (21). The concept is that athletes who do not develop this level of lactate are likely not conditioning themselves sufficiently. Those exceeding the 4-mmol/L (36-mg/dL) level are likely doing more tissue damage than positive conditioning and might be advised to reduce their workout accordingly. Using this conditioning paradigm, athletes are able, with time, to increase the duration and intensity of their exercise before they reach the 4-mmol/L (36-mg/dL) lactate level. Currently, this appears to be the most justifiable reason to consider making POCT lactate measurements available in sports medicine.

FUTURE POINT-OF-CARE TESTING IN SPORTS MEDICINE

POCT in sports medicine is an example of the "bedside to bench to bedside" concept that describes the process of expansion of medical knowledge. Often this begins with the publication of new observations on a single patient, which is followed by additional anecdotal reports of similar observations. There is a review of published reports, including clinical laboratory findings, current therapy, and outcome. Additional studies are conducted in research laboratories that further define the biochemical and molecular characteristics of the disorder. Clinical guidelines are published to assist the clinician in diagnosis and management of patients with the disorder who are usually treated in the hospital or outpatient clinic. Finally, the technology to perform the diagnostic studies becomes portable, and the standard of care becomes point-of-care testing.

An example of this process is the increase in understanding of the high-altitude disease, acute mountain sickness. This is a well-known disorder, commonly exhibiting pulmonary and cerebral edema. This disorder is often fatal. Yet the cause of the disease has not been well understood, in part due to the inability to perform the sophisticated diagnostic studies required to unravel the pathogenesis at the site where the disorder develops. In the late 1980s, a study titled Operation Everest II: Man and Extreme Altitude was conducted at the US Army Research Institute of Environmental Medicine (Natick, MA). In this study, men were put into a decompression chamber to simulate an altitude of 8840 m, the height of Mount Everest (22). Many experiments were performed to study the effects of high altitude on a number of organ systems, which helped explain the pathogenesis of acute mountain sickness. Several years later, a study of high-altitude pulmonary edema moved from the sea-level laboratory to a high-altitude research laboratory at 4559 m in the Alps (23). Alveolar and arterial blood gas analysis, doppler echocardiography, and chest radiography were performed on a group of climbers with a history of high-altitude pulmonary edema; they were randomly assigned to receive a placebo or nifedipine. The drug was found to significantly decrease pulmonary arterial pressure and prevent high-altitude pulmonary edema in these subjects.

In a few years, it would not be surprising to see a television documentary on an Everest ascent team that includes a sherpa carrying an ultrasound device to perform electrocardiography, and a biochemical analyzer, which will facilitate the early diagnosis of acute mountain sickness in climbers attempting to scale the highest mountain in the world.

REFERENCES

1. Costill DL. Sweating: its composition and effects on body fluids. Ann NY Acad Sci 1977;301:160–82.
2. Young M, Sciurba F, Rinaldo J. Delirium and pulmonary edema after completing a marathon. Am Rev Respir Dis 1987;136:737–9.

3. Wheeler K. Ross symposium on medical coverage of endurance athletic events. Columbus, Ohio: Ross Laboratories, 1987.

4. Adner M, Scarlet J, Casey J, Robinson W, Jones B. Boston Marathon medical care team: 10 years of experience. Phys Sports Med 1988;16:99–106.

5. Ayus JC, Varon J, Arieff AI. Hyponatremia, cerebral edema, and non-cardiogenic pulmonary edema in marathon runners. Ann Intern Med 2000;132:711–4.

6. Adner M, Gembarowicz R, Casey J, Kelley R, Fortin R, Calflin K, et al. Point-of-care biomedical monitoring of Boston Marathon runners. Point-of-Care 2002;1:237–40.

7. Davis D, Videen J, Marino A, Vilke GM, Dunford J, VanCamp S, et al. Exercise-associated hyponatremia in marathon runners: a two-year experience. J Emerg Med 2001;21:47–57.

8. Maron BJ. Sudden death in young athletes. N Eng J Med 2003; 349:1064–75.

9. Thompson P, Buchner D, Piña I, Balady G, Williams M, Marcus B, et al. Exercise and physical activity of in the prevention and treatment of atherosclerotic cardiovascular disease. Circulation 2003;107:3109–16.

10. Giri S, Thompson P, Kiernan F, Clive J, Frain D, Mitchel J, et al. Clinical and angiographic characteristics of exertion-related acute myocardial infarction. JAMA 1999;282:1731–6.

11. Green L, Cohen S, Kurland G. Fatal myocardial infarction in marathon racing. Ann Intern Med 1976;84:704–6.

12. Siegel A, Silverman M, Evans W. Elevated skeletal muscle creatine kinase MB isoenzyme levels in marathon runners. JAMA 1983;250:2835–7.

13. Jaffe A, Ravkilde J, Roberts R, Naslund U, Apple F, Galvani M, et al. It's time for a change to a troponin standard. Circulation 2000;102:1216–20.

14. Ng S, Krishnaswamy P, Morissey R, Clopton P, Fitzgerald R, Maisel A. Ninety-minute accelerated critical pathway for chest pain evaluation. Am J Cardiol 2001;88:611–7.

15. Schmiechen N, Han C, Milzman D. ED use of rapid lactate to evaluate patients with acute chest pain. Ann Emerg Med 1997; 30:571–7.

16. Seiler S. The lactate threshold. http://www.aemma.org/misc/lactate_threshold.htm (accessed February 2004).

17. Hue O, Coman F, Blonc S, Hertogh C. Effect of tropical climate on performance during repeated jump-and-reach tests. J Sports Med Phys Fitness 2003;43:475–80.

18. Itoh H, Ohkuwa T. Ammonia and lactate in the blood after short-term sprint exercise. Eur J Appl Physiol 1991;62:22–5.

19. Osnes J-B, Hermansen L. Acid-base after maximal exercise of short duration. J Appl Physiol 1972;32:59–63.

20. Stansbie D, Begley J. Biochemical consequences of exercise. JIFCC 1991;3:87–90.

21. Mader A, Liesen H, Heck A, Philippi R, Rost R, Schuerch P, et al. Zur Beurteilung der sportartspezifischen Ausdauerieistungsfahigkeit im Labor. Sportarzt u. Sportmed 1976;4:80–8.

22. Houston C, Sutton J, Cymerman A, Reeves J. Operation Everest II: man at high altitude. J Appl Physiol 1987;63:877–82.

23. Bärtsch P, Maggiorini M, Ritter M, Noti C, Vock P, Oelz O. Prevention of high-altitude pulmonary edema by nifedipine. N Eng J Med 1991;325:1284–9.

Chapter 31

Point-of-Care Testing in Diabetes Mellitus

Andrew J. Krentz, Rasaq Olufadi, and Christopher D. Byrne

Diabetes mellitus, already the most common endocrine problem in clinical practice, will soon attain epidemic proportions throughout the world (1, 2). Approximately 5% of populations in developed and developing countries have diabetes. In the United States, for example, there is an estimated population of ~16 million people with diabetes, the global prevalence exceeding 150 million adults (1, 2).

Type 2 diabetes, traditionally regarded as a disorder of the middle-aged and elderly, is becoming a major public health concern in adolescents and children. This appears to be largely attributable to the increasing incidence of childhood obesity, which has resulted from sociocultural changes in western societies. An aging global population, allied to adverse trends in nutrition and habitual physical activity, is projected to increase the worldwide prevalence to >350 million by 2030 (1). Along with serious morbidity associated with specific microvascular complications of diabetes (i.e., retinopathy, nephropathy, and neuropathy), diabetes is a major independent risk factor for atherosclerosis (2). Microvascular complications already present healthcare systems with an enormous and increasing burden (3); diabetic retinopathy remains the single largest cause of visual loss in the working population, while diabetic nephropathy has become the leading cause of end-stage renal failure in western societies.

It is feared that the rapidly rising incidence of diabetes—predominantly type 2 diabetes—will also detonate a time bomb of coronary heart disease, stroke, and peripheral arterial disease; developing countries with limited resources will face potentially insurmountable difficulties (2). Diabetes tends to maximally affect people in their economically productive years, which may adversely affect the economy of emerging countries (4). These considerations provide the rationale for attempts to prevent diabetes and, when established, to minimize the risk of chronic vascular complications (2, 5). Measures directed at controlling blood glucose concentrations and other major cardiovascular risk factors such as dyslipidemia and hypertension are major objectives of management. The poor prognosis of patients with diabetes who develop atherosclerosis adds further impetus to this aim (2). A firm evidence base informs the approach to the patient with diabetes—and to a lesser extent prediabetes—to which a recently expanded therapeutic armamentarium may be brought to bear (6). However, attainment of effective long-term metabolic control continues to present patients and their clinicians with challenges.

Diabetes often detracts from the quality of life. Patients with diabetes generally have to make major lifestyle adjustments, learning to live with dietary restrictions, multiple daily oral antidiabetic agents, and/or insulin injections; self-monitoring of capillary blood glucose is an increasingly important aspect of diabetes management. Intrinsic to the pursuit of glycemic control is the risk of iatrogenic hypoglycemia on one hand, and metabolic decompensation on the other.

Lifestyle changes including regular physical exercise and dietary modification play a critical role in preventing or at least delaying the development of type 2 diabetes in high-risk subjects (7). In obese subjects with impaired glucose tolerance, lifestyle measures or metformin reduced the rate of progression to diabetes in the US Diabetes Prevention Program (7). Translation of the results from such clinical trials into strategies applicable to broader populations remains a major hurdle.

EPIDEMIOLOGY

Type 1 Diabetes. Type 1 diabetes represents 5–15% of all cases of diabetes. Type 1 diabetes generally presents in childhood, the peak age for presentation being 14 years in boys and 11 years in girls. However, type 1 diabetes can occur in any age group, even nonagenarians. Approximately 5% of white individuals >65 years of age are reported to have type 1 diabetes. The incidence of type 1 diabetes is highest in northern European countries. By contrast, the incidence of type 1 diabetes in African and Asian countries is low: approximately 1 case per 100,000 per year.

Type 2 Diabetes. Type 2 diabetes accounts for 85–95% of all cases of diabetes globally. Approximately 2–4% of white populations in western societies have type 2 diabetes. In these countries, roughly 10% of the population >70 years have type 2 diabetes. Type 2 diabetes is considerably more common among Asian and African immigrants in westernized societies such as the United Kingdom. Type 2 diabetes is most commonly diagnosed in those older than 40 years, the incidence rising to a peak at 60–65 years. Type 2 diabetes shows considerable geographical variation. In rural China, for instance, the prevalence of type 2 diabetes is said to be <1%, whereas among the Pima Indians of Arizona, the prevalence exceeds 50%. The prevalence of obesity among Pima Indians is also exceptionally high, about 80% of the population having a body mass index (BMI) > 30 kg/m^2. China and India are expected to experience the greatest increase in type 2 diabetes in the coming decades.

PATHOPHYSIOLOGY

Insulin is an anabolic hormone that plays a pivotal role in the regulation and integration of carbohydrate, protein, and lipid metabolism. Insulin enhances the uptake, utilization, and storage of glucose by tissues such as liver and muscle. It inhibits lipolysis and protein catabolism and promotes electrolyte movement across cell membranes; longer-term effects include modulation of cell differentiation and growth. A detailed discourse on the actions of insulin is beyond the scope of this chapter; recent texts may be consulted for further details (8).

Diabetes mellitus is a clinical condition characterized by persistent hyperglycemia due to relative or absolute lack of insulin. Because the pathophysiology dictates the treatment, a brief discussion of the current classification is warranted (9). In contrast to earlier classifications, the 1997 revision categorizes diabetes according to the underlying pathophysiology rather than its treatment. Diabetes is currently classified as follows:

Type 1. There is an absolute lack of insulin, usually due to selective autoimmune destruction of the insulin-producing β-cells of the pancreatic islets. There is a mandatory requirement for uninterrupted insulin treatment to prevent ketoacidosis. The risk of insulin-induced hypoglycemia is ever present, severe recurrent episodes being the main obstacle to attaining near-normal long-term glycemic control (10).

Type 2. A relative lack of insulin is accompanied in most cases by obesity-related or intrinsic insulin resistance. Dietary nutrition therapy—calorie restriction being the main objective for overweight and obese subjects—is rarely sufficient to provide adequate long-term glycemic control. Accordingly, oral antidiabetic agents—secretagogues, insulin sensitizers, and α-glucosidase inhibitors— are usually required, initially as monotherapy and subsequently in logical combinations (6). For a proportion of subjects, exogenous insulin is ultimately required. There is an increasing trend toward use of a daily dose of long-duration insulin in combination with oral antidiabetic drugs, usually as a prelude to insulin monotherapy (11). This stepwise approach reflects the progressive natural history of type 2 diabetes (12). In the early phase after diagnosis, sufficient residual endogenous insulin secretion exists to enable oral antidiabetic agents to exert glucose-lowering effects; waning of this reserve is held to be the principal cause of the inexorable rise in blood glucose concentrations with time.

Type 3. Diabetes may develop secondary to other diseases (e.g., chronic pancreatitis) or chronic administration of certain drugs (e.g., high-dose corticosteroids). Oral agents or insulin may be required.

Type 4. Denotes diabetes diagnosed during pregnancy; it usually resolves post partum. Insulin is often required temporarily, being used in preference to oral antidiabetic agents.

Consistently satisfactory glycemic control has been proven, within the setting of clinical trials, in patients with type 1 or type 2 diabetes, to reduce the main microvascular and, less effectively, the macrovascular complications of diabetes (10, 12). In addition, the following drugs have been found to be useful in preventing the development or progression of atherosclerosis:

- Antihypertensive drugs
- Lipid-modifying drugs, especially statins
- Antiplatelet drugs

Current treatment strategies are unable to prevent chronic complications. In addition to the increasing use of these drugs, therefore, early detection and treatment of complications such as retinopathy and nephropathy are required. Detection and aggressive management of hypertension reduce the risks of microvascular and macrovascular complications, multifactorial interventions being necessary in many patients with type 2 diabetes (13).

As clinicians delivering ambulatory diabetes care in a UK teaching hospital, our aim here, rather than to provide an exhaustive review of the literature, is to present a clinical perspective. This is informed by the relevant literature and our own experience in the clinic and clinical biochemistry laboratory.

CLINICAL UTILITY OF POINT-OF-CARE TESTING IN DIABETES

The origin of point-of-care testing (POCT) in diabetes can, if some license is permitted, be traced as far back as 1500 B.C.; Hindus living in the Ayur Veda region recorded that flies were attracted to the urine of some people, and that this urine tasted sweet. POCT has a logical role in the management of diabetes. This is because, par excellence among chronic noncommunicable disorders, frequent biochemical monitoring is a critical component of safe and effective management.

It is clearly wildly impractical for trained personnel to visit a patient four or five times every day to test blood glucose levels. A compromise, therefore, is to train these patients on when and how to properly conduct these simple tests. The common POCT tests used to facilitate the diagnosis and, more important, the management of diabetes and its complications include fasting or random capillary blood glucose tests and spot urinalysis for glucose, ketones, albumin, cholesterol, high-density lipoprotein cholesterol (HDLc), and triglyceride concentrations.

Tests including hemoglobin A1c (HbA1c) that have traditionally been performed in clinical biochemistry laboratories are increasingly being relocated outside the laboratory. However, while POCT can offer convenience through avoidance of prior testing and immediate feedback of results to clinician and patient, they cannot be regarded as a replacement for standard laboratory investigations. Although intuitively attractive because they are cheaper and faster, the major downside remains the problem of quality control. Very often, these tests are carried out by nonlaboratory staff who have not been trained to follow the standard operating procedures (SOPs) or adhere to the minimum standards required for performing a simple laboratory test.

Although the abnormal glycation of hemoglobin has been exploited as a measure of glycemic control in diabetic patients, any protein can undergo glycation. Glycation of albumin, for example, is measured by the fructosamine reaction. The normal half-life of albumin, roughly 21 days, is far shorter than that of hemoglobin within the erythrocyte, at approximately 120 days. As a result of this shorter half-life, the fructosamine concentration reflects mean blood glucose over a relatively short period of time: 2–3 weeks on average, compared to mean blood glucose levels of 3–4 months for HbA_{1c} (6). Although measurement of fructosamine is relatively inexpensive and may be used in clinic-based POCT, issues of accuracy and precision have detracted from its widespread adoption.

Variations in Current Practice

As is the case for most UK laboratories, we use a Diabetes Control and Complications Trial (DCCT)-aligned assay for HbA1c (10).

Current practice in our university hospital diabetes clinic requires patients to present themselves for phlebotomy, either at their local surgery or at the hospital phlebotomy service, two weeks or so prior to their next clinic appointment. Clinical chemistry tests will routinely include HbA1c, along with plasma creatinine, electrolytes, and a lipid profile. Urinary albumin:creatinine ratio is also measured in selected patients (see below). At the clinic visit, urinalysis for protein, ketones, and glucose is performed immediately prior to the clinical consultation. However, this system has certain unsurprising disadvantages. In a significant proportion of patients, blood biochemistry tests are not available for the consultation. This may be because the patient ostensibly or actually managed to forget to have the blood drawn or was unable to attend for phlebotomy because of holidays, travel, or other social commitments; in addition, many patients with chronic complication are admitted to the hospital unpredictably (e.g., for acute foot problems or coronary syndromes).

Additional unforeseen problems (e.g., reduced availability of clinical staff at short notice) necessitate rescheduling of appointments, an extra layer of complexity that compounds the problem. Thus, many specialist consultations in our clinic are compromised by a lack of fundamental biochemical information, HbA1c being the gold standard for assessment of glycemic control in clinical practice. Self-collection by the patient of capillary blood into a Sarstedt tube that is then mailed to the clinical chemistry laboratory ahead of the clinic visit is a partial solution to this perennial problem, at least for HbA1c tests.

The overall aim of these investigations is to assess glycemic control, and indirectly to monitor compliance to medication. Clinical decision making is aimed at preventing acute metabolic and long-term diabetic complications. The practical issues considered by the clinician will include:

- Dose adjustment of current medications
- Stepping up treatment (e.g., transfer from oral antidiabetic agents to insulin)
- Timing of the subsequent follow-up appointment

The aforementioned practical difficulties notwithstanding, there can be little doubt that modern biochemical monitoring of patients with diabetes—inextricably allied to advances in antidiabetic medication, notably insulin regimens—provides better overall metabolic control than in past decades. A glance at a classic clinical diabetes text from the late 1960s (14) will leave the contemporary reader marveling at the definition of "good " control, based in those days on a combination of urine testing and casual blood glucose measurements. The overwhelming evidence favoring HbA1c as the best predictor of outcomes in diabetes has rendered such approaches obsolete. HbA1c levels > 7–8% are currently considered to be the threshold for considering intensification or modification of treatment with the aim of improved glycemic control; this assumes that the circumstances of the patient merit such an approach. Employing POCT in the clinic is a means of guaranteeing that HbA1c is available at the time of the consultation. This might be particularly apposite for certain high-risk groups. Adolescents with type 1 diabetes often have very poor chronic glycemic control, which is associated with worse clinical outcomes. In a longitudinal study from the United Kingdom, glycemic control, as assessed by serial HbA1c measurements, was particularly poor in females during late teenage years (15). For the entire cohort, behavioral problems at baseline were related to higher HbA1c levels during 8 years of follow-up (15).

Several assays are available for measuring HbA1c, with high-performance liquid chromatography (HPLC) being regarded as the reference method. However, the majority of these assays are technically difficult and time-consuming—the upshot being that the result may not be available in time for the patient's clinic visit. As a result, an important part of clinical decision making is not available. Consequently, results and recommended changes in therapy are communicated post hoc to the patients, usually through their general practitioners (primary care physicians). The inefficiency of this approach does not require elaboration. HbA1c can now be obtained using a benchtop analyzer (DCA 2000; Bayer, Elkhart, IN, USA) that provides accurate and reliable results (16). Desktop analyzers can determine HbA1c levels rapidly and reliably, with a cost comparable to HPLC methodology. Recommended guidelines for measuring HbA1c at the point of care include the following:

- Analyses are performed to a standard that benefits patient care by having in place:
    Appropriate quality control procedures
    Staff training programs
    Equipment maintenance programs
- The results obtained are clinically comparable to those obtained by laboratory methods.
- Unnecessary duplication of laboratory services is avoided.
- Experienced individuals are responsible for the procurement of equipment for POCT.

In a recent report from a prominent academic diabetes center in the United States, the immediate feedback provided by the benchtop analyzer was associated with a significant decrease in subsequent HbA1c in insulin-treated patients at 6- and 12-month follow-up; HbA1c did not change in a control group (16). Instant feedback of HbA1c results was thought to facilitate adjustment of insulin dosages and regimens. The improvement in glycemic control was not accompanied by an increase in episodes of severe disabling hypoglycemia, visits to the hospital emergency room, or increased use of health resources (16). We consider this aspect of POCT in more detail below. In a randomized study of the effects of immediate versus delayed availability of HbA1c results in a heterogeneous sample of African-American patients with type 2 diabetes managed by diet, oral agents, or insulin, immediate availability of results appeared to facilitate better diabetes management (17). Whether this was attributable simply to more effective dose adjustment or perhaps linked to more subjective issues about the confidence of the patients and their clinicians in the results merits further evaluation.

CAPILLARY BLOOD GLUCOSE MEASUREMENT

Self-monitoring of blood glucose offers patients the ability to fine-tune insulin treatment. For motivated, intelligent patients, medical practitioners being among the most successful in this regard, excellent long-term glycemic control is attainable with modern insulin regimens.

Improvements in bedside capillary glucose testing technology have been considerable in the past 10–15 years. The main sources of error, especially with the first generation of glucose meters, related to the need to obtain the correct quantity of blood and the requirement that the operator manually wipe the test strip clean after a specified interval. An analytical time of ~2 min has been reduced to ~45 s with modern (so-called third generation) glucose meters (18). There was also the problem of data management, because the first glucometers had no capacity for electronic recordkeeping. Apart from a few instances of very high or low glucose levels, blood glucose readings obtained using these devices show good correlations with results obtained on the same group of patients in the standard clinical laboratory. However, methodological problems, notably with inaccuracy of readings in the hypoglycemic range, seem to persist. Witness the not-infrequent scenario wherein a general practitioner suspects spontaneous or reactive hypoglycemia in an anxious nondiabetic patient with nonspecific symptoms; the patient is duly provided with a glucose meter and a few days later presents a record of blood glucose concentrations that appear to support the diagnosis. Only when rigorous laboratory-measured samples are obtained does the apparent hypoglycemia evaporate. Nonclinical or nonlaboratory staff operators can generally obtain accurate results provided that a well-monitored training and quality control program is practiced and operator competency is maintained.

Inaccuracies are perhaps more common than is recognized among hospitalized patients with diabetes (see below).

Application of this methodology in clinical practice has expanded, in part reflecting greater awareness of the morbidity associated with poor metabolic control and the high prevalence of patients with diabetes in the hospital—at least 15% on general medical and surgical wards in our institution (Betts P, personal communication, January 2003). Capillary glucose monitoring is used in variety of clinical scenarios (Table 31-1).

The issues surrounding monitoring of patients with diabetes admitted to the hospital merits further comment. This is rightly regarded as being the equivalent of a vital sign in diabetic patients (19). The UK National Service Framework for Diabetes (20) calls for improvements in managing diabetes in hospitals (Standard 8); patients should be more involved in the daily care of their diabetes when hospitalized than has traditionally been the case. In our day-to-day experience there is considerable scope for improved education of hospital nursing and medical staff, particularly on nonmedical wards (units). Data suggesting that clinical outcomes in high-risk groups can be improved through meticulous control of blood glucose concentrations (21, 22) should be a spur to focusing more attention on the critically ill patient with hyperglycemia.

Self-Monitoring of Diabetes— What Is the Benefit?

Behavioral changes required of diabetic patients are often complex, numerous, and, traditionally at least, restrictive. Self-monitoring of blood glucose is now regarded as an essential component of management for all patients treated with insulin and for selected patients with type 2 diabetes receiving oral antidiabetic drugs. There seems no realistic doubt that POCT can be beneficial to diabetic patients. Examples include:

- Ensuring adequate day-to-day glycemic control in the face of differing meal compositions, changing mealtimes, and variable physical activity levels
- Detecting and averting hypoglycemia
- Assessing and maintaining metabolic control during acute illness

Table 31-1 Clinical Indications for Capillary Blood Glucose Monitoring

Preprandial and postprandial testing to guide self-managed adjustments of insulin doses by patients with insulin-treated diabetes, e.g., in response to variations in composition or timing of meals, exercise, or intercurrent illness
Monitoring of metabolically unstable hospitalized patients, e.g., perioperatively, during treatment of hyperglycemic and hypoglycemic emergencies, acute coronary syndromes, etc.
Rapid screening for undiagnosed hyperglycemia, especially in patients admitted to the hospital with acute illnesses, e.g., pneumonia, cellulitis

However, there is still a tendency among some healthcare professionals to equate the simple fact that a patient has the capacity to monitor his or her diabetes with improved long-term clinical outcomes. Certainly, the *potential* is there if the patient has received—and has been receptive to —instruction about the key issues. All too often, though, it seems that even surrogate biochemical indicators such as HbA1c concentration fail to be favorably influenced by rigorous self-testing per se. Any diabetologist or diabetes clinical nurse specialist will attest to the frustrating experience of being presented with a list of diligently collected home blood glucose readings yet seemingly finding themselves unable to assist in improving overall glycemic control through useful advice. Thus, there is often a sizeable gap between the theoretical promise of self-monitoring and the reality of translating this into tangible benefits for the patient. The reasons for this disparity are complex and may vary from patient to patient.

A minor practical point: an unfortunate coincidence for clinicians using the *Systeme Internationale* is the numerical similarity of units of blood glucose (in mmol/L) and HbA1c (in %); this often causes confusion in the minds of patients who, incidentally, are often not aware that carbohydrate consumption in the hours prior to measurement of HbA1c does not affect the result.

Type 1 Diabetes. Is it fair to say that self-monitoring of blood glucose has failed to live up to expectations (23), or has it instead "revolutionized" management of diabetes, as the American Diabetes Association suggests (24)? The answer will depend on who is asked and what the objectives of self-monitoring were thought to be for the individual patient. Current median HbA1c values for patients with type 1 diabetes are typically ~8–8.5%. Clearly, self-monitoring is no panacea, but it undoubtedly has value in selected patients with type 1 diabetes in the quest for near-normoglycemia that characterizes the modern era of intensive insulin treatment. This was ushered in by the results of the DCCT in 1993 (10). This trial—large, expensive, and intensive in more senses than merely more daily injections—demonstrated that intensive diabetes management could reduce the risk of microvascular complications in young, intelligent, motivated patients with type 1 diabetes. Self-monitoring of blood glucose was performed at least four times daily by patients randomized to the intensified treatment group, the latter comprising ≥3 injections daily or continuous subcutaneous insulin infusion (CSII). This was backed up by frequent face-to-face contact with dedicated healthcare professionals fired by the desire to drive glucose levels down toward the nondiabetic range. While a 2% reduction in mean HbA1c concentration was achieved in the intensive treatment group—with clinically relevant reductions in the development and progression of retinopathy and other microvascular complications—this was at the expense of weight gain and a threefold increase in the risk of severe hypoglycemia (10). Thus, intensified insulin treatment was judged not suitable for all patients, the risks of hypoglycemia possibly outweighing advantages in vulnerable patients. Intensive therapy should be used with great caution in certain groups (Table 31-2).

Table 31-2 Patients with Type 1 Diabetes in Whom Intensive Therapy Is Contraindicated

Patients with a history of repeated severe hypoglycemia
Patients under the age of 13 years
Those with advanced diabetic complications including end-stage renal disease, cardiovascular disease, and cerebrovascular disease

Self-monitoring of capillary blood glucose is generally regarded as mandatory, wherever possible, for patients treated with insulin (19). Exceptions will include exceedingly frail or disabled patients (e.g., those with deforming rheumatoid disease or poststroke patients); a caregiver or healthcare professional may be able to undertake at least occasional testing. Intensified insulin regimens using multiple daily injections or CSII require that patients be prepared to test their blood glucose concentrations four or more times daily. In the United Kingdom, current interest in flexible, intensified insulin adjusted for a more relaxed diet than has been the convention (25) also demands a commitment to frequent self-testing. Anecdotally, patients are prepared to undertake more intensive self-monitoring if they perceive benefits in terms of empowerment.

It should be acknowledged that fabrication of results is a genuine—and probably underappreciated—clinical issue. For example, a small study of diabetes in pregnancy in Newcastle, UK, using a self-monitoring device to download information showed that selective recordings in patient diaries—with a tendency to omit high readings—suggested the potential for underestimating the true degree of glycemic fluctuation (26). The implication of this finding was that near-normal HbA1c concentrations might hide pathological episodic hyperglycemia, thereby offering a potential explanation for the continuing high incidence of macrosomia in diabetic pregnancies. The potential for deliberate deception occasionally attains bizarre proportions, an example being the young patient with type 1 diabetes who claims complete remission of her disease (27). There is a more general clinical issue that is rarely discussed, i.e., that HbA1c concentrations provide no useful information about the daily glycemic profiles that are necessary to guide changes in insulin doses. It should also be noted that because HbA1c provides a measure weighted toward more recent blood glucose levels, a recent episode of major hyperglycemia could exert a disproportionate influence (28).

The complementary information supplied by appropriate self-monitoring of capillary blood glucose is useful in certain commonly encountered clinical scenarios:

- *Clinical diabetic nephropathy.* In patients with uremia, reduced erythrocyte survival and erythropoietin-dependent anemia lead to underestimation of daily hyperglycemia because of false-low glycated hemoglobin concentrations; this is often not appreciated by healthcare professionals. Subclinical nephropathy—so-called microalbuminuria (see below)—is not usually associated with this problem.

- *Anemia.* Almost any cause of anemia—or recent blood transfusion—will tend to result in false-low HbA1c levels either acutely or in the longer term.
- *Hemoglobinopathies.* Certain inherited hemoglobinopathies are associated with spurious HbA1c measurements.
- *Impaired symptomatic awareness of hypoglycemia.* This is a major complication of long-duration type 1 diabetes (29); affected patients are at increased risk of recurrent severe hypoglycemia. Restoration of warning symptoms can be achieved in some patients if biochemical hypoglycemia is scrupulously avoided for several weeks; rigorous self-monitoring of blood glucose is an integral component of this intervention.
- *Asymptomatic nocturnal hypoglycemia.* This is more common than is generally appreciated and may contribute to the aforementioned syndrome of impaired symptomatic awareness of hypoglycemia. Setting the alarm clock in order to wake and self-test in the early hours of the morning may reveal asymptomatic hypoglycemia that is amenable to therapeutic manipulation (e.g., use of prolonged-duration analog before bed in place of isophane insulin).

These caveats also apply to some patients with type 2 diabetes. Because insulin is usually regarded as a treatment of last resort, an impending transfer to insulin should be prefaced by introduction to self-testing of blood glucose (30); even elderly or frail patients often find that they can successfully accomplish the task and are often interested to receive the near-instantaneous feedback that self-testing generates. Moreover, patients seem to be able to accept administering their insulin injections—which are often feared not least because of anticipated discomfort. In reality, self-testing of blood glucose by lancet tends to be somewhat less comfortable than injecting insulin using modern fine-bore needles, claims by some manufacturers of "virtually pain-free testing" notwithstanding.

Type 2 Diabetes. The United Kingdom Prospective Diabetes Study (UKPDS) demonstrated that sustained HbA1c values close to 7% were associated with a reduced likelihood of long-term microvascular complications in patients with type 2 diabetes (12). Approximately 20–30% of patients with type 2 diabetes will ultimately require insulin therapy because of progressive loss of insulin secretion, self-monitoring being the aim in the majority.

Whether routine self-monitoring of blood glucose is advantageous in most patients treated with diet or oral agents has been the subject of much debate (31). The paucity of reliable information on this point (32) has led to something of a backlash from general practitioners in the United Kingdom keen to reduce the expense associated with a perceived explosion of self-monitoring. The limitations of poorly reported studies with limited statistical power have not deterred some investigators from embarking upon meta-analysis, an approach unlikely to usefully advance knowledge given the quality of the available data (32); accordingly, the meta-analysis of Coster et al. (32) had wide confidence intervals for the reduction in HbA1c concentrations that may have obscured a benefit of self-monitoring of blood glucose.

Until such time that it is clearly demonstrated that self-monitoring by tablet-treated patients improves glycemic control, it seems reasonable to follow recommendations for 2–6 monthly measures of HbA1c in patients with type 2 diabetes, the frequency being determined by stability and level of glycemic control (33). Because dose escalation of a given oral antidiabetic agent is unlikely to produce much in the way of additional blood glucose lowering, there is perhaps some justification to this restrictive approach. When assessing the effect of adding a thiazolidinedione, for example, the genomic action of the drug means that a maximal reduction in blood glucose is unlikely to be observed for several weeks. This, however, is not to imply that there is no role for self-monitoring of blood glucose in some patients with type 2 diabetes. Patients already receiving a secretagogue who have reasonably good glycemic control prior to the addition of the thiazolidinedione may start to experience hypoglycemia a few weeks into the combination therapy. This potentially hazardous situation can be anticipated, and self-monitoring of blood glucose will provide timely warning of impending trouble well ahead of any changes in HbA1c concentration. This is another example wherein safety issues are the prime indication for self-monitoring. Having said this, it is not uncommon to encounter elderly patients with stable type 2 diabetes who are testing their capillary glucose religiously day in and day out because the ill-informed advice of an inexperienced healthcare professional has not been countered; such patients are usually grateful to be relieved of a burden that provides little useful information and contributes to the somewhat punitive connotations—real or imagined—that accompany management of type 2 diabetes.

What of patients with type 2 diabetes who are already receiving insulin? In a US study of 201 insulin-treated veterans (mean age 65 years; >90% male) with type 2 diabetes, an 8-week period of intensified self-monitoring of blood glucose—four or more times daily—was associated with a short-term improvement in glycemic control. Tests were performed before main meals, the last being performed at bedtime. A significant and sustained decrease in HbA1c was observed from the fourth week of commencing intensified blood glucose monitoring (34). The glycemic benefits of the intensified frequency of monitoring were only observed in patients with a baseline HbA1c > 8.0% whose compliance with monitoring was >75%. With the rapidly increasing global population of patients with type 2 diabetes, more data are required about how to optimize insulin therapy. These patients are increasingly younger at diagnosis and so will face decades of life with diabetes, during much of which they are likely to be treated with insulin. Concomitant obesity adds a further challenge to attaining good long-term glycemic control in these patients (35). Application of strategies to influence self-care behavior in relation to interventions such as self-monitoring of blood glucose require further evaluation in this and other groups (36).

Future Developments in Blood Glucose Monitoring

Continuous measurement of glucose using implantable (28) or noninvasive (37) sensors linked to improvements in allied information technology may offer additional benefits (e.g., alerting patients to nocturnal hypoglycemia). Examples of these technologies are entering clinical practice, and this field is likely to advance in coming years. A preliminary estimate of the cost-effectiveness of the GlucoWatch Biographer® (Cygnus, Redwood City, CA, USA) in young patients with type 1 diabetes appeared favorable, based on a model derived from the DCCT and making certain assumptions (38).

Serious infectious diseases, such as HIV and viral hepatitis, transmitted via needlestick injuries are a major occupational hazard to healthcare providers. A new method of perforating skin to obtain capillary blood uses a battery-operated laser device (39). The device uses a portable pulsed erbium: yttrium-aluminium-garnet laser. This device has been shown to be suitable for use in POCT settings while avoiding the hazard posed by the use of lancets.

KETONEMIA

Hyperglycemic emergencies in patients with diabetes cause considerable morbidity and appreciable mortality, even in highly developed health systems (40). Diabetic ketoacidosis is a common, life-threatening metabolic emergency with a mortality rate of approximately 5% (41). Hyperosmolar nonketotic hyperglycemia carries a higher fatality rate of ~15% (42).

The total cost of treating these emergencies—which invariably require hospital management—is considerable. In the mid-1990s, hospital admissions for ketoacidosis or ketosis in the United States cost an estimated $650 million per year. *Ketosis* may be defined as an increase in blood concentration of ketone bodies, which are buffered by bicarbonate. Once the buffering capacity is exceeded, frank ketoacidosis will develop rapidly without appropriate intervention. Because all cases of diabetic ketoacidosis are theoretically preventable (sufficient insulin being able to counter developing hyperketonemia), testing for ketones during intercurrent illness is a key aspect of education of the patient with type 1 diabetes. However, there is little evidence that the incidence of diabetic ketoacidosis has fallen appreciably in recent decades.

Traditionally, patients have been instructed to test regularly for urinary ketones, their presence being an indication for a temporary increase in the dose of insulin. All too often, however, the increased insulin doses associated with acute illness fail to be administered. This is sometimes a difficult task even in a controlled and supervised environment. The resulting hyperketonemia leads to vomiting and, usually in conjunction with a glucose-driven osmotic diuresis, a rapidly progressive metabolic decompensation. Significant ketosis may develop rapidly in patients with type 1 diabetes if insulin therapy is interrupted, even in the absence of intercurrent illness and pathological levels of counterregulatory hormones (43).

In patients presenting with uncontrolled diabetes or classic clinical features, rapid bedside investigation should include prompt testing for urinary ketones. If results are positive, or if urine is not available, circulating bicarbonate, glucose, and lactate concentrations are measured and the anion gap calculated; all these tests can readily be performed on a capillary or

arterial blood sample using a standard emergency department gas analyzer (44). Plasma ketones can be semiquantitatively measured in the laboratory using Ketostix® (Bayer Diagnostics, Medfield, MA, USA), but treatment should not be delayed pending the results of laboratory-based investigations.

Urinary Ketone Tests

At our institution, Multistix® or Ketostix (Bayer Diagnostics, Medfield, MA, USA) are used to test for ketonuria. Both are based on the nitroprusside reaction, providing a semiquantitative assessment of ketonuria that is near specific for acetoacetate. The main ketone bodies produced in humans are acetoacetate (with acetone formed by nonenzymatic decarboxylation) and 3-hydroxybutyrate.

3-hydroxybutyrate dehydrogenase

$$\text{Acetoacetate} + NADH + H^+ \rightarrow \text{3-hydroxybutyrate} + NAD^+$$

The inability of Ketostix to detect 3-hydroxybutyrate is rarely a major disadvantage because the blood acetoacetate–3-hydroxybutyrate ratio is generally in equilibrium. It is often stated that use of Ketostix can underestimate the severity of ketoacidosis, particularly if tissue anoxia is also present. In this likely clinical scenario, there is an increased ratio of NADH to NAD^+, resulting in a shift in the equilibrium in favor of 3-hydroxybutyrate, the ratio rising perhaps as high as 1:10 (45). Despite the obvious limitations of this test, it is regarded as a good screening test for ketoacidosis, having a high sensitivity and negative predictive value. A negative Ketostix reaction effectively excludes significant ketosis, although prolonged exposure of test strips to air or ingestion of large amounts of ascorbic acid may give false negative results. Captopril, and other free sulphydryl drugs (46), including N-acetylcysteine, may rarely give a false positive result.

POCT for Blood 3-Hydroxybutyrate

It has recently become possible to provide POCT for ketonemia using an electrochemical ketone sensor (MediSense Optium, Abbott Laboratories, Abbott Park, IL, USA) (47). The handheld sensor produces an electrical current proportional to the blood 3-hydroxybutyrate concentration; 5–10 μL of capillary blood is required, and the result is displayed within 30 s. Blood 3-hydroxybutyrate concentrations <0.5 mmol/L (<5.3 mg/dL) are accepted as normal [hyperketonemia being defined as >1.0 mmol/L (>10.2 mg/dL)] (48). Ketoacidosis may be considered to be present when blood 3-hydroxybutyrate concentration is >3 mmol/L (>30.6 mg/dL). Use of separate electrodes confers the ability to measure both 3-hydroxybutyrate and glucose. The blood 3-hydroxybutyrate concentration measured using the handheld ketone sensor correlated well with a laboratory enzymatic reference method, the POCT device having similar accuracy and precision (49). Moreover, there was no reported interference by acetoacetate during measurement of 3-hydroxybutyrate.

Self-Testing for Blood 3-Hydroxybutyrate

Many patients have a negative perception of testing urine for ketones; consequently compliance has understandably been low. The handheld sensor, with its digital display, may increase patient compliance with self-testing for ketones (49). In the way that self-monitoring of glucose by fingerstick has almost universally replaced urine glucose testing, it is tempting to speculate that electrochemical determination of 3-hydroxybutyrate might replace self-testing for urinary ketones. Clearly, patients may benefit from early warning of imminent ketoacidosis. Blood ketone testing provides more rapid diagnosis of elevated ketone levels than urine testing (49). This may be particularly important for groups recognized to be at risk of rapid development of diabetic ketoacidosis, including children (50), patients treated with CSII (49), and pregnant women with type 1 diabetes (51). Anecdotally, knowledge of rising blood 3-hydroxybutyrate concentration may encourage patients to appropriately administer more insulin (47). However, for the reasons alluded to above, whether the ability to measure blood ketones will produce a reduction in hospital admissions for diabetic ketoacidosis remains to be determined. Based on a relatively small sample of patients, Wallace et al. (48) suggested guidelines for the interpretation of blood ketone levels in patients with type 1 diabetes (Table 31-3).

Monitoring Response to Treatment of Diabetic Ketoacidosis

With adequate treatment, 3-hydroxybutyrate levels can be expected to fall by approximately $1 \text{ mmol} \cdot L^{-1} \cdot h^{-1}$ during management of diabetic ketoacidosis (48). Apparent failure to respond to treatment may necessitate an increased dose of insulin, although inadequate rehydration, obstructed venous access, or failure of the electromechanical infusion pump must be excluded (41). Ketonuria may persist for >24 hours, long after resolution of the metabolic acidosis; this reflects increased conversion of 3-hydroxybutyrate to acetoacetate. This may give an erroneous clinical impression that the patient is not responding optimally to treatment. As mentioned above, changes in blood glucose and ketone concentrations do not necessarily parallel one another. Using the handheld sensor, a

3-hydroxybutyrate concentration < 0.5 mmol/L (<5.1 mg/dL) will reassure the clinician that the ketoacidosis has resolved (48).

ALBUMINURIA

Only ~25–30% of patients with long-duration type 1 diabetes develop nephropathy (52, 53). For these patients, and for a similar proportion of those with type 2 diabetes, the clinical challenge lies in identifying those who will progress to end-stage renal failure, as well as those who will succumb to accelerated atherosclerosis along the way. Up to 50% of dialysis patients in the United States have diabetes, mainly type 2 diabetes. The incidence of end-stage renal disease also differs among various population groups. In the United States, for example, the incidence of end-stage renal disease secondary to diabetes is higher in Hispanics, African-Americans, and Native Americans compared with non-Hispanic white patients.

The DCCT demonstrated a significant reduction in risk of developing microalbuminuria in patients with type 1 diabetes randomized to intensified insulin therapy (10). This protective effect was sustained even after completion of the trial, the so-called legacy effect (54). For patients with type 2 diabetes, the UKPDS provided evidence of the renoprotective effects of improved glycemic control (12) and tight control of hypertension (55).

At diagnosis of diabetes, functional changes that have been described include renal hypertrophy and increased glomerular filtration rate; these are reversible with control of hyperglycemia. After several years' duration of diabetes, nephropathy can be detected at a relatively—and potentially retardable—early stage by the presence of so-called microalbuminuria. This somewhat inelegant term refers to the excessive excretion of albumin, albeit in quantities too small to be revealed by routine dipstick testing, i.e., 30–300 mg albumin/day (20–200 μg/min) (52). At this subclinical stage, histological features of diabetic nephropathy are already established, although glomerular filtration rate is well preserved. Microalbuminuria not only predicts progression—albeit less reliably than was originally thought, according to some reports (56)—to more advanced stages of diabetic nephropathy but also serves as a marker for atherosclerotic cardiovascular disease. It is hypothesized that microalbuminuria reflects generalized endothelial dysfunction, an early stage in the development of atherosclerosis. Consistent with this observation, diabetic patients with microalbuminuria tend to have more marked insulin resistance, as assessed using methods such as the euglycemic hyperinsulinemic clamp technique, than their counterparts with normal albumin excretion rates (57). The prevalence of dyslipidemia and hypertension rises as nephropathy progresses (Figure 31-1).

Clinical proteinuria is readily detectable using standard urine dipsticks, being defined as ≥300 mg/24 h (200 μg/min on a timed collection). When persistent proteinuria has developed, the glomerular filtration rate declines inexorably over several years unless effective antihypertensive medication is

Table 31-3   Guidelines for Interpretation of Blood Ketone Levels in Patients with Type 1 Diabetes

Check blood ketones if blood glucose is >15 mmol/L (150 mg/dL)	
Blood 3-Hydroxybutyrate, mmol/L (mg/dL)	Action
0–1.0 (0–10.2)	Treat hyperglycemia appropriately
1.1–3.0 (11.2–30.6)	Retest glucose and ketones in 1 h
>3.0 (>30.6)	Seek medical assistance

Source: Data from Wallace et al. (48).

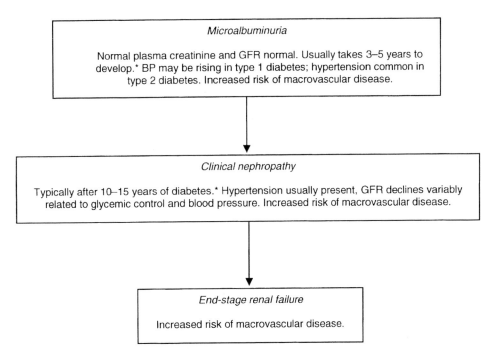

Figure 31-1   Main stages in the development of diabetic nephropathy used in clinical practice. GFR, glomerular filtration rate; BP, blood pressure. *May be present at diagnosis of type 2 diabetes due to long asymptomatic phase of hyperglycemia.

initiated. Ultimately, dialysis or renal transplantation is required.

Annual screening for microalbuminuria is recommended for patients with type 1 diabetes from age 12 years and all patients with type 2 diabetes from diagnosis (58–60).

Screening for microalbuminuria—and early introduction of drugs that block the renin-angiotensin system—is regarded as being highly cost-effective (61). Treatment of end-stage renal disease is very expensive, with estimates from the mid-1990s of ~$50,000 per year for dialysis. For the purpose of screening, first-voided morning urine is the recommended sample for determining the albumin:creatinine ratio (58–60). Alternatively, a 24-hour urine collection for albumin excretion can also be performed, although this is considerably more difficult in practice and unwieldy for screening purposes. Screening in some centers is carried out using semiquantitative dipstick testing (59, 60). Such tests, when carried out by trained personnel, reportedly have acceptable sensitivity and specificity (approximately 95% for each). However, microalbuminuria should be confirmed provided two or more consecutive urine samples are positive over a period of 3–6 months, two of three being necessary to sustain the diagnosis of microalbuminuria (Figure 31-2) (60). The thresholds for diagnosing microalbuminuria—or greater degrees of proteinuria—are:

- Men, 2.5 mg/mmol (21.9 mg/g)
- Women, 3.5 mg/mmol (30.6 mg/g)

It should be noted, however, that certain physiological and pathological conditions may transiently increase urinary albumin excretion (Table 31-4).

Good glycemic control (HbA1c < 8%), low systolic blood pressure, lower plasma lipid levels, and avoidance of cigarettes are associated with greater probability of regression of microalbuminuria, or at least delayed progression of diabetic renal disease. The prevalence of hypertension is high in patients with diabetic nephropathy and is often difficult to control (62).

DYSLIPIDEMIA

The importance of measuring lipids as part of coronary heart disease risk assessment in patients with diabetes is now well established in clinical practice. However, there is still debate as to whether diabetes should be regarded as a cardiovascular risk equivalent. Individuals with type 2 diabetes are at greater risk of cardiovascular events than individuals who do not have diabetes (63). Haffner et al. (64) showed that the risk of death from coronary heart disease (CHD) for subjects with diabetes without prior myocardial infarction was similar to that of nondiabetic subjects with prior myocardial infarction in a Finnish population. However, Evans et al. (65) found that the risk of all-cause mortality was lower among subjects with diabetes than among those with a history of myocardial infarction in both cross-sectional and cohort study designs in a Scottish population. An explanation for these apparently discrepant findings is the heterogeneity of risk in individuals with type 2 diabetes. The majority, but not all, of the individuals with type 2 diabetes also have insulin resistance and metabolic syndrome, particularly the typical pattern of dyslipidemia with reduced HDLc and increased triglyceride concentrations. The proportion of individuals with diabetes that also have this pattern of dyslipidemia is likely to vary among populations. It

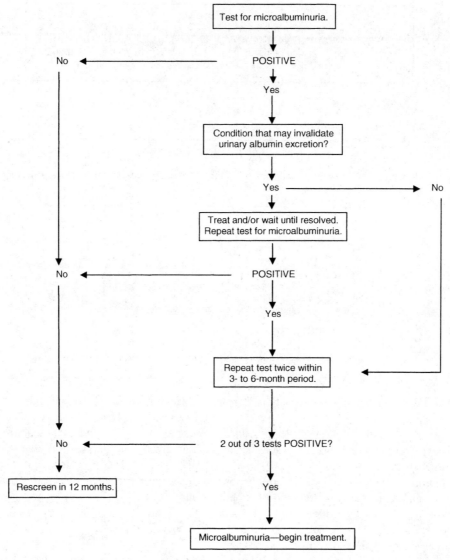

Figure 31-2 Screening for microalbuminuria. Treatment consists of intensified glycemic and blood pressure control; attention to other cardiovascular risk factors. Adapted from (60).

is possible that the presence of the metabolic syndrome, and specifically this pattern of dyslipidemia, contributes to increased risk of CHD above the risk conferred by hyperglycemia alone. Support for this notion can be found in the analysis of the data for individuals with diabetes in the National Health and Nutrition Education Survey (NHANES) III, in which the presence of the metabolic syndrome (and not the presence of

Table 31-4   Alternative Causes of Increased Urinary Albumin Excretion in Patients with Diabetes

Vigorous exercise
Urinary tract infection
Febrile illnesses
Heart failure
Acute hyperglycemic metabolic decompensation

diabetes per se) was associated with CHD in a cross-sectional analysis of the data (66).

Unlike total cholesterol or LDLc, HDLc and triglyceride levels are not targets for treatment to reduce risk of CHD despite good evidence that both are cardiovascular risk factors. Statins, through their LDLc-lowering effect, can reduce the risk of CHD and cardiovascular death by 25–33% in both primary and secondary prevention situations. To date, the best evidence for the efficacy of any lipid-lowering treatment in reducing cardiovascular events in patients with and without diabetes is for statin therapy. The National Institute for Clinical Excellence (NICE) in the United Kingdom has published guidelines for the management of lipids in type 2 diabetes, and the General Medical Services (GMS) contract for primary care in the United Kingdom has recommended treatment of total cholesterol to a target of 5.0 mmol/L (193 mg/dL) in patients with diabetes. However treatment with statins only reduces relative risk of cardiovascular events by approximately a quarter, and therefore absolute risk remains relatively high. Although there are presently no recommended targets for either HDLc or plasma triglyceride concentrations, treatment for this specific dyslipidemia should also be considered. Data from the UK Prospective Diabetes Study show that low HDLc is a risk factor for various cardiovascular disease outcomes among people with diabetes, independent of elevated LDLc, hyperglycemia, hypertension, and smoking (67). The lowest tertile of HDLc in UKPDS participants for this study was <0.95 mmol/L (<37 mg/dL). In the United States, the National Cholesterol Education Program Adult Treatment Panel III guidelines state that HDLc concentrations < 1.0 mmol/L (<39 mg/dL) for both men and women should be considered a threshold for increased coronary risk, based on expert opinion (68). Although women have higher HDLc levels, the panel decided that different cutpoints by sex would result in women at otherwise low risk being identified as eligible for LDLc-lowering drugs. A higher level of HDLc [<1.3 mmol/L (<50 mg/dL)] was defined as a marginal risk factor in women, which indicates that they would be eligible for more intensive lifestyle intervention. Treatment options for the low HDLc–high triglyceride pattern of dyslipidemia include lifestyle modifications and pharmacological interventions with fibrates, n-3 fatty acids, or nicotinic acid (niacin). Because it is accepted that an HDLc concentration < 1.0 mmol/L (<39 mg/dL) is an important CHD risk factor (see above), it is reasonable to postulate that an HDLc level ≥ 1.0 mmol/L (≥39 mg/dL) should be considered a treatment goal; therefore, it is important to consider HDLc measurement also as part of POCT in patients with diabetes. However, to date most POCT data for lipids relate to blood cholesterol.

Recent advances, in particular the development of the so-called reagent test strip, have produced a proliferation of inexpensive and convenient systems for the measurement of blood cholesterol outside the laboratory (69). Dry chemistry analyzers such as the Reflotron (Boehringer, now Roche Diagnostics, Mannheim, Germany), Cholestech (Cholestech, Hayward, CA, USA), and Ektachem DT-60 (Kodak, now Johnson and Johnson, Rochester, NY, USA) are now available to measure plasma lipids. In a comparative study of plasma and capillary venous blood from 47 fasting subjects, total HDLc and triglyceride concentrations were analyzed using these analyzers and a CDC-certified laboratory (70). Accuracy was evaluated by comparing the results of each portable analyzer against the CDC reference method. Compared to the reference method, the Ektachem and Reflotron provided significantly lower values for total cholesterol. In addition, the Cholestech and Ektachem values for HDLc were higher than the CDC values. The Reflotron and Cholestech provided higher values of triglyceride concentration than the CDC method. The Ektachem and Cholestech analyzers met the current NCEP III guidelines for accuracy in measurement of total cholesterol, while only the Ektachem met guidelines for triglyceride concentrations. In summary, all three analyzers provided a good

overall risk classification, but it was noted that values of HDLc should be used only for screening at-risk individuals.

Although the analytical performance of the reagent strips and meters can be evaluated easily in the laboratory, this information is obviously not applicable to the performance of the instrument in the hands of the individual user who lacks professional training. The establishment of a quality-control program adapted to this new approach to biochemical testing remains an important challenge, because conventional quality-control procedures with lyophilized materials or liquid ethylene glycol–based materials often are inappropriate (71).

In cost-effective population screening, extralaboratory testing by, for example, primary care clinics, pharmacies, or general practitioners could play a major part provided that their results are reliable, accurate, and reproducible. Although the accuracy and precision of high-quality POCT devices in the hands of trained laboratory technicians are excellent, little information exists on the accuracy and reproducibility of results obtained under day-to-day conditions at various point-of-care centers. In a recent study involving POCT in pharmacies (72), the analytical performance of a single point-of-care instrument and of a laboratory analyzer were compared. Between-pharmacy analytical variation was larger than between-laboratory variation (11% vs. 6.1% for cholesterol). Cholesterol assays showed a bias of −5.6 to 16.6% in pharmacies compared with −10.6 to 3.7% in laboratories. The percentage of closeness to the homeostatic set point for a single cholesterol determination performed in any pharmacy was 23.6%, and the corresponding value for the laboratories was 15.6%. Calibration bias in pharmacies may have explained the higher between-pharmacy variation than that observed between laboratories. The National Cholesterol Education Program recommends a performance of 3% CV with a 3% bias for determination of total cholesterol concentration (73, 74). This recommendation would result in a total error of 8.9% [total error = % absolute bias + (1.96 × CV_A)] vs. the true value in situations where cholesterol is determined as a single measurement affected by both systematic and random error (75). In our view it is likely that a total error of <10% would be acceptable for making treatment decisions in most cases.

Until relatively recently it was common practice to measure HDLc after serum or plasma had been pretreated with both a polyanion, such as that of phosphotungstic acid, dextran sulfate, or heparin, and a divalent metal ion (76–80). Recently, however, the practice has shifted toward assays without a pretreatment step. A direct HDLc assay is effective in reducing sample processing and reducing assay time. A large number of reagent kits are now available for large automated analyzers (81, 82). Although laboratory automation has recently been the trend, there are problems associated with this methodology, including the need for high capital investment for equipment that cannot be used for POCT (83). In addition, lipid test samples are likely to undergo denaturation during sample transportation and storage (84). In an attempt to overcome these problems, researchers have developed a dry chemistry–based assay using surfactants and have also developed a dedicated reagent (85). These investigators developed an assay system with excellent precision, dilution linearity, and inter-method comparison. This assay uses only surfactants for specificity in the direct HDLc method and may be useful for POCT in the future.

COST-EFFECTIVENESS OF POCT FOR DIABETES

Inevitably, a major concern about laboratory tests in general, including POCT, is whether this methodology and its use is cost effective (86). Tests such as HbA1c are potentially cost saving in the long term through reduced resource utilization (87, 88). Diabetes is costly to manage, and the majority of this expense is consumed in treating late-stage, potentially preventable complications. The economic costs of diabetes in the United States are estimated to be >$100 million per year (89). Intensified treatment, guided by laboratory tests and/or POCT, is an accepted principle of management that has a firm evidence base from epidemiological observations and clinical trials.

Cost–benefit analysis data for POCT are sparse in the United Kingdom, with a perceived lag of approximately a decade behind the United States (90). More broadly, it should be acknowledged that evaluation of the cost-effectiveness of POCT has not developed to the same level as the technology (91). Thorough cost accounting is essential to assess overall benefit of service against cost and may include possible savings and reduced length of hospitalization. Potential hidden costs of POCT include labor, consumables, instrument maintenance, training, recertification, and proficiency testing. However, POCT guarantees a quick turnaround time and the benefits of immediate availability of results. It should be the responsibility of the medical technologist to maintain the quality of laboratory testing and to take a lead role in managing quality control. The clinical laboratory as a whole must maintain responsibility for the development of appropriate training programs for non-laboratory personnel in the use of ancillary testing equipment, test procedures, documentation, review of test results, performance and monitoring of quality control, corrective action, proficiency testing, and equipment management. In our view, close collaboration between clinicians and clinical biochemists will help ensure that appropriate and cost-effective POCT tests are made available for patients with diabetes.

REFERENCES

1. Wild S, Roglic G, Green A, Sicree R, King H. Global prevalence of diabetes: estimates for the year 2000 and projections for 2030. Diabetes Care 2004;27:1047–53.
2. Bonow RO, Gheorghiade M. The diabetes epidemic: a national and global crisis. Am J Med 2004;116(5A):2S–10S.
3. Clark CM Jr., Lee D. Prevention and treatment of the complications of diabetes mellitus. N Engl J Med 1995;332:1210–7.
4. Narayan KM, Gregg EW, Fagot-Campagna A, Engelgau MM, Vinicor F. Diabetes—a common, growing, serious, costly, and potentially preventable public health problem. Diabetes Res Clin Pract 2000;50(Suppl 2):S77–84.
5. Gaede P, Vedal P, Larsen N, Jensen GVH, Parving H-H, Pedersen O. Multifactorial intervention and cardiovascular disease in patients with type 2 diabetes. N Engl J Med 2003;348:383–93.
6. Krentz AJ, Bailey CJ. Type 2 Diabetes in practice. London: Royal Society of Medicine Press; 2001.
7. Diabetes Prevention Program Research Group. Reduction in the incidence of type 2 diabetes with lifestyle intervention or metformin. N Engl J Med 2002;346:393–403.
8. Frayn K. Metabolic regulation: a human perspective, 2nd ed. Oxford: Blackwell Publishing; 2003.
9. American Diabetes Association. Diagnosis and classification of diabetes mellitus. Diabetes Care 2004;27(Suppl 1):S5–10.
10. Diabetes Control and Complications Research Group. The effect of intensive treatment of diabetes on the development and progression of long term complications in insulin-dependent diabetes mellitus. New Engl J Med 1993;329:977–86.
11. Riddle MC. Timely initiation of basal insulin. Am J Med 2004; 116(Suppl 3A):3S–9S.
12. UK Prospective Diabetes Study Group. Intensive blood glucose control with sulphonylureas or insulin compared with conventional treatment and risk of complications in patients with type2 diabetes (UKPDS 33). Lancet 1998;352:837–53.
13. Tuomilehto J. Controlling glucose and blood pressure in type 2 diabetes. BMJ 2000;321:394–5.
14. Malins JM. Clinical diabetes mellitus. London: Eyre & Spotiswoode; 1968.
15. Bryden KS, Peveler RC, Stein A, Neil A, Mayou RA, Dunger DB. Clinical and psychological course of diabetes from adolescence to young adulthood: A longitudinal cohort study. Diabetes Care 2001;24:1513–4.
16. Cagliero E, Levina EV, Nathan DM. Immediate feedback of HbA1c levels improves glycemic control in type 1 and insulin treated type 2 diabetic patients. Diabetes Care 1999;22:1785–9.
17. Thaler LM, Ziemer DC, Gallina DL, Cook CB, Dunbar VG, Phillips LS, et al. Diabetes in urban African-Americans: XVII. Availability of rapid HbA1c measurements enhances clinical decision making. Diabetes Care 1999;22:1415–21.
18. Lewandrowski E, Millan MC, Misiano D, Tochka L, Lewandrowski K. Process improvement for bedside capillary glucose testing in a large academic medical center: the impact of new technology on point of care testing. Clin Chim Acta 2001;307: 175–9.
19. American Diabetes Association. Bedside blood glucose monitoring in hospitals. Diabetes Care 2004;27(Suppl 1):S104.
20. National Service Framework for Diabetes: Standards. London: Department of Health; 2001. Available at http://www.publications.doh.gov.uk/nsf/diabetes/index.htm (accessed May 2004).
21. Malmberg K for the DIGAMI (Diabetes Mellitus, Insulin Glucose Infusion in Acute Myocardial Infarction) Study Group. Prospective randomised study of intensive insulin treatment on long term survival in patients with diabetes mellitus. BMJ 1997;314:1512–5.
22. Mesotten D, Van den Berghe G. Clinical potential of insulin therapy in critically ill patients. Drugs 2003;64:625–36.
23. Scobie IN, Sonksen PH. Methods of achieving better diabetic control. In: Nattrass M, Santiago JV, eds. Recent advances in diabetes. Edinburgh, UK: Churchill Livingstone; 1984:107–25.
24. American Diabetes Association. Tests of glycemia in diabetes. Diabetes Care 2004;27(Suppl 1):S91–93.

25. DAFNE Study Group. Training in flexible, intensive insulin management to enable dietary freedom in people with type 1 diabetes: dose-adjustment for normal eating (DAFNE) randomised controlled trial. BMJ 2002;325:746–9.

26. Kyne-Grzebalski D, Wood L, Marshall SM, Taylor R. Episodic hyperglycaemia in pregnant women with well-controlled type 1 diabetes mellitus: a major potential factor underlying macrosomia. Diabetic Med 1999;16:621–2.

27. Krentz AJ, Hale PJ, Albutt E, Nattrass M. Haemoglobin A$_1$ in the diagnosis of factitious remission of diabetes. Ann Clin Biochem 1988;25:150–4.

28. Pickup JC. Diabetic control and its measurement. In: Williams G, Pickup JC. Textbook of diabetes, 3rd ed. Oxford: Blackwell Publishing; 2003:1–34.

29. Heller S. Insulin-induced hypoglycaemia. In: Krentz AJ, ed. Emergencies in diabetes. Chichester, UK: John Wiley & Sons; 2004:73–93.

30. Evans A, Krentz AJ. Benefits and risks of transfer from oral agents to insulin in type 2 diabetes. In: Krentz AJ, ed. Drug treatment of type 2 diabetes. Auckland, New Zealand: ADIS Books; 2000:85–101.

31. Patrick AW, Gill GV, MacFarlane IA, Cullen A, Power E, Wallymahamed M. Home glucose monitoring in type 2 diabetes: is it a waste of time? Diabetic Med 1994;11:62–5.

32. Coster S, Gulliford MC, Seed PT, Pwrie JK, Swaminathan R. Self-monitoring in type 2 diabetes mellitus: A meta-analysis. Diabetic Med 2000;17:755–61.

33. National Institute for Clinical Excellence. Inherited guideline G: Management of type 2 diabetes. Management of blood glucose. London: National Institute for Clinical Excellence; 2002. Available at http://www.nice.org.uk/page.aspx?o=36738 (accessed May 2004).

34. Murata GH, Shah JH, Hoffman RM, Wendel CS, Adam KD, Solvas PA, et al. Intensified blood glucose monitoring improves glycemic control in stable, insulin-treated veterans with type 2 diabetes. Diabetes Care 2003;26:1759–63.

35. Rosenstock J, Wyne K. Insulin treatment in type 2 diabetes. In: Goldstein BJ, Müller-Wieland D, eds. Textbook of type 2 diabetes. London: Martin Dunitz; 2003:131–54.

36. Jones H, Edwards L, Vallis TM, Ruggerio L, Rossi SR, Rossi JS, et al. Changes in diabetes self-care behaviors make a difference in glycaemic control. Diabetes Care 2003;26:732–7.

37. Rohrschieb M, Robinson R, Eaton RP. Non-invasive glucose sensors and inproved informatics—the future of diabetes management. Diabetes Obes Metab 2003;5:280–4.

38. Eastman RC, Leptien AD, Chase HP. Cost-effectiveness of use of the GlucoWatch Biographer in children and adolescents with type 1 diabetes: a preliminary analysis based on a randomized controlled trial. Pediatr Diabetes 2003;4:82–6.

39. Fonseca V, Hinson J, Pappas A. An erbium:YAG laser to obtain capillary blood samples without a needle for point-of-care laboratory testing. Arch Path Lab Med 1997;121:685–8.

40. American Diabetes Association. Hyperglycemic crises in patients with diabetes mellitus. Diabetes Care 2001;24:154–61.

41. Krentz AJ, Holt HB. Diabetic ketoacidosis in adults. In: Krentz AJ, ed. Emergencies in diabetes. Chichester, UK: John Wiley & Sons; 2004:1–32.

42. Holt HB, Krentz AJ. Metabolic emergencies in type 2 diabetes: hyperosmolar non-ketotic hyperglycaemia, ketoacidosis and lactic acidosis. In: Goldstein BJ, Müller-Wieland D, eds. Textbook of type 2 diabetes. London: Martin Dunitz; 2003:184–98.

43. Krentz AJ, Singh BM, Wright AD, Nattrass M. Effects of autonomic neuropathy on glucose, fatty acid, and ketone body metabolism following insulin withdrawal in patients with insulin-dependent diabetes. J Diabetes Complicat 1994;8:105–10.

44. Schwab TM, Hendey GW, Soliz TC. Screening for ketonemia in patients with diabetes. Ann Emerg Med 1999;34:342–6.

45. Laffel L. Ketone bodies: A review of physiology, pathophysiology and application of monitoring to diabetes. Diabetes Metab Res Rev 1999;15:412–46.

46. Csako G. Causes, consequences, and recognition of false-positive reactions for ketones. Clin Chem 1990;36:1388–9.

47. Byrne HA, Tieszen KL, Hollis S, Dornan TL, New JP. Evaluation of an electrochemical sensor for measuring blood ketones. Diabetes Care 2000;23:500–3.

48. Wallace TM, Meston NM, Gardner SG, Matthews DR. The hospital and home use of a 30-second hand-held blood ketone meter: guidelines for clinical practice. Diabetic Med 2001;18:640–5.

49. Guerci B, Benichou M, Floriot M, Bohme P, Fougnot S, Franck P, et al. Accuracy of an electrochemical sensor for measuring capillary blood ketones by fingerstick samples during metabolic deterioration after continuous subcutaneous insulin infusion interruption in type 1 diabetic patients. Diabetes Care 2003;26:1137–41.

50. Samuelsson U, Ludvigsson J. When should determination of ketonaemia be recommended? Diabetes Technol Ther 2002;4:645–50.

51. Kamalakannan D, Baskar V, Barton DM, Abdu TA. Diabetic ketoacidosis in pregnancy. Postgrad Med J 2003;79:454–7.

52. Mogensen CE, Keane WF, Bennett PH, Jerums G, Parving HH, Passa P, et al. Prevention of diabetic renal disease with special reference to microalbuminuria. Lancet 1995;346:1080–4.

53. Hovind P, Tarnow L, Rossing P, Jensen BR, Graae M, Torp I, et al. Predictors for the development of microalbuminuria and microalbuminuria in patients with type 1 diabetes: inception cohort study. BMJ 2004;328:1105–8.

54. Writing team for the Diabetes Control and Complications Trial/ Epidemiology of Diabetes Intervention and Complications Research Group. Sustained effect of intensive treatment of type 1 diabetes mellitus on development and progression of diabetic nephropathy: the Epidemiology of Diabetes Interventions and Complications (EDIC) study. JAMA 2003;290:2159–67.

55. UK Prospective Diabetes Study Group. Tight blood pressure control and risk of macrovascular and microvascular complications in type 2 diabetes: UKPDS 38. BMJ 1998;317:703–13.

56. Perkins BA, Ficociello LH, Silva KH, Finkelstein DM, Warram JH, Krolewski AS. Regression of microalbuminuria in type 1 diabetes. N Engl J Med 2003;348:2285–93.

57. Krentz AJ. Insulin resistance. Oxford: Blackwell Publishing; 2002.

58. Bennett PH, Haffner S, Kasiske BL, Keane WF, Mogensen CE, Parving HH, et al. Screening and management of microalbuminuria in patients with diabetes mellitus. Am J Kidney Dis 1995;25:107–12.

59. National Institute for Clinical Excellence. Inherited guideline F. Management of type 2 diabetes. Renal disease—prevention and early management. London: National Institute for Clinical Excellence; 2002. Available at http://www.nice.org.uk/page.aspx?o=39385 (accessed May 2004).

60. American Diabetes Association. Nephropathy in diabetes. Diabetes Care 2004;27(Suppl 1):S79–83.

61. Rodby RA, Firth LM, Lewis EJ. An economic analysis of captopril in the treatment of diabetic nephropathy. The Collaborative Study Group. Diabetes Care 1996;19:1051–61.

62. Mogensen CE. Microalbuminuria and hypertension with focus on type 1 and type 2 diabetes. J Intern Med 2003;254:45–66.

63. Wilson PW, Kannel WB, Anderson KM. Lipids, glucose intolerance and vascular disease: the Framingham study. Atherosclerosis 1985;13:1–11.

64. Haffner SM, Lehto S, Ronnemaa T, Pyorala K, Laakso M. Mortality from coronary heart disease in subjects with type 2 diabetes and in nondiabetic subjects with and without prior myocardial infarction. N Eng J Med 1998;339:229–34.

65. Evans JM, Wang J, Morris AD. Comparison of cardiovascular risk between patients with type 2 diabetes and those who had had a myocardial infarction: cross sectional and cohort studies. BMJ 2002;324:939–42.

66. Alexander CM, Landsman PB, Teutsch SM, Haffner SM. Third National Health and Nutrition Examination Survey (NHANES III); National Cholesterol Education Program (NCEP). NCEP-defined metabolic syndrome, diabetes, and prevalence of coronary heart disease among NHANES III participants age 50 years and older. Diabetes 2003;52:1210–14.

67. Turner RC, Millns H, Neil HAW, Stratton IM, Manley SE, Matthews DR, et al. Risk factors for coronary artery disease in non-insulin dependent diabetes mellitus: United Kingdom prospective diabetes study (UKPDS 23). BMJ 1998;316:823–8.

68. Third report of the National Cholesterol Education Panel Expert Report on Detection, Evaluation, and Treatment of High Blood Cholesterol in Adults (Adult Treatment Panel III). Bethesda, MD: National Heart, Lung, and Blood Institute; National Institutes of Health NIH Publication No. 02–5215 September 2002.

69. Steinhausen RL, Price CP. Principles and practice of dry chemistry systems. In: Price CP, Alberti KGMM, eds. Recent advances in clinical biochemistry. Vol. 3. Edinburgh, UK: Churchill Livingstone; 1985:273–96.

70. Rubin DA, McMurray RG, Harrell JS, Carlson BW, Bangdiwala S. Accuracy of three dry-chemistry methods for lipid profiling and risk factor classification. Int J Sport Nutr Exerc Metab. 2003;13:358–68.

71. Forest J, Rousseau F, Carrier R, Hivon P, Gosselin M. Quality-control scheme for blood glucose measured outside the laboratory. Clin Chem 1987;33:1233–5.

72. du Plessis M, Ubbink JB, Vermaak WJ. Analytical quality of near-patient blood cholesterol and glucose determinations. Clin Chem 2000;46:8:1085–90.

73. Laboratory Standardization Panel. Recommendations for improving cholesterol measurement. A report from the Laboratory Standardization Panel of the National Cholesterol Education Program. NIH Publication No. 90–2964. Bethesda, MD: National Institutes of Health; 1990.

74. National Cholesterol Education Program. Recommendations on lipoprotein measurement from the Working Group on Lipoprotein Measurement. NIH Publication No. 95–3044. Bethesda, MD: National Heart, Lung and Blood Institute; 1995.

75. Rogers EJ, Misner L, Ockene IS, Nicolosi RJ. Evaluation of seven Cholestech LDX analyzers for total cholesterol determinations. Clin Chem 1993;39:860–4.

76. Hatch FT. Practical methods for plasma lipoprotein analysis. Adv Lipid Res 1968;6:1–8.

77. Burstein M, Scholnick HR, Morfin R. Rapid method for the isolation of lipoproteins from human serum by precipitation with polyanions. J Lipid Res 1970;11:583–95.

78. Warnick GR, Benderson J, Albers JJ. Dextran sulfate-Mg^{2+} precipitation procedure for quantitation of high-density-lipoprotein cholesterol. Clin Chem 1982;28:1379–88.

79. Warnick GR, Albers JJ. A comprehensive evaluation of the heparin-manganese precipitation procedure for estimating high density lipoprotein cholesterol. J Lipid Res 1978;19:65–76.

80. Warnick GR, Cheung MC, Albers JJ. Comparison of current methods for high-density lipoprotein cholesterol quantitation. Clin Chem 1979;25:596–604.

81. Wiebe DA, Warnick GR. Measurement of high-density lipoprotein cholesterol concentration. In: Rifai N, Warnick GR, eds. Laboratory management of lipids, lipoproteins and apolipoproteins. Washington, DC: AACC Press; 1994:91–105.

82. Sugiuchi H, Uji Y, Okabe H. Direct measurement methods for HDL-cholesterol [in Japanese]. Mod Med Lab 1996;24:303–10.

83. Tatsumi N, Okuda K, Tsuda I. A new direction in automated laboratory testing in Japan: five years of experience with total laboratory automation system management. Clin Chim Acta 1999;290:93–108.

84. Myers GL, Cooper GR, Henderson LO, Hassemer DJ, Kimberly MM. Standardization of lipid and lipoprotein measurements. In: Rifai N, Warnick GR, eds. Laboratory measurement of lipids, lipoprotein and apolipoproteins. Washington, DC: AACC Press; 1994:177–205.

85. Yamada T, Nishino S, Takubo T, Hino M, Kitagawa S, Tatsumi N. Simple high-density lipoprotein cholesterol assay based on dry chemistry. Clin Chim Acta 2002;320:79–88.

86. Goldstein DE, Little RR, Wiedmeyer HM, England JD, Rohlfing CL, Wilke AL. Is glycohemoglobin testing useful in diabetes mellitus? Lessons from the diabetes control and complications trial. Clin Chem 1994;40:1637–40.

87. Diabetes Control and Complications Research Group. Resource utilization and costs of care in the diabetes control and complications trial. Diabetes Care 1995;18:1468–78.

88. CDC Diabetes Cost-Effectiveness Group. Cost-effectiveness of intensive glycemic control, intensified hypertension control, and serum cholesterol level reduction for type 2 diabetes. JAMA 2002;287:2542–51.

89. Ettaro L, Songer TJ, Zhang P, Engelgau MM. Cost-of-illness studies in diabetes. Pharmacoeconomics 2004;22:149–64.

90. Creed GM. Point-of-care testing in the United Kingdom. Crit Care Nurs Q 2001;24:44–8.

91. St-Louis P. Status of point-of-care testing: Promise, realities, and possibilities. Clin Biochem 2000;33:427–40.

Chapter 32

Point-of-Care Testing in Prenatal Care

Tanu Singhal, Andrew H. Shennan, and Jason J. S. Waugh

Point-of-care testing (POCT) is an important part of current obstetric practice. With blood pressure and proteinuria assessments being a part of every prenatal visit for low-risk women, it is impossible for any woman to avoid contact with this form of testing (1). In other more high-risk situations there is an increasing tendency to move toward point-of-care tests, where they are available, to speed up the diagnostic process and avoid unnecessary hospital admissions for women who might otherwise be managed in the community. This chapter will review POCT in current practice and highlight where new point-of-care developments have been implemented in obstetric practice.

PRENATAL SCREENING FOR TRISOMY 21

Developments in Down syndrome screening and prenatal diagnosis have centered on the development of nuchal translucency (NT) measurement by ultrasound and first-trimester placental protein markers in maternal serum. The overall intention of these screening programs is to minimize the number of invasive procedures undertaken while maximizing the number of cases of Down syndrome identified. The provision for screening services in clinical practice has lagged behind advances in the performance of screening programs over the past decade (2). In 2003, the Serum, Urine and Ultrasound Screening Study (SURUSS) (3) concluded that for the women who choose to have screening in the first trimester, the combined test with nuchal translucency, free β–human chorionic gonadotrophin (β-hCG), and pregnancy-associated plasma protein A (PAPP-A) at 10 completed weeks of gestation was the most effective and safest method of screening. Overall, this integrated test with a second measurement of free β-hCG and inhibin-A at 14–20 weeks was deemed the most effective.

The concept of the one-stop clinic for assessment of risk (OSCAR) approach for trisomy 21 was developed in 1997, when the first rapid assays for serum-free β-hCG and PAPP-A became available at the point of care on the CIS Kryptor platform (now available from Brahms Diagnostica GmbH, Germany) (4). The 19-min homogeneous immunoassay technology (5), based on time-resolved amplified cryptate emission using chelates developed by Nobel Prize winner Jean-Marie Lehn, can be carried out in the same time that it takes a qualified sonographer to measure fetal size (crown rump length) and nuchal translucency (NT) thickness and report a mini–anomaly scan. Within 45 min a counselor can discuss this report with a woman in a post-test counseling session. If appropriate, diagnostic testing by chorionic villus sampling can be scheduled for the following day, with a quantitative polymerase chain reaction diagnostic result available within 48 h (6). The prospective review of 15,030 pregnancies at the OSCAR clinic for Down syndrome was recently presented by Bindra et al. (7). For a fixed false-positive rate of 5%, the detection rates for Down syndrome by maternal age alone was 30.5%; by maternal age and serum-free β-hCG and PAPP-A, 59.8%; by maternal age and fetal NT, 79.3%; and by maternal age, fetal NT, and serum markers, 90.2%. (See Chapter 33 for a more detailed case study.)

The recent identification of a strong relationship between the absence of the nasal bone on the 11–14 week ultrasound examination and an increased risk of trisomy 21 suggests that detection rates of 92% can be achieved (at a 5% screen-positive rate) when combined with NT thickness. When combined with maternal serum biochemistry at the same visit, expected detection rates will be on the order of 95% for a 2% screen-positive rate (8).

The identification of pregnancies at increased risk in the first trimester has several advantages. These include, for some women, an earlier diagnosis with a consequently safer and less traumatic therapeutic abortion, and for the majority of women earlier reassurance.

DIAGNOSIS OF IMMINENT PRETERM LABOR: FETAL FIBRONECTIN TESTING

Preterm birth, which occurs in up to 10% of pregnancies, remains the largest single cause of perinatal mortality and morbidity. Despite major improvements in medical care and the socioeconomic status of the population in developed countries, there has not been a decrease in the incidence of preterm births in the past 50 years. Consequently, there has been extensive research into methods of screening both low- and high-risk groups for spontaneous preterm birth (SPB). The potential benefits of screening for SPB include short-term treatment (tocolysis, transfer to an appropriate tertiary care center, the administration of maternal steroids to enhance fetal lung maturity), and the long-term prevention of preterm delivery (hospitalization for bed rest or cervical cerclage therapy). Whereas the identification of those at risk of preterm birth is an important challenge in maternal-fetal medicine, the effectiveness of interventions to prevent or arrest this process, such as cervical cerclage, remains controversial.

When fetal fibronectin is found in the cervix or vagina of women in the late second trimester who are not in established labor, it is the most potent predictor of subsequent early preterm birth yet described (9–11). Fetal fibronectin is a basement membrane protein produced by fetal and placental tissues and probably serves to adhere the placental membranes to the endometrium (12). It is distinguishable from adult fibronectin immunologically, probably because of differences in several sulfate bonds. Its frequent presence in the lower genital tract before 20 weeks' gestation is thought to be caused by the absence of a complete fusion between the fetal membranes and the decidua, whereas its rarity in the cervix or vagina after that time is believed to result from that fusion (12). The appearance in the cervix and vagina of fetal fibronectin in the late second trimester and early third trimester is thought to represent disruption of the chorion–decidua interface, which likely accounts for fetal fibronectin's powerful capability to predict spontaneous preterm birth (13).

In the Preterm Prediction Study, Mercer et al. (14) evaluated the prediction of preterm premature rupture of membranes through clinical findings and ancillary testing. Women with a positive fibronectin screen and shortened cervix had a greater risk of SPB associated with prelabor premature rupture of the membranes (PPROM) before 37 weeks [relative risk (RR) = 4.9] and before 35 weeks (RR = 13.5) than those without these risk factors. With all three risk factors, multiparae had a 31.3-fold increased risk of SPB associated with PPROM occurring before 35 weeks (14).

In 2002, Honest et al. (15) performed a quantitative systematic review of all studies published to date to test the accuracy of fetal fibronectin as a predictor of preterm labor. Sixty-four primary articles were identified, consisting of 28 studies in asymptomatic women and 40 in symptomatic women, in a total of 26,876 women. Among asymptomatic women the best summary likelihood ratio for positive results was 4.01 [95% confidence interval (CI) 2.93, 5.49] for predicting birth before 34 weeks gestation, with a corresponding summary likelihood ratio for negative results of 0.78 (95% CI 0.72, 0.84). Among symptomatic women the best summary likelihood ratio for positive results was 5.42 (95% CI 4.36, 6.74) for predicting birth within 7–10 days of testing, with a corresponding ratio for negative results of 0.25 (95% CI 0.20, 0.31) (15). If prenatal steroids were to be used for all symptomatic women at this gestation to improve fetal lung maturity without fibronectin testing, then 109 women would need to be treated with prenatal steroids to prevent one case of respiratory distress syndrome. If only those women with a positive fibronectin test result were treated, 17 would need to be treated, a figure considerably lower than that without testing. These results might enable clinicians to make a more rational approach to decision making regarding inpatient admission, administration of prenatal steroids, and in utero transfer in women with threatened spontaneous preterm birth. Their results showed the accuracy of the cervicovaginal fetal fibronec-

tin in predicting various spontaneous preterm birth outcomes. The test is most accurate in predicting spontaneous preterm birth within 7–10 days after testing among women with symptoms of threatened preterm birth before advanced cervical dilatation (15). In a recent prospective randomized controlled trial in a tertiary care center, the negative test result was associated with fewer admissions to the prepartum ward and a shorter length of stay (16).

PRENATAL CARE

The central aims of prenatal care include the identification of hypertensive disorders of pregnancy and, more controversially, gestational diabetes mellitus. Both of these groups of disorders remain significant sources of morbidity and mortality for pregnant women throughout the world. However, the value of traditional prenatal care is increasingly being questioned both by the provider and by those receiving care.

The principle criticisms focus on the social aspects of care, in that it is impersonal and that advice and information are either insufficiently or inappropriately provided. Women's criticisms of the medical aspects of their care have focused on poor communication of the results of screening tests rather than the tests themselves.

Automated technology allows multiple measurements to be taken away from the clinical environment and has addressed many of the errors associated with conventional measurements of blood pressure and proteinuria.

Hypertensive Disorders in Pregnancy

The detection of hypertension remains a cornerstone of prenatal care. The standard practice of recording the blood pressure at the first prenatal visit and then taking sequential recordings with increasing frequency toward term is now integral to the protocols of all prenatal clinics. Proteinuria detection by dipstick urinalysis is used in tandem with blood pressure measurement to screen for the disease, although it is recognized that both proteinuria and hypertension appear late in the pathophysiological process. In the United Kingdom, admissions related to hypertensive disorders in pregnancy constitute 12% to 24% of all prenatal inpatients (17), and the majority of referrals to the prenatal day care unit are for blood pressure assessment (18).

The syndrome of preeclampsia is multisystemic in nature, with both the maternal kidney and cardiovascular systems being affected. There is a clear association between both proteinuria and blood pressure and increasing perinatal mortality and morbidity (19–23). Proteinuria also correlates with the incidence of growth restriction (24), and these associations justify the inclusion of proteinuria as a defining feature of the syndrome in both research and clinical practice.

There are, however, problems with the use of hypertension and urinary protein as the sole defining features of preeclampsia. Eclampsia, which is recognized as one indication of severe disease (25), may occur without proteinuria (26, 27). Blood pressure need also not be severe in eclampsia (25), and pro- teinuria can be detected in women who become eclamptic without hypertension. Not only is blood pressure variable but, as early as 1939, Chesley (28) demonstrated that there was significant variability in protein excretion in successive 4-h periods. This chapter considers those aspects that affect the accuracy of measurement of the two key signs of preeclampsia: proteinuria and hypertension, including the potential advantages and problems associated with using new technology such as automated devices and dipstick readers.

Blood Pressure Measurement in Pregnancy

Normal pregnancy causes a decrease in blood pressure during the midtrimester or earlier (29), with a return to normal value by the third trimester. This suggests that the fall in blood pressure occurs before the low resistance shunt of the utero-placental circulation can influence the blood pressure.

Blood pressure recordings in pregnancy have traditionally been made with the mercury sphygmomanometer, and it is this device that has determined the thresholds on which we base our clinical decisions and decide the management of patients. This measurement technique has well-documented, inherent inaccuracies (30). Diurnal variation in blood pressure (31), as well as many other factors such as age (32) and race, affect within-patient variability. Even under the most controlled of circumstances, the relationship between clinic-recorded blood pressure and pregnancy outcome variables remains weak (29, 33).

Each component of the measuring system, from the observer through the stethoscope to the manometer, can lead to measurement error. Errors can be compounded by the application of poor technique with regard to patient position (34), rate of cuff deflation, and interpretation of the Korotkoff sounds (35). In addition, there has been disagreement about which Korotkoff sound should be used in pregnancy to measure diastolic blood pressure, with Korotkoff V now recommended as being more reproducible (35). There is also disagreement as to what actually constitutes an abnormal blood pressure in pregnancy (i.e., the definition of hypertensive disease) (36, 37).

Anxiety caused by the measurement itself or by the environment in which it is taken can influence blood pressure. This is sometimes referred to as the white-coat effect, and it is important, as hypertension is defined by clinic blood pressure measurements. Its prevalence is between 20% and 40%, and some investigators have found it to be more common in women (38). Some women may be susceptible to higher readings when attending hospital clinics or on visits to their obstetrician, which may lead to unnecessary investigation or inappropriate intervention. White-coat hypertension does decrease after repeated visits, due to habituation to the clinic setting or regression to the mean. Therefore, this should only be diagnosed if an individual has sustained clinic hypertension (i.e., after the second or third visit) with normal blood pressure at other times; this has to be determined using some form of home blood pressure monitoring. Clinic blood pressure readings are found to be significantly different from home readings in nearly 50% of pregnant women, the vast majority of readings being lower

at home (39). Whether white-coat hypertension is a benign condition in nonpregnant individuals is unlikely, as the risk appears to fall somewhere between those who are normotensive and those with sustained hypertension (40).

Automated blood pressure measuring devices have been available to clinicians for several years and have become established in the management of the nonpregnant patient (41). There are currently >400 automated blood pressure devices on the market. Automated devices can be divided into two distinct groups. There are ambulatory devices, which are devices that are programmed to record the blood pressure a specified number of times over a predefined time period and are worn constantly (usually for 24 h or more). These have the advantage of obtaining a 24-h profile of a patient's blood pressure, thus allowing the identification of isolated systolic or diastolic hypertension, white-coat hypertension, and nocturnal hypertension (42–45). These subdivisions of hypertensive disease are of interest in the nonpregnant population, though the role of circadian variation remains to be clarified in hypertensive disease of pregnancy (46). What is known in both the pregnant and nonpregnant patient is that 24-h ambulatory blood pressure monitoring is a better predictor of outcome as measured by cardiovascular target organ involvement in the nonpregnant population (47, 48) and the development of severe hypertension in the pregnant population (49). This makes the use of such technology attractive to clinicians and to date would also seem to be very well tolerated by the women asked to wear the devices (49, 50). The second group of machines are designed to be patient-initiated home monitors available for clinical use. These are increasingly for sale in pharmacies as well as in the hospital and GP setting.

There are 16 studies relating to validation of automated devices in pregnancy and preeclampsia (9 include data from women with preeclampsia). In total, 10 devices have sufficient data to perform a meta-analysis. The total number of subjects included in these studies was 605 in pregnancy and 206 in preeclampsia (Table 32-1). Overall average errors were not large, and although these devices do under-record in pre-eclampsia, the degree of error does not preclude their use in clinical practice. Some individual machines do have large errors and the recommendation remains that each device should be assessed for accuracy before it can be relied on. Accuracy assessment should include pregnant women with preeclampsia (51).

Proteinuria Detection in Pregnancy and Preeclampsia

The current threshold that defines significant proteinuria is based on reference data from the uncomplicated pregnant population. The determination of an upper percentile (95th to 99th) to define an "abnormal population" has previously been used (52–54). Such studies have varied in their methodology, but the consensus is that up to 300 mg protein/24 h is physiological.

Page et al. (55), in a prospective study of almost 13,000 pregnant women, found that significant proteinuria (defined as 2+ or more on dipstick analysis) was associated with an

Table 32-1   Meta-analysis of 10 Studies in Which Validation of Devices Was Carried Out in Pregnant Women With and Without Preeclampsia

| | Blood pressure difference,[a] mmHg | | | |
| | Mercury device | | Intraarterial device | |
Variable	Normal pregnancy	Preeclamptic toxemia	Normal pregnancy	Preeclamptic toxemia
Subjects, *n*	597	176	8	30
Systolic	-1.13 ± 5.80	-4.60 ± 8.04	4.11 ± 10.95	-7.76 ± 10.12
Diastolic	-1.20 ± 6.03	-5.16 ± 7.19	3.00 ± 8.00	-8.17 ± 6.59

[a] Values are means $\pm$ SD.

increase in stillbirth rates, intrauterine growth restriction, and neonatal morbidity, when associated with hypertension. Brown et al. (56) report this threshold (2+ dipstick) can be associated with up to 50% false-positive rates. As proteinuria increases, there is evidence to suggest that if it is heavy (>5 g /24 h), delivery will be necessary within 2 weeks in most cases (88%). This 5-g/24-h threshold has been advocated as one of the criteria denoting severe preeclampsia.

Studies now suggest that it is the presence of proteinuria that confers increased maternal and perinatal morbidity, not necessarily its severity. Schiff et al. (57) found that, in patients with severe disease managed conservatively, a third will have a significant increase in protein excretion (>2 g/24 h) and at least one-third of women will cross the 5-g/24-h threshold. No evidence was recorded for an increase in adverse maternal or fetal outcomes in relation to the degree of proteinuria, either absolute or percentage increase, and, as such, this suggests that the degree of proteinuria alone should not be an indication for delivery. Therefore, the threshold for proteinuria needs to be accurately defined in relation to clinical risk.

Measuring Proteinuria in Pregnancy

The laboratory measurement of proteinuria, usually based on a 24-h urine collection, has been suggested as the gold standard for proteinuria assessment in preeclampsia. Several authors have also described the close correlation between the protein–creatinine ratio in a single voided urine sample and the total protein excretion in a 24-h urine sample in both pregnant and nonpregnant women. Recently, the International Society for the Study of Hypertension in Pregnancy has advocated the use of a protein–creatinine ratio from a spot urine sample to be suitable for defining proteinuria in pregnancy (58). The use of the protein–creatinine ratio as an alternative to dipstick urinalysis is hampered in most clinical settings by the delay in obtaining a result from the laboratory where the protein and creatinine assays are performed. All studies, however, have concluded that as the degree of proteinuria increases there is a greater variation in the protein–creatinine ratio over time (59). As such, this means that the test is unable to replace total protein quantification in a 24-h sample, but at lower protein excretions (<500 mg/24 h) the correlation is excellent, making an ideal rule-in/rule-out test. Where it is possible to obtain results quickly, the improved predictive value of this test

means that it is to be recommended over dipstick urinalysis for the identification of significant proteinuria. We have found that the use of a laboratory protein:creatinine ratio [30 mg/mmol (262 mg/g)] has a positive predictive value (PPV) for proteinuria levels of 300 mg/24 h of 79%, and a negative predictive value (NPV) of 98% for determining 500 mg/24 h.

Problems with 24-h urine collection, such as inaccurate timing or incomplete collection due to ureteric dilatation, are well recognized in pregnancy. Several studies of 24-h urine volume have been published. Lindow et al. (59) quote a mean 24-h urine volume (from catheter specimens) of 2.258 L. Meyer et al. (60) defined a volume of <0.9 L as inadequate, and Boler et al. (61) discarded 37% of samples on the basis of inadequate volume (although they do not state their threshold). In our own studies, we have found up to 13% of samples to be <0.9 L. An incomplete collection may give a false-negative assessment of proteinuria, but when compared with a dipstick will increase apparent false-positive rates for the dipstick being tested. No single laboratory technique has gained wide acceptance as a standard method of assessing urinary protein excretion, and different methods have different reference intervals. Variation among protein assays has several important implications. We have shown that when two assays are compared, the prevalence of significant proteinuria (>0.3 g/24 h) varies from 70.1% (95% CI 63.1–76.4%) to 24.9% (95% CI 19.0–31.5%) with the benzethonium chloride assay in a group of women with hypertension in pregnancy. Clearly, it is difficult to compare different studies on women with preeclampsia if their urine protein levels have been quantified by different biochemical assays (62).

The choice of assay is also important when it comes to testing point-of-care urine dipsticks. The predictive value of dipstick urinalysis is highly dependent on which biochemical assay is employed as a gold standard. In our study, when dipsticks were compared with the benzethonium chloride assay, they had a sensitivity of 22.5% (95% CI 15.8–30.3%) and a specificity of 98.3% (95% CI 90.9–99.9%). The false-positive rate was only 1/32 (3%), but the false-negative rate was 107/165 (65%). When compared with the Bradford assay, dipstick urinalysis had a sensitivity of 57.1% (95% CI 42.2–71.2%) but a specificity of 97.3% (95% CI 93.2–99.3%). The false-positive rate was 4/32 (12.5%), and the false-negative rate was 21/165 (13%). The NPV differed significantly. The difference in NPV was 52.1% (95% CI, 43.7–60.5%; $P < 0.001$) (62).

The absence of agreed standards makes the enforcement of rigid thresholds suggested in guidelines difficult. Variability in standardization makes it very likely that different studies are not comparing like with like, due to a lack of harmonization in quantification.

Dipstick Urinalysis in Pregnancy

Point-of-care urinary dipstick tests remain important measures of proteinuria, both clinically and in obstetric research. Two recent reviews of the definition of preeclampsia for research purposes found that dipsticks were used to confirm the presence of proteinuria (and hence preeclampsia) in 35% of studies and were the only measure of proteinuria in 12% to 21% of studies (63, 64). This method of detecting proteinuria has been demonstrated to vary in its positive and negative predictive value in the identification of preeclampsia.

In a recent meta-analysis to compare urine dipstick tests, seven studies were identified that were methodologically suitable for analysis. Six studies compared visual urinalysis and produced a pooled positive likelihood ratio of 3.48 (95% confidence intervals 1.66, 7.27) and a pooled negative likelihood ratio of 0.6 (0.45, 0.8) for the prediction of 300 mg/24 h (65).

It should also be noted that dipsticks provide a semi-quantitative measure of protein concentration, usually measured in a random urine sample. The concentration of urinary protein, which is highly variable over time, will be influenced by contamination, exercise, posture and osmolality. As such, the urine dipstick results will vary over time, and collection of a 24-h sample of urine averages out this daytime variability; this effect is significantly reduced by using the protein:creatinine ratio. Furthermore, there is an assumption in clinical practice that a threshold for urine concentration of 300 mg/L (30 mg/dL, or 1+) is equivalent to 300 mg/24 h. This will only be the case when the urine volume is 1 L (0.3 g/L $\times$ 1000 mL/24h = 300 mg/24 h). All studies consistently report urine volumes of greater than 1300 mL, and this is likely to contribute to the false negative rate seen in these studies.

When screening for proteinuria, it has been suggested that a test should be associated with a low false-negative rate (high sensitivity) to avoid missing significant proteinuria and hence preeclampsia (66). There has always been controversy over the difficulty of interpreting "trace proteinuria." As such, the allocation of this finding as test positive or test negative has a significant effect on the sensitivities and specificities for the detection of significant proteinuria.

Lowering the threshold for dipstick proteinuria to trace, or 150 mg/L (15 mg/dL), may improve detection and reduce false-negative rates. There is also evidence that the finding of trace proteinuria in pregnant women with hypertension is associated with an increase in adverse outcome (67).

Automated Urinalysis in Pregnancy

The use of automated technology, such as automated blood pressure monitors and urinanalyzers, addresses many of the observer errors associated with these common screening tests. Automated dipstick readers offer a simple and observer-error-free reading of standard urinary dipsticks (Figure 32-1). Their accuracy with standard protein solutions has been demonstrated, as has their accuracy in pregnancy (68). The use of automated dipstick urinalysis was first reported by Saudan et al. (69). They reported a significant improvement in PPV with automated versus visual dipstick reading (47% vs. 24%) with no change in false-negative rates. We have also reported the advantages of automated dipstick readers. In a comparative study, we found significant improvements in the area under the curve of receiver-operating characteristic curves for automated dipstick urinalysis compared with visual testing. This improvement translates into an improvement in positive and negative predictive value for significant proteinuria (PPV 78% vs. 64%; NPV 84% vs. 65%). The simple patient-friendly approach means that these automated readers have the potential to both improve prenatal screening and to allow home testing, thus increasing sampling and testing in an accurate and reproducible manner. The more accurate definition of pathology may also reduce unnecessary hospitalization and have economic implications for healthcare.

In the future, the development of fully quantitative automated urinanalyzers that can be housed in clinical areas may negate the need for laboratory analysis. Such devices offer

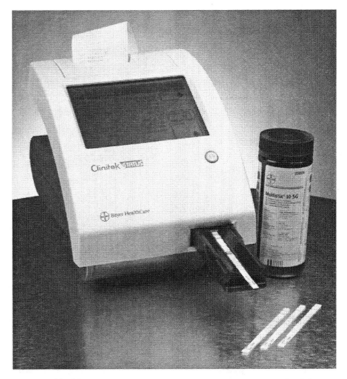

Figure 32-1 The Clinitek Status urinanalyzer. Reprinted with permission from Bayer HealthCare, Diagnostics Division.

attractive alternatives to waiting for laboratory results, which may take up to 24 h.

Microalbuminuria Testing in Pregnancy

Microalbuminuria is defined as urinary excretion of albumin that is persistently above normal, although below the sensitivity of conventional semiquantitative test strips. In the nonpregnant population, it reflects glomerular or, less commonly, tubulointerstitial dysfunction, and is considered only after structural abnormalities and infection of the renal tract have been excluded.

We have described the gestation-specific reference range for microalbuminuria in pregnancy (70) using point-of-care measurement techniques, and explored the predictive abilities of microalbuminuria techniques for clinical proteinuria. The advantage of the albumin:creatinine ratio to quantify albumin excretion is that it allows a single urine void to be tested.

Others have reported that microalbuminuria may be of benefit in screening for preeclampsia. Rodriguez et al. (71) reported that, when urinary microalbumin concentration was combined with a low calcium:creatinine ratio, the test had a sensitivity of 50% and a specificity of 99% (PPV 83%, NPV 94%) for the detection of subsequent preeclampsia in 88 low-risk nulliparous women. Similarly, Holm et al. (72) combined serum uric acid measurement with relative albumin clearance measurements in two cohorts of women at 24–41 weeks of gestation (54 normal, 14 preeclampsia). They reported a PPV of 100% and an NPV of 100%. These studies are obviously limited by small numbers and differing methodologies. Bar et al. (73) described a phase of microalbuminuria that preceded clinical proteinuria, and this test has some predictive value for severe disease. They also suggest that the accepted definition of gestational proteinuria should be reconsidered.

These studies all relied on random urine samples that were sent for laboratory analysis. Higby et al. (74) compared two point-of-care screening tests for the detection of significant proteinuria (>300 mg/24 h) in a normotensive and hypertensive pregnant population. They compared methods of urine screening against a gold-standard urine biochemical assay (rather than clinical outcomes). This assay would have defined the preeclamptic population. The microalbumin test had a sensitivity of 87%, compared with 36% for the protein test of the Multistix[®] 10SG (Bayer, Elkart, IN, USA). It also had a higher specificity, PPV, and NPV. They concluded that this is a better screening test to identify preeclampsia at point of care.

New Developments in Proteinuria Assessment in Pregnancy

As mentioned, urinalysis devices that can give fully quantitative urine protein measurements at the point of care are available. One such device is the DCA[®] 2000 (Bayer, Elkart, IN, USA) which we have studied in relation to uncomplicated pregnancy and preeclampsia. The device measures albumin and is able to detect albumin concentrations as low as 5 mg/L (0.5 mg/dL) (i.e., microalbuminuria). It also measures urinary

creatinine and gives results as an albumin:creatinine ratio. We have validated the DCA 2000 in women with uncomplicated pregnancies and hypertensive pregnancies and with urine from a variety of specimens, from early morning samples to 24-h samples. We found the device to be highly accurate and a viable alternative to a laboratory test (75).

Having validated the device and constructed a 95th-percentile reference range, we sought to test the device for proteinuria prediction in hypertensive pregnancies. The threshold for normality in the nonpregnant population is 3.4 mg/mmol (30 mg/g). As this is well above our 95th percentile, we also constructed receiver operating characteristic curves for the DCA 2000 and found that the optimal threshold was 2.0 mg/mmol (17.6 mg/g). Using this threshold, we found that the device had both a sensitivity and specificity of 94%. These results allow a highly predictive assessment of proteinuria for women with hypertension to be performed in an obstetric day unit.

Glucose Homeostasis in Pregnancy

Gestational diabetes and impaired glucose tolerance (IGT) affects 3% to 6% of all pregnancies, and both have been associated with complications. However, a lack of conclusive evidence has led clinicians to equate the greater risk of adverse perinatal outcome with preexisting diabetes rather than conditions confined to pregnancy. Consequently, women are often intensively managed, with increased obstetric monitoring, dietary regulation, and in some cases insulin therapy. However, there has been no sound evidence base to support intensive treatment. The key issue for clinicians and consumers is whether identification and treatment of gestational diabetes and IGT will improve perinatal outcome. There are insufficient data for any reliable conclusions about the effect of treatments for IGT on perinatal outcome. The difference in abdominal operative delivery rates is not statistically significant (RR 0.86, 95% CI 0.51–1.45) and the effect on special-care baby unit admission is also not significant (RR 0.49, 95% CI 0.19–1.24). Reduction in birth weight >90th percentile (RR 0.55, 95% CI 0.19 to 1.61) was not found to be significant. The Cochrane review suggests that an interventionist policy of treatment may be associated with a reduced risk of neonatal hypoglycemia (RR 0.25, 95% CI 0.07–0.86). No other statistically significant differences were detected. There are insufficient data at present for any reliable conclusions about the effects of treatments for impaired glucose tolerance on perinatal outcome (76).

Self-monitoring of blood glucose (SMBG) has become a major tool in the management of diabetes over the past decade. Various guidelines are in use for validating blood glucose meters. There are currently no analytical guidelines for validating the procedures available for noninvasive or minimally invasive blood glucose meters in pregnancy. As a result, manufacturers of these meters need to comply with different regulations in different countries with concomitant high costs. National and international organizations have now made recommendations regarding accuracy and precision for blood glucose monitors.

Many new technologies are being applied to measure blood glucose concentrations, but there is a lack of a standardized approach to evaluate the performance of these devices. Chen et al. (77) examined these elements in a multicenter study of four brands of glucose meters that are commonly used by diabetic patients. They tested control materials, spiked whole-blood specimens, and 461 heparinized whole-blood specimens in triplicate by each of the four glucose meters, and analyzed the plasma glucose concentrations of these specimens by a hexokinase (HK) method that incorporated reference materials developed by the National Institute of Standards and Technology. Testing with glucose meters was performed at three sites, with multiple operators, meters, and representative lots of reagents. They then evaluated the systematic bias, random error, and clinical significance of the glucose meter tests. Meters were precise with a coefficient of variation of <4% across a wide range of glucose concentrations. Slopes significantly different from 1.0 were observed for two meters with 11% to 13% and −11% to −13% at the 95% CI level by the linear regression of meter results versus the HK method of 33 to 26.7 mmol/L (481 mg/dL) [$r > 0.98$ and $S_{y|x} < 0.7$ mmol/L (<13 mg/dL) for both meters]. Analysis of the clinical significance of bias by the Clarke error grid showed that results of the four meters were outside the accurate zone (26.5, 2.4, 1.5, and 5.6%). Only a small number of the results showed clinically significant bias, mostly in the hypoglycemic range. Meters performed consistently throughout the study and generally were precise, although precision varied at extremely high or low glucose concentrations. Two of the glucose meters had substantial systematic bias when compared with an HK method, indicating a need for improving calibration and standardization. Analytical performance varied over the physiological range of glucose values so that separate accuracy and precision goals should be defined for hypoglycemic, normoglycemic, and hyperglycemic ranges (77).

Henry et al. (78) tested the hypothesis that the accuracy of SMBG values of patients with diabetes during pregnancy deviates substantially from reference values. Patient glucose values were measured on six different SMBG meters; reference values were from the HemoCue B glucose analyzer (HemoCue, Angelholm, Sweden). Over a 5-year period, 1973 comparisons between SMBG values and reference values were recorded during clinic visits and used for this study. Data were analyzed for the percentage of values that varied $> \pm 10.5\%$ and $\pm 15.5\%$ from the reference value. Out-of-range data at each variance level were analyzed to determine the effect on medical management if decisions were based solely on SMBG values. One-third of SMBG readings deviated significantly, which could adversely affect treatment for half of these patients if diabetes management was based on SMBG values. At the 10.5% deviation level, 34% of SMBG meter readings were out of range; 54% of these would have implied erroneous treatment. At the 15.5% deviation level, 18% were out of range; 63% of these would have implied erroneous management. They concluded that the accuracy of home meters should be verified at regular intervals and SMBG values should not be the sole criterion for diabetes management during pregnancy (78).

Ryan et al. (79) retrospectively analyzed 107 case records of subjects with gestational diabetes, each of whom had three simultaneous laboratory and glucose meter glucose tests. The results were compared using the performance goals that (a) all glucose meters should have readings within 10% of the reference value and (b) the error grid analysis in the standard format and a modified version suitable for gestational diabetes should be used. The modified version of the error grid analysis demonstrated that 39% of the values were outside the acceptable range. Within subjects, a substantial number (26%) had a range of differences that exceeded 20% difference between each other. Although the meters give reasonable results that might be acceptable for general diabetes care, the results provide some cause for concern in the management of gestational diabetes. Given the need for precision in the setting of pregnancy, particularly in making the decision on whether to start or withhold insulin therapy, caregivers need to be cognizant of these inaccuracies (79).

CONCLUSIONS

The role of point-of-care tests in the management of high- and low-risk pregnancy continues to increase. The application is ever more diverse, from screening to diagnostics and from mother to fetus. With ever-increasing demands for community-based services with better diagnostic accuracy, manufacturers are challenged to develop this exciting technology for the 21st century.

REFERENCES

1. National Collaborating Centre for Women's and Children's Health. Antenatal care: routine care for the healthy pregnant woman. London: Royal College of Obstetricians and Gynaecologists Press, 2003.
2. Wald NJ, Kennard A, Hackshaw A, McGuire A. Antenatal screening for Down's syndrome. J Med Screen 1997;4:181–246.
3. Wald NJ, Rodeck C, Hackshaw AK, Walters J, Chitty L, Mackintosh AM. First- and second-trimester antenatal screening for Down's syndrome: results of the Serum, Urine and Ultrasound Screening Study (SURUSS). Health Technol Assess 2003; 7:1–77.
4. Spencer K. Near patient testing and Down's syndrome screening. Proc UK NEQAS 1998;3:130.
5. Mathis G. Rare earth cryptates and homogeneous fluoroimmunoassay with human sera. Clin Chem 1993;39:1953–9.
6. Levett LJ, Liddle S, Meredith R. A large-scale evaluation of amnio-PCR for the rapid prenatal diagnosis of fetal trisomy. Ultrasound Obstet Gynecol 2001;17:115–8.
7. Bindra R, Heath V, Liao A, Spencer K, Nicolaides KH. One-stop clinic for assessment of risk for trisomy 21 at 11–14 weeks: a prospective study of 15,030 pregnancies. Ultrasound Obstet Gynaecol 2002;20:219–25.
8. Cicero S, Curcio P, Papageorghiou A, Sonek J, Nicolaides K. Absence of nasal bone in fetuses with trisomy 21 at 11–14 weeks of gestation: an observational study. Lancet 2001;358:1665–7.

9. Goldenberg RL, Iams JD, Mercer BM, Meis PJ, Moawad AH, Copper RL. The Preterm Prediction Study: fetal fibronectin testing and spontaneous preterm birth. Obstet Gynecol 1996;87: 643–8.

10. Goldenberg RL, Mercer BM, Iams JD, Moawad AH, Meis PJ, Das A, et al. The Preterm Prediction Study: patterns of cervicovaginal fetal fibronectin as predictors of spontaneous preterm delivery. Am J Obstet Gynecol 1997;177:8–12.

11. Goldenberg RL, Iams JD, Mercer BM, Meis PJ, Moawad AH, Copper RL, et al. The Preterm Prediction Study: the value of new vs. standard risk factors in predicting early and all spontaneous preterm birth. Am J Public Health 1998;88:233–8.

12. Lockwood CJ, Senyei AE, Dische MR, Casal D, Shah KD, Thung SN, et al. Fetal fibronectin in cervical and vaginal secretions as a predictor of preterm delivery. N Engl J Med 1991;325:669–74.

13. Feinberg RF, Kliman JH, Lockwood CJ. Is oncofetal fibronectin a trophoblast glue for human implantation? Am J Pathol 1991; 138:537–43.

14. Mercer BM, Goldenberg RL, Meis PJ, Moawad AH, Shellhaas C, Das A, et al. The Preterm Prediction Study: prediction of preterm premature rupture of membranes through clinical findings and ancillary testing. The National Institute of Child Health and Human Development Maternal-Fetal Medicine Units Network. Am J Obstet Gynecol 2000;183:738–45.

15. Honest H, Bachmann LM, Gupta JK, Kleijnen J, Khan KS. Accuracy of cervicovaginal fetal fibronectin test in predicting risk of spontaneous preterm birth: systematic review. BMJ 2002; 325:301.

16. Lowe MP, Zimmerman B, Hansen W. Prospective randomized controlled trial of fetal fibronectin on preterm labor management in a tertiary care center. Am J Obstet Gynecol 2004;190:358–62.

17. Rosenberg K, Twaddle S. Screening and surveillance of pregnancy hypertension—an economic approach to the use of daycare. Ballierers Clin Obstet Gynaecol 1990;4:89–107.

18. Anthony J. Improving antenatal care. The role of the antenatal assessment unit. Health Trends 1992;24:123–5.

19. Naeye RL Friedman EA. Causes of perinatal death associated with gestational hypertension and proteinuria. Am J Obstet Gynecol 1979;133:8–10.

20. Butler NR, Bonham DG. Toxaemia in pregnancy. In: Perinatal mortality. Edinburgh: E and S Livingstone, 1963:86–100.

21. Ferrazzani S, Caruso A, De Carolis S, Martino IV, Mancuso S. Proteinuria and outcome of 444 pregnancies complicated by hypertension. Am J Obstet Gynecol 1990;162:366–71.

22. Chua S, Redman CW. Prognosis for pre-eclampsia complicated by 5 g or more of proteinuria in 24 hours. Eur J Obstet Gynecol Reprod Biol 1992;43:9–12.

23. Moore MP, Redman CW. Case-control study of severe pre-eclampsia of early onset. BMJ 1983;287:580–3.

24. Tervila L, Goecke C, Timonen S. Estimation of gestosis of pregnancy (EPH-gestosis). Acta Obstet Gynecol Scand 1973;52: 235–43.

25. Douglas K, Redman C. Eclampsia in the United Kingdom. BMJ 1994;309:1395–400.

26. Sibai BM, McCubbin JH, Anderson GD, Lipshitz J, Dilts PV Jr. Eclampsia. I. Observations from 67 recent cases. Obstet Gynecol 1981;58:609–13.

27. Porapakkham S. An epidemiologic study of eclampsia. Obstet Gynecol 1979;54:26–30.

28. Chesley LC. The variability of proteinuria in the hypertensive complications of pregnancy. J Clin Invest 1939;18:617–20.

29. Moutquin JM, Rainville C, Giroux L, Raynauld P, Amyot G, Bilodeau R, et al. A prospective study of blood pressure in pregnancy: prediction of preeclampsia. Am J Obstet Gynecol 1985;151:191–6.

30. Littler WA, Honour AJ, Carter RD, Sleight P. Sleep and blood pressure. BMJ 1975;3:346–8.

31. Perry IJ, Wilkinson LS, Shinton RA, Beevers DG. Conflicting views on the measurement of blood pressure in pregnancy. Br J Obstet Gynaecol 1991;98:241–3.

32. Kannel WB. Role of blood pressure in cardiovascular morbidity. Prog Cardiovasc Dis 1974;17:5–24.

33. Gallery ED, Hunyor SN, Ross M, Gyory AZ. Predicting the development of pregnancy associated hypertension. The place of standardised blood pressure measurement. Lancet 1977;1: 1273–5.

34. Gellman M, Spitzer S, Ironson G, Llabre M, Saab P, De Carlo Pasin R et al. Posture, place and mood effects on ambulatory blood pressure. Psychophysiology 1990;27:544–51.

35. Shennan A, Gupta M, Halligan A, Taylor D, de Swiet M. Lack of reproducibility of Korotkoff phase IV using mercury sphygmomanometry in pregnancy. Lancet 1996;347:139–42.

36. Redman CW, Jeffries M. Revised definition of pre-eclampsia. Lancet 1988;2:809–12.

37. National High Blood Pressure Education Programme Working Group report on high blood pressure in pregnancy. Am J Obstet Gynaecol 1990;163:1691–712.

38. Khoury S, Yarows SA, O'Brien TK, Sowers JR. Ambulatory blood pressure monitoring in a nonacademic setting. Effects of age and sex. Am J Hypertens 1992;5:616–23.

39. Rayburn WF, Zuspan FP, Piehl EJ. Self-monitoring of blood pressure during pregnancy. Am J Obstet Gynecol 1984;148: 159–62.

40. Julius S, Mejia A, Jones K, Krause L, Schork N, van de Ven C, et al. "White coat" versus "sustained" borderline hypertension in Tecumseh, Michigan. Hypertension 1990;16:617–23.

41. Staessen JA, Byttebier G, Buntinx F, Celis H, O'Brien E, Fagard R. For the ambulatory blood pressure monitoring and treatment investigators. Antihypertensive treatment based on conventional blood or ambulatory blood pressure measurement. A randomized controlled trial. JAMA 1997;278:1065–72.

42. Gupta R, Sharma AK. Prevalence of hypertension and sub-types in an Indian rural population: clinical and electrocardiographic correlates. J Hum Hypertens 1994;8:823–9.

43. Lin JM, Hsu KL, Chiang FT, Tseng CD, Tseng YZ. Influence of isolated diastolic hypertension identified by ambulatory blood pressure on target organ damage. Int J Cardiol 1995;48: 311–6.

44. Fang J, Madhaven S, Cohen H, Alderman MH. Isolated diastolic hypertension. A favourable finding among young and middle aged hypertensive subjects. Hypertension 1995;26:377–82.

45. Cerasola G, D'Ignoto G, Cottone S, Nardi E, Grasso L, Zingona F, Volpe V. Blood pressure pattern importance in the development of left ventricular hypertrophy in hypertension. G Ital Cardiol 1991;21:389–94.

46. Halligan A, Shennan AH, Lambert PC, de Swiet M, Taylor DJ. Diurnal blood pressure difference in the assessment of pre-eclampsia. Obstet Gynaecol 1996;87:205–8.

47. Padfield PL, Benediktsson R. Ambulatory blood pressure monitoring: from research to clinical practice. J Hum Hypertens 1995; 9:413–6.

48. O'Brien E, Staessen J. Normotension and hypertension as defined by 24-hour ambulatory blood pressure monitoring. Blood Press 1995;4:266–82.

49. Penny JA, Halligan AWF, Shennan AH, Lambert PC, Jones DR, de Swiet M, et al. Automated, ambulatory, or conventional blood pressure measurement in pregnancy: which is the better predictor of severe hypertension? Am J Obstet Gynaecol 1998;178:521–6.

50. Peek M, Shennan A, Halligan A, Lambert P, Taylor DJ. Hypertension in pregnancy: which method of blood pressure measurement is most predictive of outcome? Obstet Gynecol 1996;88:1030–3.

51. Critchley H, MacLean A, Poston L, Walker J, eds. RCOG study group in pre-eclampsia. London: Royal College of Obstetricians and Gynaecologists Press, 2003.

52. Higby K, Suiter CR, Phelps JY, Siler-Khodr T, Langer O. Normal values of urinary albumin and total protein excretion during pregnancy. Am J Obstet Gynecol 1994;171:984–9.

53. Lorincz AB, McCartney CP, Pottinger RE, Li KH. Protein excretion patterns in pregnancy. Am J Obstet Gynecol 1961;82:252–9.

54. Kuo VS, Koumantakis G, Gallery EDM. Proteinuria and its assessment in normal and hypertensive pregnancy. Am J Obstet Gynecol 1992;167:723–8.

55. Page EW, Christianson R. Influence of blood pressure changes with and without proteinuria upon outcome of pregnancy. Am J Obstet Gynecol 1976;126:821–33.

56. Brown MA, Buddle ML. Inadequacy of dipstick proteinuria in hypertensive pregnancy. Aust N Z J Obstet Gynaecol 1995;35:366–9.

57. Schiff E, Friedman SA, Kao L, Sibai BM. The importance of urinary protein excretion during conservative management of severe pre-eclampsia. Am J Obstet Gynecol 1996;175:1313–6.

58. Brown MA, Lindheimer MD, de Swiet M, Van Assche A, Moutquin JM. The clasification and diagnosis of the hypertensive disorders of pregnancy: statement from the International Society for the Study of Hypertension in Pregnancy. Hypertension in Pregnancy 2001;20:IX-XIV.

59. Lindow SW, Davey DA. The variability of urinary protein and creatinine excretion in patients with gestational hypertension. Br J Obstet Gynaecol 1992;99:869–72.

60. Meyer NL, Mercer BM, Friedman SA, Sibai BM. Urinary dipstick protein: a poor predictor of absent or severe proteinuria. Am J Obstet Gynecol 1994;170:137–41.

61. Boler L, Zbeller EA, Gleicher N. Quantitation of proteinuria in pregnancy by use of single voided urine samples. Obstet Gynecol 1987;70:99–100.

62. Waugh J, Bell SC, Kilby M, Lambert P, Shennan A, Halligan A. Effect of concentration and biochemical assay on the accuracy of urine dipsticks in hypertensive pregnancy. Hypertens Pregnancy 2001;20:205–17.

63. Chappell L, Poulton L, Halligan A, Shennan AH. Lack of consistency in research papers over the definition of pre-eclampsia. Br J Obstet Gynaecol 1999;106:983–5.

64. Harlow FH, Brown MA. The diversity of diagnoses of pre-eclampsia. Hypertens Pregnancy 2001;20:57–67.

65. Waugh JJ, Clark TJ, Divakaran TG, Khan KS, Kilby MD. Accuracy of urianlysis dipstick techniques in predicting significant proteinuria in pregnancy. Obstet Gynecol 2004;103:769–77.

66. Halligan AWF, Bell SC, Taylor DJ. Dipstick proteinuria: caveat emptor. Br J Obstet Gynaecol 1999;106:1113–5.

67. North RA, Taylor RS, Schellenberg JC. Evaluation of a definition of pre-eclampsia. Br J Obstet Gynaecol 1999;106:767–74.

68. Bell SC, Armstrong CA, Shennan AH, Boyce T, Halligan AWF. Reliable urine analysis in the management of hypertensive pregnancies. Eur J Obstet Gynecol Reprod Biol 2000;93:181–3.

69. Saudan PJ, Brown MA, Farrell T, Shaw L. Improved methods of assessing proteinuria in hypertensive pregnancy. Br J Obstet Gynaecol 1997;104:1159–64.

70. Waugh J, Bell SC, Kilby MD, Lambert P, Blackwell CN, Shennan AH, et al. Urinary microalbumin creatinine ratio: reference range in uncomplicated pregnancy. Clin Sci 2003;104:103–7.

71. Rodriguez MH, Masaki DI, Mestman J, Kumar D, Rude R. Calcium/creatinine ratio and microalbuminuria in the prediction of pre-eclampsia. Am J Obstet Gynecol 1988;159:1542–5.

72. Holm J, Hemmingsen L, Irgens-Moller L. Diagnostic value of hyperuricemia and microalbuminuria in pre-eclampsia. Med Sci Res 1988;16:123–4.

73. Bar J, Hod M, Erman A, Friedman S, Gelerenter I, Kaplan B, et al. Microalbuminuria as an early predictor of hypertensive complications in pregnant women at high risk. Am J Kidney Dis 1996;28:220–5.

74. Higby K, Suiter CR, Siler-Khodr T. A comparison between two screening methods for detection of microproteinuria. Am J Obstet Gynecol 1995;173:1111–4.

75. Waugh J, Kilby MD, Lambert P, Bell SC, Blackwell CN, Shennan A, et al. Validation of the DCA 2000 microalbumin: creatinine ratio urinanalyser for its use in pregnancy and preeclampsia. Hypertens Pregnancy 2003;22:97–113.

76. Tuffnell DJ, West J, Walkinshaw SA. Treatments for gestational diabetes and impaired glucose tolerance in pregnancy. Cochrane Database Syst Rev 2003;3:CD003395.

77. Chen ET, Nichols JH, Duh SH, Hortin G. Performance evaluation of blood glucose monitoring devices. Diabetes Technol Ther 2003;5:749–68.

78. Henry MJ, Major CA, Reinsch S. Accuracy of self-monitoring of blood glucose: impact on diabetes management decisions during pregnancy. Diabetes Educ 2001;27:521–9.

79. Ryan EA, Nguyen G. Accuracy of glucose meter use in gestational diabetes. Diabetes Technol Ther 2001;3:91–7.

Chapter **33**

Screening at the Point of Care: Down Syndrome—A Case Study

Kevin Spencer

The natural frequency of chromosomal abnormalities at birth, in a population without any form of prenatal diagnosis, is estimated at 6 per 1000 births. Of the various types of chromosomal abnormalities, the aneuploidies represent the most frequent. The most common of the aneuploidies is the autosomal trisomy 21 (Down syndrome), with an often-quoted birth prevalence of 1 in 800. The other common autosomal trisomies include trisomy 18 (Edwards syndrome) and trisomy 13 (Patau syndrome), which occur with birth incidences of 1 in 6500 and 1 in 12,500 respectively.

TRISOMY 21

Langdon Down, in his 1866 essay "Observation of an Ethnic Classification of Idiots," first described the phenotypic expression of the syndrome that bears his name to this day (1). Although Shuttleworth (2) described the association between the syndrome and increased maternal age in 1909, it was not until the work of Lejune et al. (3) and Jacobs et al. (4) in 1959 that it was demonstrated that the condition was a result of an extra copy of chromosome 21. This extra copy of genetic material, either the whole chromosome or a segment of the long arm of chromosome 21, occurs as a result of either nondysjunction or translocation. In approximately 95% of cases of nondysjunction, the additional genetic material is of maternal origin.

The major clinical consequences of trisomy 21, apart from the learning disability with IQ scores ranging from 20 to 70, are congenital heart defects, with a reported incidence of 50% of individuals. Gastrointestinal complications occur in some 30% of cases, and visual, ear, nose, and throat problems occur in some 40–60% of affected children. The frequency of hypothyroidism is increased significantly, as is epilepsy. Also there is a three-fold increase in the incidence of leukemia in children with trisomy 21. In recent years the average life expectancy has improved considerably, with an average life expectancy now close to 50 years. However along with increased life expectancy it has been found that by 40 years of age virtually all adults with trisomy 21 have neuropathological changes similar to those seen in Alzheimer's dementia.

TRISOMIES 18 AND 13

Edwards described the condition trisomy 18 in 1960 (5), and Patau et al. described the condition trisomy 13 in 1960 (6). In both cases the median survival time is less than 1 week, with 90% of infants dying by 6 months and <5% surviving to 1 year. The characteristic in utero feature is one of retarded growth and development.

PRENATAL SCREENING PROGRAMS

The incidence of the major trisomies (13,18, and 21) increases with maternal age while those for the sex aneuploidies (45 x0, 47xxy, 47xyy) and triploidy do not (Figure 33-1). As a consequence of the change in the pattern of childbirth over the past 20 years in most developed countries, with mothers postponing childbearing until later in life, the general prevalence of trisomy 21 has increased from 1 in 740 in 1974 to 1 in 504 in 1997 in the United States (7). Thus the development of prenatal screening programs for trisomy 21 and other chromosomal anomalies has become a feature of obstetric care in many countries over the past two decades.

The aim of prenatal screening programs is to provide information with which couples can make appropriate informed choices about reproductive decisions. It is not to establish programs which will focus on disabilities and lead to their eradication.

Not only does the incidence of a specific chromosomal anomaly vary with maternal age but, due to the varying intrauterine lethality, the incidence (relative risk) varies throughout gestation (Figure 33-2). This means that at 12 weeks of gestation the number of chromosomally affected fetuses is significantly higher than at 18 weeks or at term.

The aim of prenatal screening programs is essentially to identify a subgroup of women who may be at high risk of carrying a fetus affected by trisomy 21 or one of the other major chromosomal anomalies. This subgroup of women could then be offered an invasive diagnostic test such as amniocentesis and karyotyping or chorionic villus sampling—both techniques which have a potential fetal loss rate of ~0.5–1% above the background rate.

The first prenatal screening program for trisomy 21 was based on selecting women of a specific maternal age for an invasive test. Typically, in the United States and the United Kingdom during the 1970s and 1980s, a cutoff of 35 years was used to select women for amniocentesis, thereby identifying some 30% of cases, for an invasive testing rate of 6%. The predictive value of such a screening program was poor, with

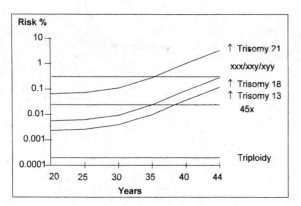

Figure 33-1 Maternal age–related risk for various chromosomal anomalies.

only one abnormal case being identified for every 125 invasive procedures. Uptake of amniocentesis among this group was also little better than 50%, so the overall program impact on birth prevalence was poor. With the changing demographics of pregnant populations in the developed world, now consisting of 15% of the pregnant female population over the age of 35 years, using maternal age would identify some 50% of cases with trisomy 21 at the expense of invasive testing for 15% of the population. Assuming a fetal loss rate of 1% due to the invasive procedure, such screening would result in the loss of three normal fetuses for every two cases identified—a loss rate that cannot be considered acceptable. Fortunately, in most jurisdictions other than the United States, offering invasive testing to women over 35 years of age has been superseded by developments over the past two decades. The entire pregnant population is now screened by maternal serum biochemical markers in the second trimester or by a combination of maternal serum biochemical markers and ultrasonography in the first trimester, increasing detection rates to 75% in the second trimester and 90% in the first. All this for the same 5% invasive testing rate.

Second-Trimester Maternal Serum Biochemical Screening

Second-trimester screening protocols have been developed over the past 15 years based on observations that, on average, levels of maternal serum α-fetoprotein (AFP) and unconjugated estriol (UE3) are lower in pregnancies complicated by fetal trisomy 21, and levels of maternal serum free β-hCG, total hCG, and dimeric inhibin-A are higher than normal. Because the absolute levels of each of these fetal, placental, or fetoplacental products vary with gestational age, it is not possible to define specific concentration cutoffs or reference ranges. To take into account gestational age variation, the measured marker level is expressed as a ratio of the median expected value in normal pregnancy of the same gestational age. This value, the multiple of the median (MoM), is reduced to ~0.7 for AFP and UE3 in trisomy 21 pregnancies and is ~2.0 for free β-hCG, total hCG, or dimeric inhibin-A. In

pregnancies with trisomy 18, on average the UE3, free β-hCG, and total hCG are reduced to 0.4, while AFP and dimeric inhibin-A are reduced to 0.65 and 0.87, respectively (8). In other anomalies no clear pattern of markers is evident.

In addition to gestational age, many other maternal factors can affect marker levels, and some, particularly maternal weight, smoking, and fetal number, may be worth correcting. Further information on such factors and their correction can be found in published work (8–10).

When expressed as MoMs, the biochemical markers generally follow a Gaussian distribution in both the normal and affected populations after the MoM has been $\log_{10}$ transformed. Unfortunately, with all markers there is a significant overlap of the normal and affected populations, and to use the marker information effectively a likelihood ratio is calculated. At any one marker MoM, the ratio of the heights of the distributions in the affected and unaffected populations is the likelihood ratio. To calculate the patient-specific risk, the a priori maternal age risk is then multiplied by the likelihood ratio. Thus in a 30-year-old woman the age risk is 1 in 600; assuming a likelihood ratio for Trisomy 21 of 3, the revised risk would be 3 in 600 or 1 in 200.

No one individual marker alone has sufficient clinical discrimination, and a more efficient screening program can be obtained in practice by combining information from more than one marker. If markers are independent, then the likelihood ratios for each marker can simply be multiplied to obtain the combined ratio. In practice, markers are correlated to varying degrees or provide similar information, and these factors must be corrected for by complex mathematical and statistical procedures (11).

Expected screening performance using various marker combinations can be modeled from data in retrospective case control studies. A disparity exists in estimates of detection and false-positive rates in the various studies due to a variety of factors including sample size, sample (pre) selection, assay methodology, analyte stability, risk algorithms, estimation of gestational age, marker distribution, marker correlation, marker truncation, and correction for covariables. In general terms, model predictions for second-trimester markers would suggest detection rates for trisomy 21 of 65–70% using a

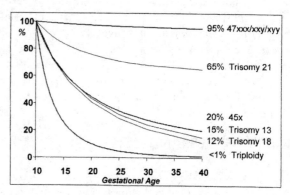

Figure 33-2 Gestational age–related risk for various chromosomal anomalies compared with the incidence at 10 weeks.

2-marker (AFP and free β-hCG or total hCG) or a 3-marker protocol (AFP, free β-hCG or total hCG, and UE3) at a 5% false-positive rate (9). The addition of inhibin A increases the detection by a further 3–5%. For trisomy 18 the 2- or 3-marker protocols give detection rates of ~50–60% at a 0.5–1% false-positive rate (12, 13).

First-Trimester Maternal Serum Biochemical Screening

In the first trimester, only two maternal serum biochemical markers are of value in screening for chromosomal anomalies (8). In cases of trisomy 21, levels of free β-hCG average ~2 MoM (14), whereas in trisomies 13 and 18 the levels are significantly reduced (0.5 and 0.3, respectively) (15–17). Unlike in the second trimester, total hCG is a very poor discriminator for trisomy 21 in the first trimester (18). The only other biochemical marker of value is pregnancy-associated plasma protein-A (PAPP-A), which is reduced to approximately 0.5 MoM in trisomy 21 (14) and to 0.2 MoM in trisomies 13 and 18 (15–17). Because of its changing clinical discrimination throughout pregnancy, this marker looses all clinical discrimination by week 17 and is of no value in screening in the second trimester (19, 20).

As in the second trimester, markers can be combined to make effective use of the information each provides. However, the two biochemical markers together in the first trimester have detection rates no better than 65% at a 5% false-positive rate (14), making the combination poorer than second-trimester biochemical screening.

Ultrasound in the First Trimester

The major marker of fetal aneuploidy is the first-trimester ultrasonographic marker fetal nuchal translucency thickness (NT) (21). An echogenic area of fluid exists in all fetuses between the fetal skin and the soft tissue overlying the cervical spine. Initial studies of high-risk populations identified an association between increased NT thickness and the presence of a fetal chromosomal anomaly (22). Because the measurement is small (1–2.5 mm in normal pregnancies) it is necessary to use a standardized approach to measurement; the Fetal Medicine Foundation approach to training, sonographer/obstetrician certification, and audit has become an almost-universal standard in this area (23). The NT measurement can be taken at the same time as the early pregnancy dating scan between 10 and 14 weeks, and in most experienced hands such examinations can be achieved within a 15-minute examination period. In studies that have used the Fetal Medicine Foundation protocol, detection rates for trisomy 21 of 70–75% for a 5% false-positive rate have been achieved (24).

Combined Ultrasound and Biochemical Screening in the First Trimester

Combining maternal serum biochemistry and NT measurement in the first trimester is an effective screening procedure because

the two modalities are not correlated (14). In a large-scale retrospective study of more than 200 cases with trisomy 21, 89% of cases were detected at a 5% false-positive rate. In addition, this combination can identify pregnancies complicated by trisomy 13 (16), trisomy 18 (15), Turner syndrome, other sex aneuploidies (25), and triploidy types I and II (26). It has been estimated that 90% of chromosomal anomalies other than trisomy 21 can be detected for an additional 1% false positive rate.

The identification of pregnancies at increased risk in the first trimester has a number of advantages. For some women, these advantages include an earlier diagnosis with a consequent safer and less traumatic therapeutic abortion; the majority of women obtain an earlier reassurance. While improvements in screening performance have in the past been measured by increased detection rates, little attention or research has focused on service delivery and counseling or how this affects maternal and family anxiety and stress at a time when families should be celebrating a new family addition.

Screening necessarily causes anxiety because it identifies individuals with a high risk of having a baby with a serious disorder. An "increased-risk" result makes the awareness of the risk real and personal at a particularly poignant time because of the strong emotions associated with pregnancy. The screening service should be provided in such a way that the general environment of screening, including appropriate information and personal support, causes no more than temporary and minimal anxiety, thus helping women and their partners to make the decisions that they feel are appropriate for them.

Screening should not be confined to simply performing tests and reporting risks. Women and couples need appropriate knowledge of the screening test, along with its limitations, so that they can decide whether to be screened. They need to consider their possible action if a screening result suggests that a diagnostic procedure is indicated and if an anomaly is diagnosed. It is important for them to understand that "increased risk" (or "screen positive," to use a common but confusing phrase) does not necessarily mean the pregnancy is affected. Equally important, "not at increased risk" does not provide absolute reassurance that there is no risk. With first-trimester screening, 9 in 10 cases with trisomy 21 will be identified, but 1 in 10 will be missed. Equally, of those identified as being at risk, 29 in 30 will not be trisomy 21, and 9 in 10 will have no chromosomal abnormality.

It is self-evident that the service must provide a well-informed, compassionate response that respects the wishes of individuals. Unfortunately, in many centers this is often not considered. A few limited studies have examined women's experiences and some have examined the health professionals who provide the service. Most have found that screening does cause anxiety in women and that sometimes this is made worse by how the service is delivered and by health professionals who are ill-informed.

Conventional screening programs based on second-trimester screening usually rely on sending a blood sample to a central laboratory, with a typical report turnaround of 3 days.

Women who are found to be at increased risk are required to attend the clinic for counseling regarding an offer of amniocentesis, which could take a further 3 days to arrange. Amniocentesis and conventional karyotyping will mean a further 2- to 3-week delay. Thus a final diagnosis of risk in the pregnancy is available some 4 weeks after the first screening test, with mothers having to wait anxiously for results and having to contemplate termination at ~20 weeks. With first-trimester screening, the same wait for laboratory results, the same wait for organization of counseling and chorionic villus sampling (CVS), and a further week for karyotyping means a total waiting period of 2 weeks, with termination being considered before the 14th week. An alternative screening program proposed recently (27, 28) argues that integrating prenatal screening across a 5-week period, measuring markers at 10, 11, and 15 weeks gestation with nondisclosure of the earlier screening test results, brings about improved detection (92% detection at a 5% screen-positive rate)—but at what cost to patient anxiety and stress during the 10-week screening period from initial test to diagnosis, not to mention the moral and ethical issues of nondisclosure of the earlier results, which could have identified 90% of the cases by the 14th week?

ONE-STOP CLINIC FOR ASSESSMENT OF RISK FOR FETAL ANOMALIES

Fortunately, with the advent of new diagnostic technologies it becomes possible to look at screening service delivery in a different way, which may result in reduced family anxiety, more informed choice, and a more efficient use of healthcare professionals' time. Rapid immunoassay systems suitable for point-of-care testing (POCT) are a further step that will allow the development of more widespread one-stop clinics for the assessment of risk for fetal anomalies (OSCAR) in the first trimester.

One-stop clinics have developed over the past decade in a number of clinical areas ranging from breast cancer screening through cardiovascular risk clinics and one-stop surgical clinics. These services all have in common the integration of a range of clinical and diagnostic services, which allow for a better use of clinical time and improved diagnostic efficiency. They aim to maximize patient satisfaction by reducing the number of patient visits, minimizing patient travel costs, and minimizing patient anxiety and stress. In the context of prenatal screening for chromosomal anomalies, the integration of counseling, ultrasound, biochemistry, midwifery, and obstetrics in a one-stop clinic does seem to be acceptable to women and, while offering maximum utilization of hospital outpatient resources, provides a high diagnostic efficiency and potentially allows for a more informed choice.

The concept of the OSCAR approach was developed in 1997 (29), when the first rapid assays for serum free β-hCG and PAPP-A became available on the CIS Kryptor platform (Brahms AG, Berlin, Germany). The 19-min homogeneous immunoassay technology (30), based on time-resolved amplified cryptate emission using chelates developed by Nobel Prize winner Jean-Marie Lehn, can be carried out in the same time that it takes a qualified sonographer to measure the fetal size (crown rump length) and nuchal translucency thickness and report a mini–anomaly scan. More recently other manufacturers have developed similar systems, such as the PerkinElmer Delfia Express system (PerkinElmer, Wellesley, MA) and the Aio! system (Innotrac Diagnostics, Turku, Finland) (31). The technology of such systems is outlined in Chapter 3.

With rapid testing technology it became possible to consider locating the testing within the antenatal clinic and organizing a clinic in such a way that the mother presents to the clinic at a specified appointment time for a 1-h visit (Table 33-1). In 65% of cases in the United Kingdom, the mother is initially seen in the community (either at home or in the general practitioner's office) by a member of the community midwifery team who will discuss all aspects of pregnancy care. At this stage an appointment will have been made for the mother to attend the OSCAR clinic when she is 12 weeks pregnant, based on the best estimate of her gestation at the time, and she will also have received an information leaflet regarding what screening tests she may be offered. When she attends the clinic, the first step is further pre-test counseling with a midwife counselor. If she so wishes, she can then (with informed consent) proceed to the clinic phlebotomy station to have blood collected and passed to the adjacent laboratory. The mother then proceeds to the ultrasound suite, and while the ultrasound scan is being performed, the free β-hCG and PAPP-A levels in her blood are measured. Following the ultrasound examination, a patient-specific multimarker risk assessment can be made, and within 45 min of attending the clinic, this report can be discussed with the mother in a post-test counseling session. If appropriate, diagnostic testing by chorionic villus sampling can be scheduled for the following day, with a quantitative PCR diagnostic result available within 48 h (32). The clinic is thus dependent upon a range of professional interactions in order to succeed, and such interdisciplinary teamwork has much to benefit staff working in this environment (Figure 33-3).

Such clinics have been in operation in two centers in the United Kingdom since 1998. The results of the first 3 years of screening women of all maternal ages in these centers have been reported, with detection rates of 92% for trisomy 21 and 96% for all aneuploidies, and a false positive rate of <5% (33, 34). The 5-year summary data from these two centers are

Table 33-1   OSCAR Clinic Flow

Patient Booked for a 1300 Appointment with 15-min Intervals

Time	Activity
1300	Pre-test counseling
1315	Blood samples taken
1320	Patient taken for NT/CRL and anomaly scan
1325	Samples on Kryptor for free β-hCG and PAPP-A
1345	Free β-hCG, PAPP-A, NT, and CRL results available
1350	Composite report available
1355	Post-test counseling

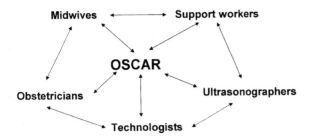

Figure 33-3 Professional interactions in the one-stop clinic for the assessment of risk for fetal anomalies.

shown in Table 33-2. Patient acceptance of offers of screening was high (97%), indicating that early one-stop screening was acceptable to women. Even screening twin pregnancies with such a procedure seems to be clinically effective in identifying 3 of 4 cases in twins discordant for trisomy 21 (10, 35). For the 8% of women who present too early for NT, i.e., ultrasound examination shows them to be prior to 11 weeks 0 days (crown rump length 45 mm), it is a simple task to reschedule a new visit at the appropriate gestation time. For the 5% of women presenting too late for NT, i.e., beyond 13 weeks 6 days (crown rump length 84 mm), second-trimester biochemical screening can be performed in the same time scale.

The introduction of such a service was fairly straightforward in a routine NHS setting. Ultrasound had been used since 1992 for the diagnosis of neural tube defects in our clinic. Therefore, the decision to dispense with second-trimester maternal serum biochemical screening for neural tube defects was made easier by the fact that ultrasound in our hands was considered an effective tool for diagnosis and screening for neural tube defects. The laboratory had provided second-trimester screening for trisomy 21 since 1991, and at that time clinic-based phlebotomy was already well established. Also early (12-week) booking and dating scans had been introduced in 1992, and by 1995, 80% of pregnancies were being booked and scanned at 12 weeks. In 1995 our ultrasound department became part of the Fetal Medicine Foundation NT project (21), which was carried out with no further staffing or equipment but was accomplished by reorganizing scanning time. In late 1997 a business plan was proposed to the hospital board to develop the OSCAR service, for which the only additional staff required was a dedicated midwife counselor and the location of a room to house the small screening laboratory, along with one biomedical scientist and one clerical officer. A decision was made in the spring of 1998 and the service went live on June 1, 1998, serving a local clinic population of ~5000 pregnant women.

As with many one-stop clinics, a full and accurate economic appraisal is often difficult to carry out. Certainly our services have developed along these lines because of our research involvement, and to translate the costs of our service to other sites that may not have had the benefits of our developed infrastructure would be totally wrong. Indeed, when others have carried out economic appraisal of breast cancer clinics, some have argued that the costs saved in the reduction in the frequency of outpatient visits are more than offset by those associated with the same-day reporting of diagnostic tests (36). However, others have argued that such crude economic assessments, which only take into account hospital costs and which take no account of patient costs, or indeed increased costs in primary care due to increased patient anxiety, should not be part of any evidenced-based approach (37–39).

In an attempt to provide some cost argument for the OSCAR service, we have examined what additional costs would be incurred by not providing the immediate service and compared this with the additional costs incurred for providing such a service. We have used the costs derived in a respected health economic study of ultrasound screening (40), adjusted for the Retail Price Index between the 1998–1999 study period and 2003 (1.113). If women were not provided with results within the 1-h visit, those whose results suggested that they were not at increased risk could be given their results at the next clinic visit (some 8 to 10 weeks later), or they could telephone the clinic for their results. In the latter case this would occupy additional midwifery time estimated at 10 min per client at a total cost of £10,313 ($17,532) for 4500 women. Those 500 women (5%) who were identified as being at increased risk, rather than being counseled in the clinic at the time of screening, would need to be telephoned by the counselor and then brought back to the clinic for a consultation with a fetal medicine specialist and the midwife counselor. This

Table 33-2 Prospective Performance of Combined Ultrasound and Maternal Serum Biochemical Screening in Two OSCAR Centers over a 5-year Period

Result	Spencer (33)	Year 4 and 5 (Spencer, unpublished)	Bindra (34)	Total
Screened	12,030	19,959	14,383	46,372
At increased risk	577 (5.2%)	767 (3.8%)	1096 (7.6%)	2440 (5.3%)
T21 detected/total	23/25 (92%)	47/52 (90%)	75/81 (92%)	145/158 (92%)
T18 detected	11	7	21	39
T13 detected	4	6	10	20
45× detected	4	7	10	21
Triploidy detected	5	4	7	16
Others detected	2	3	6	11

visit would invariably also include both partners. The additional visit costs to the patients would be £6911 ($11,749). The additional clinic administration cost for these visits would be £518 ($881), and the additional midwifery and clinical time cost would be £11,459 ($19,480). The estimated additional hospital costs of such visits would be £11,977 ($20,361), and £18,888 ($32,110) when taking into account patient costs. The costs of providing the one-stop service over and above the normal clinic operating costs are related to the fact that the laboratory provides a full-time equivalent biomedical scientist when only half of the time is associated with the analysis of 4500 specimens. Thus, the hospital savings of £11,977 ($20,361) is reduced by the need to fund the additional half-time laboratory post (£8815) ($14,986), making a net gain to the hospital of approximately £3162 ($5374). When patient costs are taken into account, the OSCAR services produce an overall savings on the order of £10,000 ($17,000) per annum.

New developments such as these, which are made possible by innovative health technologies, also must be assessed in a social context. One such program in the United Kingdom, the Innovative Health Technologies Program (www.york.ac.uk/res/iht), jointly sponsored by the Economic and Social Research Council and the Medical Research Council, has been running for ~3 years. The program aims to bring together researchers with experience in social science, medicine, and health research to examine innovative health technologies, investigating the mutual shaping of science, technology, and society through theoretical and empirical research. The projects under investigation in this program have a considerable genetics influence and aim to evaluate and compare the existing and new models of service delivery (such as OSCAR) and to assess the effects on patient anxiety and stress and the social management of pregnancy. The results of this study, which is comparing conventional service delivery (second-trimester laboratory-based screening) with an OSCAR first-trimester service, are just coming together. Preliminary results suggest that women who have been screened in an OSCAR setting are more knowledgeable about screening and the disorders being screened for than their counterparts who have undergone second-trimester screening. Also, anxiety scores postscreening were lower in women screened in the OSCAR clinic. Women in either system felt they were given enough time for decision making, something that was of concern when the OSCAR service was first planned. The fact that results are available quickly does not mean that women and couples cannot take as long as they need to make decisions at the various stages of the screening process.

In summary, 5 years of experience in an OSCAR clinic has shown the feasibility and benefits of delivering prenatal screening in a point-of-care environment. The fact that 97% of women who were offered such screening accepted demonstrates how pregnant mothers view such a service. Further evidence of what women want has been found in a recent survey of >1000 women at six hospital sites (41). At four of the sites women were routinely offered second-trimester screening, while at one site they routinely had first-trimester

screening with results provided some 3 to 4 days later, and at the last site women had the opportunity of using the OSCAR service. Women were given four screening options, indicating the time it would take for them to get the results and the detection rate of the test (at a fixed 5% false-positive rate), with the options including second-trimester testing, first-trimester testing results in 3 days, first-trimester OSCAR, and integrated screening between 11 and 16 weeks. Seventy-five percent of women selected a first-trimester test as their first choice, with 68.2% expressing a preference for the OSCAR approach. Only 1% expressed a preference for second-trimester screening, and only 24% thought that the perceived 3% increased detection with the integrated test was worth the prolonged wait of 5 to 6 weeks for a screening result. The timing and rapid reporting of results appear to influence women's preferred choice of a screening test. Such preferences must be taken into account when formulating screening policy.

The benefits of a one-stop approach using rapid testing technology may have applications in other areas, such as oncology clinics, where it would be possible to have biomarker testing prior to a consultation with an oncologist for review or revision of therapies.

REFERENCES

1. Down JL. Observations on an ethnic classification of idiots. Lond Hosp Rep 1866;3:259–62
2. Shuttleworth GE. Mongoloid imbecility. BMJ 1909;2:661–5.
3. Lejeune J, Gautier M, Turpin R. Etudes des chromosomes somatiques de neuf enfants mongoliens. C R Acad Sci 1959;248: 1721–2.
4. Jacobs PA, Baikie AG, Court Brown WM, Strong JA. The somatic chromosomes in mongolism. Lancet 1959;1:710.
5. Edwards JH, Harnden DG, Cameron AH, Crosse VM, Wolff OH. A new trisomic syndrome. Lancet 1960;1:787–90.
6. Patau K, Smith DW, Therman E, Inhorn SL, Wagner HP. Multiple congenital anomaly caused by an extra autosome. Lancet 1960;1:790–93.
7. Egan JF, Benn P, Borgida AF, Rodis JF, CampbellWA, Vintzileos AM. Efficacy of screening for fetal Down's syndrome in the United States from 1974 to 1997. Obstet Gynecol 2000;96: 979–85.
8. Aitken DA, Crossley JA, Spencer K. Prenatal screening for neural tube defects and aneuploidy. In: Rimoin DL, Connor JM, Pyeritz RE, Korf BR, eds. Emery and Rimoin's principles and practice of medical genetics. London: Churchill Livingstone, 2002; 763–801.
9. Wald NJ, Kennard A, Hackshaw A, McGuire A. Antenatal screening for Down's syndrome. Health Technol Assessment 1998;2:1–112.
10. Spencer K. Non-invasive screening tests. In: Blickstein I, Keith L, eds. Multiple pregnancy: epidemiology, gestation and perinatal outcome. London: Parthenon, 2004 [in press].
11. Reynolds T, Penney M. The mathematical basis of multivariate risk analysis: with special reference to screening for Down syndrome associated pregnancy. Ann Clin Biochem 1990;27:452–58.
12. Spencer K, Mallard AS, Coombes EJ, Macri JN. Prenatal screening for trisomy 21 with free beta human chorionic gonadotrophin as a marker. BMJ 1993;307:1455–8.

13. Palomaki GE, Haddow JE, Knight GJ, Wald NJ, Kennard A, Canick JA, et al. Risk based prenatal screening for trisomy 18 using alpha-fetoprotein, unconjugated estriol and human chorionic gonadotropin. Prenat Diagn 1995;15:713–23.

14. Spencer K, Souter V, Tul N, Snijders R, Nicolaides KH. A screening program for trisomy 21 at 10–14 weeks using fetal nuchal translucency, maternal serum free β-human chorionic gonadotropin and pregnancy-associated plasma protein-A. Ultrasound Obstet Gynecol 1999;13:231–7.

15. Tul N, Spencer K, Noble P, Chan C, Nicolaides KH. Screening for trisomy 18 by fetal nuchal translucency, maternal serum free β-hCG and PAPP-A at 10–14 weeks of gestation. Prenat Diagn 1999;19:1035–42.

16. Spencer K, Ong C, Skentou H, Liao AW, Nicolaides KH. Screening for trisomy 13 by fetal nuchal translucency thickness and maternal serum free β-hCG and PAPP-A at 10–14 weeks. Prenat Diagn 2000;20:411–6.

17. Spencer K, Nicolaides KH. A first trimester trisomy13/trisomy 18 risk algorithm combining fetal nuchal translucency thickness, maternal serum free β-hCG and PAPP-A. Prenat Diagn 2002;22: 877–9.

18. Spencer K, Berry E, Crossley JA, Aitken DA, Nicolaides KH. Is maternal serum total hCG a marker of trisomy 21 in the first trimester of pregnancy? Prenat Diagn 2000;20:311–7.

19. Spencer K, Crossley JA, Aitken DA, Nix ABJ, Dunstan FDJ, Williams K. Temporal changes in maternal serum biochemical markers of trisomy 21 across the first and second trimester of pregnancy. Ann Clin Biochem 2002;39:567–76.

20. Spencer K, Crossley JA, Aitken DA, Nix ABJ, Dunstan FDJ, Williams K. The effect of temporal variation of biochemical markers of trisomy 21 across the first and second trimester of pregnancy on the estimation of individual patient-specific risks and detection rates for Down's syndrome. Ann Clin Biochem 2003;40:219–31.

21. Snijders RJM, Noble P, Sebire N, Souka A, Nicolaides KH. UK multicentre project on assessment of risk of trisomy 21 by maternal age and fetal nuchal-translucency thickness at 10–14 weeks of gestation. Lancet 1999;18:519–21.

22. Pandya PP, Snijders RJM, Johnson SJ, Brizot M, Nicolaides KH. Screening for fetal trisomies by maternal age and fetal nuchal translucency thickness at 10–14 weeks of gestation. Br J Obstet Gynaecol 1995;102:957–62.

23. Nicolaides KH, Sebire NJ, Snijders RJM. The 11–14 weeks scan—the diagnosis of fetal abnormalities. London: Parthenon Publishing, 1999.

24. Nicolaides KH. Screening for chromosomal defects. Ultrasound Obstet Gynecol 2003;21:313–21.

25. Spencer K, Tul N, Nicolaides KH. Maternal serum free β-hCG and PAPP-A in fetal sex chromosome defects in the first trimester. Prenat Diagn 2000;20:390–4.

26. Spencer K, Liao AWJ, Skentou H, Cicero S, Nicolaides KH. Screening for triploidy by fetal nuchal translucency and maternal serum free β-hCG and PAPP-A at 10–14 weeks of gestation. Prenat Diagn 2000;20:852–3.

27. Wald NJ, Watt HC, Hackshaw AK. Integrated screening for Down's Syndrome based on tests performed during the first and second trimesters. N Engl J Med 1999;341:461–7.

28. Wald NJ, Rodeck C, Hackshaw AK, Walters J, Chitty L, Mackinson AM. First and second trimester antenatal screening for Down's syndrome: the results of the Serum, Urine and Ultrasound Screening Study (SURUSS) [Special issue]. Health Technol Assess 2003;7(11).

29. Spencer K. Near patient testing and Down's Syndrome screening. Proc UK NEQAS 1998;3:130.

30. Mathis G. Rare earth cryptates and homogeneous fluoroimmunoassay with human sera. Clin Chem 1993;39:1953–9.

31. Qin Q-P, Christiansen M, Pettersson K. Point-of-care time-resolved immunofluorometric assay for human pregnancy-associated plasma protein A: use in first-trimester screening for Down syndrome. Clin Chem 2002;48:473–83.

32. Hulten MA, Dhanjal S, Pertl B. Rapid and simple prenatal diagnosis of common chromosome disorders: Advantages and disadvantages of the molecular methods of FISH and QF-PCR. Reproduction 2003;126:279–97.

33. Spencer K, Spencer CE, Power M, Dawson C, Nicolaides KH. Screening for chromosomal abnormalities in the first trimester using ultrasound and maternal serum biochemistry in a one stop clinic: a review of three years prospective experience. Br J Obstet Gynaecol 2003;110:281–6.

34. Bindra R, Heath V, Liao A, Spencer K, Nicolaides KH. One stop clinic for assessment of risk for trisomy 21 at 11–14 weeks: a prospective study of 15,030 pregnancies. Ultrasound Obstet Gynecol 2002;20:219–25.

35. Spencer K, Nicolaides KH. Screening for trisomy 21 in twins using first trimester ultrasound and maternal serum biochemistry in a one stop clinic: a review of three years experience. Br J Obstet Gynaecol 2003;110:276–80.

36. Dey P, Bundred N, Gibbs A, Hopwood P, Baildam A, Boggis C, et al. Costs and benefits of a one stop clinic compared with a dedicated breast clinic: Randomised controlled trial. BMJ 2002; 324:507–10.

37. Rapid responses to Dey et al. http://bmj.bmjjournals.com/cgi/eletters/324/7336/507 (assessed June 2004).

38. Jefferson TO, Demicheli V. Quality of economic evaluations in health care. BMJ 2002;324:313–4.

39. Thorne AL, Yiangou C. Fast track breast clinics: Do they have a future ? Eur J Surg Oncol 2001;27:782.

40. Henderson J, Bricker L, Roberts T, Mugford M, Garcia J, Neilson J. British National Health Service's and women's costs of antenatal ultrasound screening and follow-up test. Ultrasound Obstet Gynecol 2002;20:154–62.

41. Spencer K, Aitken DA. Options for prenatal screening for chromosomal abnormalities—what women want. Prenat Diagn 2004;24 [in press].

Chapter 34

Point-of-Care Testing in Pediatrics

Franke N. Gill and Michael J. Bennett

The principles of point-of-care testing (POCT) in the pediatric population are much the same as in any adult population. There are, however, instances in which the rationale for use of POCT methods is driven by inherent physiological differences between pediatric and adult patients.

The increasing availability of testing methods that are portable, easy to use, require a small sample size, do not require sample preparation, and deliver rapid results is providing the momentum for increased POCT. The idea of instant results at the bedside is so seductive to clinicians and other caregivers that the economic factors are often discounted. The clinical justification for instant testing is not well documented for many currently available bedside methods. Even though outcomes data indicating the benefit of bedside testing are largely absent, there are a number of compelling reasons for performing bedside tests in a pediatric setting.

PHYSIOLOGICAL DIFFERENCES BETWEEN CHILDREN AND ADULTS

Infants and children can exhibit more rapid changes in clinical status than adults for a variety of reasons. During the neonatal period the oxygen consumption per kilogram of weight is 180 to 279 $mL \cdot min^{-1} \cdot m^{-2}$ as opposed to adult rates (after ~ 10 years of age) of 122 to 220 $mL \cdot min^{-1} \cdot m^{-2}$ (1). Although the oxygen delivery in neonates and young children is higher than in adults, the rate nears maximal levels because of the limitations of heart rate and cardiac output of the extremely young child. This dearth of oxygen reserve may contribute to rapid cardiorespiratory deterioration in response to increased oxygen demand, as in the case of cold, stress, infection, or pain or when decreased oxygen delivery results from pulmonary or cardiac disease (2, 3). In addition, infants are more susceptible to respiratory failure than adults because of immature respiratory function (4, 5). Faster metabolism causes greater demand on the relatively inefficient lungs, which contributes to rapid deterioration of optimum blood gas status. Respiratory muscles, central nervous system control of respiratory functions, and cartilage and elastic tissues are not as developed in the child as they are in adults (6). All of these contribute to an increased likelihood of respiratory failure in children experiencing respiratory distress as compared with adults. These factors spur the use of point-of-care blood gas measurement for monitoring the rapid respiratory changes in the pediatric population.

In addition, fluid and electrolyte balance needs to be monitored rapidly in children (7). Young children may become dehydrated or experience fluid overload rapidly because of evaporation as a result of their relatively large surface area to mass ratio. The highly permeable skin of the preterm infant and use of open warmers exacerbate this problem. Homeostatic mechanisms are not as well developed in children as they are in adults, especially in preterm infants. The renal function of preterm infants is immature. Concentrating and diluting ability is limited, resulting in an inability to compensate for hemoconcentration caused by insensible water losses (8). Premature infants exhibit sodium wasting, and children up to 1 year of age may develop metabolic acidosis because of ineffective excretion of acid and lower renal threshold for bicarbonate reabsorption. In infants with pyloric stenosis, vomiting may cause large amounts of chloride to be lost. Thus the ready ability to monitor pH and electrolytes is necessary to assess metabolic status and to aid in correction of the electrolyte imbalances in children.

Hypoglycemia is frequently seen in young children. Infants have little glycogen storage and immature gluconeogenic capacity (9). Stress episodes and even moderate caloric restriction associated with reduced food intake can quickly result in hypoglycemia (10). Glucose levels must be evaluated frequently, both for the possibility of hypoglycemia and for prevention of hyperglycemia during cardiopulmonary and trauma resuscitation, an event associated with poor neurologic outcome. Children may present with hypoglycemic and acidotic symptoms caused by metabolic disorders, which are often severe and life threatening. Immediate intervention in these cases is essential, again making a strong case for the rapid turnaround time provided by bedside testing.

Furthermore, children often exhibit markedly abnormal laboratory values that are not predicted by the apparent condition of the patient. Because of the young child's inability or unwillingness to communicate, often the only indication of a pediatric patient's condition is whether he or she "looks good," and small children tend to look good even though they are rapidly becoming unstable. Often, by the time they begin showing overt clinical signs they are already critically ill. (In contrast, adults tend to demonstrate their condition more appropriately; that is, when they feel bad, they look bad.)

Unfortunately, the inability or unwillingness of young children to communicate makes assessment of status more difficult than in adults. Children with developmental delay may also have difficulty communicating their fears or discomforts.

Even older children may fear the staff and be unwilling to communicate. They may also feel that the symptoms or the treatment are a type of punishment and refuse to cooperate. Children, especially adolescents, may also deny symptoms or conditions such as pregnancy, drug use, or sexually transmitted disease when in the presence of their parents, thus making diagnoses more difficult and the use of laboratory tests even more necessary. Children, having less experience with illness than adults, may not comprehend that they are ill. They may not be asked the correct questions or may not be asked in the most effective manner to ascertain their health status. Thus, objective measurements of status are even more necessary in children than in adults.

PHYSICAL CONSIDERATIONS

Reference Intervals

The inherent differences between adults and children place a burden on instrumentation manufacturers with regard to the development of age-related dynamic ranges of the instruments. Also, there is a need for the development of systems to alert the user to age-specific reference intervals. There are considerable differences in the reference intervals of some analytes when the age of the patient is considered. Emergency procedures that require rapid determination of blood gases are precisely the situations in which reliance on memory for reference ranges is most dangerous. Use of incorrect reference ranges may lead to inappropriate treatment.

Reference intervals for pH and Po_2 for infants appear in Table 34-1 (11, 12).

Specimen Size

Most POCT devices require small specimen volumes, making POCT in pediatric patients particularly advantageous. Excessive blood loss is a chronic problem when children face extended hospital stays. Blood volume is quickly depleted, especially in very small infants, when multiple tests are ordered. Guidelines for the maximum amounts of blood to be drawn on pediatric patients are summarized in Table 34-2.

Plasma volume remains relatively constant at 4% to 5% of body weight. In an infant weighing approximately 1.5 kg, the total volume of plasma is approximately 70 mL. The total blood volume of a 1-kg infant is so small that 1 mL of blood

Table 34-1   Age-Specific Reference Intervals for pH and Po_2

Age (begin)	pH	Po_2, mmHg
0 min	7.11–7.36	8–24
5 min	7.09–7.30	33–75
10 min	7.21–7.38	31–85
30 min	7.26–7.49	55–80
60 min	7.29–7.45	54–95
2 days	7.35–7.45	83–108

Table 34-2   Maximum Amount of Blood to Be Drawn on Pediatric Patients

Patient weight		Maximum volume per 24 h, mL	Maximum total vol per hospital stay (<1 month), mL
lb	kg		
<2	<0.9	1	8
2–4	0.9–1.8	1.5	12
4–6	1.8–2.7	2.0	17
6–8	2.7–3.6	2.5	23
8–10	3.6–4.5	3.5	30
10–15	4.5–6.8	5	40
16–20	7.3–9.1	10	60
21–25	9.5–11.4	10	70
26–30	11.8–13.6	10	80
31–35	14.1–15.9	10	100
36–40	16.4–18.2	10	130
41–45	18.6–20.5	20	140
46–50	20.9–22.7	20	160
51–55	23.2–25.0	20	180
56–60	25.5–27.3	20	200
61–65	27.7–29.5	25	220
66–70	30.0–31.8	30	240
71–75	32.3–34.1	30	250
76–80	34.5–36.4	30	270
81–85	36.8–38.6	30	290
86–90	39.1–40.9	30	310
91–95	41.4–43.2	30	330
96–100	43.6–45.5	30	350

Adapted with permission from data from Hermann Hospital Clinical Laboratories, Houston, TX.

would be equivalent to 70 mL of blood in an average adult. Blood transfusions may become necessary in infants when >10% of the blood volume is withdrawn in less than 2 to 3 days. Withdrawing as little as 8 mL from a 0.75-kg infant may necessitate transfusion (13). For patients weighing 2.5 to 3.5 kg the maximum amount to be drawn during a 24-h period should be limited to 2.5 mL; the volume withdrawn for a hospital stay of <1 month should total no more than 23 mL. Even for a child who weighs approximately 10 to 15 kg, the maximum withdrawal allowed during any one 24-h period is 10 mL (14). In view of the myriad of tests ordered on severely ill patients, many of which cannot be performed on small amounts of blood, it is essential whenever possible to employ the methods that use the smallest volumes.

Sampling technique is equally important. Venipuncture is not recommended in very small children, and it may be almost impossible in neonates. The stress of procuring specimens from cranial veins or arterial punctures may produce more problems than obtaining laboratory results alleviates. Performing venipuncture on very small children is traumatic to the child and to the parents. In addition, venipuncture is not efficient: It has been observed that as much as 10% of blood loss caused by sampling for laboratory tests is hidden in syringe dead space and the tubing of butterfly sets (15). Obtaining blood from a fingerstick or heelstick is much less stressful, and proper technique can be mastered fairly quickly by ancillary staff. This allows for better utilization of the skills of professionals at the bedside.

Current technology makes it possible to perform a single glucose measurement on 5 μL of blood. Multiple analytes—including blood gas, electrolytes, glucose, blood urea nitrogen (BUN), and ionized calcium—can be determined using 65 μL of blood. A blood gas may also be added to these tests, boosting the total sample to 95 μL.

Certain instruments available for use at the point of care can perform prothrombin time and activated partial thromboplastin time tests on a single drop of blood from a fingerstick sample (in contrast to the minimum volume of 1.8 mL required for methods used in most hospital laboratories). Recent developments have produced devices capable of using extremely small samples to determine activated clotting time, cholesterol, and even platelet function. Screening for blood lead is possible using a few drops of blood from a fingerstick. Glycated hemoglobin can be determined using 5 μL of blood, and total hemoglobin is available on 10 μL. A complete blood count, including a three-part differential count, can be performed on 12 μL of blood using an instrument with a small footprint. Although some of these tests are not necessary at the bedside and some are of limited use in a pediatric setting, the availability of tests using small sample sizes complicates decision making in regard to whether to perform tests at the point of care or in the central laboratory.

REASONS FOR PERFORMING TESTS AT THE POINT OF CARE

Rapid Turnaround Time

The most obvious reason for performing tests at the point of care is to obtain rapid results. Providing rapid turnaround time for test results becomes more beneficial the faster the change in condition is likely to occur. Obtaining results quickly would allow for the treatment of the patient while the values obtained are still indicative of the patient's status.

Intuitively, one assumes that POCT produces rapid turnaround times. In actuality, the turnaround time for test results is difficult to measure (16). If one considers the turnaround time to be the total time from the point the physician decides that the test should be performed until the result is seen by that physician, it would include the time necessary for the order to be placed by the physician, transcription by a secretary, collection by phlebotomist, and delivery to laboratory before the test can be performed. The testing itself includes receipt of the sample into the laboratory system, sample preparation, and instrument testing time along with the posting of the result to the patient's chart. Once the result is posted, although it is available to the ordering physician, there is often lag time before the result is seen and acted on. This is in contrast to the POCT turnaround time. Included in this is the order by the physician, the collection of the specimen by personnel presumably already at the bedside or nearby, performance of the test at the bedside, and posting of the results to the chart or

notification of the physician. Ideally, the total time should be so short that the physician is able to obtain the results and make clinical decisions immediately rather than proceeding to other patients or tasks while waiting for test results

Parent Satisfaction

It is difficult to imagine a more fervent desire for rapid test results than that of parents waiting for the diagnosis or treatment for their child. Several needs have been identified in dealing with parents of sick children, some of which include having questions answered honestly, knowing the child's prognosis, participating in their child's care, and knowing that their child is receiving the best possible care (17).

Many of these needs may be ameliorated by the use of bedside testing methods. The parent is present during the testing; the results are apparent and can be explained or acted on at that time. Seeing the test performed can give the parents greater confidence in the results and their utilization, contributing to greater trust and assurance that their child is receiving good care. As one parent of a child in ICU being treated for Reye's syndrome reported, "There were times when I would see something change, and I would call the doctor or nurse and feel particularly good if they did something or adjusted something that would bring that number back down. . ." (18). Children receiving venipuncture and their parents display less distress if the parent is present for the procedure. The presence of children's parents has little effect on the comfort level of the health professionals involved in the procedures (19). In fact, the majority of parents would prefer to be present and report that it makes them feel better (20). Both rapid results and the ability to use small specimen volumes are appreciated by parents and contribute to the push toward use of bedside testing.

APPLICATIONS OF POCT

Extracorporeal Membrane Oxygenation

One therapy largely restricted to use in pediatric populations is extracorporeal membrane oxygenation (ECMO). Used for the treatment of patients with acute respiratory failure (ARF), it is most effective in patients who have reversible lung disease. Neonates presenting with persistent pulmonary hypertension or meconium aspiration often display critical ARF in the first days of life, which may resolve as pulmonary vascular resistance decreases. Our institution and others also use ECMO to manage pediatric respiratory failure and to effect cardiac support, especially for postsurgical cardiac failure. ECMO was used at our hospital in a recent case of a 2-year-old with life-threatening endocarditis that resolved subsequent to ECMO therapy (personal observation). Patients awaiting heart transplants may also be maintained for a time using ECMO.

This procedure suggests several opportunities for the use of POCT, including measurement of blood gas and activated clotting time in patients receiving ECMO therapy. Blood gases must be measured frequently on the patient and the associated circuitry. These results are used to monitor the progress of the treatment not only during the steady-state period but also, and more important, during the initiation of therapy and the critical intervals when the patient is weaned from the ECMO circuit. During the weaning periods it is often necessary to obtain blood gas values on various parts of the circuit at 5- to 15-min intervals. Access to a rapid method of determining the blood gas result is critical, and having one that uses less than 0.1 mL of blood is even more desirable. In our institution the laboratory maintains and provides quality assurance for a mobile blood gas analyzer that is made immediately available for use by trained respiratory therapists for ECMO patients. When the instrument is taken to the ICU it is interfaced with the hospital information system; thus the tests are ordered, performed, and read at the bedside. Hemoglobin measurement is available with blood gas measurements on some instruments and is available separately using POC devices.

Because of the heparinization of the circuit it is necessary to monitor the activated clotting time (ACT) frequently. ACT is an example of a test that can be performed only at the point of care. ACT is performed on fresh, whole blood without any added anticoagulant. The sample begins to clot as soon as it is withdrawn from the patient and the test must be initiated as quickly as possible. As a result of these constraints, it is not possible to transport the sample any great distance from the patient.

The combined use of ECMO and POCT has reduced the mortality and morbidity of neonates enormously.

Surgery and Postoperative Management

Lactate measurement is now available using POCT instruments. Blood lactate may be used as an indicator of circulatory impairment and oxygenation state of patients. In surgical patients lactate levels measured after surgery show the extent of oxygen debt incurred during surgery, and subsequent measurements may be used to guide therapy (21). Blood lactate level has been shown to be of use in determining the need for instituting ECMO treatment and for monitoring its course (22). Because lactate is moderately unstable once collected, measurement of lactate at the bedside becomes even more desirable (23).

Diabetes Management

Management of pediatric diabetic patients is greatly enhanced using point of care instruments; the most obvious is the glucose meter. Studies have shown that diabetic patients maintain better control and have fewer long-term complications with self-monitoring of glucose on a continuing basis (24, 25). This is especially important in pediatric patients who have many years during which potential complications can arise. Hypoglycemia, for instance, is an important acute side effect of insulin therapy. Children have more active counter-regulatory responses to hypoglycemia than do adults, but diabetic children may lose their glucagon responses to plunging glucose yet retain the vigorous catecholamine, cortisol, and growth hor-

mone responses. This, combined with the natural insulin resistance during puberty, may lead to unstable diabetes control. Counter-regulatory response defects may result from recurrent episodes of hypoglycemia, thus increasing the risk of life threatening hypoglycemia and ketoacidosis. In addition, the ability of younger children to experience or express autonomic symptoms such as sweating, shaking, feeling anxious, and palpitations, which would alert adolescent or adult diabetics, may not be well developed, thus increasing the risk of severe episodes (26). Using glucose meters on diabetic units in the hospital is advantageous because it gives the staff the opportunity to educate the patient in device use. It also increases the perceived reliability of the results obtained because the glucose values the physician uses while the patient is in the hospital are obtained from the same device that the patient uses in the home.

Measurement of glycated hemoglobin as a monitor of long-term metabolic control can be performed on 5 μL of blood. The protocol for diabetic patients seen in our endocrine clinic includes a glycated hemoglobin every 3 months and determination of microalbumin in the urine once per year. Laboratory determined glycated hemoglobin requires a sample of at least 0.5 mL and approximately 2 days to collect, process, and transport the specimen (from the clinic location to the laboratory, a distance of approximately 1 mile); and to perform the test, which is run in batches on alternate days. One option that has been tried is to have patients come to the main hospital phlebotomy area to have their blood drawn before their clinic visit. We found that because of the complexity of this system some patients would get lost and either forget to go to the laboratory first or never make it to the endocrine clinic. A third option, performing the HbA$_{1C}$ on a POCT instrument in the clinic, seems to have provided the best solution to these problems. If performed on the POCT device, the test takes 5 μL of blood and is completed in 6 min using the same fingerstick as the glucose test. The principal advantage of obtaining the results while the patient is still in the clinic is the opportunity for the physician to educate the patient about noncompliance issues. Patients tend to adhere to the program more faithfully when the physician and diabetes educator are present to discuss the laboratory findings with the patient.

The microalbumin is measured using urine test strips. This test is a screening device and if it is positive, the patient is given the materials necessary to collect a 24-h urine at that time for quantitation of microalbumin. Using urine test strips to measure glucose and ketones is also carried out at the bedside while patients are hospitalized, thus helping to educate them in using the strips at home.

Trauma

Emergency care for children is a prime setting for POCT. Children, especially those who live in urban environments, are at high risk for illness and injury that requires emergency care. The nation's highest rates of violent injury, whether deliberate or not, occur in urban settings. These children also display higher morbidity rates from chronic diseases such as asthma and diabetes owing to lack of access to primary care (27). Access to care is also an issue for rural patients. Primary healthcare is often lacking and emergency centers are employed as outpatient clinics. POCT is increasingly being used to expedite treatment of these patients in community-based clinics, physicians' offices, and emergency transport.

Tests that screen for drugs of abuse in urine samples, for example, are available as POC tests. Drugs of abuse may be found in children as a result of accidental ingestion of either illegal or prescription drugs used by adults in their homes. Point-of-care screening tests are increasingly worthwhile in pediatric emergency medicine, community outreach clinics, and physician offices as an indicator of drug abuse in the pediatric population.

Transport

Because of the previously discussed factors driving rapid assessment of children's healthcare status, it is also advantageous to utilize POCT devices in transport situations. Glucose meters and instruments that analyze blood gas and electrolytes are becoming standard in transport. The hand-held blood gas analyzers used by our transport team are certified for use in ground transport, fixed wing aircraft, and helicopters. Clearly, small instruments are essential both because of vehicle space limitations and for the transport team's convenience.

Clinics

There are several areas in which POCT is of value in pediatric clinics or physician's offices:

1. Prothrombin times and partial thromboplastin times performed in a clinic location are valuable in monitoring hemostasis in cardiac patients.
2. Rapid streptococcus screens are now available as POC tests that make it possible to determine quickly if antibiotic therapy should be started. In the past it was necessary to wait for the results of cultures before starting treatment for streptococcal infections.
3. Pregnancy tests, sadly, are often required for pediatric patients in cases of suspected child abuse, the differential diagnosis of abdominal pain, or prior to various surgical or radiological procedures.
4. Lead testing is now available on fingerstick samples and can be performed with a small instrument that may be used in a clinic. In a study of more than 1000 children, 30 patients exhibited elevated lead levels; subsequent confirmatory testing identified nine true positives. Fingerstick testing was found to be a convenient and cost-effective alternative to direct venous testing for lead in children (28). Because children are particularly prone to the devastating neurological effects of lead poisoning, this is a very positive addition to the POC repertoire.

ORGANIZATION AND MANAGEMENT OF POCT

Regulating POCT

One provision of the Clinical Laboratory Improvement Amendment (CLIA) was to organize tests by complexity and to apply regulations based on the difficulty of performing the test and the possible consequences of erroneous results. For our institution it seemed advisable to group the tests using the CLIA complexity categories and to place the various groups under separate regulating authorities. These are summarized in Table 34-3.

The waived tests are grouped under one CLIA number with a Certificate of Waiver. These tests are under the authority of the laboratory, and the director of our laboratory is also listed as the director on this certificate. The moderate- and high-complexity tests are grouped together under a Certificate of Accreditation. While all of the testing remains under the authority of the laboratory, grouping the tests using separate CLIA numbers makes it possible to employ different criteria for managing the testing. In this manner the waived tests can be validated by Joint Commission on Accreditation of Healthcare Organizations (JCAHO) on the 3-year hospital survey, and the moderate- and high-complexity tests are inspected by the Laboratory Accreditation Program of the College of American Pathologists (CAP) during the routine biennial review of the laboratory. Another CLIA certificate was obtained for offsite clinic locations such as the endocrine clinic, which performs moderate-complexity tests. This required that the facility be inspected by HCFA on a 2-year rotation. CLIA certificates for Physician Performed Microscopy have been obtained for two clinics within our institution. These certificates are under the directors of the respective clinics and not the laboratory director. Regulations for waived tests under JCAHO are less stringent than those of CAP. It is possible, using the JCAHO guidelines, to determine a frequency and manner of performing quality control on waived tests that are appropriate for each institution. If there is no recommendation by the manufacturer, the institution is expected to devise the most suitable system for its facility.

Quality Control

Quality control is an essential element of all laboratory tests. This has been a point of contention as the laboratory transi-

Table 34-3 Categories of CLIA Complexity and Accrediting Agencies for Laboratory Testing

Accrediting agency	CLIA complexity	Location
JCAHO	Waived	Hospital and outlying clinics
CLIA	Moderate	Outlying clinics
CAP	Waived, moderate, high	Main laboratory

tioned to supervising ancillary testing. Whereas laboratory personnel regard performing quality control as second nature, physicians and the nursing staff do not. In our experience, most nonlaboratory personnel believe that quality-control testing is an unwarranted use of their time and that it should be done by the laboratory staff.

Many POCT instruments in use in hospital settings today have "QC lockout," which is a system designed to prevent testing of patient samples if the daily quality control is not performed. The systems have varying amounts of success at locking out patient testing. *We strongly recommend only systems with adequate lockout be used, thus ensuring compliance with the standards.*

We are relying on education of the POCT personnel to improve performance of quality control for instruments that do not have data management or lockout features and for manual tests.

Our approach to education includes a lecture and practical session given to each new nurse during his or her week of orientation, and annual retraining of the existing staff at skills days. Lecture sessions address the reasons for performing quality control, including the fact that documentation of quality-control results could be evidence in court indicating proper test performance and equipment operation. Most staff are more willing to do quality control when you can make clear to them how the patient benefits.

INDIVIDUAL POINT-OF-CARE TESTS

Urine Reagent Strips

Urine reagent strips are prone to production of erroneous results when the bottle is left open. This deterioration can occur rapidly in humid conditions. To prevent use of substandard strips we have developed an approach that we think seems reasonable to users, thereby helping foster compliance with the quality-control program.

Although in the main laboratory the strips are checked daily against two levels of control solution, we felt that this was not necessary when the strips were being used only sporadically on the nursing units. We determined that a frequency of once per week would be sufficient to assure adequate performance of the reagent strips.

Since the strips are used in so many locations in the hospital, it was necessary to devise different methods of checking them, depending on the location. Some areas have refrigerators that are used for storage of patient samples. These "dirty" refrigerators may be used to store the urine control solutions, which are in dropper-top bottles of 12 mL and are stable until the manufacturer's expiration date when kept refrigerated. When the bottle is empty, a new supply is obtained from the laboratory and stored in the refrigerator on the unit.

For locations that have no storage facilities, we keep a supply of control material in a specific refrigerated location in the main laboratory. The person performing the quality control on the strips for that week comes to the laboratory and takes the solutions to their location. The person checks all bottles of strips that are in use on their unit, documents the results, and returns the bottles of control solution to the laboratory.

The diabetes unit within our hospital preferred not to maintain a floor stock of urine reagent strips but to obtain individual bottles for each patient. They were used for patient testing while the patient was in the hospital and for education of that patient in performing the urine tests at home. The strips were then sent home with the patient and did not remain on the unit for more than a week. These strips are distributed by the laboratory, and each lot is checked by laboratory personnel using the previously described urine control solutions. The diabetes unit may then request a bottle of the strips by sending an order with the patient information to the laboratory. The strips are sent to the unit from the laboratory and charged to the patient.

Documentation of the quality control activities described in the preceding is accomplished by recording the results on log sheets kept on the units where the strips are being used. Log sheets are collected monthly and retained in the laboratory. Because many bottles have the same expiration date and lot number, and there are no marks differentiating bottles, we quickly determined that it was impossible to tell whether a specific individual bottle had been tested. To remedy this problem we printed custom labels and affix them to each bottle of strips when the original quality control is performed. The person performing the quality control dates and initials the label. Thus, anyone who uses that bottle of strips can easily observe the last time they were checked. The label is shown in Figure 34-1.

Occult Blood

Occult blood test cards incorporate quality control into the test procedure. Each card has a positive and negative area that must perform correctly before the patient test result is accepted.

In our institution, we ascertained that no record of the quality-control results was being made by the nursing staff when this test was performed. We realized that it was counterproductive to require the person performing the test to document that the controls worked correctly each time that the test results were recorded. We thought it might also be visually confusing to record the result of the positive control and the negative control and then to record the patient result all in a very small area. We decided that documenting the results of the occult blood quality control weekly on a log sheet would suffice. The same "QC Done" label that is used on the urine strips is used for the boxes of occult blood cards.

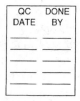

Figure 34-1 Quality control label designed for use on bottles of reagent strips.

Gastric samples may need to be tested for occult blood. A separate test designed for this purpose is available. Note that, as stated on the card and in the package insert, the cards used for stool samples must not be used for gastric samples. In our institution the stool occult blood cards were frequently used with inappropriate sample types. Both tests are in the CLIA waived category and are equally simple to perform but the cards and developer solution are different for the two tests. To prevent confusion, we decided to allow stool occult blood testing on the units but to limit testing of other types of samples to the central laboratory.

Glucose

For glucose meters the frequency for performing quality control is determined by the manufacturer's recommendation of two levels of control every 24 h. Many features facilitate monitoring meter usage and performance of quality control. Most meters have data management systems that require entering the patient identification and operator identification before testing is performed. These meters also have options for entering reagent lot numbers, quality control ranges, and expiration dates of reagents and quality control materials.

Using software provided by the manufacturers, reports of quality control data, user data, and a multitude of other data configurations are recorded. A recent development is downloading these data to laboratory or hospital information systems, making it possible to enter the results electronically in patient charts, and to assign charges patients for bedside tests in much the same manner that laboratory charges are generated. Most glucose meters in use in hospital settings today have QC lockout to prevent testing of patient samples if the daily quality control is not performed. The systems have varying degrees of success at locking out patient testing. *We strongly recommend only systems with adequate lockout be used, thus ensuring compliance with the standards.*

Hemoglobin

Hemoglobin can be measured very accurately on some current POCT instruments. We recently performed a 20-patient study comparing hemoglobin values obtained concurrently from two POCT instruments and our laboratory instrument. We found very good correlation between the laboratory values and one POCT device but poor correlation with the other POCT instrument (unpublished study). We no longer use the second POCT device for hemoglobin measurements. Quality control is defined by the manufacturer as two levels every 24 h. The control material for the instrument used in our institution must be refrigerated but has a shelf life of several months if stored properly. These instruments now have data management capabilities and can accept user identification, patient identification, control ranges and lot numbers, and cuvette lot numbers. These data are available to the user on the instrument screen, or they may be retrieved using software that can be installed on most PCs. Prior to institution of the data management form of the

meters, we maintained a log sheet for recording the quality control and maintenance for these instruments.

Pregnancy Tests

Several available pregnancy test systems have CLIA waived status. These kits contain procedural controls; that is, during the performance of the test certain indicators show that the test is performing correctly. The manufacturers have FDA approval for the kits used in this manner. We believe that external controls should be used as well to ensure result reliability. Currently, we check each kit with positive and negative controls upon opening it. We record these results on a log sheet and review them monthly. The same reagent kit is used in the laboratory and the clinic locations, making it possible to order larger amounts of the same lot number and to share between locations if the tests are used infrequently.

Rapid Streptococcus Tests

Primary care clinics and emergency centers find streptococcus screening useful in treating their patients. Waived tests are available for streptococcus screening. Many of the test kits include procedural controls, and external controls are available for testing of each kit. Although, as with pregnancy kits, the manufacturer allows patient testing without recommending any external controls, we feel that testing of each kit is a minimum requirement. Results should be logged and checked monthly by the laboratory. With both streptococcus and pregnancy test kits, the frequency of controls may be adjusted depending on the volume of testing conducted. In large clinics or where large numbers of tests are being performed, it may be reasonable to assay controls only with each shipment and with new lot numbers.

Prothrombin Time

Prothrombin time (PT) is a valuable POC measurement in a cardiology clinic. Monitoring PT in the clinic location is convenient for the patients visiting the clinic, as the results are available while they are there. The physician also has access to the results and is able to adjust treatment immediately rather than wait for results from the laboratory, which may take several hours or even days. When choosing an instrument, consider that a waived instrument requires less stringent monitoring, and some PT instruments are FDA approved to be sent home with patients who live in outlying areas. Although selection of patients who are good candidates for self-testing is problematic, some patients are quite able to perform tests accurately and can be trusted to communicate well with the physician. This is especially true when the patient is a child and self-testing will save the parent a trip back to the clinic. Requirements for quality control differ depending on the instrument chosen. At the very least, controls should be performed on every shipment of reagents and on each new lot number.

Glycated Hemoglobin

The system that we use for POC glycated hemoglobin measurement requires that quality control be performed daily. The instrument has limited memory, and information retrieval is tedious. Because there is no printer capability, quality-control and patient results are recorded on a log sheet. At the clinics, a hospital information system interface is available for ordering and entering test results. Clinic personnel are instructed in performing these tasks.

The quality-control results are also logged in the computer. Thus, the technical consultant (TC) for the laboratory can review the results from the main laboratory and advise the clinic staff if there are any problems. The lot numbers and ranges for the controls are entered into the computer by the TC. The laboratory oversees proficiency testing. Proficiency material is ordered and received in the laboratory and delivered to the appropriate clinic location on a rotating basis. Results are available on the computer and are retrieved by the TC, who sends them to the regulating agency. Performance evaluations are returned to the TC in the laboratory and are routed through the review process. Everyone who is involved with the process has an opportunity to study the evaluations, and any issues are addressed. After the final review by the laboratory director, the evaluation is stored in the laboratory for at least 2 years.

Blood Gases and Electrolytes

Most point-of-care blood gas analyzers today are small countertop instruments. They are too large to be conveniently carried from one patient to another.

We perform POCT of blood gases along with electrolytes, BUN, glucose, and ionized calcium on a handheld analyzer. The instrument is a microprocessor-controlled electromechanical device designed to measure electrical signals generated by sensors on individual cartridges. All of the reagents needed for the tests are contained in the individual cartridge. Calibrating solution is also present within the cartridge, and calibration is effected on each cartridge before patient testing is performed. The signals produced by the sensors in response to the calibrant solution are measured. A message is displayed if calibration fails for any one of the analytes on the cartridge and that test is not performed on the patient sample.

Internal electronic quality control is performed automatically every 8 h. It is also possible to perform an external electronic control on the instrument if error messages are produced by the internal quality control function.

Cartridges may be left at room temperature for only 2 weeks. To ensure the integrity of the reagents, we order the cartridges and keep them in the laboratory refrigerators and each shipment or lot number of cartridges is quality controlled by laboratory personnel.

Cartridges are manufactured with various combinations of analytes. Some analytes are measured directly whereas others are calculated from the measured values. Table 34-4 shows a list of the analytes currently available on this system.

Table 34-4 Typical Range of Analytes Available at the Point of Care in a Pediatric Setting

Measured	Calculated
pH	Oxygen saturation
P_{CO_2}	HCO_3
P_{O_2}	Base excess
Sodium	Total CO_2
Potassium	Anion gap
Chloride	Hemoglobin
Ionized calcium	
Hematocrit	
Glucose	
Urea nitrogen	
Lactate	
Activated clotting time	
Prothrombin time	

We use the cartridge that includes blood gas and glucose testing for patients who present with diabetic ketoacidosis. Glucose measurements from this instrument compare well with our laboratory glucose values. We find this method is more accurate than bedside glucose meters, especially so for patients in ketoacidosis.

Results from these analyzers are downloaded at remote locations within the hospital and are transmitted to a computer in the POC coordinator's office. The system automatically logs the tests into the hospital computer and places the results on the patient's electronic chart. Thus, results are readily available to caregivers at any location in the hospital.

In the patient transport area blood gases are performed using these instruments but they are not downloaded to the hospital system. Results are printed and the printout is placed on the transport record.

In addition to the blood gas instruments previously mentioned, a hemoximeter is used in the cardiac catheterization suite. Most of the time, measurement of oxygen saturation is sufficient for the staff's purposes. Using this instrument, oxygen saturation can be measured with 0.3 mL of blood. The results are available in <1 min. Despite the accessibility of a tube system, this arrangement is more efficient than ordering an O_2 saturation test from the laboratory. In actuality, permitting the cardiac catheterization laboratory staff to perform this test themselves also allows the laboratory to handle the urgent blood gas tests that are sent from other areas in the hospital more effectively.

ACT/Heparin Management

There are three different methods in use in our institution for ACT testing. In the dialysis unit, the test is performed by nurses using glass-activated plastic tubes that require only 0.5 mL of sample. CLIA requires two levels of quality control every 8 h. The manufacturer has recently introduced quality-control material in a self-contained dropper vial comprised of an ampoule of lyophilized sample surrounded by a premeasured volume of diluent. The operator crushes the ampoule within the vial to reconstitute the control material. This eliminates measuring, mixing, and accidental needle sticks. In a two-year period at a local hospital it was found that failure of controls to fall within acceptable ranges was entirely attributable to the inability of the users to reconstitute control material correctly. Not one control failure was traced to reagent or instrument problems. For this reason liquid control material is used in this system only for each new box of ACT tubes.

Many hospitals have chosen to analyze liquid controls only on new shipments or lot numbers of tubes. While we feel that this is adequate validation of reagents when lots and shipments can be monitored, our current system of reagent delivery requires that we verify each box. In addition to the liquid control material, electronic controls are now available for many ACT instruments. These simulate the behavior of the tubes with liquid control and thus confirm the instrument performance. Electronic controls that produce numerical results have been judged acceptable to HCFA and more recently to CAP. Two levels of electronic controls per 8-h shift meet the CLIA requirement.

We had been using the glass bead method during cardiac catheterization procedures, for our ECMO patients, and for patients undergoing continuous veno-venous hemodialysis (CVVH). We recently began performing ACTs using 0.4 mL of blood on the same handheld device we use for blood gas and electrolyte measurements. The results are transmitted directly to the patient charts, and a charge is generated for each test performed. We had been unable to find an efficient way to charge the patients for ACT tests using the previous system.

In surgery two units that measure ACT and heparin concentration are available. These tests are performed by perfusionists who are trained and monitored by the laboratory. After a 3-mL syringe is filled and clamped into the dispenser assembly, the instrument automatically dispenses the correct volume into each channel of the cartridge selected. ACTs are run in duplicate and use 0.4 mL of sample in each channel. Heparin dose-response cartridges have six channels and use 0.35 mL in each. The heparin assay uses only 0.2 mL in each of four channels. Electronic quality control is performed each day of use for this unit. The perfusionists who are performing the patient tests also perform the quality control. The lyophilized control material is reconstituted in one step and usually produces results that fall within published ranges, but the occasional out-of-range result is seldom related to reagent or instrument failure. The results are stored in the instrument memory and are downloaded and reviewed by the POC coordinator. Very little maintenance is required on these instruments, but it is critical that the temperature within the instrument be kept constant. The instrument can display the temperature continuously or may be set to display only on request. Monthly maintenance includes verification of the temperature with an external probe. Instrument maintenance is recorded in a log book.

Recent software upgrades have made it possible to keep electronic records of the lot numbers and expirations of re-

agents used on these instruments. It is also possible to prevent use of the instrument when quality control tests have not been performed. Unfortunately, the current software does not allow enough flexibility in quality control schedules for our purposes and we have chosen not to use the lockout feature at this time.

Platelet Function

Since 1910, the bleeding time test has been used to attempt to identify disorders of primary hemostasis. The results of this test are highly subjective. The test is also labor intensive and may be traumatic for the patient. Even if the test provided useful results, it would be advantageous to devise a test that was less traumatic and less dependent on the skill of the person performing the test. One platelet function analysis system uses 0.8 mL of blood to determine the platelet function in less than 5 min. Because citrated blood is used for this system it is not necessary to perform the test at the bedside; however, the instrument is small and easy to use and could be a welcome addition in a surgery stat laboratory.

BENEFITS OF POCT

POCT is not an either/or proposition. In most cases the same tests performed in the main laboratory are performed at the bedside. The decision is not whether to perform these tests at the bedside but to what extent and in which instances.

It is necessary to consider all of the factors mentioned previously—rapid results, sample size, outcomes, economics, and customer satisfaction—when determining the best approach to testing.

When considering rapid results it is not enough to determine the time required to receive the results. It is also necessary to determine whether obtaining those results more quickly would benefit the patient. In an evaluation of the possible effects of more rapid results obtained from a handheld blood analyzer in an emergency room setting, physicians were blinded to the results from the handheld analyzer and later asked whether there would have been a different or earlier treatment. The physicians indicated that in 9.5% of the cases, a different or earlier therapeutic approach would have ensued (29). However, none of the physicians indicated that the final outcome would have been affected.

Another attempt at determining the benefits of POCT involved comparison of the length of stay (LOS) of patients visiting the emergency department in a five-week period before use of the POCT device, a five-week period using the device, and a three-week control period following use of the POCT instrument. Even though at least one test was ordered for almost one-third of the patients that was available on the POCT instrument, there was no difference in the LOS during the experimental period in which the POCT device was used (30).

Improved turnaround times also assume that there is someone available at the bedside who is trained to perform the tests being ordered. For instance, if only respiratory therapists are trained to use handheld blood gas instruments, the test could not be performed until the therapist was available. Constructing good models for assessing the health benefits resulting from the use of POCT is very difficult, and little evidence is available in the literature that substantiates or even claims measurably improved outcomes resulting from the use of bedside testing.

The cost of performing tests at the bedside is also difficult to determine. Many studies with varying conclusions have been published; however, several investigators have found that tests performed in the central laboratory were less costly than bedside testing and that the cost per test for POCT increased as the volume of testing decreased (31, 32). If the health benefits of bedside testing were compelling, the higher cost could be justified (33); however, much bedside testing does not replace but is performed in addition to central laboratory tests (34). In our institution, a tertiary care pediatric hospital of 350-bed capacity, 73,000 glucose strips were purchased in a 1-year period. Assuming that the number of strips involved in quality control, wastage, repeat testing, and routine diabetic control and education amounts to 75% of the total strips used, we are still left with >18,000 instances in which it was deemed necessary to obtain a glucose value at the bedside. It is doubtful that a large portion of these tests were used for critical situations.

We have determined that it is more efficient to perform most of the urinalysis and occult blood tests in the main laboratory. The physicians and nursing staff in the ICU were consulted regarding the necessity for rapid results for these two tests. A pneumatic tube system connects the ICU with the central laboratory and, if necessary, a 15-min turnaround time is possible for these tests. The ICU staff decided to discontinue use of these two tests at the bedside. Clearly, this option will not be available for institutions without good pneumatic tubing systems in which the need for rapid turnaround will increase POCT usage.

Occasionally the mechanism described earlier of obtaining a bottle of strips for a particular patient is still used, if the situation warrants. Thus far, there have been no reports of adverse effects for ICU patients resulting from the transfer of these tests to the central laboratory. We have saved approximately $8500 per year on testing supplies alone in the 2 years since beginning this program. Additional resources are saved, both in disposables and nursing time, by not performing quality control on each unit. Previously, these tests did not generate revenue for the hospital. They are now charged to the patient. After observation of the success of this method in ICU, several other departments have decided to discontinue these tests at the bedside.

The decision to discontinue these tests has also alleviated another disadvantage resulting from easy access to testing materials: excessive use. Determination of occult blood in the stool may be of value one time or even once per day in certain circumstances, but it is difficult to justify performing this test on every stool produced.

Table 34-5 summarizes the locations in which certain POC tests are recommended. Other uses of these tests need further

Table 34-5 Recommended Uses of Point-of-Care Tests

POC test	Recommended uses
Urine test strips	Diabetes wards, trauma
Occult blood	Trauma
Glucose	Diabetes wards, trauma
Rapid strep screen	Clinics, physicians' offices
Blood gases	Transport, trauma, codes
Electrolytes	Transport, trauma, codes
Lactate	Postop ICU
Oxygen saturation	Cardiac catheterization
CBC	Clinics, physicians' offices
Hemoglobin	Trauma, surgery
Pregnancy tests	Clinics, physicians' offices
HbA$_{1c}$	Diabetes clinics
Microalbumin	Diabetes clinics
Prothrombin time	Cardiology clinics, home use
ACT/heparin	Surgery, ECMO, dialysis
Platelet function	Surgery, postop ICU

study to determine whether they are of benefit either clinically or operationally. This applies both to the institution of a new test and evaluation of testing currently in use.

OUTCOMES

Constructing good models for assessing the health benefits resulting from use of POCT is very difficult, and little evidence is available in the literature that substantiates or even claims measurably improved outcomes resulting from the use of bedside testing in pediatric or adult medicine.

Recently in a landmark study of goal-directed therapy based on prospective POC lactate measurement, Rossi and Khan (35) demonstrated improved outcome for pediatric patients following surgery for congenital heart disease. There was a significant reduction in mortality in a cohort of children in whom therapy was directed by the lactate level compared to historical data from the same institution. The reduction in mortality was particularly significant for the neonatal population and those undergoing the highest-risk surgery.

CONCLUSIONS

It is impossible to make generalizations about all types of tests based on any one set of criteria. Customer satisfaction (physician, patient, or parent) at being able to derive immediate results that impact diagnosis and treatment is a clear and general benefit from POCT.

The need for rapid results may be the driving force for performing one test while the requirement for using fresh, whole blood without anticoagulants makes another POC test advantageous. The existence of a test for cholesterol that takes only a few microliters of blood, a few minutes of time, and a small investment in materials does not mandate the performance of this test as a bedside test. If the result of the test is not going to have an effect on the treatment of the patient, it is not necessary to perform the test at the bedside to obtain the results rapidly.

On the other hand, another justification for performing a test at the bedside is that the test specimen cannot be transported. In the case of ACT, for example, the test requires fresh whole blood without any anticoagulant. It would be impossible to obtain accurate results if this test were performed at any distance from the patient.

POCT clearly has a place in pediatric healthcare; however, care should be taken to justify its use. The burden of proof should lie with those requesting it.

We should perform POCT not because it is possible, but because it is best.

REFERENCES

1. Hazinski MF. Anatomic and physiologic differences between children and adults. In: Levin DL, Morriss FC, eds. Pediatric intensive care, 2nd ed. New York: Churchill Livingstone, 1997: 1116.

2. Hirschl RB. Oxygen delivery in the pediatric surgical patient. Curr Opin Pediatr 1994;6:341–7.

3. Rudolph AM. Fetal circulation and cardiovascular adjustments after birth. In: Rudolph AM, ed. Pediatrics, 20th ed. East Norwalk, CT: Appleton & Lange, 1996:1409–13.

4. Davis GM, Bureau MA. Pulmonary mechanics in newborn respiratory control. Clin Perinatol 1987;14:551–9.

5. Chernick V, Avery ME. The functional basis of respiratory pathology. In: Kendig EL, ed. Disorders of the respiratory tract in children. Philadelphia: WB Saunders, 1977:3–61.

6. Agostoni E, Mognoni P, Torri G. Relation between changes of rib cage circumference and lung volume. J Appl Physiol 1965;20: 1179–86.

7. Myers A. Fluid and electrolyte therapy for children. Curr Opin Pediatr 1994;6:303–9.

8. Edelman CM Jr, Barnett HL, Troupka V. Renal concentrating mechanisms in newborn infants. J Clin Invest 1960;39:1062–9.

9. Williams AF. Hypoglycaemia of the newborn: a review. Bull WHO 1997;75:261–90.

10. Shelley HJ. Carbohydrate reserves in the newborn infant. Br Med J 1964;1:273–5.

11. Tietz NW, ed. Clinical guide to laboratory tests, 3rd ed. Philadelphia: WB Saunders, 1995:460.

12. Children's Medical Center of Dallas. Historical data.

13. Kaplan LA, Tange SM, eds. Standards of laboratory practice: guidelines for the evaluation and management of the newborn infant. National Academy of Clinical Biochemistry. Washington DC: AACC Press, 1998:6–7.

14. Adapted from Hermann Hospital Clinical Laboratories, Houston, TX, with permission.

15. Blanchette VS, Zipursky A. Assessment of anemia in newborn infants. Clin Perinatal 1984;11:489–516.

16. Nosanchuk JS, Keefner R. Cost analysis of point-of-care laboratory testing in a community hospital. Clin Chem 1994;103: 240–3.

17. Renick J. The needs of patents with a child in pediatric intensive care [Thesis]. University of Toronto, 1998.

18. Levin DL, Morriss FC, eds. Pediatric intensive care, 2nd ed. New York: Churchill Livingstone, 1997:1050–5.

19. Wolfram RW, Turner ED. Effects of parental presence during children's venipuncture. Acad Emerg Med 1996;1:58–64.

20. Bauchner H, Vinci R, Waring C. Pediatric procedures: do parents want to watch? Pediatrics 1989;84:907–9.

21. Abramson D, Scalea TM, Hitchcock R, Trooskin SZ, Henry SM, Greenspan J. Lactate clearance and survival following injury. J Trauma 1993;35:584–9.

22. Tofaletti J, Hansell D. Interpretation of blood lactate measurements in paediatric open-heart surgery and in extracorporeal membrane oxygenation. Scand J Clin Lab Invest Suppl 1995;55: 301–8.

23. Tofaletti J, Hammes ME, Gray R, Lineberry B, Abrams B. Lactate measured in diluted and undiluted whole blood and plasma: comparison of methods and effect of hematocrit. Clin Chem 1992;38:2430–4.

24. American Diabetes Association: Consensus statement on self-monitoring of blood glucose. Diabetes Care 1995;18:47–52.

25. The Diabetes Control and Complications Trial Research Group. The effect of intensive treatment of diabetes on the development and progression of long-term complications in insulin-dependent diabetes mellitus. N Engl J Med 1993;329:977–86.

26. Amiel SA. Studies in hypoglycaemia in children with insulin-dependent diabetes mellitus. Horm Res 1996;45:285–90.

27. Foltin GL. Critical issues in urban emergency medical services for children. Pediatrics 1995;96:174–9.

28. Schonfeld DJ, Rainey PM, Cullen MR, Showalter DR, Cicchetti DV. Screening for lead poisoning by fingerstick in suburban pediatric practices. Arch Pediatr Adolesc Med 1995;149:447–50.

29. Sands VM, Auerbach PS, Birnbaum J, Green M. Evaluation of a portable clinical blood analyzer in the emergency department. Acad Emerg Med 1995;2:172–8.

30. Parvin CA, Lo SF, Deuser SM, Weaver LG, Lewis LM, Scott MG. Impact of point of care testing on patients' length of stay in a large emergency department. Clin Chem 1996;42:711–7.

31. Greendyke RM, Gifford FR. Testing blood glucose at the bedside in a chronic care hospital. Lab Med 1997;28:63–7.

32. Jacobs E. Is point-of-care testing cost effective? Clin Lab News 1996 Jun;32–34.

33. Winkelman JW, Wybenga DR, Tanasijevic MJ. The fiscal consequences of central vs. distributed testing of glucose. Clin Chem 1994;40:1628–30.

34. Lee-Lewandrowski E, Laposata M, Eschenbach K, Camooso C, Nathan D, Godine JE, et al. Utilization and cost analysis of bedside capillary glucose testing in a large teaching hospital: implications for managing point of care testing. Am J Med 1994;97:222–30.

35. Rossi AF, Kahn D. Point-of-care testing: improving pediatric outcomes. Clin Biochem 2004 [in press].

Chapter 35

Point-of-Care Testing in the Community

Roger E. H. Kirkbride

In the United Kingdom, ~6 million people visit a community pharmacy every day and >2.3 million prescriptions are dispensed. Eighty percent of the income of the majority of pharmacies comes from the National Health Service (NHS), yet community pharmacies are generally seen as operating outside the NHS (1). The role that the community pharmacy fulfills—supplying medicines to patients according to doctor prescriptions—has changed little since the inception of the NHS. However, the skills and knowledge needed for compounding, interpreting the prescription, ensuring appropriate dosage, and avoiding interactions between drugs have been replaced by original package dispensing and computer technology. New skills and roles have been developed in hospital pharmacy, but these have been slow to translate to community pharmacies. However, they are now regarded as the most underutilized resource available to the NHS, and a substantial change in the role of both the pharmacy and the pharmacist is under way. This chapter explores the way in which these roles are changing and the part that point-of-care testing (POCT) is playing in supporting that change.

THE CHANGING ROLE OF THE PHARMACIST

The underutilization of community pharmacists has been recognized for some time, and policymakers have been taking steps to enable their skills to be used more effectively (2). Benefits are seen as reducing the workload of general practitioners (GPs), improving access to healthcare for patients, giving greater prominence to public health, and generating better value for money (3).

The Profession's Perspective

In 1995, the Royal Pharmaceutical Society of Great Britain (RPSGB) began a process of engaging pharmacists in defining how the roles of pharmacists would have to change to meet the challenges ahead. *Pharmacy in a New Age* involved widespread consultation with pharmacists, patients, and other professionals and planners (4). In 1997, the RPSGB identified five themes that would form the core of the role of pharmacists in the future (5). These were:

- The management of prescribed medicines
- The management of long-term conditions
- The management of common ailments

- The promotion and support of healthy lifestyles
- Advice and support for other healthcare professionals.

Subsequent development of the roles that pharmacists could play in the delivery of healthcare has been based on these themes.

The Government's Perspective

In July 2000, the Secretary of State introduced the NHS Plan, which was designed to reform the NHS and redesign the provision of services around the patient (6). A separate document was introduced for pharmacy (7), detailing the government's vision for the place of pharmacy in the new NHS. Helping patients to get the best from their medicines and redesigning services around patients were key themes in this document. The concept of a new contract for pharmacy, based on the quality of services provided rather than the volume of prescriptions dispensed, was introduced.

In July 2003, ten key roles for pharmacy were identified by the chief pharmaceutical officer of the Department of Health (8). These included:

- Being the first point of contact with health services in the community
- Providing medicine management services, especially for people with enduring illness
- Contributing to seamless and safe medicine management throughout the patient journey
- Prescribing medicines and monitoring clinical outcomes.

This document went on to illustrate the kind of services that were envisioned. They included monitoring patients and recommending alteration of dosage of medicines that require careful monitoring, such as warfarin or lithium; and diagnostic or monitoring services as part of an integrated local service.

The new pharmacy contract, due to come into effect in late 2004, will allow primary care organizations to commission services from a pharmacy on the basis of local need. These will be paid for from locally controlled budgets (9) and will begin to move pharmacy toward a service-based remuneration system and away from one based almost completely on volume. Primary care organizations will be able to contract with pharmacies to provide screening, monitoring, and disease management services, many of which will require tests to be carried out within the pharmacy.

THE CLINICAL CONTEXT FOR PHARMACY-BASED POCT

Pharmacy-based POCT will take place in the context of pharmacists providing new services to patients on behalf of primary care organizations; they are a means to an end—interaction with a patient—not an end in themselves. POCT will be carried out for three purposes: (*i*) as part of the treatment of long-term conditions, (*ii*) as part of a screening program, or (*iii*) prior to treatment of a specific condition.

Long-Term Conditions

Long-term conditions account for a large part of NHS and social care spending. It is estimated that 17.5 million people in the United Kingdom may be living with a long-term condition and that up to 75% of people over 75 years of age suffer from a chronic condition (10). By 2030, the estimate is that the incidence of chronic disease in people over 65 will double and that almost half of these will have more than one condition. These patients already account for >80% of GP consultations. The growth in the number of people with a long-term condition, coupled with higher standards of care being set for them through national service frameworks (NSFs) will result in a substantial increase in GP workload. NSFs have been set for coronary heart disease (11), diabetes (12), mental health, cancer, and for older people (13). These lay out standards of care that the NHS should achieve, and these standards have been used to establish the quality indicators in the new general medical services (GMS) contract (14), the contract under which GPs are judged for payment.

The Prescription Pricing Authority has identified that the conditions covered by the NSFs account for 40% of prescriptions written in England and that implementing the standards would result in a 5.6% increase in total prescription costs (15), indicating a substantial increase in workload, not only for GPs, but also for laboratories processing samples taken in GP health centers.

The GMS contract stipulates the outcomes that need to be demonstrated to trigger the payments rewarding achievement of quality targets. Primary care organizations also have targets relating to the NSFs that they are expected to achieve; both GPs and primary care organizations have flexibility in how they achieve their targets. GPs may contract pharmacies to manage groups of patients on their behalf. Similarly, primary care organizations may purchase services from pharmacies if there is underprovision of general medical services in the area or if they believe that additional or alternative provision is required.

Cardiovascular Disease. Cardiovascular disease is the main cause of death in the United Kingdom; half of cardiovascular disease deaths are attributable to coronary heart disease (CHD) and about a quarter to stroke (16). To comply with NSF standards, every GP practice should have a CHD risk register and protocols for systematic assessment, treatment, and follow-up for patients on the register. Quality measures

reflect these standards and include targets for blood pressure measurement, cholesterol levels, and anticoagulant therapy.

There is a real opportunity here for pharmacy-based monitoring and dose adjustment for patients with raised blood pressure or cholesterol levels and those on anticoagulant therapy.

Equipment to measure blood pressure in the pharmacy is available and adequate for the task; the RPSGB issued practice guidance on blood pressure measurement in the pharmacy in January 2003 (17), and this details equipment that has been formally validated against mercury sphygmomanometry. Modified treatment will come through locally driven protocols agreed upon by the primary and secondary care teams or through supplementary prescribing arrangements.

Monitoring and managing cholesterol levels are tasks that could be delegated to pharmacies; the RPSGB produced guidance on cholesterol testing in June 2003 (18). The quality indicator in the GMS contract calls for records of patients' total cholesterol and sets targets for total cholesterol levels. Although the requirement is to monitor only total cholesterol, equipment is available to give total cholesterol, HDL, triglycerides, and an estimate of LDL cholesterol; an assessment of liver function can be made through an alanine aminotransferase test (19). Any service established within a primary care organization may require tests at this level of detail to comply with local protocols.

Diabetes. Diabetes accounts for 5% of total NHS resources and up to 10% of hospital inpatient resources. Over 1.3 million people in the United Kingdom have been diagnosed with diabetes; 85% of these have type 2 diabetes, and many hundreds of thousands more may be living with type 2 diabetes without realizing it (12). The number of prescription items dispensed for insulin and oral hypoglycemic drugs reached 3.8 million in 2003, an increase of 80% over 5 years. The growth in prescriptions written for oral hypoglycemic agents between 2001 and 2003, at 26%, was higher than that for insulin, demonstrating the growth in diagnosed type 2 diabetes (20).

The National Institute for Clinical Excellence has issued a number of guidelines for the management of people with diabetes, the complications that occur with diabetes, and the issues of comorbidity associated with it. They require monitoring a range of clinical indicators including HbA1c, total cholesterol, HDL cholesterol, LDL cholesterol, triglycerides, creatinine, microalbuminuria, proteinuria, and liver function (21–23). Most of these parameters are reflected in the GMS contract quality indicators. POCT devices exist for all of these analytes, and their measurement is possible within a community pharmacy setting. However, conducting the full range of tests is more likely to take place within the context of an annual review, a process that is more suited to a secondary care setting or primary care specialist clinic, where retinal screening and other physical checks can be carried out. Routine measurement of HbA1c is most likely to be undertaken in the pharmacy as it is a good indicator of glycemic control and would be used as the basis of a medicine management protocol to adjust oral hypoglycemic or insulin dosage.

Other Long-Term Conditions. Although cardiovascular disease and diabetes represent by far the greatest number of patients who may receive POCT as a part of increased care through the pharmacy, there are other significant diseases that may also be suitable for pharmacy management. Monitoring patients taking medication for a thyroid condition and those taking lithium therapy is possible and may be desirable for certain groups. Monitoring patients taking disease-modifying antirheumatic drugs is more complex, but regular monitoring of liver function and renal function in the pharmacy may form part of the shared care plan for people with severe rheumatoid arthritis.

Screening

Given the high level of usage of the pharmacy, participation in screening programs for conditions that are substantial public health issues is likely to be effective in identifying people with those conditions. Such screening is likely to involve the use of simple POCT and protocols. Screening programs for CHD and for type 2 diabetes are being considered.

A national screening program for chlamydia infection is being established in the United Kingdom (24). This relies primarily on the opportunistic screening of sexually active women under the age of 25 who attend GP health centers, family planning clinics, or genitourinary medicine clinics. However, 70% of women with chlamydia infection are asymptomatic, and the screening program does not specifically target men. Pharmacies are likely to be the most frequently used healthcare resources of the target screening groups and could form part of the network of screening access points. A number of POCT devices are available that would allow rapid assessment of chlamydia status. Specificity, sensitivity, and ease of use are less than ideal and would currently limit their potential. However, a number of companies are developing new generations of tests, and the potential for small scale rapid PCR-based testing is growing.

Prior to Treatment

There are a number of infectious conditions for which a definitive diagnosis is beneficial before treatment is initiated. The drug of choice may differ, depending on the causative organism, or the treatment may be dependent on a definitive diagnosis. Point-of-care tests coupled with patient group directions (PGDs; i.e., written instructions for the sale, supply, and administration of named medicines in an identified clinical situation) (25), provide an opportunity to offer better patient care, reduce GP workload, and avoid overuse of antibiotics, thus reducing the rate of growth of antibiotic resistance.

The eradication of *Helicobacter pylori* infection is recommended for patients with duodenal or gastric ulcers where *H. pylori* is present. Testing from the GP health center often requires referral to secondary care facilities or the collection and sending away for analysis of ^{13}C labeled breath specimens. Both of these involve a second trip to the GP center to obtain results and the passage of some days or weeks before a result

is known. Portable ^{13}C breath analyzers are now available, opening up the potential for the GP to reduce workload, shortening the time taken to initiate eradication treatment, and reducing unnecessary prescribing. The GP may refer a patient directly to the pharmacy for a ^{13}C breath test with eradication following a PGD.

Epidemics of influenza cause massive increases in workload not just for GPs but also for secondary care facilities. In 2003, the UK National Institute for Clinical Excellence issued guidance on the use of zanimivir and oseltamivir for the treatment of influenza (26). Later that year, Roche prepared a draft PGD for oseltamivir, which was then tailored by a number of primary care organizations anticipating an epidemic. This would have allowed treatment to be initiated by pharmacists rather than GPs. However, in a presentation made to an SMi Group conference on point-of-care diagnostics in February 2004, S. Wayne Kay (of Quidel) pointed out that only one-third of patients with influenza-like symptoms actually have influenza. In the United States, where there was a substantial and early epidemic of influenza in the winter of 2003–2004, physicians were encouraged to use POCT for influenza prior to treatment. A similar process could be implemented in pharmacies in the United Kingdom, speeding up diagnosis and treatment, reducing overprescribing of antiviral agents, and potentially saving costs. Whether cost savings are achievable may be debatable; studies in the United States have shown conflicting conclusions (27, 28), although the contexts of the studies and that of the UK healthcare model are different.

DEVELOPING PHARMACY INVOLVEMENT IN POCT

The previous section describes the potential for POCT in community pharmacies as opposed to the situation that we see now. If primary care organizations and community pharmacies invest in a strategy that encourages the development of increased chronic disease management and increased speed of access to services, and POCT forms part of these services, not all pharmacies will choose to participate equally. We should expect them to develop a degree of specialization in one condition or another, or in one field or another, e.g., diabetes or CHD, chronic condition management or minor ailments.

A survey conducted in 2002 (29) showed that the majority—73%—of UK pharmacies offered some kind of POCT. In the majority of these, the only test offered was pregnancy testing (157 out of 161 respondents), with 21% offering blood pressure monitoring. Other services included cholesterol screening, glucose measurement, and allergy testing. Independently owned pharmacies were more likely to offer POCT than were national chains.

However, since then, the provision of services that utilize POCT has begun to develop as pharmacies begin to embrace the new roles that are emerging and anticipate the services that may be possible under the new pharmacy contract. The larger chains are also beginning to participate more; for example

Lloyds' pharmacies (a chain of almost 1400 pharmacies throughout the United Kingdom) offer free diabetes screening in 1000 of their stores, a service that was launched in 2003. The initiation of over-the-counter statins in the second half of 2004 is likely to result in an expansion of pharmacy-based POCT for cholesterol measurement and CHD risk assessment.

There are a number of anticoagulant clinics already established in community pharmacies; anticoagulation services are well established in the northeast of England and are beginning to be introduced in other areas, including Sheffield and northern London. A survey of primary care organizations in 2002 showed that almost half were considering establishing community-based anticoagulant monitoring and that almost 60% of these were likely to involve pharmacists (30). The authors conclude that the relatively low response rate of primary care organizations (26%) to the survey means that the results cannot be extrapolated to the whole of the United Kingdom; however, they do provide a useful indicator of future community-pharmacy involvement.

Pharmacies within each primary care organization are represented by a local pharmaceutical committee (LPC) whose role is to promote the interests and roles of pharmacists within the primary care organization and to respond to issues and opportunities presented. The Dorset LPC has proposed frameworks for managing hypertension, coronary heart disease, anticoagulation, and diabetes in the community pharmacy. Under the hypertension framework, newly diagnosed patients would receive their initial medication from the pharmacist following a protocol agreed to by the patient's GP. Monitoring would then take place in the pharmacy at regular intervals. Under the CHD framework, pharmacists would carry out a full lipid profile and a liver function test for patients referred from a GP. The proposals form part of a 5-year plan proposed to the Strategic Health Authority to embrace the new roles for pharmacists emerging under the new contract (31).

The Rationale for Pharmacy-Based POCT

The rationale for the development of POCT goes beyond what is possible and may be desirable from the perspective of the pharmacy profession. For pharmacy-based POCT to develop, there has to be benefit to the patient and the health system in which it operates. Patient benefits may be qualitative, but system benefits are more often viewed in terms of economic impact.

Patient Benefits. A number of models of care exist in the United Kingdom, depending on the condition that the patient has and the protocols used between primary care, secondary care, and laboratory services in the area where he or she lives.

Some patients attend secondary care clinics where their condition is monitored and their treatment regime is modified. The modifications often take effect only when the patient returns to their GP for a repeat prescription that they then have to take to a pharmacy to be dispensed. In this scenario, the patient has to make multiple trips to a number of locations,

incurring travel expenses and using substantial amounts of time. Furthermore, the elapsed time between the decision to change medication and the implementation of that change can be many days or even weeks.

When a greater degree of care is managed through the GP health center, samples for analysis are still sent away to large centrally located laboratories. The patient is spared the inconvenience of attending a secondary care clinic but still has to make multiple visits to the GP health center. The time elapsed between a decision to adjust a medication and its dispensation may still be several days. Even where the GP utilizes POCT, the health center may not be open at times convenient to the patient, and the prescription still has to be collected and then filled at a pharmacy.

Once a patient has a clear diagnosis, has stabilized, and has a well-defined care plan, managing the patient's condition at the pharmacy can result in considerable savings to the patient in time and transportation costs. A single visit can be made at a time to suit the patient, and this may include evenings and weekends. Any tests can be taken while the patient is in the pharmacy utilizing POCT, and any dosage adjustment can be made according to protocols set within local guidelines and agreed to by pharmacist and the patient's GP.

Similarly, the treatment of certain infectious conditions can be made more certain and more rapid through the application of POCT and a suitable PGD to the benefit of the patient, the people with whom the patient may come into contact, and the health service.

System Benefits. The health system benefits of pharmacy-based POCT are difficult to measure. Clearly, cost-effectiveness is required, but how is this measured? Microeconomic cost analysis of POCT has consistently shown POCT to be more expensive than laboratory testing (32), but looking only at the cost of providing the test does not take in to account the true economic impact of POCT. The benefits of faster decision making, more rapid intervention, better control of a patient's condition, reduced waste, and other factors should also be taken into account. Patients who are persistent nonattenders of GP or secondary care clinics may well find the accessibility of a community pharmacy attractive. These patients may, as a consequence of better care, experience better control of their condition and thus reduce their use of secondary care.

The UK government has set out an agenda that requires more patient care to take place in the community and for work to move from hospitals to GP health centers. GPs may develop a special interest in specific conditions or therapeutic areas where secondary care provision is scarce or subject to long waiting lists, for example, in minor surgery or dermatology. Managing groups of patients with chronic conditions through the pharmacy may create the capacity in the GP's health center to allow these areas of special interest to be exploited. However, assessing the indirect benefits of pharmacy management of chronic conditions, and use of POCT as part of that process, may prove complex.

THE EVIDENCE FOR PHARMACY-BASED POCT

If there are theoretical or potential benefits for chronic conditions to be managed through the pharmacy, what evidence is there that pharmacists can perform the roles that are suggested for them? In a study published in 2003, Anderson et al. (33) concluded that there is clear evidence of the potential for the pharmacist to contribute more; the review drew on research conducted throughout the world, much of it from the United States, where medicine management by pharmacists is more established. It looked at many different areas of activity, including smoking cessation, lipid management, screening for CHD risk factors, anticoagulation, weight management, skin cancer prevention, drug misuse, emergency hormonal contraception, and diabetes. The review did not look specifically at whether POCT plays an important part in these new roles. However, other published material indicate a growing body of evidence to suggest that the use of POCT assists with achieving positive outcomes.

Lipid Management

There are studies looking at the management of cholesterol by pharmacists in the community; many of them show clinical benefits resulting from pharmacists measuring cholesterol levels and providing patient education and recommending additional physician intervention.

Madejski et al. (34) conducted a study to investigate whether the community pharmacy is an appropriate site for identifying patients with hypercholesterolemia. They recruited 539 individuals and identified that 78% had abnormal cholesterol levels. Eighty-three percent of these reported lifestyle modifications, 81% requested diet information, and 23% accepted an offer to rescreen. They concluded that a community pharmacy is an easily accessible, well-accepted, and effective site for cholesterol screening.

Nola et al. (35) showed that patients allocated to a community pharmacy lipid management program achieved LDL reduction, whereas the control group saw their LDL increase. Both groups experienced HDL increases and triglyceride level decreases. A total of 32% of the study group achieved their cholesterol goals, compared with 15% in the control group. Furthermore, the treatment group's hyperlipidemia knowledge scores increased significantly, and patient satisfaction scores were favorable toward the pharmacist.

Project ImPACT (36) showed a positive impact on cholesterol levels across a population of 397 patients and 26 community-based pharmacists. Patients had their cholesterol measured at an initial consultation with the pharmacist and were then monitored each month for the first three months of the study; thereafter, they returned every 3 months to be retested and have their condition reviewed. Patients were followed up for an average of 24.6 months. A total of 62.5% of patients reached and maintained their lipid goals. Observed rates for persistence and compliance with medication therapy were 93.6% and 90.1%, respectively. Other studies have shown

that as few as one-third of patients take their lipid lowering medication and that after 2 years as many as 85% have discontinued treatment (37).

Tsuyuki et al. (38) reported on a Canadian study where patients were randomized to a pharmacist intervention program that included cholesterol measurement, education, and regular follow-ups. The clinical benefit was clear, with 57% of patients reaching the primary endpoint versus 31% in the control group, resulting in the external monitoring committee recommending early termination of the study.

Diabetes

A number of studies show that pharmacists can manage care for people with type 2 diabetes; most of these involve pharmacists operating in a hospital or primary care clinic settings rather than community pharmacies. However, there are some examples of community pharmacy managed care for type 2 diabetes.

Warmeille et al. (39) reported on a study in Scotland involving four community pharmacies. Pharmacists assessed medical records and conducted face-to-face interviews with patients, and from this initial assessment a clinical care plan was developed. At the end of the study, patients' HbA1c levels and blood pressure had fallen and their knowledge of their oral hypoglycemic control had increased.

A long-term study of type 2 diabetics in North Carolina showed good results in glycemic control and workdays lost. The Ashville Project (40) was a 5-year study following patients on to a community pharmacy–based diabetes management program. Community pharmacists provided education, clinical assessment, monitoring, and collaborative drug therapy management with physicians. Mean HbA1c decreased at all follow-ups, with more than 50% of patients demonstrating improvements at each time. Total medical costs decreased by $1200, and sick days decreased every year.

Anticoagulant Monitoring

Anticoagulant monitoring is probably the best-established pharmacy service utilizing POCT. Hospital pharmacists have been managing anticoagulant therapy for some time, and there are numerous examples of well-run services in the community.

Yamreudeewong et al. (41) demonstrated that monitoring international normalized ratio (INR) values utilizing POCT was similar to conventional laboratory methods and that patients receiving warfarin therapy can be monitored and managed effectively by pharmacists. In this case, the clinic was located within a hospital rather than the community.

Macgregor et al. (42) showed that a pharmacist conducting a clinic in a GP surgery was effective and that it had several benefits to the patient and the health service. Control of INR was comparable with hospital clinics; attendance at the surgery clinic cost less for 48% of patients and more for only 4%; travel time was less for 64% and greater for 20%; and patients were seen within 10 min of their appointed time, whereas hospital waiting time routinely exceeded 1 h.

Holden et al. (43) showed that pharmacists managing INR through an anticoagulant clinic in a community pharmacy setting were at least as effective as GPs. Results from their study showed a trend toward better control, with patients spending less time outside their target INR range, although statistically the difference between GP-managed patients and pharmacist-managed patients was found to be not significant.

Other Clinical Areas

Anticoagulant monitoring and lipid clinics are the most common services provided by pharmacists; management of type 2 diabetes is less common but has been shown to be effective. Pharmacist management of other conditions has been reported; these include management of hypertension, asthma, lithium therapy, anticonvulsant therapy, and eradication of *H. pylori*.

FURTHER DEVELOPMENT OF PHARMACIST'S MANAGEMENT OF MEDICINES UTILIZING POCT

Given the desire of both government and the pharmacy profession in the United Kingdom for a widening of the roles that pharmacists in the community can perform, it is probable that we will see an increase in the number and variety of medicine management services provided. Many of these will require monitoring of biochemical parameters, and this will be carried out utilizing POCT. However, before services become widespread, a number of issues have to be addressed.

Training

Pharmacists will require additional training in the management of the conditions that they become involved in, the principles of the tests used to monitor the patient's condition, and the details of the specific tests to be used.

Although the core of every pharmacist's training is the understanding of disease processes and the therapeutic use of drugs to modify biochemical process and treat disease, the management of patients goes beyond the conditions that they have. Furthermore, treatment protocols are not necessarily standardized and are subject to local variation. Pharmacists will need to learn about patient management and what protocols pertain to their area from other healthcare professionals, including GPs, nurses, and consultants in secondary care departments.

Clinical tests vary in terms of accuracy, precision, sensitivity, and specificity between tests used for different conditions; between laboratories for the same tests; between point-of-care tests and laboratory tests; and between different types of POCT for the same condition. Pharmacists need to be cognizant of the differences, and they need to understand the significance of the results on which their decisions are based. The RPSGB has launched a series of CPD articles on clinical testing (44). However, in developing any service, pharmacists would benefit from additional training, perhaps from clinical

biochemists in the laboratory that is part of the local health system.

Operational Requirements

Managing a patient's condition will require the pharmacist to spend some time with the patient, performing tests, talking about the patient's condition, and modifying therapy as required. It is unlikely that any patients would be happy for this to take place over-the-counter, so a consultation room will be required. Few pharmacies currently possess such a facility, but elements of the new pharmacy contract will require all pharmacies to have suitable consultation space.

Arrangements for the quality control of the tests and the pharmacist's ability to perform them properly and consistently will have to be put in place. At the inception of a service, it is reasonable to assume that correct operation of the equipment and the pharmacist's competence will be ensured. However, over time, equipment may require recalibration, or it may begin to malfunction, producing invalid results. Also, the pharmacist's practices may begin to drift away from those initially established. Quality control of the tests and the operator are needed to ensure that the service continues to operate correctly and that patients continue to be managed safely and effectively.

Pharmacies have operated largely in isolation from the rest of the health system in the United Kingdom. When providing patient services on behalf of the GP or under contract to the primary care organization, it is essential that the pharmacist is seen to be part of the team delivering healthcare and that communication between the pharmacist and the other members of the team is effective. Pharmacists will have to provide patient management information to other team members and will need to have effective support and referral pathways. The NHS is investing substantial amounts of money in an information technology system to allow for a single patient medical record. Access to this record will facilitate certain aspects of record keeping and communication, but developing relationships with other members of the team will also be required.

Evidence Base

We have seen that there is a desire for pharmacists to develop new services and that there is some evidence that they can deliver these effectively. However, the evidence base for pharmacy services involving POCT is not extensive and rarely explores the health economic aspects. If pharmacists want to develop new roles and want to be paid fairly for those services, they will have to provide evidence of effectiveness from both a clinical perspective and an economic perspective. This will require a much greater participation in research than pharmacists are used to.

CONCLUSIONS

There is a strong desire to see more patients with long-term conditions managed through pharmacies. The key drivers are the growth in the number of people with long-term conditions and the resulting increase in workload for the NHS, the need for the government to find alternative ways of providing care to those patients, and the desire of the pharmacy profession to utilize the skills of pharmacists in a wider role. POCT will play an important part in enabling and supporting disease management in the pharmacy.

There is a rationale for the development of new pharmacy services, and there is evidence that pharmacists can achieve good clinical outcomes using POCT, particularly in lipid management and oral anticoagulant therapy. However, there are a number of issues that have to be addressed in developing medication management services involving POCT. Integration of the pharmacist with the rest of the healthcare team is vital; cooperation and collaboration with clinical biochemists, GPs, nurses, and other practitioners will be required for the pharmacist to develop the requisite skills and support framework.

REFERENCES

1. Department of Health: A vision for pharmacy in the new NHS. London: Department of Health, 2003.
2. Murdock A. The consultant pharmacist and pharmacist technician in primary care. In: Lissauer R, Kendall L, eds. New practitioners in the future health service. London: Institute for Public Policy Research, 2002;13–20.
3. Taylor D, Carter S. Realising the promise: community pharmacy in the new NHS. London: University of London, School of Pharmacy, 2003.
4. Parkin B. Pharmacy in a new age: the road to the future. Tom Pharm 1999;October:58–60.
5. Royal Pharmaceutical Society of Great Britain. Building the future: a strategy for a 21st-century pharmaceutical service. London: Royal Pharmaceutical Society of Great Britain, 1997.
6. Department of Health. The NHS Plan. A plan for investment. A plan for reform. London: Department of Health, 2000.
7. Department of Health. Pharmacy in the future—implementing the NHS plan. London: Department of Health, 2000.
8. Department of Health. A vision for pharmacy in the NHS. London: Department of Health, 2003.
9. Department of Health. Framework for a new community pharmacy contract. London: Department of Health, 2003.
10. Department of Health. Improving chronic disease management. London: Department of Health, 2004.
11. Department of Health. National service framework for coronary heart disease. London: Department of Health, 2000.
12. Department of Health. National service framework for diabetes. London: Department of Health, 2001.
13. Department of Health. National service framework for older people. London: Department of Health, 2001.
14. Department of Health. Investing in general practice. The new general medical services contract. London: Department of Health, 2003.
15. Prescription Pricing Authority. Pharmaceutical directorate: update on growth in prescription volume and cost year to December 2003. London: Prescription Pricing Authority, 2004.
16. Prescription Pricing Authority. PACT centre pages: cardiovascular prescribing. London: Prescription Pricing Authority, Jan–Mar 2002.
17. Royal Pharmaceutical Society of Great Britain. Practice guidance on blood pressure monitoring. London: Royal Pharmaceutical Society of Great Britain, 2003.
18. Royal Pharmaceutical Society of Great Britain. Practice guidance on cholesterol testing: London: Royal Pharmaceutical Society of Great Britain, 2003.
19. Cholestec Corporation. Test cassettes and accessories. http://www.cholestech.com/products/cassettes.asp (accessed March 2004).
20. Prescription Pricing Authority. PACT centre pages: drugs used in diabetes. London: Prescription Pricing Authority, Apr–Jun 2003.
21. National Institution for Clinical Excellence. Management of type 2 diabetes—management of blood pressure and blood lipids (guideline H). London: National Institution for Clinical Excellence, 2002.
22. National Institution for Clinical Excellence. Management of type 2 diabetes—management of blood glucose (guideline G). London: National Institution for Clinical Excellence, 2002.
23. National Institution for Clinical Excellence. Management of type 2 diabetes—renal disease, prevention and early management (guideline F). London: National Institution for Clinical Excellence, 2002.
24. Department of Health. New moves to improve sexual health: press release reference number 2004/0017. London: Department of Health, 2004.
25. Royal Pharmaceutical Society of Great Britain. Fitness to practice and legal affairs directorate fact sheet 10, patient group directions. London: Royal Pharmaceutical Society of Great Britain, 2004.
26. National Institute for Clinical Excellence. Guidance on the use of zanamivir, oseltamivir and amantadine for the treatment of influenza. London: National Institute for Clinical Excellence, 2003.
27. Rothberg MB, Bellantonio S, Rose DN. Management of influenza in adults older than 65 years of age: cost-effectiveness of rapid testing and antiviral therapy: Ann Int Med 2003;139:321–9.
28. Hueston WJ, Benich JJ. A cost-benefit analysis of testing for influenza A in high-risk adults. Ann Fam Med 2004;2:33–40.
29. Dhoot A, Rutter PM. The provision of diagnostic and screening services by community pharmacies. Int J Pharm Pract 2002;10(Suppl):R51.
30. Khan A, Rutter PM. The provision of anticoagulant services by primary care groups and trusts. Has community pharmacy a role to play? Int J Pharm Pract 2002;10(Suppl):R50.
31. De Mont A. Wide-ranging roles sought in Dorset five-year plan. Chemist & Druggist 2004;261:5.
32. Jacobs E. Is point-of-care testing cost effective? Clin Lab News 1996;22:32, 34, 51.
33. Anderson C, Blenkinsop A, Armstrong M. The contribution of community pharmacy to improving the public's health. London: Pharmacy HealthLink and the Royal Pharmaceutical Society of Great Britain, 2003.
34. Madejski RM, Madejski TJ. Cholesterol screening in a community pharmacy. J Am Pharm Assoc 1996;36:243–8.
35. Nola KM, Gourley DR, Portner TS, Gourley GK, Solomon DK, Elam M, et al. Clinical and humanistic outcomes of a lipid management programme in the community pharmacy setting. J Am Pharm Assoc 2000;40:166–73.
36. Bluml BM, McKenney JM, Cziraky MJ. Pharmaceutical care services and results in project ImPACT: hyperlipidemia. J Am Pharm Assoc 2000;40:57–65.
37. Carter S, Taylor D, Levenson R. A question of choice—compliance in medicine taking. London: Medicines Partnership, 2003.

38. Tsuyuki RT, Johnson JA, Teo KK, Simpson SH, Ackman ML, Biggs RS, et al. A randomized trial of the effect of community pharmacist intervention on cholesterol risk management; the study of cardiovascular risk intervention by pharmacists (SCRIP). Arch Int Med 2002;162:1149–55.

39. Wermeille J, Bennie M, Brown I, McKnight J. Pharmaceutical care model for patients with type 2 diabetes: integration of the community pharmacist into the diabetes team pilot study. Pharm World Sci 2004;26:18–25.

40. Cranor CW, Bunting BA, Christensen DB. The Ashville Project: long-term clinical and economic outcomes of a community pharmacy diabetes care program. J Am Pharm Assoc 2003;43:173–84.

41. Yamreudeewong W, Johnson JV, Cassidy TG Berg JT. Comparison of two methods for INR determination in a pharmacist-based oral anticoagulation clinic: Pharmacotherapy 1996;16:1159–65.

42. Macgregor SH, Hamley JG, Dunbar JA, Dodd TR, Cromarty JA. Evaluation of a primary care anticoagulation clinic managed by a pharmacist. BMJ 1996;312:560.

43. Holden K, Holden J. A comparative study of pharmacist and GP management of anticoagulant therapy following deviation from the target international normalised ratio. Int J Pharm Pract 2001;R24.

44. Mason P. Basic concepts in clinical testing. Pharmaceut J 2004;272:384–6.

Chapter 36

Infectious Diseases and Point-of-Care Testing

James W. Gray

INTRODUCTION

Worldwide, utilization of point-of-care testing (POCT) for diagnosis of infectious diseases varies depending partly on the nature of clinical services and the availability of local laboratory services. In developing countries, there may be no alternative to using POCT, some of which offer relatively poor sensitivity and specificity, and the World Health Organization regularly publishes advice on the bedside diagnosis of infectious diseases in developing countries (1). POCT for the diagnosis of infectious diseases has been slow to develop in industrialized countries, mainly because of the limitations of currently available tests for infections where there would be most clinical benefit from rapid diagnosis. Nevertheless, there is a growing clinical need for rapid diagnosis of infectious diseases, especially to guide the rational use of antibiotics and the new antiviral drugs. Rapid progress in adapting new technologies, especially molecular biology, for POCT may herald a new era for POCT in diagnosis of infectious diseases.

TESTS FOR DIAGNOSIS OF INFECTION AND THEIR APPLICABILITY TO POCT

Three broad categories of tests may be used to assist in the diagnosis of infection. The most commonly used methods involve detection of pathogenic microorganisms or their components in clinical samples. Techniques include microscopy, culture, antigen detection, and molecular biology. Infections with a specific pathogen can also be diagnosed by demonstration of a specific immune response to that agent, usually by antibody detection. Finally, there is a range of tests that can provide nonspecific evidence of an infective (or at least inflammatory) process. These tests may be applied, with variable success, to determine whether or not a patient has an infection, to distinguish between localized and systemic infections, or to distinguish between bacterial and viral infections.

Culture

Culture is the mainstay of laboratory diagnosis of the majority of bacterial and fungal infections. It is relatively inexpensive,

readily detects a wide range of different pathogens, and provides important additional information, including a full range of antimicrobial susceptibilities, which is not obtainable with any other technique. Culture does not generally lend itself to POCT, not least because there is an inherent delay, usually of at least one day, before even a preliminary result is available; with standard culture techniques, further manipulation, and still further delay, is required in order to identify isolates. There are also safety issues in handling and disposing of microbial cultures at the bedside. Selective indicator broth-culture media selectively promote the growth of specific pathogens, which is detected concurrently through a color change in the media. These media can be readily adapted for safe inoculation and incubation at the bedside and can give positive results in as little as 2 to 3 h (2). However, the rate of detection is dependent on the number of bacteria present in the original sample, and a negative result cannot be confidently determined for much longer. This delay is still too long for culture to be useful for POCT in most circumstances, while the versatility of standard culture methods in being able to detect a wide range of pathogens is lost. Despite these drawbacks, broth culture as a POCT may occasionally be useful in situations where large numbers of samples require processing in settings where laboratory access is restricted.

Microscopy

Microscopy allows direct visualization of microorganisms in clinical material, but it is a relatively insensitive technique and gives limited information on the identity of the microorganisms seen. It is most useful for examination of specimens that are normally sterile (where the presence of any microorganisms is abnormal) or where pathogenic microorganisms have distinctive morphology. Microscopy can also demonstrate the presence of white blood cells, which is another pointer to infection. Microscopy is rapid and, with conventional light microscopy, requires little in the way of specialized equipment. The drawbacks of microscopy for POCT are that preparations may need to be stained and that subjective interpretation is required, placing a demand for training and experience of the microscopist such that microscopy is only viable as a POCT in settings where there is a regular and high throughput of specimens.

Antigen Detection and Molecular Techniques

The technology behind antigen detection systems is fundamentally more compatible with POCT. Most early applications of POCT used insensitive methodologies (usually latex agglutination) that were originally developed for identification of pure laboratory cultures of microorganisms (3–5). Not surprisingly, these performed poorly when used directly on clinical material, and they have now been largely superseded by more sophisticated immunoassays, such as enzyme or optical immunoassays. Further refinements have seen amalgamation of the antigen extraction and detection stages to minimize hands-on time, and to facilitate more clear-cut differentiation of positive and negative results. Until very recently, molecular biological methods would have been considered too complex and time-consuming to be viable for POCT. DNA probe technology has occasionally been used for POCT (6, 7), but the most promising breakthrough in molecular biology to date is the development of real time nucleic acid amplification technology, which can realistically provide results in under 2 h (8). Further developments in reaction vessels and thermocyclers now permit nucleic acid extraction, amplification, and detection to be undertaken in a closed system that minimizes both hands-on time and the risk of contamination. This technology is already being widely used outside the laboratory for agricultural and military purposes (9), and the first clinical applications of real-time nucleic acid amplification techniques for POCT are currently being evaluated.

Antibody Detection

Antibody detection technology is relatively easily transferable to the POCT setting, with the proviso that testing is conventionally undertaken on serum or plasma. However, methods have been developed that allow antibody detection in whole blood, saliva, or urine. The main limiting factor for POCT is that serodiagnosis is mainly used for infections for which there is often little clinical benefit from rapid results turnaround.

CLINICAL NEED FOR POCT IN THE DIAGNOSIS OF INFECTIOUS DISEASES

Benefits of POCT for Infectious Diseases

In order to be worthwhile undertaking any POCT, the test must be able to offer some tangible clinical benefit. There are some occasions when immediate knowledge of microbiology results is essential for optimal clinical management. However, the majority of patients with suspected life-threatening infections can be effectively managed empirically until laboratory results become available, while therapeutic decisions for patients with less serious infections can, at least in theory, be delayed until results from the laboratory are available. However, POCT has several potential advantages for diagnosis of infectious diseases (Table 36-1). More rapid availability of results can facilitate earlier and more rational use of antibiotics. This can

Table 36-1   Possible Benefits and Limitations of Point-of-Care Testing for Infectious Diseases

Possible benefits of point-of-care testing

Facilitation of lifesaving treatment
Direction of appropriate antibiotic therapy
Limitation of antibiotic use
Improved diagnostic yield
Decreased laboratory workload
Facilitation of infection control decisions
Improved client satisfaction
Reduced clinical workload through avoidance of follow-up
  appointments
The location of testing at offsite clinics
Improved cost per episode

Possible limitations of point-of-care testing

Inferior sensitivity
Inferior specificity
Risk of transmission of infection to tester (but also in the
  central laboratory)
Risk of transmission of infection to other patients
Possibility of unreliable results due to the complexity of test or
  the need for subjective assessment
Antibiotic susceptibilities not available
Only a limited number of infections can be tested for
Infrequent clinical need for many tests
Limited clinical value of the test per se

help to ensure prompt antibiotic treatment where it is required, with the facility to conclude outpatient consultations at the first visit, or to reduce the length of stay of hospitalized patients. Of increasing importance is the potential to control antibiotic use, both by identifying patients in whom antibiotic therapy is not indicated and allowing targeted narrow spectrum therapy for others. Limiting antibiotic use in this way may reduce prescribing costs, but it is also important in view of the growing concern about the relationship between large-scale antibiotic use, both in hospitals and in the community, and the emergence and spread of antibiotic resistance (10). By permitting earlier identification of patients with infections that are readily transmissible in hospitals, POCT might also be useful in preventing healthcare-associated infections.

Although culture is the current reference standard for diagnosis of the majority of bacterial and fungal infections, a significant proportion of patients with a clinical diagnosis of infection will have negative cultures. Potential reasons for this include recent antibiotic therapy, loss of viability of pathogens, or overgrowth of contaminants during transit to the laboratory. POCT that is not dependent on the viability of the target microorganisms has the potential to circumvent all of these problems and might be of particular value in primary care, where the diagnostic value of specimens sent to the laboratory for culture (in terms of yield and results turnaround) is sometimes so low that samples for microbiological examination are not even collected. Not only can POCT in this situation assist in clinical management, it might also afford valuable epidemiological information on the pattern of infections in the community.

POCT can reduce laboratory workload, either through its use as a substitute for laboratory testing or by filtering out negative specimens that do not require laboratory investigation.

Limitations of POCT for Infectious Diseases

Tests for infectious diseases may be used in three clinical settings: (*i*) to investigate patients with equivocal signs of infection, where tests can help determine whether infection is likely and therefore whether antibiotic therapy is indicated; (*ii*) in investigating patients with clinical signs of infection in order to identify the etiological agent; and (*iii*) for testing asymptomatic individuals with risk factors for a specific infection. There are many drawbacks with currently available POCT for infectious diseases (Table 36-1). The main problem with tests in the former category is with the clinical value of the results they provide rather than their adaptability to POCT. For tests in the latter two categories, sensitivity and specificity are important considerations.

Many point-of-care tests offer inferior sensitivity or specificity compared with reference tests. However, the reasons for undertaking POCT for infectious diseases are far more complex than for many other areas of POCT, and in some situations tests offering inferior sensitivity or specificity may still be clinically useful. For example, a relatively low sensitivity might be acceptable for a test that is used primarily for infection control purposes if patients with the highest microbial burdens, and therefore the most infectious, are detected. Problems with a low sensitivity might also be acceptable in other situations, especially if samples that test negative are sent to a laboratory for further testing. Despite this, evaluation of POCT has tended to focus on straightforward comparisons of the sensitivity and specificity of the tests against a reference standard (which is usually culture), rather than examining the impact of POCT on clinical outcomes (11). Sometimes evaluation of the test kits is even undertaken in the laboratory, rather than in a point-of-care setting, meaning that there has been little or no consideration of either the accuracy or feasibility of undertaking POCT. Also, very few studies have examined the cost-effectiveness of testing, which is an important consideration for tests that are not immediately lifesaving.

The inability of point-of-care tests to demonstrate important phenotypic characteristics of microorganisms, including antimicrobial susceptibilities, is an important drawback that means that if POCT is to be used as the basis for instituting treatment, then the antimicrobial susceptibilities of the agent tested for must be relatively predictable. It is investigation of infected patients to determine the etiological agent that is least amenable to POCT, because few infectious syndromes are pathognomic of infection with a single microorganism, and currently no point-of-care test can approach the versatility of laboratory-based culture in detecting a wide range of pathogens. This largely limits the use of these tests to the infectious conditions where the clinical presentation points to one, or at least a small number of, potential pathogens.

For POCT for any infection to be viable in any clinical setting, there must be sufficient need for that test to ensure both that users retain sufficient experience in performing and interpreting the test, and that there is not excessive waste of unused date-expired kits. Another very important consideration in POCT for infectious diseases is the health and safety aspects of handling clinical samples that might contain large numbers of readily transmissible pathogens (12). There is a potential risk to staff from microorganisms such as *Mycobacterium tuberculosis* in respiratory secretions or verocytotoxin-producing *Escherichia coli* in feces that may make examination of these specimen types inappropriate. There is also a risk of health-care-associated infections where the tester may move from handling a contaminated sample to caring for another patient without washing his or her hands.

CLINICAL USES OF POCT FOR DIAGNOSIS OF INFECTIOUS DISEASES

Investigation of Patients with Equivocal Signs of Infection

The term *systemic inflammatory response syndrome* (SIRS) refers to a systemic inflammatory response that may be due to infection (sepsis) or to a range of noninfective insults, including trauma, burns, surgery, hemorrhage, hypothermia, and pancreatitis (13). Among patients with less severe and/or localized infections, it is often clinically impossible to distinguish between bacterial infections (which require antibiotic therapy) and viral infections (which do not). In both these clinical situations, there is a theoretical risk that antibiotic therapy of patients with bacterial infections will be delayed, but the more likely scenario is that antibiotics are overprescribed. Immense effort has been directed into investigating tests, or combinations of tests, that can reliably distinguish sepsis from noninfective causes of SIRS, or distinguish between bacterial and viral infections. While none has yet proved to be the panacea for determining indications for antibiotic therapy, these tests are widely used in the laboratory and at the point of care for assessment of patients.

Hematology and Clinical Biochemistry Tests. Various hematological and biochemical tests may be helpful in the initial evaluation and monitoring of the patient with suspected infection. These are described briefly here; for a more detailed description, see the relevant chapters.

There is a correlation between absolute and neutrophil leucocytosis and the presence of bacterial or fungal infection; however, the positive predictive value of these findings is low, especially in children (14). Leukopenia, and especially neutropenia, can both predispose to sepsis and be secondary to severe sepsis. Thrombocytopenia may occur as an isolated defect in patients with sepsis, or in the course of a disseminated intravascular coagulopathy (DIC). Prolongation of prothrombin and partial thromboplastin times, hypofibrinogenemia and the presence of fibrin degradation products or D-dimers, are all consistent with DIC. Fibrinogen is an acute phase reactant and may be increased in sepsis without DIC; however, this increase is rarely high enough to be of diagnostic value (15).

In the early phase of sepsis, arterial blood gases show a mixed respiratory alkalosis and metabolic acidosis, but as the septic state progresses, metabolic acidosis predominates due to the accumulation of lactic acid (16). Measurement of serum lactic acid is a good reflection of tissue oxygenation and has prognostic value in severe sepsis and septic shock (17).

Measures of the Inflammatory Response. The erythrocyte sedimentation rate (ESR) is still widely used as a measure of the acute phase response. It reflects the plasma concentration of acute phase proteins of large molecular size. From a practical point of view, it is easy to perform and inexpensive. However, in POCT there are safety issues related to handling relatively large blood volumes in an office or ward setting, and to the potential for incorrect results arising through nonstandardization of test conditions or reading errors (18). The biggest drawback of the ESR is that it is of very limited value in assessing patients for infection. There is considerable intersubject variability in both the initial ESR result and in the rate of decline during convalescence. The ESR is of more value in assessing patients with noninfective conditions, especially temporal arteritis and polymyalgia rheumatica.

C-reactive protein (CRP) concentrations exhibit less variability than the ESR, and concentrations also fall more rapidly and predictably in response to treatment. As a result, CRP measurement has now superseded ESR in many hospitals for the assessment of patients with suspected sepsis. However, CRP is still a nonspecific maker of inflammation and is still not a particularly sensitive or specific means of assessing patients with SIRS, or of distinguishing between patients with bacterial and viral infections (19–21). The limitations of CRP have in turn led to evaluation of other markers, including TNF and IL-6. Of these, the one that shows most promise is procalcitonin (PCT) (22–23).

PCT is a prohormone of calcitonin that may mediate the inflammatory response to sepsis in humans and play a role in the development and progression of multiorgan failure (22, 23). Plasma concentrations in health are generally <0.1 ng/mL, and systemic infections are unlikely with a concentration of <0.5 ng/mL. Plasma concentrations of 2–10 ng/mL are seen in bacterial infections with a systemic element, while concentrations of >10 ng/mL indicate severe bacterial infection (24, 25). Although many studies suggest that PCT estimation may be a better marker of sepsis than other measures of the acute phase response, the sensitivity and specificity may still be unacceptably low because plasma concentrations are also elevated to some degree in patients following trauma or with multiorgan failure for other reasons. Compared with CRP, concentrations of PCT increase and decrease more rapidly in response to insults and are less age dependent (19). The degree of elevation of PCT concentration may be proportional to the severity of organ failure and predictive of mortality in patients with septic shock, while a rapid decline in PCT concentration

following therapy may be a indicator of favorable prognosis (19, 21, 23, 26).

Studies on both pediatric and adult intensive care units have shown that PCT concentrations are markedly elevated on the first day of bacterial sepsis (19, 21, 23, 26). However, because the difference in PCT concentrations between noninfective and infective causes of SIRS may be small, the greatest value may be from prospective monitoring of patients at risk of infection so that the magnitude of any increase can be gauged. Diagnosis of infection in patients with cardiogenic shock following cardiac surgery can be particularly difficult. Following uncomplicated cardiac bypass surgery, PCT concentrations peak within 24 h and return to normal values within 3 days, whereas CRP concentrations take up to 5 days to return to normal values (27–28). PCT concentrations remain elevated in patients with postoperative cardiogenic shock and multiorgan failure in the absence of sepsis, but it has been reported that the magnitude of this elevation is substantially less than that usually seen in sepsis.

PCT has also been evaluated in the neonatal intensive care unit (29–33). The problem here is that PCT concentrations in the first 72 hours of life may be influenced by factors such as maternal illness and labor complications (30). In some studies, PCT has been found to offer better sensitivity than CRP (typically 70% to 80%, compared with 35% to 65%) (30, 32, 33), whereas others have found little or no difference (29, 31). The most consistent finding is the high negative predictive value (>90%) of a low PCT measurement (29, 31, 33). However, PCT may not offer any significant advantage over traditional tests in this respect (29).

PCT estimation has also been evaluated in assessing patients with equivocal signs of infection outside the intensive care unit, where it has been reported to be superior to CRP in distinguishing between bacterial and viral infections (34, 35), and between invasive and noninvasive bacterial infections (36, 37).

Diagnosis of Urinary Tract Infections

Urinary tract infection (UTI) is accompanied by the presence of bacteria (bacteriuria) and white cells (pyuria) in urine. UTI is usually diagnosed in the laboratory by microscopy and semiquantitative culture. Although UTIs are common, up to 90% of urine samples sent for microbiological examination are culture negative. This high negativity rate underlines the unreliability of clinical diagnosis of UTI, and also means that processing negative urine samples constitutes a substantial proportion of the workload of many microbiology laboratories. Another disadvantage of laboratory diagnosis of UTI is that urine samples begin to deteriorate after collection, especially through the overgrowth of contaminants.

Point-of-care tests are widely used to investigate suspected UTIs and can be useful in both guiding the immediate clinical management of patients with suspected UTI and reducing the workload of microbiology laboratories. However, application of POCT for UTI needs to take account of the differing diagnostic challenges and clinical significance of UTI in different patient groups.

Microscopic examination of urine at the bedside is still used in some centers to investigate patients with suspected UTI. However, microscopy requires a degree of subjective interpretation that requires a level of training and ongoing experience that makes it viable only in clinical settings where large numbers of urine samples are examined. In most settings, microscopy has been superseded by test strips that detect leukocyte esterase (LE) and nitrite. LE is produced by segmented neutrophils, and its presence in urine correlates well with leukocyte counts of 10 or fewer per high-powered field. The sensitivity of LE strips means that large numbers of urine samples with low levels of pyuria that are culture negative are detected. False positives can also occur due to ascorbic acid or albumin in urine. Detection of nitrite is based on the fact that most urinary pathogens reduce nitrate to nitrite. False positives can occur in old specimens. False negatives can be due to patients taking a vegetable-free diet, drug interference, and infection with non–nitrite producing bacteria (e.g., enterococci). However, the most important cause of false-negative results is because urine collected shortly after a previous voiding may not have had sufficient time for the nitrite concentration to increase.

A combination of LE and nitrite test results has generally been found to give the best compromise between sensitivity and specificity (38). In adults with suspected UTI, most studies have reported sensitivities >90%, but the most consistent finding has been of a high negative predictive value when both tests are negative (38–41). This can be used to reduce the number of urine specimens sent to the laboratory by at least 25% (39), although this means that a large number of negative urines are still sent for culture. POCT performs less well for specific patient groups. Up to 5% of women in early pregnancy have asymptomatic bacteriuria (ASB), of whom, without treatment, up to 30% will develop symptomatic UTI during pregnancy. Screening for ASB is therefore part of routine antenatal care in many countries. Point-of-care screening could obviate the need to recall women with infection, as well as substantially reduce laboratory workload. However, in this patient group the sensitivity may be as low as 33.3% (42, 43), probably because women with ASB often have low-level or absent pyuria. Some adult (44) and pediatric (45) patients have urinary symptoms associated with low bacterial counts of 10^4 to 10^5 per mL, or even less. Unsurprisingly, nitrite testing performs poorly in these patients, meaning that the sensitivity of combined LE and nitrite testing may be as low as 25% (38). Sensitivity can be improved, at the expense of specificity, by considering only the LE result. Although dipstick testing has been reported to be useful in an urodynamics clinic (46), it is probably inadvisable to use it as a replacement for culture in specialist urology or urogynecology clinics. UTI in infants and young children is an important diagnosis, because investigation for underlying anatomical abnormality may be indicated. However, the difficulty of collecting urine specimens from these subjects presents unique diagnostic challenges. Noninvasive collection methods, such as bags, may lead to contamination of urine with perineal or fecal bacteria, whilst invasive methods such as suprapubic aspiration and catheterization require interpretation of the significance of small numbers of bacteria. Differences in specimen type may be one explanation for the conflicting results in pediatric studies. Some authors have reported successful use of dipsticks in children (47, 48), while some have found the sensitivity too poor to be of value (49). Others have found that despite less than optimal sensitivity, the negative predictive value is sufficiently high to make clinical decisions based on negative results (50).

Given the lack of consensus in the literature about the reliability of dipstick testing as a substitute for culture, especially in specialist patient groups, it is advisable that protocols should be based on local experience of the sensitivity, specificity, and negative and positive predictive values of dipstick testing.

Diagnosis of Genital Tract Infections

Despite public education programs, sexually transmitted infections (STIs) such as chlamydia remain a major public health problem in many countries. Patients with STIs often fail to return to clinics in a timely manner; therefore, the facility to conclude a consultation with diagnosis and treatment of STIs in one visit is highly attractive. This is particularly the case with opportunistic screening of young people outside the genitourinary (GU) medicine clinic setting, which is increasingly being used as a means of controlling STIs. While the potential benefits of POCT may seem clear, there are two important caveats. First, the sensitivities surrounding a diagnosis of STI require that only tests that provide high levels of accuracy are suitable. Second, in high-throughput clinics, even result turnaround times of 30 min have been found to be unworkable (51).

Microscopy can be a valuable tool in assessing patients with suspected genital tract infections. Pathogens such as *Treponema pallidum, Trichomonas vaginalis,* and candida have sufficiently distinctive morphologies to allow a presumptive microscopic diagnosis. The same is true of sexually transmitted infections such as chancroid and donovanosis, which are uncommon in Western countries. Microscopic examination of samples for Gram-negative cocci, typical of *Neisseria gonorrhoeae,* is also useful. In women, the microscopic appearance of vaginal fluid is one of the key components of diagnosis of bacterial vaginosis, while the presence of leukorrhea may point to cervical infection with gonorrhoea or chlamydia. Point-of-care microscopy is a key element of GU medicine services, where the throughput of patients is sufficient to justify providing suitable laboratory facilities and trained personnel to undertake microscopy. For situations where microscopy is unavailable or unsuitable, a variety of alternative POCT devices are now available.

Chlamydial Infection. *Chlamydia trachomatis* is the most common sexually acquired bacterial infection in most industrialized countries. Infection in both sexes is frequently subclinical, yet is associated with substantial long-term morbidity in females, including pelvic inflammatory disease, ectopic pregnancy, and tubal infertility. Currently available kits suitable for POCT are immunoassays that can give results in under 30 min. These tests have been reported to offer sensitivities comparable to laboratory-based immunoassays on female endocervical swabs and male urine samples (51–55). However, immunoassays for the detection of *C. trachomatis* have been largely superseded in the laboratory by molecular techniques that can detect at least 40% more cases. DNA amplification techniques offer the additional benefit for screening programs in that less invasive specimen types from females can be used, such as urines and self-collected vulval or low vaginal swabs. At present, therefore, POCT cannot be regarded as a substitute for laboratory-based molecular testing, but in some circumstances it might be justified as an adjunct in the screening of high-prevalence populations.

Syphilis.   Syphilis is now uncommon in industrialized countries, but it remains common in some developing countries, especially in sub-Saharan Africa, where prevalence rates are as high as 10% to 15%. Untreated, syphilis progresses through primary and secondary stages, when large numbers of treponemes are present in mucocutaneous lesions, followed by an asymptomatic latent phase of many years, after which the characteristic manifestations of tertiary syphilis may develop. A pregnant woman with symptomatic or early latent syphilis may transmit the infection via the placenta to her fetus. Identification and treatment of infected women during the first half of pregnancy virtually ensures that the baby will be unaffected.

Early syphilis can be diagnosed by detection of treponemes with characteristic motility by dark ground microscopy performed on material collected from the lesions of primary and secondary syphilis. This technique has to be undertaken at the bedside, because *T. pallidum* rapidly dies away from the body. However, now that patients rarely present with the mucocutaneous lesions of primary or secondary syphilis, the investigation of syphilis is usually based on serological testing. Serology can be used to diagnose symptomatic syphilis, but it is much more widely used to screen asymptomatic populations such as pregnant women or GU clinic attendees. Two types of serological test are available. Nontreponemal tests can give a result in under 30 min, but they have a relatively high rate of biological false positives, so that all positives have to be confirmed by at least one treponemal test. The rapid plasma regain (RPR) card test is a long-established nontreponemal test that is suitable for POCT, albeit that it requires plasma or serum. Recently, a hemagglutination inhibition test has been developed that uses whole blood rather than serum (56). Treponemal tests are more specific, but in general are less suitable for use outside the laboratory. However, a commercially available latex agglutination test using cloned treponemal antigens is now available that allows point-of-care testing in under 3 min. In a limited number of published studies, this test has been shown to offer comparable sensitivity and specificity to the usual laboratory treponemal tests (57).

In countries where syphilis is uncommon and there is ready access to laboratories there are few, if any, advantages to

point-of-care serological testing for syphilis. There might be greater potential benefit in developing countries, but even here POCT has not been found to increase treatment rates or reduce perinatal mortality where access to laboratory facilities is available (58).

Gonorrhea.   Microscopic examination of Gram-stained preparations is currently the mainstay of rapid presumptive diagnosis of gonorrhea. The sensitivity is highest on male urethral swabs (>80%), but is only ~50% in endocervical and rectal swabs. Infections with some serovars of *N. gonorrhoeae* appear to be less likely to be detected by microscopy (59). Several gonococcal antigen detection kits have been marketed over the years, most of which have subsequently been withdrawn because of poor sensitivity and specificity. Among the currently available immunoassays, the GC OIA® (ThermoBiostar™, Boulder, CO, USA) detects a novel ribosomal protein marker that is unique to *N. gonorrhoeae* and is claimed to give superior sensitivity and specificity. Tests on endocervical swabs from women and urine from men can be completed in <30 min. However, at the time of writing there were no published studies on this product. As with chlamydia, the greatest potential for POCT for gonorrhea would be in opportunistic screening, where the utility of currently available tests is limited by the requirement for endocervical swabs from women. The inability to determine antibiotic susceptibilities in the face of increasing antibiotic resistance in *N. gonorrhoeae* is another significant drawback of current POCT devices.

Bacterial Vaginosis.   Bacterial vaginosis (BV) is a condition associated with replacement of the normal predominant lactobacilli in the vaginal flora by characteristic aerobic and anaerobic bacteria, including *Gardnerella vaginalis, Mobiluncus* species, and mycoplasmas. It is the most common cause of malodorous vaginal discharge, but up to half of women with this condition do not report symptoms. BV has been associated with serious maternal and fetal pregnancy-related morbidity, including spontaneous abortion, premature rupture of the membranes, and postpartum endometritis. However, in the absence of clear evidence that treatment influences pregnancy outcome, screening, certainly of low-risk women, is not currently recommended (60). Presence of BV preoperatively has also been reported to be associated with postoperative complications such as endometritis in nonpregnant women undergoing genital tract surgery. Preoperative screening could be used to direct appropriate antibiotic prophylaxis.

The diagnosis of BV is usually based on Amsel's clinical criteria (vaginal discharge, vaginal pH >4.5, the presence of volatile amines after addition of 10% KOH, and the presence of clue cells) (61), and/or on the appearance of Gram-stained vaginal smears, using a scoring system such as that devised by Nugent (62). Microscopic examination of wet mounts may be more suitable for POCT and may be at least as accurate as Gram staining (63). The drawback of microscopy is the degree of subjective assessment required.

A number of alternative POCT devices are commercially available that circumvent the need for microscopy. The

FemExam® test card system (Cooper Surgical™, Trumbull, CT, USA) uses two cards. The first card measures pH and amines, and the second determines proline iminopeptidase (a marker enzyme for BV) activity (64). Taking the results of these tests together, the sensitivity may be as high as 90%, but the specificity is only ~60%. The BVBlue® system (Gryphus Diagnostics, Birmingham, AL, USA) is a chromogenic test that detects elevated concentrations of sialidase (another marker enzyme) in vaginal fluid (65). Results are available within 10 min. Compared with examination of Gram-stained smears, the BVBlue test is claimed by the manufacturers to have a sensitivity of 90% and specificity of at least 95%.

The Affirm™ VPIII Test (BD™, Franklin Lakes, NJ, USA) is a DNA probe method that is claimed to identify *Candida* species, *Gardnerella vaginalis*, and *T. vaginalis* within 45 min, with less than 2 min of hands-on time required (7). For detection of GV, the test is relatively insensitive (2 × 10^5 bacteria), which is claimed to reduce the possibility of false-positive results from women with low-level colonization but who do not have BV.

While the limited published data on these tests suggest that they perform reasonably well in comparison with microscopy, at the present time it is not clear whether there is any real clinical benefit from point-of-care diagnosis of BV.

Detection of Colonization with Group B Streptococcus

Without intervention, the group B streptococcus (GBS) is the commonest cause of serious neonatal sepsis in most industrialized countries. Administration of antibiotics during labor can prevent up to 80% of early-onset neonatal disease. At present, one of two approaches is used to determine which women should receive antibiotics. The US Centers for Disease Control and Prevention endorse the screening-based approach, which entails culturing vaginal and rectal swabs at 35–37 weeks gestation (66). Earlier screening is unreliable because maternal colonization with GBS may be transient. The disadvantage of this approach is that screening misses preterm deliveries, which are associated with the highest risk of neonatal GBS disease. The alternative risk-based approach currently favored in the United Kingdom (67) entails administration of antibiotics to women with risk factors for neonatal GBS disease. This has the disadvantage that a large number of women will receive antibiotics unnecessarily, while other women with GBS will not receive antibiotics.

The definitive means of determining which women should receive intrapartum antibiotics would be POCT during labor. Two possible approaches are currently available, but neither has been fully evaluated either for its performance as a point-of-care test, or to determine the impact of testing on clinical outcomes. The only antigen test that is approved by the FDA is an optical immunoassay (Strep B OIA®, ThermoBiostar, Boulder, CO, USA). Using culture as the gold standard, widely differing sensitivities of 37% to 82.5% have been reported for this test (68–73). A real-time PCR for detection of GBS (IDI StrepB™, Cepheid, Sunnyvale, CA, USA) has recently become commercially available. As yet there is limited experience with this test, but early work suggests that a sensitivity approaching that of culture should be attainable (8, 74).

Diagnosis of Viral Respiratory Tract Infections

In hospitals with an onsite virology department, a wide range of respiratory virus infections can be diagnosed reasonably rapidly by immunofluorescent staining of respiratory secretions. While this technique permits simultaneous screening for most common respiratory viruses, the time taken to obtain a result is measured in hours rather than minutes. POCT devices for two common respiratory viruses, influenza viruses and respiratory syncytial virus (RSV), are widely used in order to guide both therapeutic and infection control management. These tests can give results in ~15 min. Specific therapies are now available for both RSV (ribavirin) and, more recently, influenza (the neuraminidase inhibitors); rapid diagnosis of these viral infections is important in directing prompt and appropriate antiviral therapy for these conditions. Establishing a diagnosis early might also help reduce antibiotic prescribing and demand for radiological and other laboratory investigations. Viral respiratory tract infections are readily transmissible from patient to patient in hospitals; therefore, it is advisable that hospitalized patients with these infections be isolated. However, during seasonal epidemics, it is not usually feasible to isolate individual patients in single cubicles. Instead, it is common practice to cohort patients identified as having the same infection by rapid testing. Logistically, this works reasonably well, provided that it is understood that a negative POCT result does not exclude RSV, or indeed any other respiratory virus that merits isolation (75, 76). However, there is little evidence that this approach, as opposed to cohort isolation of symptomatic cases, reduces rates of hospital-acquired RSV infection (77, 78). Indeed it is theoretically possible that increased waiting time in the admissions area, where infection control measures are often basic, may actually increase the risk of nosocomial transmission.

Another problem with POCT for respiratory virus infections is obtaining samples containing sufficient numbers of virus particles. Nasopharyngeal aspirates are preferable to swabs, but they can only be obtained easily from infants and young children. This probably explains why many studies have shown that the sensitivities of POCT devices are significantly lower in adults than in children (79, 80).

Influenza. Influenza is the most serious of the common respiratory tract infections; however, it cannot be distinguished from other respiratory infections on clinical grounds. Not only is influenza treatable with the new generation of neuraminidase inhibitor drugs, but the facility to diagnose influenza rapidly became even more important with the emergence of SARS during 2002.

A wide variety of immunoassays are currently available as POCT devices for influenza. Most of these detect both influenza A and influenza B, although there is an increasing number of diagnostic kits that either detect only influenza A or can distinguish between the virus types. Distinction between influenza A and B is important, because the latter tends to be a less serious condition, for which antiviral therapy is not usually indicated. Typically, sensitivities of 60% to 80% have been reported for detection of all influenza cases, with specificities of >95% (80–85). In general, the tests have been found to be more sensitive for detection of influenza A than influenza B. Sensitivity is directly related to viral load (86), underlining the importance of good specimen quality.

The use and impact of POCT for influenza has been investigated in a number of clinical settings. In making therapeutic decisions, there is general agreement that testing can be cost-effective. During an epidemic it has been suggested that empiric therapy based on clinical signs may suffice (87), whereas others have suggested that even in an epidemic setting a clinical case definition provides insufficient specificity or positive predictive value (85). Early diagnosis of influenza has also been reported to decrease antibiotic prescribing and laboratory and radiographic investigations (88, 89).

Respiratory Syncytial Virus. The RSV is the most important respiratory pathogen in infants, causing bronchiolitis and pneumonia. Epidemics occur each year, peaking in late autumn and early winter, resulting in large numbers of infants being admitted to hospital. RSV has also been reported to be an important cause of life-threatening respiratory illness in immunocompromised patients of all ages. Probably the main reason for rapid RSV testing is for infection control purposes, although as indicated earlier, evidence of the clinical impact of this is lacking. Rapid preadmission RSV testing of infants with bronchiolitis waiting in assessment units has been reported to have a sensitivity of 70% to 80% compared with laboratory-based direct immunofluorescence or culture (75, 76, 90, 91).

Rapid RSV testing can also be used to guide the use of ribavirin therapy. Ribavirin has limited efficacy, but may be used for patients of all ages at risk of severe or complicated RSV infection. However, for patients outside infancy the sensitivity of rapid RSV testing may be as low as 10% to 25% (79).

Diagnosis of Infectious Mononucleosis

In industrialized countries, up to one-third of adolescents and young adults will acquire a primary EBV infection. Of these, around half develop the syndrome of infectious mononucleosis (IM), characterized by the triad of sore throat, lymphadenopathy, and fever. Rapid confirmation of the diagnosis of IM may be useful because it can provide immediate reassurance that the patient does not have a more serious condition, and it can help avoid the prescription of antibiotics (especially of ampicillin and amoxicillin, which when prescribed in IM are associated with a high risk of skin rashes).

The diagnosis of IM is confirmed by serological tests that may detect either heterophile antibodies or specific anti-EBV antibodies. Heterophile antibodies are found in 90% of EBV infections in adolescents and young adults, but in a much smaller proportion of young children. Early tests for heterophile antibodies were based on agglutination of animal red

cells. However, more accurate results that require less subjective assessment are obtainable using purified or selected antigens. Various latex agglutination and immunoassays are available that can provide results from plasma, serum, or whole blood within 15 min (92), but there are few published data on the use of these in POCT settings.

Diagnosis of Pharyngitis Due to Group A Streptococcus (*Streptococcus pyogenes*)

The majority of sore throats are self-limiting and viral in etiology. The group A streptococcus (GAS) is the commonest cause of bacterial sore throat, accounting for up to 30% of cases of pharyngitis presenting to medical services. This is clinically important because it can be associated with serious side effects that are preventable by early antimicrobial therapy, and because it can spread very rapidly from person to person, including from health care worker to patient. Clinical history and physical examination cannot reliably identify patients with GAS sore throats (93). Rapid tests for GAS might therefore be useful in identifying individuals for whom antibiotic therapy is indicated, or in aiding hospital infection control. Tests based on antigen detection have been reported by some to have a low sensitivity of <60% (94), but when applied only to throat swabs from patients with clinical symptoms commonly associated with GAS pharyngitis, the sensitivity can exceed 95% (95, 96). Nevertheless, the American Academy of Pediatrics still recommends that negative tests be backed up by culture (97).

Rapid tests for GAS streptococci now give good specificity (usually >95%) on samples from patients with sore throats. However, the specificity may be considerably lower on throat swabs from asymptomatic individuals. Pseudo-outbreaks associated with false-positive results have been reported where POCT has been used to test asymptomatic individuals during epidemiological investigations (98).

Rapid testing for GAS has been reported to be cost-effective compared with empiric antibiotic prescribing, but at normal prevalence rates is more expensive than culture (99). In children, modeling has been used to suggest that rapid testing may be the most cost-effective strategy to prevent acute rheumatic fever (100).

Diagnosis of Infection with *Helicobacter pylori*

Helicobacter pylori is associated with chronic gastritis, peptic ulcer disease, and gastric carcinoma. While the definitive diagnosis of *H. pylori* infection is based on biopsy specimens obtained at endoscopy, numerous noninvasive methods are available both for diagnosis and confirmation of cure (101). The noninvasive "test and treat" strategy for uninvestigated dyspepsia, especially in patients under 50 years of age, is an effective alternative to prompt endoscopy that is less invasive and less expensive (102, 103). Antibody detection in serum, urine, or saliva is a reliable indicator of *H. pylori* infection, but cannot discriminate between active and recent past (3 years) infections (104–110). Stool antigen testing is less reliable as a diagnostic test but may be useful in confirmation of cure. However, testing needs to be deferred for six to eight weeks to confirm eradication. The urea breath test is the gold standard noninvasive test for diagnosis of active infection with *H. pylori* and as a test of cure. The basis of the test is that intragastric hydolysis of urea by *H. pylori* leads to a change in the isotopic ratio ($^{13}CO_2/^{12}CO_2$) in the breath. All of these methods can be used for POCT, although the benefits of POCT are not always clear-cut, and one of the drivers for POCT may have been the inability of local laboratories to meet the requirements of their users (111). Antibody screening can be readily undertaken by POCT with sensitivities comparable to laboratory-based testing (110), but probably the only advantage of doing so is that it allows therapy to be commenced at the initial consultation. Stool antigen testing requires patient compliance with specimen collection (112) and is effectively a send-out test rather than a true point-of-care test. The ^{13}C-UBT has been simplified and shortened by the use of a citric acid test meal and elimination of the need for a 4-h fast. Together with the use of infrared spectrophotometry in place of the more traditional gas isotope ratio mass spectrometry, this means that POCT is feasible (113, 114). The benefits of wider availability of this gold standard test have not yet been fully assessed.

A systematic review of the literature concluded that serological testing was useful where the probability of infection was neither exceptionally high nor low. Where the pre-test probabilities of a positive test were >80% or <20%, negative and positive results, respectively, were too unreliable (115). This is a particular problem in children, where the prevalence of infection is low (116).

Diagnosis of Gastrointestinal Tract Infections

Quite apart from the lack of suitable tests, there are two important disincentives to using POCT for diagnosing gastrointestinal tract infections. First, most common infections, including viral gastroenteritis, salmonellosis, and campylobacter infection, resolve without antibiotic treatment, and there is often little clinical advantage in making a rapid diagnosis. Second, there are significant hazards associated with handling feces samples that may contain dangerous and highly transmissible pathogens such as *Salmonella typhi* or verotoxin-producing *E. coli* (VTEC).

However, some of the antigen detection tests intended primarily for laboratory diagnosis of infection with *Clostridium difficile* (117–120) and rotavirus (121) could readily be used for POCT, giving results in as little as 10 min. By coincidence, these are two infections that frequently present infection control challenges in hospitals, so that there may be real clinical benefit from rapid diagnosis. Early diagnosis of *C. difficile* infection might also guide prompt antibiotic therapy, thereby reducing the risk of progression to life-threatening pseudo-membranous colitis. Moreover, because these infections occur mainly in specific patient groups (rotavirus in children and the elderly; *C. difficile* following antibiotic expo-

sure), it would be feasible to devise test protocols to help prevent testing of higher-risk samples.

Diagnosis of Blood-Borne Virus Infections

The diagnosis of blood borne virus (BBV) infections, such as hepatitis B and HIV, requires the highest level of accuracy and is normally confirmed only after repeat testing of the original sample and a second sample. While diagnosis of these infections is often urgent, in most situations there is sufficient time for a result to be obtained from the laboratory; many laboratories are geared to providing a same day, or even more rapid, results service. POCT for these infections requires special consideration of issues of patient consent (so that patients are informed that a positive POCT result can only be regarded as a provisional result), quality assurance, and safety.

HIV. Rapid tests for antibodies to HIV-1 offer results in as little as 20 min (122), but the first POCT devices had the disadvantage that plasma or serum was required. The OraSure® and OraQuick® rapid HIV-1 tests (OraSure Technologies, Bethlehem, PA, USA) are, respectively, undertaken on saliva and whole blood obtained by finger prick. Early trials of these tests have been reported to provide 100% sensitivity and >99% specificity. It has been reported that false negatives may occur in HIV-infected subjects who have received early highly active antiretroviral therapy, but it is unlikely that this would cause problems in POCT (123).

Routine HIV testing has been recommended by the the US Centers for Disease Control and Prevention for patients attending hospitals and health care clinics with a high prevalence of HIV (124). POCT may be useful in such settings, especially in outreach clinics, and where there is a high rate of subjects failing to return (125). There are few situations where diagnosis of HIV is a true emergency. One such instance is testing women, during labor, who have not been tested earlier in pregnancy. Diagnosis of maternal HIV infection at this stage still allows interventions that significantly reduce the risk of mother-to-infant transmission. POCT was evaluated in three Chicago hospitals, where the staff undertaking testing was expected to continue with their other duties while awaiting development of the test results. The median results turnaround time in these hospitals was 45 min, compared with 210 min in a fourth hospital, where samples were tested urgently by an on-site laboratory (123).

Another possible important use of POCT for HIV is in the assessment of the sources of needle-stick injuries (126). For maximum efficacy, it is recommended that postexposure prophylaxis (PEP) with antiretroviral drugs should be commenced for the recipient of a needle-stick injury from an HIV-positive source as soon as possible, and ideally within 1 h. This means that recipients of injuries usually have to decide whether to commence PEP before the results of source HIV testing available from the laboratory; POCT could facilitate informed decision making and would be particularly valuable in settings with a high prevalence of HIV.

Direct detection of viral genome is increasingly being used as an additional screening test for HIV, especially to detect early infections during the window period before seroconversion. It would be feasible to use PCR as a POCT to screen for HIV infection. A quantitative PCR could have the additional benefit of facilitating the monitoring of patients receiving highly active antiretroviral therapy. Simultaneous detection of HIV and other retroviruses (HTLV1 and 2) (127) or blood-borne hepatitis viruses (128) using DNA chip-based assays has recently been reported. With the development of user-friendly work stations such as the Nanochip® Molecular Biology Workstation (Nanogen,® San Diego, CA, USA) there is the potential for point-of care-screening of at-risk individuals for the whole range of blood-borne virus infections.

Hepatitis B. There are various serological markers of hepatitis B infection. Hepatitis B surface antigen (HBsAg) is simply a marker of infection, whereas HBeAg is a marker of infectivity. Rapid disposable tests for HBsAg are readily available, although there has been little published evaluation of these for POCT (12). POCT for HBsAg alone might be useful for screening in some situations. However, knowledge of the HBeAg status of HBsAg-positive subjects is urgently required in some clinical situations, for example, in determining the management of needle-stick injuries from an HBsAg-positive source, or of babies born to hepatitis B–infected mothers. A new 10-min test for both HBsAg and HbeAg (NOW® ICT Hepatitis B sAg/eAg, Binax, Portland, ME, USA) suitable for use with whole blood, is user friendly and has been shown to be sensitive and specific in a laboratory-based evaluation (129).

Detection of Methicillin-Resistant *Staphylococcus aureus*

Methicillin-resistant *Staphylococcus aureus* (MRSA) are strains of *S. aureus* that are resistant to β-lactam antibiotics and often to several other antibiotic classes. Without control measures, MRSA can spread rapidly in hospitals. Rapid detection of MRSA could be useful in ensuring that infected patients receive prompt treatment with appropriate antibiotics and that infection control measures are implemented early. Real-time PCR has been successfully used to directly detect MRSA in clinical samples within 1 h, with a sensitivity of >90% compared with culture (130, 131). This test could feasibly be undertaken by POCT, but it is doubtful whether there could be sufficient clinical need.

CONCLUSION

POCT for infectious diseases is currently far less well established than in disciplines such as clinical chemistry and hematology. Central to the reasons for this are that, the most commonly used microbiology laboratory technologies are not transferable to POCT, that most infections are comparatively uncommon, and that currently POCT cannot offer the versatility of laboratory-based culture. However, we may be on the threshold of a new era in POCT for infectious diseases with the advent of new technologies such as the electronic nose (132;

see also Chapter 5) and, especially, molecular biology (DNA chip), methods that allow simultaneous testing for several different pathogens and/or characteristics such as common antibiotic resistances. Although immediate knowledge of microbiology results is rarely lifesaving, rapid diagnosis of infectious diseases by POCT has considerable potential to streamline clinical care through optimization of antimicrobial therapy and infection control practices, avoidance of unnecessary investigations, and reductions in clinical visits or duration of hospital stay.

REFERENCES

1. World Health Organization. http://www.who.int (accessed May 2004).
2. Reardon EP, Noble MA, Luther ER, Wort AJ, Bent J, Swift M. Evaluation of a rapid method for the detection of vaginal group B streptococci in women in labor. Am J Obstet Gynecol 1984; 148:575–8.
3. Baker CJ. Inadequacy of rapid immunoassays for intrapartum detection of group B streptococcal carriers. Obstet Gynecol 1996;88:51–5.
4. Harrison LH, Steinhoff MC, Sridharan G, Castelo A, Khallaf N, Ostroff SM, et al. Monovalent latex agglutination reagents for the diagnosis of nonmeningitic pneumococcal infection. Diagn Microbiol Infect Dis 1996;24:1–6.
5. Winn HN, McLennan M, Amon E. Clinical assessment of the rapid latex agglutination screening test for group B *Streptococcus*. Int J Gynaecol Obstet 1994;47:289–90.
6. Rosa C, Clark P, Duff P. Performance of a new DNA probe for the detection of group B streptococcal colonization of the genital tract. Obstet Gynecol 1995;86:509–11.
7. Witt A, Petricevic L, Kaufmann U, Gregor H, Kiss H. DNA hybridisation test: rapid diagnostic tool for excluding bacterial vaginosis in pregnant women with symptoms suggestive of infection. J Clin Microbiol 2002;40:3057–9.
8. Ke D, Menard C, Picard FJ, Boissinot M, Ouellette M, Roy PH, et al. Development of conventional and real-time PCR assays for the rapid detection of group B streptococci. Clin Chem 2000; 46:324–31.
9. Perdue ML. Molecular diagnostics in an insecure world. Avian Dis 2003;47(Suppl):1063–8.
10. Standing Medical Advisory Committee Subgroup on Antimicrobial Resistance. The path of least resistance. London: Department of Health, 1998.
11. Price CP. Point of care testing. BMJ 2001;322:1285–8.
12. Bevan VM, Bullock DG, Haeney M, Dhell J. The application of near patient testing to microbiology. Comm Dis Pub Health 1999;2:14–21.
13. BalcI C, Sungurtekin H, Gurses E, Sungurtekin U, Kaptanoglu B. Usefulness of procalcitonin for diagnosis of sepsis in the intensive care unit. Crit Care 2003;7:85–90.
14. Cornbleet PJ. Clinical utility of the band count. Clin Lab Med 2002;22:101–36.
15. Toh CH, Dennis M. Disseminated intravascular coagulation: old disease, new hope. BMJ 2003;327:974–7.
16. Iverson RL. Septic shock: a clinical perspective. Crit Care Clin 1988;4:215–28.
17. Kobayashi S, Gando S, Morimoto Y, Nanzaki S, Kemmotsu O. Serial measurement of arterial lactate concentrations as a prog-

nostic indicator in relation to the incidence of disseminated intravascular coagulation in patients with systemic inflammatory response syndrome. Surg Today 2001;31:853–9.

18. Tabuchi T, Tominaga H, Tatsumi N. Problems related to rapid methods for erythrocyte sedimentation rate test and their solution. Southeast Asian J Trop Med Public Health 2002;33(Suppl 2):151–4.

19. Casado-Flores J, Blanco-Quiros A, Asensio J, Arranz E, Garrote JA, Nieto M. Serum procalcitonin in children with suspected sepsis: a comparison with C-reactive protein and neutrophil count. Pediatr Crit Care Med 2003;4:190–5.

20. Jaye DL, Waites KB. Clinical applications of C-reactive protein in pediatrics. Pediatr Infect Dis J 1997;16:735–46.

21. Luzzani A, Polati E, Dorizzi R, Rungatscher A, Pavan R, Merlini A. Comparison of procalcitonin and C-reactive protein as markers of sepsis. Crit Care Med 2003;31:1737–41.

22. Carrol ED, Thomson AP, Hart CA. Procalcitonin as a marker of sepsis. Int J Antimicrob Agents 2002;20:1–9.

23. Hatherill M, Tibby SM, Turner C, Ratnavel N, Murdoch IA. Procalcitonin and cytokine levels: relationship to organ failure and mortality in pediatric septic shock. Crit Care Med 2000;28:2591–4.

24. Chirouze C, Schuhmacher H, Rabaud C, Gil H, Khayat N, Estavoyer JM, et al. Low serum procalcitonin level accurately predicts the absence of bacteremia in adult patients with acute fever. Clin Infect Dis 2002;35:156–61.

25. Hubl W, Krassler J, Zingler C, Pertschy A, Hentschel J, Gerhards-Reich C, et al. Evaluation of a fully automated procalcitonin chemiluminescence immunoassay. Clin Lab 2003;49:319–27.

26. Han YY, Doughty LA, Kofos D, Sasser H, Carcillo JA. Procalcitonin is persistently increased among children with poor outcome from bacterial sepsis. Pediatr Crit Care Med 2003;4:21–5.

27. Beghetti M, Rimensberger PC, Kalangos A, Habre W, Gervaix A. Kinetics of procalcitonin, interleukin 6 and C-reactive protein after cardiopulmonary-bypass in children. Cardiol Young 2003;13:161–7.

28. Geppert A, Steiner A, Delle-Karth G, Heinz G, Huber K. Usefulness of procalcitonin for diagnosing complicating sepsis in patients with cardiogenic shock. Intensive Care Med 2003;29:1384–9.

29. Blommendahl J, Janas M, Laine S, Miettinen A, Ashorn P. Comparison of procalcitonin with CRP and differential white blood cell count for diagnosis of culture-proven neonatal sepsis. Scand J Infect Dis 2002;34:620–2.

30. Chiesa C, Pellegrini G, Panero A, Osborn JF, Signore F, Assumma M, et al. C-reactive protein, interleukin-6, and procalcitonin in the immediate postnatal period: influence of illness severity, risk status, antenatal and perinatal complications, and infection. Clin Chem 2003;49:60–8.

31. Guibourdenche J, Bedu A, Petzold L, Marchand M, Mariani-Kurdjian P, Hurtaud-Roux M-F, et al. Biochemical markers of neonatal sepsis: value of procalcitonin in the emergency setting. Ann Clin Biochem 2002;39:130–5.

32. Kordek A, Giedrys-Kalemba S, Pawlus B, Podraza W, Czajka R. Umbilical cord blood serum procalcitonin concentration in the diagnosis of early neonatal infection. J Perinatol 2003;23:148–53.

33. Resch B, Gusenleitner W, Muller WD. Procalcitonin and interleukin-6 in the diagnosis of early-onset sepsis of the neonate. Acta Paediatr 2003;92:243–5.

34. Fernandez Lopez A, Luaces Cubells C, Garcia Garcia JJ, Fernandez Pou J; Spanish Society of Pediatric Emergencies. Procalcitonin in pediatric emergency departments for the early diagnosis of invasive bacterial infections in febrile infants: results of a multicenter study and utility of a rapid qualitative test for this marker. Pediatr Infect Dis J 2003;22:895–903.

35. Galetto-Lacour A, Zamora SA, Gervaix A. Bedside procalcitonin and C-reactive protein tests in children with fever without localizing signs of infection seen in a referral center. Pediatrics 2003;112:1054–60.

36. Prat C, Dominguez J, Rodrigo C, Gimenez M, Azuara M, Jimenez O, et al. Elevated serum procalcitonin values correlate with renal scarring in children with urinary tract infection. Pediatr Infect Dis J 2003;22:438–42.

37. Smolkin V, Koren A, Raz R, Colodner R, Sakran W, Halevy R. Procalcitonin as a marker of acute pyelonephritis in infants and children. Pediatr Nephrol 2002;17:409–12.

38. Semeniuk H, Church D. Evaluation of the leukocyte esterase and nitrite urine dipstick screening tests for detection of bacteriuria in women with suspected uncomplicated urinary tract infections. NJ Clin Microbiol 1999;37:3051–2.

39. Holland DJ, Bliss KJ, Allen CD, Gilbert GL. A comparison of chemical dipsticks read visually or by photometry in the routine screening of urine specimens in the clinical microbiology laboratory. Pathology 1995;27:91–6.

40. Preston A, O'Donnell T, Phillips CA. Screening for urinary tract infections in a gynaecological setting: validity and cost-effectiveness of reagent strips. Br J Biomed Sci 1999;56:253–7.

41. Moore KN, Murray S, Malone-Lee J, Wagg A. Rapid urinalysis assays for the diagnosis of urinary tract infection. Br J Nurs 2001;12:995–1001.

42. Tincello DG, Richmond DH. Evaluation of reagent strips in detecting asymptomatic bacteriuria in early pregnancy: prospective case series. BMJ 1998;316:435–7.

43. McNair RD, MacDonald SR, Dooley SL, Peterson LR. Evaluation of the centrifuged and Gram-stained smear, urinalysis, and reagent strip testing to detect asymptomatic bacteriuria in obstetric patients. Am J Obstet Gynecol 2000;182:1076–9.

44. Kunin CM, White LV, Hua TH. A reassessment of the importance of "low-count" bacteriuria in young women with acute urinary symptoms. Ann Intern Med 1993;119:454–60.

45. Hansson S, Brandstrom P, Jodal U, Larsson P. Low bacterial counts in infants with urinary tract infection. J Pediatr 1998;132:180–2.

46. Nunns D, Smith AR, Hosker G. Reagent strip testing urine for significant bacteriuria in a urodynamic clinic. Br J Urol 1995;76:87–9.

47. Lohr JA, Portilla MG, Geuder TG, Dunn ML, Dudley SM. Making a presumptive diagnosis of urinary tract infection by using a urinalysis performed in an on-site laboratory. J Pediatr 1993;122:22–5.

48. Newman TB, Bernzweig JA, Takayama JI, Finch SA, Wasserman RC, Pantell RH. Urine testing and urinary tract infections in febrile infants seen in office settings: the Pediatric Research in Office Settings' Febrile Infant Study. Arch Pediatr Adolesc Med 2002;156:44–54.

49. Yuen SF, Ng FN, So LY. Evaluation of the accuracy of leukocyte esterase testing to diagnose pyuria in young febrile children: prospective study. Hong Kong Med J 2001;7:5–8.

50. Sharief N, Hameed M, Petts D. Use of rapid dipstick tests to exclude urinary tract infection in children. Br J Biomed Sci 1998;55:242–6.

51. Hopwood J, Mallinson H, Gleave T. Evaluation of near patient testing for *Chlamydia trachomatis* in a pregnancy termination service. J Fam Plann Reprod Health Care 2001;27:127–30.

52. Arumainayagam JT, Matthews RS, Uthayakumar S, Clay JC. Evaluation of a novel solid-phase immunoassay, Clearview Chlamydia, for the rapid detection of *Chlamydia trachomatis*. J Clin Microbiol 1990;28:2813–4.

53. Lauderdale TL, Landers L, Thorneycroft I, Chapin K. Comparison of the PACE 2 assay, two amplification assays, and Clearview EIA for detection of *Chlamydia trachomatis* in female endocervical and urine specimens. J Clin Microbiol 1999;37:2223–9.

54. Pate MS, Dixon PB, Hardy K, Crosby M, Hook III EW. Evaluation of the Biostar chlamydia OIA assay with specimens from women attending a sexually transmitted disease clinic. J Clin Microbiol 1998;36:2183–6.

55. Stratton NJ, Hirsch L, Harris F, de la Maza LM, Peterson EM. Evaluation of the rapid CLEARVIEW Chlamydia test for direct detection of chlamydiae from cervical specimens. J Clin Microbiol 1991;29:1551–3.

56. Meyer MP, Baughn RE. Whole-blood hemagglutination inhibition test for Venereal Disease Research Laboratory (VDRL) antibodies. J Clin Microbiol 2000;38:3413–4.

57. Fears MB, Pope V. Syphilis fast latex agglutination test, a rapid confirmatory test. Clin Diagn Lab Immunol 2001;8:841–2.

58. Myer L, Wilkinson D, Lombard C, Zuma K, Rotchford K, Karim SS. Impact of on-site testing for maternal syphilis on treatment delays, treatment rates, and perinatal mortality in rural South Africa: a randomised controlled trial. Sex Transm Infect 2003;79:208–13.

59. Manavi K, Young H, Clutterbuck D. Sensitivity of microscopy for the rapid diagnosis of gonorrhoea in men and women and the role of gonorrhoea serovars. Int J STD AIDS 2003;14:390–4.

60. Lamont RF. Infection in the prediction and antibiotics in the prevention of spontaneous preterm labour and preterm birth. BJOG 2003;110(Suppl 20):71–5.

61. Hellberg D, Nilsson S, Mardh PA. The diagnosis of bacterial vaginosis and vaginal flora changes. Arch Gynecol Obstet 2001;265:11–5.

62. Nugent RP, Krohn MA, Hillier SL. Reliability of diagnosing bacterial vaginosis is improved by a standardized method of gram stain interpretation. J Clin Microbiol 1991;29:297–301.

63. Schmidt H, Hansen JG. Validity of wet-mount bacterial morphotype identification of vaginal fluid by phase-contrast microscopy for diagnosis of bacterial vaginosis in family practice. APMIS 2001;109:589–94.

64. Myziuk L, Romanowski B, Johnson SC. BVBlue test for diagnosis of bacterial vaginosis. J Clin Microbiol 2003;41:1925–8.

65. West B, Morison L, van der Loeff MS, Gooding E, Awasana AA, Demba E, et al. Evaluation of a new rapid diagnostic kit (FemExam) for bacterial vaginosis in patients with vaginal discharge syndrome in the Gambia. Sex Transm Dis 2003;30:483–9.

66. Schrag S, Gorwitz R, Fultz-Butts K, Schuchat A. Prevention of perinatal group B streptococcal disease. Revised guidelines from CDC. MMWR Recomm Rep 2002;51:1–22.

67. Brocklehurst P. Green top guideline "Prevention of early onset neonatal group B streptococcal disease." London: Royal College of Obstetricians and Gynaecologists, 2003.

68. Baker CJ. Inadequacy of rapid immunoassays for intrapartum detection of group B streptococcal carriers. Obstet Gynecol 1996;88:51–5.

69. Carroll KC, Ballou D, Varner M, Chun H, Traver R, Salyer J. Rapid detection of group B streptococcal colonization of the genital tract by a commercial optical immunoassay. Eur J Clin Microbiol Infect Dis 1996;15:206–10.

70. Nguyen TM, Gauthier DW, Myles TD, Nuwayhid BS, Viana MA, Schreckenberger PC. Detection of group B streptococcus: comparison of an optical immunoassay with direct plating and broth-enhanced culture methods. J Matern Fetal Med 1998;7:172–6.

71. Park CH, Ruprai D, Vandel NM, Hixon DL, Mecklenburg FE. Rapid detection of group B streptococcal antigen from vaginal specimens using a new optical immunoassay technique. Diagn Microbiol Infect Dis 1996;24:125–8.

72. Samadi R, Stek A, Greenspoon JS. Evaluation of a rapid optical immunoassay-based test for group B streptococcus colonization in intrapartum patients. J Matern Fetal Med 2001;10:203–8.

73. Thinkhamrop J, Limpongsanurak S, Festin MR, Daly S, Schuchat A, Lumbiganon P, et al. Infections in international pregnancy study: performance of the optical immunoassay test for detection of group B streptococcus. J Clin Microbiol 2003;41:5288–90.

74. Bergeron MG, Ke D, Menard C, Picard FJ, Gagnon M, Bernier M, et al. Rapid detection of group B streptococci in pregnant women at delivery. N Engl J Med 2000;343:175–9.

75. Mackenzie A, Hallam N, Mitchell E, Beattie T. Near patient testing for respiratory syncytial virus in paediatric accident and emergency: prospective pilot study. BMJ 1999;319:289–90.

76. Mackie PL, Joannidis PA, Beattie J. Evaluation of an acute point-of-care system screening for respiratory syncytial virus infection. J Hosp Infect 2001;48:66–71.

77. Mlinaric-Galinovic G, Varda-Brkic D. Nosocomial respiratory syncytial virus infections in children's wards. Diagn Microbiol Infect Dis 2000;37:237–46.

78. Karanfil LV, Conlon M, Lykens K, Masters CF, Forman M, Griffith ME, et al. Reducing the rate of nosocomially transmitted respiratory syncytial virus. Am J Infect Control 1999;27:91–6.

79. Casiano-Colon AE, Hulbert BB, Mayer TK, Walsh EE, Falsey AR. Lack of sensitivity of rapid antigen tests for the diagnosis of respiratory syncytial virus infection in adults. J Clin Virol 2003;28:169–74.

80. Reina J, Padilla E, Alonso F, Ruiz De Gopegui E, Munar M, Mari M. Evaluation of a new dot blot enzyme immunoassay (directigen flu A + B) for simultaneous and differential detection of influenza a and B virus antigens from respiratory samples. J Clin Microbiol 2002;40:3515–7.

81. Cazacu AC, Greer J, Taherivand M, Demmler GJ. Comparison of lateral-flow immunoassay and enzyme immunoassay with viral culture for rapid detection of influenza virus in nasal wash specimens from children. J Clin Microbiol 2003;41:2132–4.

82. Dunn JJ, Gordon C, Kelley C, Carroll KC. Comparison of the Denka-Seiken INFLU A. B-Quick and BD Directigen Flu A + B kits with direct fluorescent-antibody staining and shell vial culture methods for rapid detection of influenza viruses. J Clin Microbiol 2003;41:2180–3.

83. Poehling KA, Griffin MR, Dittus RS, Tang YW, Holland K, Li H, et al. Bedside diagnosis of influenzavirus infections in hospitalized children. Pediatrics 2002;110:83–8.

84. Quach C, Newby D, Daoust G, Rubin E, McDonald J. QuickVue influenza test for rapid detection of influenza A and B viruses in a pediatric population. Clin Diagn Lab Immunol 2002;9:925–6.

85. Ruest A, Michaud S, Deslandes S, Frost EH. Comparison of the Directigen flu A + B test, the QuickVue influenza test, and clinical case definition to viral culture and reverse transcription-PCR for rapid diagnosis of influenza virus infection. J Clin Microbiol 2003;41:3487–93.

86. Landry ML, Ferguson D. Suboptimal detection of influenza virus in adults by the Directigen Flu A + B enzyme immunoassay and correlation of results with the number of antigen-positive cells detected by cytospin immunofluorescence. J Clin Microbiol 2003;41:3407–9.

87. Sintchenko V, Gilbert GL, Coiera E, Dwyer D. Treat or test first? Decision analysis of empirical antiviral treatment of influenza virus infection versus treatment based on rapid test results. J Clin Virol 2002;25:15–21.

88. Bonner AB, Monroe KW, Talley LI, Klasner AE, Kimberlin DW. Impact of the rapid diagnosis of influenza on physician decision-making and patient management in the pediatric emergency department: results of a randomized, prospective, controlled trial. Pediatrics 2003;112:363–7.

89. Sharma V, Dowd MD, Slaughter AJ, Simon SD. Effect of rapid diagnosis of influenza virus type A on the emergency department management of febrile infants and toddlers. Arch Pediatr Adolesc Med 2002;156:41–3.

90. Abels S, Nadal D, Stroehle A, Bossart W. Reliable detection of respiratory syncytial virus infection in children for adequate hospital infection control management. J Clin Microbiol 2001;39:3135–9.

91. Subbarao EK, Dietrich MC, De Sierra TM, Black CJ, Super DM, Thomas F, et al. Rapid detection of respiratory syncytial virus by a biotin-enhanced immunoassay: test performance by laboratory technologists and housestaff. Pediatr Infect Dis J 1989;8:865–9.

92. Bruu AL, Hjetland R, Holter E, Mortensen L, Natas O, Petterson W, et al. Evaluation of 12 commercial tests for detection of Epstein-Barr virus-specific and heterophile antibodies. Clin Diagn Lab Immunol 2000;7:451–6.

93. Woods WA, Carter CT, Schlager TA. Detection of group A streptococci in children under 3 years of age with pharyngitis. Pediatr Energ Care 1999;15:338–40.

94. Uhl JR, Adamson SC, Vetter EA, Schleck CD, Harmsen WS, Iverson LK, et al. Comparison of LightCycler PCR, rapid antigen immunoassay, and culture for detection of group A streptococci from throat swabs. J Clin Microbiol 2003;41:242–9.

95. Gieseker KE, Mackenzie T, Roe MH, Todd JK. Comparison of two rapid *Streptococcus pyogenes* diagnostic tests with a rigorous culture standard. Pediatr Infect Dis J 2002;21:922–7.

96. Johansson L, Mansson NO. Rapid test, throat culture and clinical assessment in the diagnosis of tonsillitis. Fam Pract 2003;20:108–11.

97. Gieseker KE, Roe MH, MacKenzie T, Todd JK. Evaluating the American Academy of Pediatrics diagnostic standard for *Streptococcus pyogenes* pharyngitis: backup culture versus repeat rapid antigen testing. Pediatrics 2003;111:666–70.

98. Karchmer TB, Anglim AM, Durbin LJ, Farr BM. Pseudoepidemic of streptococcal pharyngitis in a hospital pharmacy. Am J Infect Control 2001;29:104–8.

99. Neuner JM, Hamel MB, Phillips RS, Bona K, Aronson MD. Diagnosis and management of adults with pharyngitis: a cost-effectiveness analysis. Ann Intern Med 2003;139:113–22.

100. Ehrlich JE, Demopoulos BP, Daniel KR Jr., Ricarte MC, Glied S. Cost-effectiveness of treatment options for prevention of rheumatic heart disease from Group A streptococcal pharyngitis in a pediatric population. Prev Med 2002;35:250–7.

101. Megraud F. Diagnostic modalities for the detection of *Helicobacter pylori*. Drugs Today (Barc)1999;35:419–27.

102. Gatta L, Ricci C, Tampieri A, Vaira D. Non-invasive techniques for the diagnosis of *Helicobacter pylori* infection. Clin Microbiol Infect 2003;9:489–96.

103. Ladabaum U, Fendrick AM, Glidden D, Scheiman JM. Helicobacter pylori test-and-treat intervention compared to usual care in primary care patients with suspected peptic ulcer disease in the United States. Am J Gastroenterol 97:3007–14, 2002.

104. Adachi K, Kawamura A, Ono M, Masuzaki K, Takashima T, Yuki M, et al. Comparative evaluation of urine-based and other minimally invasive methods for the diagnosis of *Helicobacter pylori* infection. J Gastroenterol 2002;37:703–8.

105. Breslin NP, Lee JM, Buckley MJ, Balbirnie E, Rice D, O'Morain CA. Validation of serological tests for *Helicobacter pylori* infection in an Irish population. Ir J Med Sci 2000;169:190–4.

106. Delaney BC, Holder RL, Allan TF, Kenkre JE, Hobbs FD. A comparison of Bayesian and maximum likelihood methods to determine the performance of a point of care test for *Helicobacter pylori* in the office setting. Med Decis Making 2003;23:21–30.

107. Fujisawa T, Kaneko T, Kumagai T, Akamatsu T, Katsuyama T, Kiyosawa K, et al. Evaluation of urinary rapid test for *Helicobacter pylori* in general practice. J Clin Lab Anal 2001;15:154–9.

108. Wong WM, Lam SK, Xia HH, Tang VS, Lai KC, Hu WH, et al. Accuracy of a new near patient test for the diagnosis of *Helicobacter pylori* infection in Chinese. J Gastroenterol Hepatol 2002;17:1272–7.

109. Wu DC, Kuo CH, Lu CY, Su YC, Yu FJ, Lee YC, et al. Evaluation of an office-based urine test for detecting *Helicobacter pylori*: a prospective pilot study. Hepatogastroenterology 2001;48:614–7.

110. Langhorst J, Heuer S, Drouven FU, Schwobel HD, Reichenberger S, Neuhaus H. Evaluation of a new immunochromatogrpahic based whole near patient test for the diagnosis of *Helicobacter pylori* infection. Z Gastroenterol 2002;40:389–93.

111. Luman W, Ng HS. Survey of dyspepsia management in the community. Singapore Med J 2001;42:206–9.

112. Cullen KP, Broderick BM, Jayaram J, Flynn B, O'Connor HJ. Evaluation of the *Helicobacter pylori* stool antigen (HpSA) test in routine clinical practice-is it patient-friendly? Ir Med J 2002;95:305–6.

113. Hegedus O, Ryden J, Rehnberg AS, Nilsson S, Hellstrom PM. Validated accuracy of a novel urea breath test for rapid *Helicobacter pylori* detection and in-office analysis. Eur J Gastroenterol Hepatol 2002;14:513–20.

114. Opekun AR, Abdalla N, Sutton FM, Hammoud F, Kuo GM, Torres E, et al. Urea breath testing and analysis in the primary care office. J Fam Pract 2002;51:1030–2.

115. Roberts AP, Childs SM, Rubin G, de Wit NJ. Tests for *Helicobacter pylori* infection: a critical appraisal from primary care. Fam Pract 2000;17(Suppl 2):S12–20.

116. Day AS Sherman PM. Accuracy of office-based immunoassays for the diagnosis of *Helicobacter pylori* infection in children. Helicobacter 2002;7:205–9.

117. Barbut F, Mace M, Lalande V, Tilleul P, Petit JC. Rapid detection of *Clostridium difficile* toxin A in stool specimens. Clin Microbiol Infect 1997;3:480–3.

118. O'Connor D, Hynes P, Cormican M, Collins E, Corbett-Feeney G, Cassidy M. Evaluation of methods for detection of toxins in specimens of feces submitted for diagnosis of *Clostridium difficile*–associated diarrhea. J Clin Microbiol 2001;39:2846–9.

119. Vanpoucke H, De Baere T, Claeys G, Vaneechoutte M, Verschraegen G. Evaluation of six commercial assays for the rapid detection of *Clostridium difficile* toxin and/or antigen in stool specimens. Clin Microbiol Infect 2001;7:55–64.

120. Yucesoy M, McCoubrey J, Brown R, Poxton IR. Detection of toxin production in *Clostridium difficile* strains by three different methods. Clin Microbiol Infect 2002;8:413–8.

121. Pai CH, Shahrabadi MS, Ince B. Rapid diagnosis of rotavirus gastroenteritis by a commercial latex agglutination test. J Clin Microbiol 1985;22:846–50.

122. Centers for Disease Control and Prevention. Approval of a new rapid test for HIV antibody. JAMA 2002;288:2960.

123. Centers for Disease Control and Prevention (CDC). Rapid point-of-care testing for HIV-1 during labor and delivery—Chicago, Illinois, 2002. MMWR Morb Mortal Wkly Rep 2003;52:866–8.

124. Centers for Disease Control and Prevention. Routinely recommended HIV testing at an urban urgent-care clinic—Atlanta, Georgia, 2000. MMWR Morb Mortal Wkly Rep 2001;50:538–41.

125. Keenan PA, Keenan JM. Rapid HIV testing in urban outreach: a strategy for improving post-test counselling rates. AIDS Educ Prev 2001;13:541–50.

126. Burrage J Jr. HIV rapid tests: progress, perspective and future directions. Clin J Oncol Nurs 2003;7:207–8.

127. Seifarth W, Spiess B, Zeilfelder U, Speth C, Hehlmann R, Leib-Mosch C[b]. Assessment of retroviral activity using a universal retrovirus chip. J Virol Methods 2003;112:79–91.

128. Wen JK, Zhang XE, Cheng Z, Liu H, Zhou YF, Zhang ZP, et al. A visual DNA chip for simultaneous detection of hepatitis B virus, hepatitis C virus and human immunodeficiency virus type-1. Biosens Bioelectron 2004;19:685–92.

129. Clement F, Dewint P, Leroux-Roels G. Evaluation of a new rapid test for the combined detection of hepatitis B virus surface antigen and hepatitis B virus e antigen. J Clin Microbiol 2002;40:4603–6.

130. Fang H, Hedin G. Rapid screening and identification of methicillin-resistant *Staphylococcus aureus* from clinical samples by selective-broth and real-time PCR assay. J Clin Microbiol 2003;41:2894–9.

131. Grisold AJ, Leitner E, Muhlbauer G, Marth E, Kessler HH. Detection of methicillin-resistant *Staphylococcus aureus* and simultaneous confirmation by automated nucleic acid extraction and real-time PCR. J Clin Microbiol 2002;40:2392–7.

132. Guernion N, Ratcliffe NM, Spencer-Phillips PT, Howe RA. Identifying bacteria in human urine: current practice and the potential for rapid, near-patient diagnosis by sensing volatile organic compounds. Clin Chem Lab Med 2001;39:893–906.

Chapter 37

Point-of-Care Testing for Cardiac Markers: An Outcome-Based Appraisal

Robert H. Christenson and Paul O. Collinson

Real-time provision of biochemical marker measurements is important for the clinical workup of patients suspected of having active cardiovascular disease including cardiac ischemia, myocardial infarction (MI), and heart failure (HF). This testing is important because "heart attack" is the biggest killer in the Western world, responsible for ~500,000 deaths each year in the United States alone. Analytes including myoglobin, creatine kinase-MB (CK-MB), and, most importantly, cardiac troponin I (cTnI) or cardiac troponin T (cTnT) are essential for assessing suspected MI patients. Congestive heart failure (CHF) is also a major healthcare issue, and is increasing as the median age of populations increases. HF is responsible for the deaths of 250,000 Americans annually. Analytes including B-type natriuretic peptide (BNP) and its metabolic counterpart NT-proBNP are useful for HF diagnosis and monitoring. The purpose of this chapter is to describe the clinical need and context for biochemical markers of acute heart disease and to use an outcome-based approach to examine the potential benefits of measurements provided at the point of care.

CARDIAC ISCHEMIA AND MYOCARDIAL INFARCTION: THE ACUTE CORONARY SYNDROMES

As we mature from birth through old age, formation of fatty streaks occurs in our coronary arteries that can be detected as early as the teenage years. These fatty streaks may develop into coronary plaques depending on a complex interaction of risk factors including genetic predisposition; living habits such as diet, tobacco use, exercise, and ethanol intake; and comorbidities including diabetes mellitus, hypertension, and the metabolic syndrome. Progression of coronary plaque and cardiovascular disease results in the narrowing of coronary arteries. Extensive narrowing can result in an inadequate supply of oxygen and nutrients to cardiac tissue for meeting physiological demand. This supply–demand mismatch may cause a constellation of clinical symptoms that can include severe pain in the chest, jaw, or elsewhere; dyspnea; and fatigue. If plaque has narrowed the artery, but is stable, then this supply–demand mismatch is referred to as "stable angina." With rest and/or administration of vasodilators such as nitroglycerin, the symptoms of stable angina usually resolve in a short time.

The sturdy plaque associated with stable angina is neither an activator of platelets nor thrombogenic. On the other hand, when plaque becomes destabilized, eroded, and/or ruptured, collagen and the plaque's contents are exposed to circulating platelets, coagulation proteins, and other factors, which results in a volatile clinical state that is termed "unstable angina" (UA). Unstable plaque associated with UA causes platelet activation and puts the patient at considerable risk for intravascular thrombosis, occlusion, ischemia, and cell death. Unstable plaque is a key pathophysiological trigger of a group of conditions termed "acute coronary syndromes" (ACS), a spectrum of disease that spans from UA and reversible cell injury to MI with extensive necrosis.

Management of suspected ACS patients must be considered a medical emergency because there is high risk of adverse outcomes such as myocardial necrosis and death. Traditionally, initial risk assessment has been based on patient history, clinical signs and symptoms, and the electrocardiogram (ECG). More recently, seven indicators for classifying high-risk ACS patients have been combined to calculate a thrombolysis in myocardial infarction (TIMI) risk score (1). TIMI risk score variables include age > 65 years; ≥3 risk factors for coronary artery disease; prior coronary stenosis > 50%; ST deviation on the ECG; ≥2 anginal events in previous 24 h; aspirin use in past 7 days; and elevated cardiac markers. For scoring, patients are assigned 1 point for each indicator; over the next year a continuum of risk for death/MI/urgent revascularization spans from 4.7% for a score of 0 or 1 to an event rate of almost 40% with a TIMI risk score of 6 or 7 (1).

ACS is a heterogeneous disease state that can be conveniently classified according to ECG results (2). The ECG is considered a tool for assessing cardiac ischemia, and characteristic abnormalities can evolve rapidly, as soon as a few minutes following onset of symptoms. However the conventional ECG has a diagnostic sensitivity of only ~50% for ischemia and is dependent on the anatomic location of the thrombus, nature of the ischemic event, and other factors.

Figure 37-1 shows that the ECG can be used to classify ACS patients by ST elevation (STE) or no ST elevation (NSTE). The diagnosis of STE myocardial infarction (STEMI) is dependent on the appearance of specific changes on the ECG. As indicated in Figure 37-1, the finding of STE implies that the thrombus is rich in fibrin and is likely to be totally occlusive of the infarct-related artery (3). This affects treat-

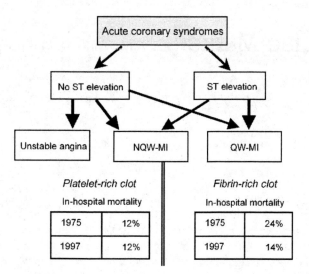

Figure 37-1 The continuum of acute coronary syndromes (ACS) can be divided into no ST elevation (NSTE) and ST elevation (STE) based on results of the electrocardiogram. NSTE ACS can be either unstable angina; non–Q-wave myocardial infarction (NQW-MI), which is usually not totally occlusive of the infarct-related artery; or Q-wave myocardial infarction (QW-MI). In the majority of cases, STEMI is associated with QW-MI and is frequently totally occlusive of the infarct-related artery. NSTE ACS is associated with platelet-rich thrombus and mortality in the majority of cases, as shown. Thrombus with STEMI is fibrin-rich in the majority of cases, and mortality has been reduced dramatically over the past 20 years due to advances in fibrinolytic therapy and interventional cardiology.

ment choice because STEMI patients benefit from fibrinolytic therapy administered within the first 12 h after onset of symptoms. Also, these patients are frequently referred for angioplasty or percutaneous coronary intervention and stent placement within 90 min of hospital presentation. In the United States, these effective treatment strategies, along with improved primary prevention efforts, have reduced the in-hospital mortality from STEMI by nearly half, from 24% in 1977 to 14% in 1997 (Figure 37-1). STEMI occurs in only about 15% of patients presenting with ACS. Biochemical markers have prognostic importance in STEMI patients (4), but point-of-care testing (POCT) is of modest value for diagnosis and treatment because acute clinical decisions are based on symptoms at presentation and ECG findings. In contrast, biochemical markers play a fundamental role for diagnostic and clinical decisions in NSTEMI and UA, which affect the majority of ACS patients.

UA and NSTEMI patients represent ~85% of ACS patients. The diagnosis of UA and NSTEMI is inherently more complicated, mainly because there is currently no widely accepted early tool for detection of myocardial ischemia analogous to the ECG for STEMI. Also, the majority of UA and NSTEMI patients are older and present with vague signs and symptoms that are common to many other conditions; these symptoms may include breathlessness, diaphoresis, nausea, and "atypical" pain. Presentation with vague symptoms serves to confound the pre-test probability of UA and NSTEMI in the acutely ill emergency medicine population. However, because

the potential outcome of ACS is dire, even patients having relatively low pre-test probability of the condition must be considered at substantial risk until proven otherwise. Further, data indicate that 1–3% of high-risk ACS patients are released from care inappropriately (5). Together, these factors have led to a paradigm shift toward a need for risk stratification as the means of detecting and managing cardiovascular disease during the acute presentation. There is clear evidence that abnormal positive cTnT or cTnI results confer a higher risk profile among both STE and NSTE patients; meta-analyses show that positive troponin translates to a 2.5- to 8.0-fold greater risk of adverse outcomes including (re)infarction and death in ACS patients (4, 6).

Biochemical markers have become an essential part of risk stratification strategies in the treatment of UA and NSTEMI, along with the other TIMI risk factors (1). A Class I recommendation of clinical guidelines for UA and NSTEMI from the American Heart Association (AHA) and the American College of Cardiology (ACC) states that cardiac markers (i.e., cTnI or cTnT, CK-MB, and myoglobin) should be available for initial assessment of UA and NSTEMI patients (7).

The pathophysiology of NSTE ACS contrasts with that of STEMI (3). NSTE patients generally have thrombus that does not totally occlude the infarct-related artery. Also, the clot composition in UA and NSTE is predominately platelet rich rather than fibrin rich as with STEMI. Fibrinolytic therapy is not efficacious for treating platelet-rich thrombus, and these drugs are associated with untoward side effects; therefore fibrinolytic therapy is contraindicated in NSTE ACS. For treatment of UA and NSTE, a meta-analysis has compiled evidence that indicates a 15% decrease in adverse events following treatment with antagonists targeting the glycoprotein (GP) IIb/IIIa receptor on platelets (8). Evidence also indicates that treatment with low-molecular-weight heparin is effective for NSTE ACS (9).

NSTE ACS patients having positive cTnT or cTnI results are a subset for whom treatment with GP IIb/IIIa inhibitors and low-molecular-weight heparin has been shown to be particularly beneficial (8, 9). In fact, no outcome benefit was apparent in patients with negative troponin values (8, 9). This evidence provides the basis for guiding treatment with these drugs in NSTE ACS patients having positive cTnT or cTnI results. AHA/ACC guidelines include a Class I recommendation that lists positive troponin results as a high-risk indicator (7). An early invasive strategy, such as percutaneous coronary intervention, within 48 h of onset of symptoms and stent placement is recommended for high-risk UA and NSTEMI without serious comorbidity (7).

COMPROMISED MYOCARDIAL FUNCTION: CONGESTIVE HEART FAILURE

Although current strategies for the management of ACS patients have significantly improved survival, this success has produced a patient cohort with impaired ventricular function that frequently progresses to cardiac failure. This patient cohort presents the challenge of managing the sequelae of myocardial remodeling that follows cell death. This remodeling is caused by the need for the heart to compensate for dysfunctional myocardial regions. There are numerous risk factors for developing HF, many of which are shared with risk of ACS. Some HF risk factors include hypertension, renal insufficiency, diabetes, tobacco use, ethanol use, obesity, and hyperlipidemia.

Although the heart has long been recognized as an exquisitely engineered pump, it is also an active endocrine organ that responds quickly to stress on the cardiovascular system. Fluid overload is a major heart stress; in response, cardiac hormones are released to correct fluid imbalance by acting on the kidney, systemic vasculature, and myocardium. In this way, release of heart hormones compensates for stresses resulting from hypertension, myocardial scarring after MI, fluid overload in renal insufficiency, or other factors, all in an effort to maintain normal myocardial function. This compensatory system is painless and functions well for maintaining cardiac output and normal activity, even though the heart is failing. The disease is insidious because most patients remain asymptomatic well into the progression of their disease. However the myocardial remodeling is irreversible and progresses to a frank HF without treatment.

HF is the most common discharge diagnosis in patients over 65 years of age; there are 400,000 to 700,000 new cases diagnosed annually in the United States. Table 37-1 lists the most commonly used criteria for HF classification that were developed by the New York Heart Association. It is noteworthy that one-third of all HF patients are Class I and asymptomatic. By the time patients present with symptoms, their disease has substantially progressed. The mortality of HF from time of diagnosis has a median survival of 3.2 years, and the 5-year mortality is greater than for many cancers, at 70%. It is estimated that cardiac failure will become the single most important health burden in the next 20 years, at an annual cost of $30 billion in the United States alone. HF is notoriously difficult to diagnose, and it has been estimated that 50% of referrals to secondary care with a diagnosis of HF are incorrect. Effective treatments are available; diuretics, angiotensin-converting enzyme inhibitors (ACE-I), angiotensin II receptor blockers (A2 blockers), and beta-blocking drugs have all been shown in clinical trials to improve quality of life and survival.

Biochemical Cardiac Markers of Acute Coronary Syndromes and Congestive Heart Failure

Figure 37-2 shows the typical rise and fall of biochemical markers after myocardial necrosis. There is nearly universal agreement that quantitative rather than qualitative results are desirable because they allow monitoring of the dynamic release (increase) and clearance (decrease) of cardiac markers. Although biochemical markers are of modest value for diagnosis of STE ACS, measurement of cTnI or cTnT is useful for risk stratification and monitoring the CK-MB pattern for a second peak can be useful for assessing reinfarction or infarct extension in both STE and NSTE ACS (10). POCT technologies available for measurement of cardiac markers have recently been reviewed (11). BNP and NT-proBNP testing has a number of possible applications in clinical practice including HF diagnosis, screening for left ventricular dysfunction, risk stratification and prognostication, and treatment monitoring.

Table 37-1   Heart Failure Classifications and Definitions[a]

Class I (35%, 1.68 million)

No symptoms. No limitation of physical activity. No shortness of breath, fatigue, or heart palpitations with ordinary physical activity.

Class II (35%, 1.68 million)

Symptoms on ordinary exertion. Slight limitation of activity. Shortness of breath, fatigue, or heart palpitations with ordinary physical activity, but patients are comfortable at rest.

Class III (25%, 1.20 million)

Symptoms with less than ordinary exertion. Marked limitation of activity. Shortness of breath, fatigue, or heart palpitations with less than ordinary physical activity, but patients are comfortable at rest.

Class IV (5%, 240,000)

Symptoms at rest. Severe to complete limitation of activity. Shortness of breath, fatigue, or heart palpitations with any physical exertion and symptoms appear even at rest.

[a] Criteria were developed by the New York Heart Association (NYHA). The proportion and approximate number of individuals affected in the United States are also listed.

Preinfarction Markers (Acute Myocardial Ischemia)

The assessment and determination of a thrombotic state or myocardial ischemia, prior to or in the absence of cell death and release of the necrosis markers displayed in Figure 37-2, is an important component of clinical decision making. No biomarker currently has widespread acceptance, but several markers have been proposed and may prove useful, particularly if available as POCT. One such marker that has achieved FDA clearance is ischemia-modified albumin (IMA). Mechanistically, it is believed that IMA is formed by an ischemia-induced pH decrease, which causes release of copper from ceruloplasmin (12). The unbound copper activates a free radical–mediated mechanism that induces a structural modification in the N-terminal region of albumin to form IMA (12). The assay for IMA, called the Albumin Cobalt Binding Test (ACB,™ Ischemia Technologies, Denver, CO, USA), detects a binding difference between IMA and native albumin for the metal cobalt. The specificity of the ACB test has not been completely defined. However, IMA measurement, along with the standard

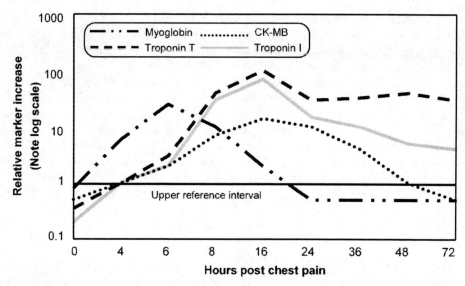

Figure 37-2   Temporal profiles of myocardial necrosis biomarkers. Note the log scale and that the *x*-axis is not linear.

tools of ECG and troponin, has been found to have a high negative predictive value in the range of 96% (12). Table 37-2 lists other information regarding IMA. At present there is no point-of-care test available for IMA.

Potential early markers of myocardial ischemia that are less developed commercially are Nourin-1 (13), free fatty acid (14), myeloperoxidase (15), whole blood choline (16), and soluble CD40L (17). Nourin-1 offers promise because it is a potent leukocyte chemotactic factor that is released within 5 min by cardiac tissues in response to both reversible and irreversible ischemic injury. Free fatty acids are a chief energy source for myocardial cells, and the myocardial ischemia causes release of high levels of these acids. Myeloperoxidase is a leukocyte enzyme and is considered an inflammatory marker that is released when plaques are unstable and vulnerable to forming thrombus. Whole blood choline is increased in patients with ischemia; whole blood choline is measured by nuclear magnetic resonance. Elevated plasma levels of soluble CD40L reportedly identified ACS patients who were at increased risk of death and recurrent MI (17). Of note, soluble CD40L complemented cTnI prognostic information for death and MI (17). All of these markers are in relatively early stages of development and characterization, and presently there are no POCT systems available for their measurement.

Markers of Myocardial Infarction

Myoglobin. Table 37-2 shows the characteristics of myoglobin, the earliest-appearing necrosis marker that is routinely available for assessment of ACS patients. Meta-analysis has shown that the clinical sensitivity of myoglobin exceeds 90% with serial sampling at presentation and then 2–6 h later (18). Myoglobin's amino acid sequence is the same in both cardiac and skeletal muscle, so clinical specificity may be compromised with skeletal muscle injury and also with renal insufficiency due to decreased clearance. The negative predic-

tive value of myoglobin is in the range of 96% when chest pain onset is acute. Although many clinicians are skeptical about the added contribution of myoglobin measurements to CK-MB or troponin, evidence from the CHECKMATE study (19) and the TACTICS analysis (20) indicates that myoglobin significantly contributes to other markers for predicting an outcome of death or MI.

Creatine Kinase-MB (CK-MB).   Cytoplasmic CK is dimeric, composed of M and/or B subunits that associate to form CK-MM, CK-MB, and CK-BB isoenzymes. Figure 37-2 shows that the first increase in CK-MB after MI occurs 4–6 h after onset of symptoms and that serial sampling over a period of 8–12 h yields high sensitivity for myocardial injury. However specificity is an issue because skeletal muscle has higher total CK activity per gram of tissue, which may be made up of up to 3% CK-MB. CK-MB mass assays were considered the gold standard for MI diagnosis through the 1980s until the mid-1990s, having a sensitivity of 97% and specificity of 90% (21). Although CK-MB has lost its gold-standard status to cTnT and cTnI measurement (Table 37-2), CK-MB mass measurement is still a sound tool that is useful in the evaluation of MI. POCT methods utilize two-site immunoassays, or mass assays. These CK-MB mass assays are automated, highly sensitive (<1 μg/L), and specific, and have a rapid turnaround time (as low as 7 min).

Proteins of the Troponin Complex.   The troponin complex is located on the thin filament of striated skeletal and heart muscle and consists of three subunits: TnT, TnI, and TnC. Separate TnT and TnI isoforms are encoded by different genes that are activated in cardiac or skeletal muscle. These protein isoforms have distinct amino acid sequences that allow production of antibodies for specific recognition of the cardiac isoforms. Because the amino acid sequence in both skeletal and cardiac tissues is identical, TnC has no potential as a cardiac-specific marker.

As indicated in Table 37-2, cTnT and cTnI are the preferred markers of cardiac necrosis (22). Several hours are required for cTnT or cTnI to rise above detectable limits after onset of acute cardiac ischemia (Figure 37-2). For this reason, cTnT or cTnI are not early necrosis markers. For high sensitivity and specificity, guidelines recommend sampling at patient presentation, at 6–9 h, and at 12–24 h if clinical suspicion is high and earlier results were negative (22). Elevation of cTnI and cTnT after necrosis is prolonged (Figure 37-2), which allows utilization for diagnosis many days after MI has occurred. The precise pattern of troponin release is unpredictable, so cTnT and cTnI are less useful for assessing reocclusion or for utilization in infarct sizing.

Standardization of cTnI assays is a substantial issue in both laboratory and clinical medicine. This problem is complicated because there are both systematic (reference value) and assay-specific (antibody and reagent) issues. Systematic issues take the form of value assignment for a reference material; assay-specific differences result because different cTnI epitopes are targeted by the various assays. This situation is far less complex for cTnT because a single manufacturer produces all the commercial assays. At present there can be a 30-fold difference between cTnI assays, which may be resolved, in part, by defining a cTnI reference material (23). The American Association of Clinical Chemistry has formed a committee to address cTnI standardization; this committee has designated a reference material and strategy for harmonization of cTnI assays.

NATRIURETIC PEPTIDES

The physiology and clearance of the natriuretic peptides atrial natriuretic peptide (ANP) and BNP have been reviewed recently (24). The stimuli for secretion of ANP and BNP are myocardial stretch, ventricular dilation, and/or increased filling pressures. Investigations have shown that BNP is preferentially produced and secreted in the ventricles and is more diagnostically useful than ANP, as is its metabolic counterpart NT-proBNP. Human BNP is derived from the 134-aa precursor preproBNP. Upon stimulation by ventricular stretch, a 26-aa signal peptide sequence is cleaved from the N-terminus of preproBNP to produce $proBNP_{1-108}$. During release into the circulation, the $proBNP_{1-108}$ prohormone is further cleaved by a membrane-bound serine protease, called a corin, into an N-terminal pro-BNP_{1-76} fragment and the active 32-peptide BNP hormone. BNP and NT-proBNP are released in a 1:1 molar ratio and both are important diagnostic markers (Table 37-2). Table 37-2 presents a listing and summary of the biochemical characteristics of natriuretic peptides.

Clinical Application of the Natriuretic Peptides

The central laboratory can now offer measurements of BNP or NT-proBNP. BNP/NTpBNP quantification has been shown to be a useful aid to clinical assessment, ECG, and chest radiog-raphy for initial detection and assessment of ventricular dysfunction (25). There is a growing body of evidence that indicates that natriuretic peptides can be used for monitoring response to treatment, with drug dose titration determined by BNP levels (25). In the acute hospital setting, BNP or NT-proBNP measurements can be used for the differential diagnosis of dyspnea from the diagnosis of heart failure (25), and there is evidence that measurements are useful for risk stratification of ACS patients that provides independent additive prognostic information to troponin measurement (26–29).

Technical Measurement of Biochemical Markers of Acute Coronary Syndromes and Heart Failure

Table 37-3 displays the key characteristics of technologies available for measurement of biochemical markers of ACS and HF at the point of care. The analytical goals for these measurements are driven mainly by the day-to-day variability of the marker and evidence showing that a defined decision point is clinically important. For myoglobin and CK-MB, clinical interpretation involves either use of a decision limit (cutoff) near the upper reference limit or a doubling of myoglobin over a period of 2 h after presentation (30). A day-to-day CV of 5% appears to be adequate for this purpose. For cTnT or cTnI, a joint committee of the European Society for Cardiology and the American College Cardiology (ACC) has proposed the ambitious analytical goals of a day-to-day CV of 10% at the 99th percentile value of a reference control population (22). Current technologies, either central laboratory or POCT, have not yet met this imprecision goal (31).

Availability of POCT for the natriuretic peptides has been limited to BNP, although systems for providing NT-proBNP measurements at the point of care are in development (see Table 37-3). The day-to-day CV for the POCT BNP assay is in the range of 10%. However this imprecision is adequate because the intra-individual day-to-day biological variability is substantially greater for BNP (and NT-proBNP), in the range of 30–40% (32). Together the analytical and biological CV yields a least significant change of approximately 100% for the natriuretic peptides (32). Clinically, this translates to the fact that at least a twofold change in the natriuretic peptide is necessary in serial measurements to overcome expected biological variability and confer clinical significance. This is an important consideration when interpreting the evolving literature on the use of BNP by POCT for monitoring patients (25).

POTENTIAL BENEFITS AND CLINICAL AND ECONOMIC OUTCOMES OF POINT-OF-CARE TESTING

Measurement of cardiac markers is essential for the diagnosis, monitoring, and treatment of ACS and CHF patients, and these measurements are integrated into clinical guidelines (2, 7, 33). In the context of UA and NSTEMI, markers are used in combination with a number of clinical indictors and ECG

Table 37-2 Biochemical Markers of the Acute Coronary Syndromes and Congestive Heart Failure

Biochemical marker	Point-of-care test available?	Molecular weight, g/mol	Cardiac specific?	Advantage	Disadvantage	Duration of elevation	Diagnostic performance, comments
				Myocardial ischemia			
Ischemia modified albumin	Not at present	65,000	Unknown	Biochemical marker would be helpful because myocardial ischemia is difficult to diagnose.	No ischemia gold standard, agreed reference clinical standard, or biochemical test for myocardial ischemia.	Preliminary data suggest 6–8 h	Clinical trials pending.
Glycogen phosphorylase-BB	No	177,000	Yes +++	Biochemical marker would be helpful because myocardial ischemia is a difficult diagnosis.	Inability to reproduce initial results.	8 h	Initial data promising, but unable to be reproduced.
				Myocardial necrosis[a]			
Myoglobin	Yes	18,000	No	High sensitivity and negative predictive value. Useful for early detection of MI and reperfusion.	Low specificity in presence of skeletal muscle injury and with renal insufficiency. Rapid clearance after necrosis.	12–24 h	2–6 h after presentation: Sensitivity: 90% (CI: 88–93%)[b] Specificity: 86% (CI: 85–87%) Negative predictive value: 96%
CK-MB, mass assays	Yes	85,000	Yes +++	Ability to detect reinfarction. Large clinical experience. Previous gold standard for myocardial necrosis.	Lowered specificity in concombinant skeletal muscle injury.	24–36 h	Two serial values above 99th percentile of control reference population in the setting of ischemia is benchmark for myocardial necrosis.
Cardiac troponin T	Yes	37,000	Yes ++++	Tool for risk stratification. Detection of MI up to 2 weeks. High specificity for cardiac tissue.	Not an early marker of myocardial necrosis. Limited ability to detect reinfarction.	10–14 days	A single value above 99th percentile of control reference population is surrogate of myocardial necrosis in setting of myocardial ischemia.

Natriuretic peptides[c]

Cardiac troponin I	Yes	23,500	Yes ++++	Tool for risk stratification. Detection of MI up to 7 days. High specificity for cardiac tissue.	Not an early marker of myocardial necrosis. No analytical reference standards. Limited ability to detect reinfarction.	4–7 days	A single value above 99th percentile of control reference population is surrogate of myocardial necrosis in setting of myocardial ischemia.
B-Type natriuretic peptide (BNP)	Yes	5,200	Yes +++	Tool for diagnosis of CHF[c] versus other causes of dyspnea in ED populations. Potential tool for risk stratification in CHF and acute coronary syndrome.	Also elevated in cor pulmonale and right-sided heart failure. Reference intervals vary with sex and age differences.	20-min half-life	Physiologically active hormone. For diagnosis of CHF in an ED population, 95% sensitivity and 80% specificity.
NT-proBNP	No	12,000	Yes +++	Tool for diagnosis of CHF. Potential tool for risk stratification in CHF and ACS.	Also elevated in cor pulmonale and right-sided heart failure. Reference intervals vary quite dramatically with sex and age, and it is necessary to report different reference intervals.	Half-life unknown with certainty, although substantially longer than BNP. 90- to 120-min half-life accepted.	Physiologically inactive counterpart to BNP from cleavage of preproBNP. Presently, diagnostic differences between BNP and NT-proBNP are dwarfed by similarities.

[a] Time of first increase for the markers are 1–3 h for myoglobin, 3–4 h for CK-MB mass, 3–4 h for cardiac troponin T, and 4–6 h for cardiac troponin I.
[b] CI = 95% confidence interval.
[c] CHF = congestive heart failure.

Table 37-3 Characteristics of Currently Available Technologies for POC Testing of Cardiac Markers

Device	Cardiac marker	Suggested cutoff	Manufacturer's claim	Turnaround time, min	Specimen type and volume
i-STAT cTnI Assay and Cartridge	CTnI	Based on 99th percentile URL and 10% CV: 0.1 ng/mL *or* laboratory's equivalent cutoff for AMI	Aid in the diagnosis of AMI and risk stratification	10	Heparin whole blood or plasma, 16 μL
Roche Cardiac T® Rapid Assay	CTnT	0.1 ng/mL[a]	Myocardial damage is detected	12	Heparin whole blood, 150 μL
Roche Cardiac™ M Rapid Assay	Myoglobin	Male: 76 ng/mL Female: 64 ng/mL	Above normal range	8	Heparin whole blood, 150 μL
Cardiac STATus™ device[b] (Spectral Diagnostics)	CK-MB Myoglobin	5 ng/mL (Abbott method) 50 ng/mL (Behring Diagnostics method)	Aid in the diagnosis of cardiac ischemia	15	Serum or heparinized whole blood or plasma, 200 μL
Stratus® CS STAT Fluorometric Analyzer (Dade Behring)	CTnI CK-MB Myoglobin	1.5 mL (Dade Stratus II Method) 3.5 ng/mL Male: 98 ng/mL Female: 56 ng/mL	All markers: Aid in the diagnosis of AMI	14 min to first result, 4 min for each additional result	Whole blood (lithium or sodium heparin), 3 mL Plasma (lithium or sodium heparin), 200 μL for first test, 100 μL for each additional test on the same run
Triage® Cardiac Panel (Biosite Diagnostics)	CTnI CK-MB Myoglobin CTnI BNP	0.06 ng/mL 10.0 ng/mL 170.0 ng/mL 1.0 ng/mL 5.0 pg/mL	cTnI: Risk stratification Aid in the diagnosis of MI/cTnI risk stratification Aid for diagnosis of CHF	~15	Heparinized whole blood or plasma, 250 μL
RAMP Reader (Response Biomedical)	Myoglobin CK-MB CTnI	99.3 ng/mL 3.74 ng/mL 0.12 ng/mL	Aid in the diagnosis of AMI	~15	EDTA whole blood, 70 μL
NT-proBNP[c] (Nexus Dx™)	NT-proBNP	Not available	Aid for the diagnosis of heart failure	Not available	Not available

[a] Values <0.05 ng/mL indicate negative TnT; values from 0.05 to <0.1 ng/mL indicate low TnT and test should be repeated within 1 h with a fresh blood sample; values from 0.1 to 2.0 ng/mL indicate myocardial damage; values >2.0 ng/mL indicate massive myocardial damage.

[b] This assay yields qualitative results.

[c] This assay is not commercially available at press time.

information, i.e., variables in the TIMI Risk score (1), and the paradigm has clearly shifted from diagnosis only to risk assessment and management. The highest-risk group for in-hospital adverse outcome is patients presenting with STEMI, but their initial assessment does not require biomarker measurement. Biomarkers function to audit diagnosis and provide supplementary information for subsequent risk stratification in STEMI patients; however, they do not affect their immediate management, hence POCT is unlikely to be useful.

A major issue with interpretation of biochemical markers is that the population must be defined and a setting of myocardial ischemia and an acute coronary syndrome must be established (22). This is because all of the diagnostic, prognostic, and treatment information is based on patients within the continuum of ACS. Thus the significance and interpretation of biomarker elevations with other causes such as chest trauma, renal insufficiency, surgery, electrocution, and so on, is largely unknown. Management is aimed at rapid confirmation of infarction for intervention (rule in) or rapid exclusion of disease (rule out).

The natriuretic peptides are useful for HF diagnosis, particularly in symptomatic patients presenting to the emergency medicine service. There are also data indicating that natriuretic peptides may be useful for screening patients for whom more extensive assessment of cardiac dysfunction is warranted (25). Early studies on the use of these markers for applications such as therapeutic monitoring and guiding therapy appear to be promising but must be considered preliminary at this time.

The issue to be addressed here is whether there is a need for speed; i.e., is there evidence that providing measurements of cardiac markers by POCT makes a difference in important outcomes? There are three questions regarding the impact of POCT on outcomes that will be considered. The first involves treatment and management of patients, the second involves administration and costs, and the third involves physician and patient satisfaction. Table 37-4 summarizes selected studies that will be referred to as evidence to address these questions.

How Quickly Are Results Needed?

Traditionally in laboratory medicine, turnaround time has reflected the duration from receipt of the patient specimen in the central laboratory to reporting of the result via the laboratory computer (or other) system. However, this laboratory dwell time is not relevant to caregivers because they consider laboratory delay in a more global sense, from specimen collection at the patient bedside to when they have knowledge of the result for interpretation. This global time can be referred to as the "vein-to-brain" time; laboratorians must be keenly aware of the clinician's perspective and strive to minimize the front-end transport time from the patient's bedside to the central laboratory, and the back-end time of result delivery to the caregiver. Minimizing or eliminating the specimen transport and result delivery time-components of the vein-to-brain time is perhaps the biggest advantage of POCT.

A key question regarding POCT is: If the laboratory medicine result is needed rapidly, then what is the timeframe in which having results affects the outcome? Is there a measurable outcome difference if the results are available in 10 min versus 30 min? One hour versus three hours? It must be realized that assessment of ACS and HF is a multivariate process that requires many pieces of information in addition to cardiac markers. Thus it will be obvious that the design of controlled studies for a randomized, evidence-based approach to the need for speed for cardiac markers in isolation is easily confounded. In addition to faster results, process changes and action plans must be implemented. Indeed, there is evidence that the vein-to-brain time for cardiac markers in clinical practice is more rapid by POCT (see Table 37-4), but there is little direct evidence of outcome benefit. In addition, the analytical technology for POCT may not perform as well as laboratory-based analyses in all cases. In the low-risk group, strategies are mainly aimed at exclusion of acute MI to prevent inappropriate discharge of MI patients, a figure that stands at 1–3% (5). BNP or NT-proBNP testing may assist in diminishing the overlap between medium- and low-risk ACS groups in rule-out strategies (26, 27). These lower-risk patients may be managed by transfer from coronary care to step-down units or observed in emergency departments or in chest pain units to avoid a hospital admission. The problems (and justifications) are common with the major protocol differences arising while the patient is held before exclusion of acute MI is complete. This is typically from 4 to 12 h, with a longer time used when probability of ACS is highest. There is evidence that the use of structured decision-making rule-out protocols is effective, both clinically and with regard to cost (Table 37-4). There is also evidence that more rapid biochemical testing translates into a shorter stay (Table 37-4), but to date there is little evidence that POCT has an essential role if the central laboratory is able to provide rapid turnaround and good communication. Although expert consensus is the predominant evidence for POCT of cardiac markers, there are Class I recommendations, i.e., that testing is safe and effective (7), regarding need for a rapid vein-to-brain time for assessment and treatment of ACS (2, 7). Guidelines are in development for biomarkers in the context of HF (25).

Consensus guidelines from the AHA/ACC group on UA and NSTEMI state that "When the central laboratory is used, results should be available within 60 minutes, preferably within 30 minutes." It is important to reiterate that this guideline measures result availability as the vein-to-brain time, not laboratory dwell time. This same guideline advocates POCT by stating:

> POCT systems. . .have the advantage of reducing delays in transportation and processing. . .and can reduce delays at all hours. . . .(2)

This 30- to 60-min Class I target derived from expert consensus is consistent with the 60 min stated in the Standards of Laboratory Practice from the National Academy of Clinical Biochemistry (NACB) (34), as well as the 30-min time frame for data availability quoted by the National Heart Attack Alert Program. However a recent Q-Probe survey conducted by the

Table 37-4 Studies Involving Point-of-Care Measurements for Acute Coronary Syndromes and Congestive Heart Failure

Reference	Aim/objective	Study population	n	Study design	Comments
42	Evaluate accuracy, practicality, turnaround time, and accuracy of ED cardiac marker testing.	All patients with chest pain in ED over 16 days	205	Single center prospective observational	POC decreased TAT by 55% relative to central laboratory (37 vs. 39 min) with 100% sensitivity and 100% specificity. ACS-negative patients were at high-risk for future cardiac events.
43	Determine TAT, accuracy, relevance, and justification for POCT.	Patients enrolled in CCU	177 male, 86 female	Prospective randomized controlled trial in which POC testing was compared to center to central laboratory	TAT was 72 min in central laboratory group and 20 min in POC testing group. Analytical and clinical accuracy was equivalent in two groups. In low risk patients, non-CCU stay (145.25 vs. 79.5 h) and hospital stay was reduced. (209 vs. 140 h)
44	Evaluate if multimarker POC strategy can exclude acute MI in ≤3 h.	Consecutive ED patients	817	Prospective diagnostic test study	By 90 min, sensitivity was 96.9% and specificity was 99.6%. Median time from sampling to reporting of results was 71.0 min for laboratory and 24.0 min for POC device.
45	Determine clinician satisfaction, TAT, and confidence in results of POCT satellite in ED.	ED chest pain patients	158 male, 211 female	Prospective diagnostic test; before/after implementation of satellite laboratory	TAT and ED stay decreased; excellent satisfaction with test accuracy and TAT. 41-min difference in ED bed time for laboratory cost of $16.26. POC testing may have been factor in lowering ED diversion-hours by 27%.
49	Compare diagnostic efficacy of two rapid tests: CK-MB + myoglobin, and CTnT. Test reliability of bedside diagnosis by CCU nurse.	Consecutive patients with acute chest pain admitted to CCU	151	Retrospective comparative diagnostic study	Central laboratory results were not available before 1 or more h, whereas POC tests were ready in 20 min. Bedside diagnoses by CCU nurse with CK-MB + myoglobin or cTnT are reliable diagnostic methods with same efficacy as quantitative laboratory tests.
50	Determine effects on laboratory cost and length of stay from availability of STAT CK-MB testing for patients with MI or chest pain.	Medicare patients admitted to hospitals	82	Retrospective comparative diagnostic	For MI, a CK-MB testing policy that produces shorter TAT may be justified because of an association with reduced length of stay and overall laboratory costs.

#	Objective	Population	N	Study type	Conclusion
51	Determine sensitivity and specificity of POC cTnT assay for MI, likelihood ratios of + and − cTnT results, and relative risk for serious cardiac events with + POC cTnT result on admission.	Patients admitted for evaluation of chest pain	100	Cohort, physicians blinded to POC cTnT results	POC cTnT is a simple and efficient test that provides is a useful tool for evaluation of chest pain patients.
52	Compare the analytical and diagnostic performance of a TropT rapid test to quantitative troponin T ELISA and CK-MB mass determinations.	Patients with suspected ACS	203	Comparison prospective diagnostic test	Diagnostic sensitivity of the rapid test for detection of high risk unstable angina pectoris patients w/myocardial damage was nearly the same as for trop T ELISA. Major advantage of the rapid test is ease of use and 20 min TAT, which facilitates detection of elevated trop T at alternate sites.
53	Determine the sensitivity and specificity of the Triage Cardiac Panel including cTnI, CK-MB, and myoglobin	Patients with suspected ACS	192	Prospective diagnostic study	The Triage POC analysis of multiple cardiac markers provides clinical sensitivity and specificity for the detection of acute MI comparable to central laboratory methods.
54	Evaluate each component of a cardiac multimarker panel for detection of acute MI in patients with chest pain across a spectrum of renal dysfunction. Looking for accuracy and consistency of markers in renal insufficiency patients.	Consecutive ED patients evaluated for possible MI, split into spectrum of kidney function	817	Prospective diagnostic test	The use of cTnI based POC cardiac biomarker strategy is applicable and superior to myoglobin and CK-MB in evaluating chest pain patients with renal dysfunction.
55	To evaluate the speed and accuracy for an accelerated critical pathway that used clinical history, ECG, and testing of CK-MB, myoglobin, cTnI for diagnosing MI within 90 min.	Consecutive ED patients with symptoms of cardiac ischemia	1285	Prospective observational study	A simple, inexpensive critical pathway that utilizes high-risk features from clinical history, ECG changes, and POC testing of myoglobin, CK-MB, and cTnI allows for accurate triaging of chest pain patients within 90 min of ED presentation.

Table 37-4 (Continued)

Reference	Aim/objective	Study population	n	Study design	Comments
41	Assess whether the immediate availability of serum markers would increase the appropriate use of thrombolytic therapy.	6352 patients enrolled	6352	Randomized controlled clinical trial	The availability of 0- and 1-h myoglobin and CK-MB results after ED evaluation had no effect on the use of thrombolytic therapy for patients presenting with MI, and slightly increased the number of patients admitted to the hospital who had no evidence of acute myocardial necrosis.
40	Determine the role of admission cTnT on the efficacy of percutaneous coronary interventions (PCI) in inferior MI.	Consecutive patients with inferior ST-segment MI	159	Prospective observational diagnostic test	A positive admission cTnT is associated with lower success rates of direct PCI and higher rates of cardiac events over the short and long term.
56	Evaluate diagnostic sensitivity and specificity of a whole blood analyzer for detection of MI.	Patients initially presenting to the ED with chest pain were evaluated for MI using modified WHO criteria	369 total patients; 89 (24%) diagnosed with MI	Prospective diagnostic test	A quantitative, whole blood POC testing device, operated by either laboratory or nursing personnel, was comparable to central laboratory for measuring cardiac markers for detection of MI.
48	Evaluate the sensitivity of a POC qualitative assay for serum cTnT for the detection of acute MI in the ambulance and assessed the predictive value of a positive prehospital cTnT test for death and MI.	Consecutive patients with suspected acute MI	158	Prospective diagnostic test	A positive prehospital POC cTnT result was an objective marker for a worse outcome in patients presenting with suspected acute MI.
57	Rule out acute MI on the basis of rapid assays for myoglobin, CK-MB, and cTnT.	Consecutive patients presenting with chest pain at the ED	309	Prospective observational	Myoglobin is a better marker for ruling out MI in the ED than CK-MB or cTnT, 3–6 h after the onset of symptoms. However, the maximal NPV reaches only 89%. All three markers increased earlier in patients with large infarcts, and differences in reported values of sensitivity and specificity in the literature may be explained by differences in infarct size.

	Objective	Population	N	Study type	Findings
58	Evaluate the cost effectiveness of using CK-MB and troponin tests in diagnosis of myocardial ischemia.	Patients admitted with chest pain	1066	Retrospective diagnostic	Measurement of CK-MB mass plus early exercise testing is a cost-effective initial strategy for younger patients, and those with a low to moderate probability of MI. cTnI measurement can be a cost-effective second test in higher-risk subsets of patients if the CK-MB level is normal and early exercise testing is not an option. Routine use of both troponin I and CK-MB assays is not a cost-effective strategy in guiding triage decisions for suspected MI patients.
59	Determine the cost vs. clinical effectiveness of an automated cTnI assay to current cardiac panel (CK-MB, myoglobin, CK-MB activity). Assessed length of stay, time to catheterization, and hospital/laboratory costs.	Chest pain patients	—	Prospective cohort study	Adding cTnI to the testing regimen decreased length of stay. Patients classified as low-risk for MI experienced statistically and clinically significant shorter length of stays and lower total and variable hospital costs; for patients with UA, there was an increase (though not statistically significant) in laboratory costs.
60	Evaluate if an emergency department based protocol for rapidly ruling out myocardial ischemia would reduce hospital time and expense but maintain diagnostic accuracy.	Low-risk suspected ACS patients	100	Prospective randomized study; 50 in rapid rule-out protocol, 50 in routine hospital-based care.	No diagnoses were missed within 30 days. Hospital stay was shorter and hospital charges were lower for rapid rule-in group ($P = 0.0001$). In low-risk patients who present with chest pain, the rapid rule-out protocol ruled out MI and UA more quickly and cost-effectively than routine hospital care.

Table 37-4 (Continued)

Reference	Aim/objective	Study population	n	Study design	Comments
25	Issue guidance regarding POC vs central laboratory testing for BNP and NT-proBNP in various clinical applications.	Heart failure patients, symptomatic patients presenting the ED, heart failure management	—	Expert opinion	At present, acute treatment decisions rarely depend on natriuretic peptide results, so central laboratory may be preferred. For emergency care patients, POC testing is justified if the central laboratory cannot provide results within 1 h of collection on a 24-h basis. POC testing will be used increasingly in cardiology because it offers rapid results and rapid adjustment in therapy. POC offers better organized patient care as all management decisions are made in a single visit.
29	Examine association of NT-proBNP with other biochemical markers and clinical risk indicators. Examine the independent contribution of NT-proBNP as prognostic indicator of 1-year death and MI.	ACS patients enrolled in GUSTO-IV	6809	Retrospective cohort study.	Increasing quartiles of NT-proBNP were related to short- and long-term mortality at 1 year. Of independent variables including cTnT, CRP, heart rate, ECG changes and creatinine clearance, NT-proBNP and creatinine clearance provided the best prediction with 1-year mortality.
26	Evaluate BNP for risk assessment and clinical decision-making, alone and in combination with cTnl.	NSTE patients enrolled in TACTICS-TIMI 18	1676	Prospective cohort study.	Elevated BNP at presentation identifies NSTE patients at 3.3-fold higher risk of death at 6 months and fivefold of developing CHF by 30 days. BNP adds independent prognostic information to cTnl measurements. Of note, cTnl negative, but BNP positive ACS patients are at 6.9-fold increased risk of mortality at 6-months.

	Aim	Population	n	Study design	Results
61	Evaluate sensitivity, accuracy, and NPV of cTnI and cTnT qualitative POC assays using 30-day endpoints of mortality and MI.	Consecutive patients with NSTE acute chest pain of <12 h duration	773	Prospective diagnostic study	POC tests were highly sensitive for detection of myocardial necrosis. The NPV of cTnT and cTnI was very high and (the authors say) can allow safe discharge of patients from the emergency department.
36	Test the hypothesis that a diagnostic strategy guided by rapid BNP measurement would improve the evaluation and care of patients with acute dyspnea who presented to the ED and thereby reduce the time to discharge and total treatment cost.	Patients presenting to the emergency department with acute dyspnea	452 patients; 225 assigned to a diagnostic strategy with rapid BNP testing and 227 assessed in standard manner	Prospective, randomized, controlled study	Used in conjunction with other clinical information, rapid BNP measurement in the emergency department improved the evaluation and treatment of patients with acute dyspnea and thereby reduced the median time to discharge by 3 days (8 days vs. 11 days) and the total cost of treatment by $1854 ($5410 versus $7264).
62	Compare costs associated with standard strategy that included serial ECG and CK-MB versus this standard evaluation plus serial troponin T.	Suspected myocardial ischemia patients presenting to the emergency department	856 patients randomized to standard strategy or standard strategy plus cTnT	Prospective randomized study.	Patients in the standard strategy plus cTnT has shorter lengths of stay (3.6 vs 4.7; $P = 0.01$). Reduced costs were also observed for cTnT group having acute coronary syndrome ($15,004 vs $19,202; $P = 0.01$) and those without ACS ($4487 vs $6187; $P = 0.17$). Utilization of cTnT in emergency department patients improves hospital resource utilization and reduces cost.

College of American Pathologists identified an apparent disconnect between the expectations of laboratorians and clinicians and what was actually measured. Clinicians believed the vein-to-brain time should be <1 h, laboratorians were striving for a 1-h laboratory dwell time, and the actual 90th percentile for the vein-to-brain time was 90 min (35). Clearly there is a need for better communication and consensus between laboratorians and clinicians regarding this point.

POCT has demonstrated utility in the emergency care setting, and there is increasing evidence that BNP or NTpBNP levels can be used to monitor treatment response in cardiac failure on an outpatient basis (25). Here the argument turns on convenience, reimbursement, and cost effectiveness. Ideally, patients arriving at the clinic would have their BNP or NTproBNP measured and then have treatment adjusted; again, this would require a fast turnaround time if a central laboratory service was used.

There is compelling evidence indicating that availability of BNP measurements reduces the total treatment cost of patients presenting to the emergency department with dyspnea (36) (Table 37-4). A prospective, randomized trial examined the impact of a strategy that included rapid BNP measurement compared to assessment using the standard method (36). This study demonstrated that rapid measurement of BNP in the emergency department decreased the median time to discharge by 3 days (8 days vs. 11 days), which translated into a mean cost savings of over $1850 per patient.

Overall, a vein-to-brain time of 30–60 min is the Class I recommendation for availability of biochemical markers of ACS. An NACB committee is now examining the issue of vein-to-brain needs for natriuretic peptides in the context of dyspnea and HF. Although no recommendations are yet established, evidence from diagnostic studies (37) indicates that the natriuretic peptides can aid in the diagnosis of CHF in patients with dyspnea, and a randomized trial indicates that cost savings can be realized in symptomatic patients compared to standard care (36).

Does Point-of-Care Testing of Cardiac Markers Improve the Ability of Caregivers to Treat and Monitor Patients Earlier and Lead to Improved Outcomes?

For rapid assessment tools to make a difference in outcome, the treatments to be directed by measurements must be time dependent. In the context of UA and NSTEMI, there is no evidence that very earlier treatment results in improved outcomes (38). One randomized trial, the EARLY pilot study (39), was conducted to investigate whether administration of a GP IIb/IIIa inhibitor on presentation would lead to better outcomes that included smaller enzymatic infarct size. The study group of UA and NSTEMI patients was randomized to receive the treatment later, from 12 to 16 h after presentation. The EARLY pilot was a negative trial, as there were no outcome differences between the study and control groups in the modest 300-patient cohort. Although the trial was undersized and the logistics

difficult, the fact remains that there is no evidence that earlier treatment of UA and NSTEMI patients with a GP IIb/IIIa inhibitor leads to better clinical outcomes.

In a small interventional trial, cTnT was measured in patients with inferior MI who were undergoing percutaneous coronary intervention (40). It was determined that patients who had positive cTnT had better outcomes after stent placement, suggesting that the test might be used to identify patients who would particularly benefit from this treatment. This study did not show that timing was critical, and therefore any POCT implications are strictly inferential.

Another approach to real-time use of biochemical markers was examined in the SMART trial (Table 37-4) (41). Here myoglobin data at enrollment and one hour later were used to trigger reexamination of the ECG for identifying thrombolytic-eligible STEMI patients who may have been missed on initial reading by emergency medicine physicians who were less well-trained than cardiologists in interpreting ECGs. This trial was negative, as the 1-h time frame designated for myoglobin increase apparently did not provide sufficient sensitivity.

The TACTICS TIMI-18 trial investigated the benefit of conservative versus aggressive interventional therapy for the treatment of UA and NSTEMI, and these data were incorporated into clinical guidelines (7). A combined outcome of death and (re)infarction clearly showed that these patients benefit from an urgent interventional strategy. However the timing of revascularization associated with benefit was 48 h after presentation. This timing does not imply that rapid POCT of cardiac markers is necessary for identification and guiding treatment of these patients.

Identification of HF patients in the emergency department is aided by measurement of BNP (25, 37). Detection of asymptomatic cardiac failure by measurement of BNP or NTproBNP has been shown to be diagnostically efficient (25). Treatment of asymptomatic disease with ACE inhibitors is evidence-based. While the fact that disease is detected at an asymptomatic stage does not necessarily support the need for POCT, patient and caregiver convenience and cost effectiveness rather than speed are the issues. But there is no evidence that rapid measurement by POCT improves the treatment or outcomes of these patients compared to central laboratory measurement.

Does Cardiac Marker Testing by Point-of-Care Testing Facilitate Patient Disposition and Reduce Costs?

A number of the studies listed in Table 37-4 show that the turnaround time for cardiac markers can be reduced dramatically by POCT, although many studies did not express this variable in terms of vein-to-brain time (42–44). Just having results available does not implicitly translate into an action that will save resources. The variety of payment and reimbursement methods in the United States and around the world, pressures on healthcare systems such as availability of in-patient beds, and so on make broad statements about the equivalence of reduced vein-to-brain time and saved resources unreliable. Clearly POCT *alone* will not facilitate patient disposition and reduce costs. Implementation of POCT for cardiac markers must be integrated into well-defined care pathways for ACS and HF that spells out actions to be taken. It is also important to audit performance and modify the care pathways based on best practice and new evidence.

Cost saving from utilizing cTnT in addition to the standard evaluation tools of serial ECG and CK-MB in a broad spectrum of emergency department patients was demonstrated in a prospective randomized trial conducted by Zarich et al. (62). The patients who had cTnT in addition to the standard evaluation strategy had hospital stays that were significantly shorter, leading to significant savings in treating patients with ACS (Table 37-4). Although this study did not specifically address the issue of POCT measurement of the markers, it does provide evidence for advocating troponin measurement in an emergency medicine environment.

Does Point-of-Care Testing Improve Satisfaction of Caregivers?

It seems intuitive, and is anecdotally reported, that thoughtful implementation of POCT or satellite testing for cardiac markers will yield substantial customer-relations benefits with local caregivers, particularly physicians. This is true even in the absence of hard evidence because there is immediate reward for clinicians in having critical laboratory results available during the episode of care. The availability of such data precludes having to refocus on the individual patient some hours later. The collateral benefit of this instant gratification is that the cardiac marker results are available for integration in calculating the post-test probability of ACS or HF; results available later can only confirm or refute the provisional diagnosis.

The study by Lewandowski et al. (45) made a particularly important contribution because they systematically surveyed emergency medicine personnel after implementation of POCT, finding excellent results from respondents (Table 37-4).

Additional Potential Opportunities for Point-of-Care Testing

The need for speed in the field of biochemical markers of coronary heart disease has evolved from performance in batches 5 days per week, through multiple scheduled runs per day, to STAT availability of results and POCT. It is rational to believe that the growth of cardiac marker testing at the point of care will increase, as the evidence base for patient benefit, administrative advantages, and improved consumer services increases. The following are a few areas of potential for POCT.

Define the role and interpretation of natriuretic peptides in ACS. The natriuretic peptides are useful for triage of acutely ill patients with dyspnea (25), but compelling data also indicate that the BNP and NT-proBNP are very powerful indicators of risk in ACS patients (26–29). In particular, there are data indicating that the natriuretic peptides identify a subset of troponin-negative ACS patients who are at high risk for adverse events. Thus POCT of the natriuretic peptides will enhance the ability to risk-stratify ACS patients and enhance their timely disposition.

Full integration of POCT results into risk stratification. Despite the defined role of cardiac markers for risk stratification in guidelines and the TIMI risk score, biochemical markers are infrequently incorporated into risk stratification decisions, whereas less-sensitive tools such as the ECG are virtually always utilized. There are numerous reasons for this omission, but one fundamental cause may be that biochemical markers are not readily available during the episode of acute care, and the data must be retrieved later from an information system or from the laboratory. If POCT were available for instant review, expenditures would be reduced for suspected ACS patients who are negative for troponin and who have low natriuretic peptide values because they would be identified as extremely low risk and perhaps spared the need for an immediate intervention.

Guidance of heart failure therapy with natriuretic peptides. There are good preliminary data indicating that release of the natriuretic peptides with acute treatment of decompensated heart failure allows appropriate guidance of treatment (25). Although preliminary, use of POCT for guiding heart failure therapy in some cases may be a more cost-effective strategy of care compared with use of interventional strategies.

Multiple-marker strategies. A number of studies have shown that various biochemical markers contribute independent information, both to each other and to clinical variables (46, 47). Knowledge regarding the possible contribution of ischemia markers, markers of inflammation, and indicators of plaque instability may be combined with the current tools to more quickly assess a patient's pre-test probability of disease and risk. The largest clinical impact of these tools will be realized with POCT.

Ambulance (prehospital) testing. Prehospital testing of patients suspected of ACS or HF prior to reaching the hospital environment would allow more rapid, accurate, and efficient triage upon patient arrival (48) (Table 37-4). This already occurs in some institutions in the context of urgent patient transport, and the technologies available for POCT could be easily adapted to this testing venue.

General practitioner testing. Many ACS and suspected HF patients are seen by their primary care physician, usual health plan doctor, or general practitioner (depending on the healthcare system) before seeking emergency care. It has been estimated that only 50% of primary care diagnoses of HF are correct. POCT in the primary care setting would ensure that primary care patients are referred efficiently to appropriate care. European Cardiac Society guidelines (33) as well as recommendations from UK national healthcare standards bodies include measurement of BNP as part of the workup to determine if referral to secondary care is appropriate. Long-term risk stratification (i.e., in the 5- to 10-year range) for primary prevention was not the focus here, but POCT for total cholesterol, HDL, triglyceride, and high-sensitivity CRP may also have value in the general practitioner environment. This is particularly the case for the possible identification and guidance of effective lipid-lowering agents such as the statins.

Home testing for ischemia and other markers. Despite the efforts of groups involved with prevention and care, 50% of the individuals who die from heart attacks never reach the hospital setting. Further, a majority of these patients have preinfarction angina, indicating that ischemia occurred prior to their sentinel event. Home testing of markers that could indicate (or rule out) cardiac ischemia as the cause of symptoms may cause patients to seek appropriate care before the crash occurs.

CONCLUSION

Expert consensus-based evidence indicates that rapid availability of cardiac markers including myoglobin, CK-MB, and, in particular, cTnT or cTnI is important for risk stratification and treatment decisions, as reflected in clinical and laboratory medicine guidelines. The first POCT system for BNP was made available in 2000 and has demonstrated utility for testing in the emergency care setting, particularly when HF specialists are not readily available. European-based guidelines indicate that BNP or NT-proBNP is useful in heart failure practice. However the need for speed is not clearly established, and the evolution of guidelines for rapid availability of the natriuretic peptides in the context of cardiovascular disease is still evolving. Patient and clinician convenience is enhanced substantially by POCT, as the results are available in a more timely fashion to facilitate disposition and treatment. The design goals for POCT systems used in the context of ACS are challenging because the analytical characteristics must be the same as for central laboratory instrumentation. For BNP and NT-proBNP, analytical performance is driven by intraindividual variability. There are many opportunities for POCT that will spring from development of biomarkers that are elevated before myocardial necrosis.

REFERENCES

1. Antman EM, Cohen M, Bernink PJ, McCabe CH, Horacek T, Papuchis G, et al. The TIMI risk score for unstable angina/non-ST elevation MI: A method for prognostication and therapeutic decision making. JAMA 2000;284:835–42.
2. Braunwald E, Antman EM, Beasley JW, Califf RM, Cheitlin MD, Hochman JS, et al. ACC/AHA guidelines for the management of patients with unstable angina and non-ST-segment elevation myocardial infarction: a report of the American College of Cardiology/American Heart Association Task Force on Practice Guidelines (Committee on the Management of Patients With Unstable Angina). J Am Coll Cardiol 2000;36:970–1062.
3. Mizuno K, Satomura K, Miyamoto A, Arakawa K, Shibuya T, Arai T, et al. Angioscopic evaluation of coronary-artery thrombi in acute coronary syndromes. N Engl J Med 1992;326:287–91.
4. Ottani F, Galvani M, Nicolini FA, Ferrini D, Pozzati A, Di Pasquale G, et al. Elevated cardiac troponin levels predict the risk of adverse outcome in patients with acute coronary syndromes. Am Heart J 2000;140:917–27.
5. Pope JH, Aufderheide TP, Ruthazer R, Woolard RH, Feldman JA, Beshansky JR, et al. Missed diagnoses of acute cardiac ischemia in the emergency department. N Engl J Med 2000;342:1163–70.
6. Heidenreich PA, Alloggiamento T, Melsop K, McDonald KM, Go AS, Hlatky MA. The prognostic value of troponin in patients with non-ST elevation acute coronary syndromes: A meta-analysis. J Am Coll Cardiol 2001;38:478–85.
7. Braunwald E, Antman EM, Beasley JW, Califf RM, Cheitlin MD, Hochman JS, et al. ACC/AHA guideline update for the management of patients with unstable angina and non–ST-segment elevation myocardial infarction—2002: a report of the American College of Cardiology/American Heart Association Task Force on Practice Guidelines (Committee on the Management of Patients With Unstable Angina) [Summary article]. Circulation 2002;106:1893–900.
8. Boersma E, Harrington RA, Moliterno DJ, White H, Theroux P, Van de Werf F, et al. Platelet glycoprotein IIb/IIIa inhibitors in acute coronary syndromes: A meta-analysis of major randomised clinical trials. Lancet 2002;359:189–98.
9. Lindahl B, Venge P, Wallentin L. Troponin T identifies patients with unstable coronary artery disease who benefit from long-term antithrombotic protection. Fragmin in Unstable Coronary Artery Disease (FRISC) Study Group. J Am Coll Cardiol 1997;29:43–8.
10. Muller JE, Rude RE, Braunwald E, Hartwell TD, Roberts R, Sobel BE, et al. Myocardial infarct extension: occurrence, outcome, and risk factors in the Multicenter Investigation of Limitation of Infarct Size. Ann Intern Med 1988;108:1–6.
11. Azzazy HM, Christenson RH. Cardiac markers of acute coronary syndromes: is there a case for point-of-care testing? Clin Biochem 2002;35:13–27.
12. Christenson RH, Duh SH, Sanhai WR, Wu AH, Holtman V, Painter P, et al. Characteristics of an albumin cobalt binding test for assessment of acute coronary syndrome patients: a multicenter study. Clin Chem 2001;47:464–70.
13. Elgebaly SA, Masetti P, Allam M, Forouhar F. Cardiac-derived neutrophil chemotactic factors: preliminary biochemical characterization. J Mol Cell Cardiol 1989;21:585–93.
14. Kleinfeld AM, Prothro D, Brown DL, Davis RC, Richieri GV, DeMaria A. Increases in serum unbound free fatty acid levels following coronary angioplasty. Am J Cardiol 1996;78:1350–4.
15. Brennan ML, Penn MS, Van Lente F, Nambi V, Shishehbor MH, Aviles RJ, et al. Prognostic value of myeloperoxidase in patients with chest pain. N Engl J Med 2003;349:1595–604.
16. Danne O, Mockel M, Lueders C, Mugge C, Zschunke GA, Lufft H, et al. Prognostic implications of elevated whole blood choline levels in acute coronary syndromes. Am J Cardiol 2003;91:1060–7.
17. Varo N, de Lemos JA, Libby P, Morrow DA, Murphy SA, Nuzzo R, et al. Soluble CD40L: risk prediction after acute coronary syndromes. Circulation 2003;108:1049–52.
18. Christenson RH, Duh SH. Evidence-based approach to practice guides and decision thresholds for cardiac markers. Scand J Clin Lab Invest 1999;59(Suppl 230):90–102.
19. Newby LK, Storrow AB, Gibler WB, Garvey JL, Tucker JF, Kaplan AL, et al. Bedside multimarker testing for risk stratification in chest pain units: the chest pain evaluation by creatine kinase-MB, myoglobin, and troponin I (CHECKMATE) study. Circulation 2001;103:1832–7.
20. de Lemos JA, Morrow DA, Gibson CM, Murphy SA, Sabatine MS, Rifai N, et al. The prognostic value of serum myoglobin in patients with non–ST-segment elevation acute coronary syn-

dromes. Results from the TIMI 11B and TACTICS-TIMI 18 studies. J Am Coll Cardiol 2002;40:238–44.

21. Wu AH, Lane PL. Meta-analysis in clinical chemistry: Validation of cardiac troponin T as a marker for ischemic heart diseases. Clin Chem 1995;41:1228–33.

22. Alpert JS, Thygesen K, Antman E, Bassand JP. Myocardial infarction redefined—a consensus document of the Joint European Society of Cardiology/American College of Cardiology Committee for the redefinition of myocardial infarction. J Am Coll Cardiol 2000;36:959–69.

23. Christenson RH, Duh SH, Apple FS, Bodor GS, Bunk DM, Dalluge J, et al. Standardization of cardiac troponin I assays: round robin of ten candidate reference materials. Clin Chem 2001;47:431–7.

24. Azzazy HM, Christenson RH. B-type natriuretic Peptide: physiologic role and assay characteristics. Heart Fail Rev 2003;8: 315–20.

25. Cowie MR, Jourdain P, Maisel A, Dahlstrom U, Follath F, Isnard R, et al. Clinical applications of B-type natriuretic peptide (BNP) testing. Eur Heart J 2003;24:1710–8.

26. Morrow DA, de Lemos JA, Sabatine MS, Murphy SA, Demopoulos LA, DiBattiste PM, et al. Evaluation of B-type natriuretic peptide for risk assessment in unstable angina/non-ST elevation myocardial infarction: B-type natriuretic peptide and prognosis in TACTICS-TIMI 18. J Am Coll Cardiol 2003;41:1264–72.

27. de Lemos JA, Morrow DA, Bentley JH, Omland T, Sabatine MS, McCabe CH, et al. The prognostic value of B-type natriuretic peptide in patients with acute coronary syndromes. N Engl J Med 2001;345:1014–21.

28. Omland T, Persson A, Ng L, O'Brien R, Karlsson T, Herlitz J, et al. N-terminal pro-B-type natriuretic peptide and long-term mortality in acute coronary syndromes. Circulation 2002;106: 2913–8.

29. James SK, Lindahl B, Siegbahn A, Stridsberg M, Venge P, Armstrong P, et al. N-terminal pro-brain natriuretic peptide and other risk markers for the separate prediction of mortality and subsequent myocardial infarction in with unstable coronary artery disease: a Global Utilization of Strategies to Open Occluded Arteries (GUSTO)-IV substudy. Circulation 2003;108:275–81.

30. Davis CP, Barrett K, Torre P, Wacasey K. Serial myoglobin levels for patients with possible myocardial infarction. Acad Emerg Med 1996;3:590–7.

31. Panteghini M, Pagani F, Yeo KT, Apple FS, Christenson RH, Dati F, et al. Evaluation of imprecision for cardiac troponin assays at low-range concentrations. Clin Chem 2004;50:327–32.

32. Wu AH, Smith A, Wieczorek S, Mather JF, Duncan B, White CM, et al. Biological variation for N-terminal pro- and B-type natriuretic peptides and implications for therapeutic monitoring of patients with congestive heart failure. Am J Cardiol 2003;92: 628–31.

33. The Task Force for the Diagnosis and Treatment of Chronic Heart Failure, European Society of Cardiology. Guidelines for the diagnosis and treatment of chronic heart failure. Eur Heart J 2001; 22:1527–60.

34. Wu AH, Apple FS, Gibler WB, Jesse RL, Warshaw MM, Valdes R Jr. National Academy of Clinical Biochemistry Standards of Laboratory Practice: recommendations for the use of cardiac markers in coronary artery diseases. Clin Chem 1999;45: 1104–21.

35. Novis DA, Jones BA, Dale JC, Walsh MK. Biochemical markers of myocardial injury test turnaround time: a College of American Pathologists Q-Probes study of 7020 troponin and 4368 creatine kinase-MB determinations in 159 institutions. Arch Pathol Lab Med 2004;128:158–64.

36. Mueller C, Scholer A, Laule-Kilian K, Martina B, Schindler C, Buser P, et al. Use of B-type natriuretic peptide in the evaluation and management of acute dyspnea. N Engl J Med 2004;350: 647–54.

37. Maisel AS, Krishnaswamy P, Nowak RM, McCord J, Hollander JE, Duc P, et al. Rapid measurement of B-type natriuretic peptide in the emergency diagnosis of heart failure. N Engl J Med 2002;347:161–7.

38. Ryan TJ, Antman EM, Brooks NH, Califf RM, Hillis LD, Hiratzka LF, et al. 1999 update: ACC/AHA guidelines for the management of patients with acute myocardial infarction. A report of the American College of Cardiology/American Heart Association Task Force on Practice Guidelines (Committee on Management of Acute Myocardial Infarction). J Am Coll Cardiol 1999;34:890–911.

39. Roe MT, Christenson RH, Ohman EM, Bahr R, Fesmire FM, Storrow A, et al. A randomized, placebo-controlled trial of early eptifibatide for non–ST-segment elevation acute coronary syndromes. Am Heart J 2003;146:993–8.

40. Giannitsis E, Lehrke S, Wiegand UK, Kurowski V, Muller-Bardorff M, Weidtmann B, et al. Risk stratification in patients with inferior acute myocardial infarction treated by percutaneous coronary interventions: the role of admission troponin T. Circulation 2000;102:2038–44.

41. Gibler WB, Hoekstra JW, Weaver WD, Krucoff MW, Hallstrom AP, Jackson RE, et al. A randomized trial of the effects of early cardiac serum marker availability on reperfusion therapy in patients with acute myocardial infarction: the serial markers, acute myocardial infarction and rapid treatment trial (SMARTT). J Am Coll Cardiol 2000;36:1500–6.

42. Caragher TE, Fernandez BB, Jacobs FL, Barr LA. Evaluation of quantitative cardiac biomarker point-of-care testing in the emergency department. J Emerg Med 2002;22:1–7.

43. Collinson PO. The need for a point of care testing: An evidence-based appraisal. Scand J Clin Lab Invest 1999;230(Suppl):67–73.

44. McCord J, Nowak RM, McCullough PA, Foreback C, Borzak S, Tokarski G, et al. Ninety-minute exclusion of acute myocardial infarction by use of quantitative point-of-care testing of myoglobin and troponin I. Circulation 2001;104:1483–8.

45. Lee-Lewandrowski E, Corboy D, Lewandrowski K, Sinclair J, McDermot S, Benzer TI. Implementation of a point-of-care satellite laboratory in the emergency department of an academic medical center: impact on test turnaround time and patient emergency department length of stay. Arch Pathol Lab Med 2003;127: 456–60.

46. Sabatine MS, Morrow DA, de Lemos JA, Gibson CM, Murphy SA, Rifai N, et al. Multimarker approach to risk stratification in non-ST elevation acute coronary syndromes: simultaneous assessment of troponin I, C-reactive protein, and B-type natriuretic peptide. Circulation 2002;105:1760–3.

47. James SK, Armstrong P, Barnathan E, Califf R, Lindahl B, Siegbahn A, et al.; GUSTO-IV-ACS Investigators. Troponin and C-reactive protein have different relations to subsequent mortality and myocardial infarction after acute coronary syndrome: a GUSTO-IV substudy. J Am Coll Cardiol 2003;41:916–24.

48. Schuchert A, Hamm C, Scholz J, Klimmeck S, Goldmann B, Meinertz T. Prehospital testing for troponin T in patients with

suspected acute myocardial infarction. Am Heart J 1999; 138:45–8.

49. Sylven C, Lindahl S, Hellkvist K, Nyquist O, Rasmanis G. Excellent reliability of nurse-based bedside diagnosis of acute myocardial infarction by rapid dry-strip creatine kinase MB, myoglobin, and troponin T. Am Heart J 1998;135:677–83.

50. Wu AH, Clive JM. Impact of CK-MB testing policies on hospital length of stay and laboratory costs for patients with myocardial infarction or chest pain. Clin Chem 1997;43:326–32.

51. Antman EM, Grudzien C, Sacks DB. Evaluation of a rapid bedside assay for detection of serum cardiac troponin T. JAMA 1995;273:1279–82.

52. Collinson PO, Gerhardt W, Katus HA, Muller-Bardorff M, Braun S, Schricke U, et al. Multicentre evaluation of an immunological rapid test for the detection of troponin T in whole blood samples. Eur J Clin Chem Clin Biochem 1996;34:591–8.

53. Apple FS, Christenson RH, Valdes R Jr., Andriak AJ, Berg A, Duh SH, et al. Simultaneous rapid measurement of whole blood myoglobin, creatine kinase MB, and cardiac troponin I by the triage cardiac panel for detection of myocardial infarction. Clin Chem 1999;45:199–205.

54. McCullough PA, Nowak RM, Foreback C, Tokarski G, Tomlanovich MC, Khoury NE, et al. Performance of multiple cardiac biomarkers measured in the emergency department in patients with chronic kidney disease and chest pain. Acad Emerg Med 2002;9:1389–96.

55. Ng SM, Krishnaswamy P, Morissey R, Clopton P, Fitzgerald R, Maisel AS. Ninety-minute accelerated critical pathway for chest pain evaluation. Am J Cardiol 2001;88:611–7.

56. Apple FS, Anderson FP, Collinson P, Jesse RL, Kontos MC, Levitt MA, et al. Clinical evaluation of the first medical whole blood, point-of-care testing device for detection of myocardial infarction. Clin Chem 2000;46:1604–9.

57. de Winter RJ, Koster RW, Sturk A, Sanders GT. Value of myoglobin, troponin T, and CK-MBmass in ruling out an acute myocardial infarction in the emergency room. Circulation 1995; 92:3401–7.

58. Polaczyk CA, Kuntz KM, Sacks DB, Johnson PA, Lee TH. Emergency department triage strategies for acute chest pain using creatine kinase-MB and troponin I assays: A cost-effectiveness analysis. Ann Intern Med 1999;131:909–18.

59. Anderson FP, Fritz ML, Kontos MC, McPherson RA, Jesse RL. Cost-effectiveness of cardiac troponin I in a systematic chest pain evaluation protocol: Use of cardiac troponin I lowers length of stay for low-risk cardiac patients. Clin Lab Manage Rev 1998; 12:63–9.

60. Gomez MA, Anderson JL, Karagounis LA, Muhlestein JB, Mooers FB. An emergency department-based protocol for rapidly ruling out myocardial ischemia reduces hospital time and expense: results of a randomized study (ROMIO). J Am Coll Cardiol 1996;28:25–33.

61. Hamm CW, Goldmann BU, Heeschen C, Kreymann G, Berger J, Meinertz T. Emergency room triage of patients with acute chest pain by means of rapid testing for cardiac troponin T or troponin I. N Engl J Med 1997;337:1648–53.

62. Zarich S, Bradley K, Seymour J, Ghali W, Traboulsi A, Mayall ID, et al. Impact of troponin T determinations on hospital resource utilization and costs in the evaluation of patients with suspected myocardial ischemia. Am J Cardiol 2001;88:732–6.

Chapter 38

Point-of-Care Testing in Nephrology

Christopher P. Price and Edmund J. Lamb

Diseases involving the kidneys are a major health problem throughout the world, including conditions in which renal function is impaired as a secondary complication of another disease (e.g., diabetes mellitus) as well as primary renal diseases such as polycystic kidney disease. In the United States, of the patients with end-stage renal disease (ESRD or kidney failure), 34.6% had diabetes mellitus as their primary renal diagnosis, 22.9% hypertension, and 19.9% either glomerulonephritis or cystic disease (1). In 2000, >375,000 Americans were treated for ESRD; of these, about 275,000 were on dialysis and 100,000 had a functioning renal transplant. On average, each year 90,000 new patients are registered with kidney failure (1). When lesser degrees of renal impairment are included, it is estimated that the prevalence of chronic kidney disease (CKD) overall in the United States is about 11.2%, representing a total of 19.2 million patients (2). The annual cost of treating renal failure in the US is estimated to be about $17.9 billion. The estimated incidence of ESRD is 291 per million population in the United States, 140 per million population in Canada, and 89 to 160 per million population across Europe (3). In the United Kingdom, >33,000 patients are on renal replacement therapy (treatment with dialysis and transplantation) (4); this figure is likely to double in the next 20 years, with a similar expectation being noted in the United States (5). Reasons for the increasing number of patients on treatment include the increased age of patients accepted into transplant programs and the increased prevalence of type 2 diabetes.

Despite all of the advances in diagnostic and treatment regimens, the prognosis for patients with renal disease is still poor. As noted previously, there is a much higher prevalence of early-stage kidney disease than ESRD (1). Such patients are at high risk for developing cardiovascular disease. Early detection of deteriorating kidney function and intervention can improve outcomes, for example, in the case of diabetic nephropathy by delaying the onset of complications through improved glycemic control, and in the case of hypertension by closer management and treatment with angiotensin-converting enzyme inhibitors (ACEIs) The most important risk factors for development of ESRD are the presence of diabetes, hypertension, and older age (Table 38-1) (6). Consequently, recent guidelines suggest regular monitoring of proteinuria or albuminuria in individuals at greatest risk of developing kidney disease (7–9).

THE ROLE OF LABORATORY MEDICINE

Renal disease can clearly be a multifactorial disorder. The clinician is faced with investigation and management of both primary renal disease and secondary disease. Some of the main laboratory findings in patients with renal disease are shown in Table 38-2. The investigation of renal dysfunction focuses not only on the diagnosis and monitoring of the kidneys but also on the impact that renal dysfunction might have on other comorbidities (e.g., cardiovascular disease, bone disease, endocrine function, and drug dosage and elimination). A summary of some of the key roles that the laboratory medicine service can play in the detection, diagnosis, and management of renal disease is provided in the following paragraphs, and then consideration of the potential benefits from the provision of the service at the point of care is discussed.

At-Risk Testing and Early Detection

Measurement of serum creatinine and estimation of the glomerular filtration rate (GFR) can be used to detect a reduction in renal function; however, in a large primary care study, Cockcroft and Gault estimated GFRs <50 mL/min were common in patients with normal serum creatinine (10). The discordance was most pronounced in older age groups (e.g., discordance between normal serum creatinine and reduced GFR was observed in 47% of patients ≥ 70 years of age, compared with 1.2% of patients 40 to 59 years of age) (10), confirming a long-held view on the limited utility of serum creatinine as a measure of GFR (7). Measurement of serum cystatin C may provide an earlier indication of a reduced GFR than serum creatinine (11). It is generally considered that an increase in urine protein excretion occurs in the disease progression before any significant increase in serum creatinine is observed. Measurement of urine protein has therefore also been used as a means of detecting renal dysfunction, although urine albumin is now the preferred test. In specific situations, other proteins have been suggested as indicators of disease. Urine α_1-microglobulin (12) and *N*-acetyl-β-glucosaminidase (13) have been used to detect the presence of tubular damage as a consequence of substances known to be toxic to the kidney (e.g., drugs, heavy metals, and industrial chemicals). Hematuria (blood in the urine) and the detection of hemoglobin in the urine are also signs of kidney disease.

Table 38-1 Prevalence of Advanced Renal Failure in the United Kingdom[a]

Age, years	Rate per million population
0–19	6
20–49	58
50–59	160
60–69	282
70–79	503
≥80	588

[a] Advanced renal failure defined as serum creatinine > 500 μmol/L (4.5 mg/dL).
Data from (6).

There are now a number of guidelines and proposals that recommend the regular measurement of urine albumin for the early detection of renal disease, specifically in association with diabetes mellitus (7) and hypertension (14), and more broadly in at-risk populations (8). There is considerable clinical and economic benefits to early detection of reduced kidney function, which can lead to earlier clinical intervention (15, 16).

Diagnosis and Assessment of Disease Severity

The biochemical tests referred to in the previous section, in particular serum creatinine, together with measurements of the electrolytes (i.e., sodium, potassium, bicarbonate, phosphate, and calcium) play an important role in the diagnosis and assessment of the severity of renal disease. Serum urea has also been used in addition to creatinine, but is generally regarded as less specific, because urea levels are influenced by a number of nonrenal factors. In addition, imaging of the kidneys and the urogenital tract may help in the differential diagnosis of renal disease. Invariably, in the case of primary renal disease, the definitive diagnosis will be made by histological examination following biopsy. The investigations at the time of diagnosis will also include assessment of the status of any primary disease (e.g., diabetes) and of the status of secondary disease [e.g., cardiovascular disease (cholesterol and triglycerides), metabolic bone disease (parathyroid hormone, bone alkaline phosphatase, phosphate, and calcium), and anemia (hemoglobin, hematocrit, transferrin saturation, and ferritin)].

In addition, these tests can be used to determine how certain medications are affecting renal function, especially if the kinetics of the drug are influenced by kidney function and/or if renal toxicity is of concern. This may be particularly pertinent in young children and older patients. In these situations, serum creatinine tests may have insufficient sensitivity, and clearance studies may be more useful (e.g. inulin, ^{51}Cr EDTA, or iohexol); although there are technical and practical limitations to the use of renal clearance tests (17).

Monitoring Disease Management

The two main parameters used to monitor renal function are serum creatinine (as a surrogate for assessment of GFR) and urine protein or albumin. These will be complemented by tests to assess other comorbidities as referred to earlier. In the case of patients requiring renal replacement therapy (i.e., dialysis and transplantation), additional tests are used to assess the efficacy of the replacement therapy. These include dialysis efficiency, through the use of urea elimination kinetics; assessing bone loss; assessing erythropoietin therapy; and monitoring for early signs of transplant rejection.

Prognosis

Both elevated serum creatinine (18) and increased urine albumin excretion (19) are associated with a higher risk of cardiovascular disease. In addition, low baseline GFR, proteinuria, and low serum albumin are all associated with a faster rate of progression of kidney disease (20). Some studies suggest that hyperlipidemia and anemia are also associated with a faster rate of progression (8).

Point-of-Care Testing for Early Detection of Kidney Disease

Although most of the early point-of-care testing (POCT) systems for renal dysfunction were based on the use of a urine

Table 38-2 Key Laboratory Test Changes Common in Patients with Kidney Disease

Retained nitrogenous metabolites in blood
   Increased blood concentrations of urea, creatinine, uric acid
Fluid, acid-base, and electrolyte disturbances
   Hyperkalemia
   Hypo- or hypernatremia
   Metabolic acidosis (decreased blood pH, bicarbonate)
   Hyperchloremia
   Hypocalcemia
   Fixed urine osmolality
   Hyperphosphatemia
   Hypermagnesemia
Carbohydrate intolerance
   Insulin resistance (hypoglycemia may also occur) with plasma insulin normal or increased
Abnormal lipid metabolism
   Hypertriglyceridemia
   Decreased high-density lipoprotein cholesterol
   Hyperlipoproteinemia
Altered urinary protein handling
   Proteinuria
   Albuminuria
   Low molecular weight proteinuria
Altered endocrine function
   Secondary hyperparathyroidism (increased parathyroid hormone and alkaline phosphatase)
   Hypovitaminosis D (decreased 1,25-dihydroxy vitamin D)
   Decreased erythropoietin production (decreased hemoglobin)
   Altered thyroxine metabolism
   Gonadal dysfunction (increased prolactin and luteinizing hormone, decreased testosterone)

protein test (21), there have been devices described for the measurement of urine albumin (22) and serum creatinine (23, 24). One of the limitations of these devices has been the diurnal variation in urinary excretion and the poor reliability and impracticality of 24-h urine collection. The latter problems can be overcome by the use of either the protein or albumin result as a ratio to the creatinine concentration. Newman et al. (25) showed a significant reduction in the within-day variation of the protein and albumin excretion when the ratio was used, whereas several authors have demonstrated a good correlation between both the total protein:creatinine ratio and albumin: creatinine ratio with the respective 24-h collection (26–28). POCT devices that are capable of assessing the protein:creatinine ratio or albumin:creatinine ratio enable the use of such a test in the point-of-care setting (29–31). The National Kidney Foundation–Kidney Disease Outcomes Quality Initiative (NKF–K/DOQI) clinical practice guidelines indicate that a dipstick test for proteinuria is adequate, but that the protein:creatinine ratio may be more reliable (7). The NKF recommends a confirmatory test following a positive dipstick test.

In Montana, Harwell et al. (32) audited the availability of the albumin:creatinine ratio and found the test was not available universally; furthermore, a number of different units were used for reporting as well as a different range of cutoff values. Hostetter (33), in a paper questioning whether laboratories were contributing to the problems of early detection of CKD, suggested that primary care physicians would be responsible for diagnosing most CKD, as patients with diabetes and hypertension constituted the majority of individuals at risk of developing renal disease. Also, these patients will not necessarily be referred to nephrologists. He argued that the rationale for early detection of disease was strong, because of drugs such as ACEIs and angiotensin II receptor blockers (A2RBs), which reduce the rate of onset of more severe albuminuria and kidney injury (34). Hostetter also argued that much of the detection and care of renal disease would have to be delivered in the primary care setting. The potential for POCT in the primary care setting is implied in these findings. An added benefit would be greater accessibility for patients.

Guthrie and Lott (35), who reported on urinalysis in a family practice setting, argued the case for regular dipstick monitoring for proteinuria in patients with diabetes and hypertension. In an audit of case notes in 12 primary care practices, Kissmeyer et al. (36) found a high prevalence of renal insufficiency in hypertensive and diabetic patients, using either plasma creatinine or proteinuria in their assessment Therefore, in primary care settings, they have advocated regular testing for proteinuria in patients with hypertension and/or diabetes. Also, the NKF–K/DOQI clinical guidelines (7) have recommended testing for proteinuria in the at-risk population.

Using systematic review and meta-analysis methods, Craig et al. (37) examined the feasibility of mass screening for proteinuria and the value of the detection of early kidney disease. In Australia, of the estimated 1500 individuals who developed ESRD each year, they found two-thirds were >50 years of age (~200 patients per million population per year). In

addition, proteinuria conferred a 15-fold increased risk for ESRD. The use of ACEIs could reduce the risk of ESRD by ~30% over a 2- to 3-year period. The authors argued that with opportunistic at-risk testing, 20,000 individuals > 50 years of age would need to be tested to prevent one case of ESRD; of these, 100 would be treated with ACEIs and 1000 would need the confirmatory urine test (24-h urine collection), of which 700 results would be false positives. They concluded that this approach would save health resources, although there remained some important unanswered questions (e.g., the effects of drug therapy on those people who tested positive and the effects of the testing on the individual), and a trial would be required to prove the model. The authors also felt that the use of the protein:creatinine ratio or albumin:creatinine ratio for screening would improve the results of the study.

Boulware et al. (38) analyzed the cost-effectiveness of annual screening compared to no screening (usual care) for proteinuria at age 50 years, and then, if indicated, treatment with an ACEI or an A2RB. The authors used Markov decision analytical modeling to compare the strategies. For persons who did not have hypertension or diabetes, the cost-effectiveness ratio for screening compared to no screening was unfavorable (~$282,000/quality-adjusted life year). However, selective testing beginning at age 60 years yielded a more favorable ratio (~$53,000/quality-adjusted life year). For persons with hypertension, the cost-effectiveness ratio was highly favorable (~$19,000/quality-adjusted life year, which represented an improvement from 0.0022 to 0.03 quality-adjusted life year/person). The authors concluded that broad testing for early detection of urine protein to slow progression of CKD and decrease mortality was not cost-effective, unless selectively directed toward high-risk groups (older persons and persons with hypertension) or unless conducted at an infrequent interval of every 10 years.

Garg et al. (39) studied the prevalence of albuminuria and renal insufficiency (using serum creatinine values) in the population covered by the third National Health and Nutrition Examination Survey (NHANES III). They found that it would be necessary to test three individuals with diabetes, seven nondiabetic hypertensives, or six individuals > 60 years of age to identify one case of albuminuria. They also noted that about one-third of the individuals with reduced GFR (calculated as <30 mL $\cdot$ min$^{-1} \cdot 1.73$ m^{-2}) showed no albuminuria. More than 8.0% of the study population had microalbuminuria and 1.0% had macroalbuminuria. Several studies have reported on screening programs for proteinuria. Thus, Iseki et al. (40, 41) have reported on a mass screening program of over 100,000 adults in Japan and found that proteinuria was a strong independent risk factor for ESRD. There has been a program of screening school children in Japan for several years (42). In one of these studies, Pugia et al. showed that the use of a dipstick test with the protein:creatinine ratio led to an improvement in results (43). The screening program is considered to have led to a reduction in the number of patients entering renal replacement therapy programs (40). Similar programs have been undertaken in Korea and Taiwan (44, 45).

The differential diagnosis of hematuria is broad, and includes urinary tract malignancy, urinary tract stones, urinary tract infection, and glomerulonephritis. Hematuria is either frank (macroscopic) or occult (microscopic or detectable by stick testing only). Although hematuria has long been considered pathological, there is in fact considerable debate concerning the significance of asymptomatic microscopic hematuria. The yield from investigation of asymptomatic patients displaying microscopic hematuria is very small, and the benefit of earlier detection of any urological tumors thus discovered, compared to limiting investigation to patients with macroscopic hematuria, is uncertain (46, 47). Current evidence does not support the use of urinalysis as a screening tool for urological malignancy (48).

POINT-OF-CARE TESTING DURING HEMODIALYSIS

There are a number of biochemical and hematological parameters that are monitored at the time of hemodialysis; some of these may affect the immediate hemodialysis protocol, whereas others are more associated with the long-term management of the patient (Table 38-3). Over the years, dialysis practice has changed with improvements to dialysis technique. For example, there is less need to assess the acid–base status of the patient during dialysis or to monitor the ionized calcium fraction. Invariably, there will be a blood specimen collected at the commencement of dialysis, and then another specimen taken at the end of the session, which primarily checks the adequacy of the dialysis session, and checks against any aberration of electrolyte status. In an intervention study to improve the adequacy of hemodialysis care in a single ESRD network, McClellan et al. (49) randomly assigned 42 treatment centers to feedback alone or intensive intervention; the latter showed

the greatest improvement, including a greater increase in the urea reduction ratio (a benchmark used in the ESRD network).

Point-of-Care Testing for Assessing the Adequacy of Hemodialysis

Several factors are known to affect dialysis adequacy, which is an important determinant of clinical outcome (50). There is considerable intraindividual variation (51). The adequacy of hemodialysis has been the subject of many studies over the years. Predominantly, the practice is based on urea kinetic modeling and the total urea clearance distribution volume ratio (K_t/V parameter) (17); this requires both predialysis and postdialysis urea measurements. Others have advocated multiple measurements; however, there can be problems with the effects of rebound on post-treatment specimens (52). Alternative approaches to measure urea online in either blood or dialysis fluid or to use other surrogate markers have been proposed (53). An early application used a urease-based biosensor to measure urea in the extracorporeal arterial stream (54). Fernandez et al. (55) described a neural network linked to a dialysate-side urea monitoring system, while Olesberg et al. (56) and Eddy and Arnold (57) described in-line measurement systems for urea in dialysis fluid using Fourier-transform and near-infrared spectroscopy, respectively. Fridolin et al. (58) and Uhlin et al. (59) described a similar approach using ultraviolet absorption spectrophotometry. Arrigo et al. (60) used an in-line urea biosensor, which produced some differences in the estimation of urea clearance compared with the reference method, but these were not statistically significant. Lindsay et al. (61) described ionic dialysance using in-line conductivity measurements and showed that it can give an accurate indication of effective urea clearance; Katopodis and Hoenich (62) and Kuhlmann et al. (63) produced similar findings. Hernandez-Herrera et al. (64) showed that an online urea monitoring system could be used to

Table 38-3   Some Laboratory Parameters Measured in Patients on Hemodialysis

Application	Test
Complications, acute	
Dialysis disequilibrium	Plasma electrolytes
Pyrexia	C-reactive protein
Bleeding	Clotting factors
Complications, chronic	
Anemia	Hemoglobin, ferritin
Septicemia/peritonitis	C-reactive protein
	Culture and sensitivity
Malnutrition	Albumin, prealbumin
Cardiovascular disease	Lipid profiles
Amyloidosis	Serum β_2-microglobulin
Osteodystrophy	Ca^{2+}, PO_4^-, bone alkaline phosphatase, intact parathyroid hormone, aluminium
Adequacy of dialysis	
Urea kinetic modeling (URR and K_t/V)	Pre- and postdialysis urea
Weekly creatinine clearances	Pre- and postdialysis creatinine

URR, urea reduction ratio.

assess the length of hemodialysis required to achieve the target dose of dialysis.

Alternative approaches that have been described include the measurement of dialysate creatinine using micellar electro-kinetic chromatography on samples of postdialysis fluid (65) and the use of a lacrimal urea measurement (66). The latter method uses arginase as a reagent, an enzyme also found in tears and blood; however, a reasonable correlation between lacrimal and blood urea concentration was still observed, providing the opportunity for a less invasive assessment of urea kinetics. It is presumed that other urea sensor technologies could be used.

Assessment of Hemodynamic Status

Intradialytic monitoring of hemodynamic parameters has attracted considerable interest in recent years, because of the concerns over hypotensive episodes during dialysis and the associated morbidity and mortality (67). Dialysate sodium monitoring is used as a surrogate measure of the plasma volume (the higher the sodium, the lower the plasma volume); this measure together with blood pressure, plasma volume, and thermal balance might be used in a biofeedback algorithm to guide antihypertensive medication and reduce hypotensive episodes (68). Santoro et al. (69) tested such an algorithm and found a 30% reduction in intradialytic hypotensive events.

Schroeder et al. (70) studied the ultrafiltration rate and plasma refill rate using continuous monitoring of the hematocrit with automated blood volume controlled dialysis machines and found that changes in these parameters were associated with hypotensive episodes, indicating a means of modifying the dialysis process to reduce these events. Goldstein et al. (71) evaluated the use of a hematocrit monitoring system to assess the frequency of fluid overload/hypertension in children receiving dialysis and found a dramatic reduction in hospitalization (from 64 to 2 days/year), while maintaining acceptable blood pressure control and minimizing antihypertensive medication requirements.

Assessment of Anemia Status

Anemia is known to affect 60–80% of patients with renal impairment, with a reduction in the quality of life and risk of early death. Initially the main treatment option was blood transfusion, but over the last two decades erythropoietin has become the treatment of choice (72–74). A meta-analysis of several trials showed that better mortality was observed in patients with chronic renal failure treated with erythropoietin when the hemoglobin level was maintained above 140 g/L (14 g/dL) (72). Lower hemoglobin levels were associated with a higher incidence of seizures, but a lower risk of hypertensive episodes. Despite this, Horl et al. (75) found a high level of anemia in a cohort of patients on dialysis and a low level of usage of erythropoietin. Hematocrit and hemoglobin measurements have been the mainstay of anemia status evaluation, and Marooney (76) has shown that the hemoglobin measurement is a more reliable indicator than the centrifuged hematocrit at the point of care. Agarwal and Heinz (77) showed that the HemoCue B-hemoglobin assay system (HemoCue AB, Angelholm, Sweden), when operated by patients, gave results within 10 g/L (1.0 g/dL) 96% of the time, when compared with a laboratory reference method. The authors pointed out the importance of proper training, especially in specimen collection, to ensure reliable results. Lacson et al. (78) pointed out that the hemoglobin level fluctuates in patients with ESRD over time. They also pointed out that variability in laboratory assays, biological factors, and therapeutic response affected the hemoglobin variability observed. Turco (79) and Frankenfield et al. (80) have suggested that pharmacists can play a valuable role in monitoring laboratory values and drug utilization, which may be made easier by access to POCT systems for hemoglobin measurement. The goal would be to reduce the variability in target outcome markers and increase the number of patients achieving their treatment goals (80). Balshaw-Greer and Casey (81) have advocated the self-adminstration of erythropoetin.

Assessment of Coagulation Status

Thrombotic and hemorrhagic complications do affect cardiovascular morbidity and mortality in hemodialysis patients. The choice of anticoagulation is mainly between heparin and citrate. There is a risk of thrombocytopenia when using heparin (82, 83). Holt et al. studied the use of the international normalized ratio, activated partial thromboplastin time, and platelet and thromboelastographic measurements in relation to the longevity of continuous replacement circuits and found that although the latter more closely predicted circuit longevity, there was no real clinical benefit (84). Bommer and Schwab (85) studied the use of the CoaguChek Pro (Roche Diagnostics, Mannheim, Germany) for measuring the activated clotting time in dialysis and found the results agreed well with the reference Hemochron system (International Technodyne, Edison. NJ, USA) and concluded that it could be used for monitoring heparin administration during dialysis. Furuhashi et al. (86) studied the Sonoclot coagulation analyzer (Sienco, Wheat Ridge, CO, USA), correlating the activated clotting time, clot rate, time-to-peak amplitude, and peak amplitude with conventional coagulation variables, platelet count, and fibrinogen. Both clot rate and peak amplitude correlated with platelet count and fibrinogen, and all of the Sonoclot variables except for peak amplitude were correlated with heparin dose. The authors concluded that the system could be used to monitor coagulation status and determine heparin dose during hemodialysis.

Point-of-Care Testing and Peritoneal Dialysis

Infection, in particular peritonitis, is the most common complication of peritoneal dialysis, accounting for 30–50% of treatment failures. Typically this will be apparent as a cloudy dialysate, with laboratory culture and sensitivity confirming the diagnosis; although in the early stages of infection dialysate may be clear. Leukocyte esterase reagent strips have been used in a POCT setting to facilitate earlier detection of peritonitis in patients on peritoneal dialysis (87). In this study, the stick test was found to have 100% sensitivity and 96% specificity for detecting peritonitis.

Point-of-Care Testing and Organ Procurement

There is a worldwide shortage of kidney and other organ donors, and there are many suggestions as to how the situation might be improved (88). One approach is to use a strict donor management protocol and to expand the criteria for acceptable donor organs. Rosendale et al. (89) showed how such an approach led to an increased availability of donors. Baier et al. (90) demonstrated that introduction of a POCT system for measuring the donor blood electrolytes, glucose, creatinine, and hematocrit in a protocol for donor procurement achieved a faster turnaround time and enabled the procurement protocol to operate more efficiently.

Monitoring the Secondary Complications of Renal Failure

Reference has already been made to several of the secondary complications of renal failure, including anemia and coagulation defects. Because renal dysfunction is considered a risk factor for cardiovascular disease, management of the other risk factors must be taken into account. Many patients on hemodialysis are placed on statin therapy. Viola et al. (91) reviewed the experience with a multidisciplinary hyperlipidemia program in which a pharmacist was responsible for monitoring of laboratory parameters, patient counseling, and dosage adjustment. The authors found that initiation of the program led to an increase in the number of patients achieving target LDL cholesterol values over a 6-month period from 58% to 88%. Among 26 patients, there were 15 drug dosage adjustments, eight adverse incidents (two involving discontinuation of the drug), and eight alerts to the physician for potential drug–drug interactions. As the management of chronic disease is increasingly transferred to the community setting, this style of patient management with POCT support will become more evident.

Metabolic bone disease is an important complication of renal failure and there are established guidelines (92) for its assessment, using predominantly biochemical and imaging tools. There is little evidence to date that any of this monitoring is translating to the point-of-care setting, presumably because there are few data to indicate that patient compliance with modifications to drug, diet, or lifestyle has any effect on bone density, beyond what is achieved as part of the regular dialysis and clinic review portfolio.

Impaired renal function can play an important part in pharmacokinetics and therefore must be taken into account, especially when prescribing drugs with a narrow therapeutic window and the potential for renal toxicity. This is particularly true for children and older patients. Measurement of serum creatinine is the most practical way of assessing the GFR on a regular basis in these patients; ideally, this should be combined with an estimated GFR, for example, using a palmtop GFR calculator.

CONCLUSIONS

Renal failure is a major health burden for society. There is increasing evidence of the need to screen for early signs of disease and to institute therapy as soon as possible, as well as to make every effort to mitigate the complications of the disease. There is a large repertoire of laboratory markers that play a crucial role in screening for disease as well as in diagnosis and monitoring of management. There is already evidence that POCT can play a role in improving outcomes, and this trend is likely to increase. Screening for early signs of disease is likely to be undertaken in the primary care setting, which satisfies the needs of convenience for both patient and caregiver. Monitoring, as part of a chronic disease management protocol, will also be delivered more often at the point of care, which is convenient and improves compliance with the care strategy.

REFERENCES

1. US Renal Data System. USRDS 2003 annual data report: atlas of end stage renal disease in the United States. Bethesda, MD: NIH, National Institute of Diabetes and Digestive and Kidney Diseases, 2003.
2. Coresh J, Astor BC, Greene T, Eknoyan G, Levey AS. Prevalence of chronic kidney disease and decreased kidney function in the adult US population: Third National Health and Nutrition Examination Survey. Am J Kidney Dis 2003;41:1–12.
3. International Federation of Renal Registries: European database. http://www.ifrr.net/ifrr-light/id_europa.htm (accessed March 25, 2002).
4. UK Renal Registry Report 2002. http://www.renalreg.com/home.htm (accessed March 25, 2004).
5. Brown WW, Collins A, Chen SC, King K, Molony D, Gannon MR, et al. Identification of persons at high risk for kidney disease via targeted screening: the NKF Kidney Early Evaluation Program. Kidney Int 2003;(Suppl):S50–5.
6. Feest TG, Mistry CD, Grimes DS, Mallick NP. Incidence of advanced chronic renal failure and the need for end stage renal replacement treatment. BMJ 1990;301:897–900.
7. National Kidney Foundation. K/DOQI clinical practice guidelines for chronic kidney disease: evaluation, classification and stratification. Am J Kidney Dis 2002;39(Suppl 1):S1–S266.
8. Keane WF, Eknoyan G. Proteinuria, albuminuria, risk, assessment, detection, elimination (PARADE): a position paper of the National Kidney Foundation. Am J Kidney Dis 1999;33:1004–10.
9. American Diabetes Association. Clinical practice recommendations 2001. Diabetes Care 2001;24:S69–S72.
10. Duncan L, Heathcote J, Djurdjev O, Levin A. Screening for renal disease using serum creatinine: who are we missing? Nephrol Dial Trans 2001;16:1042–6.
11. Price CP, Finney H. Developments in the assessment of glomerular filtration rate. Clin Chim Acta 2000;297:55–66.
12. Mantur M, Kemona H, Dabrowska M, Dabrowska J, Sobolewski S, Prokopowicz J. Alpha-1-microglobulin as a marker of proxi-

mal tubular damage in urinary tract infection in children. Clin Nephrol 2000;53:283–7.

13. Lybarger JA, Lichtveld MY, Amler RW. Biomedical testing of the kidney for persons exposed to hazardous substances in the environment. Ren Fail 1999;21:263–74.

14. Hemmelgarn BR, Zarnke KB, Campbell NR, Feldman RD, McKay DW, McAlister FA, et al. The 2004 Canadian Hypertension Education Program recommendations for the management of hypertension: part I. Blood pressure measurement, diagnosis and assessment of risk. Can J Cardiol 2004;20:31–40.

15. Borch-Johnsen K, Wenzel H, Viberti GC, Mogensen CE. Is screening and intervention for microalbuminuria worthwhile in patients with insulin dependent diabetes? BMJ 1993;306:1722–5.

16. Trivedi HS, Pang MM, Campbell A, Saab P. Slowing the progression of chronic renal failure: economic benefits and patients' perspectives. Am J Kidney Dis 2002;39:721–9.

17. Newman DJ, Price CP. Renal function and nitrogen metabolites. In: Burtis CA, Ashwood ER, eds. Tietz textbook of clinical chemistry, 3rd ed. Philadelphia: WB Saunders, 1999: 1204–70.

18. Mann JF, Gerstein HC, Pogue J, Bosch J, Yusuf S. Renal insufficiency as a predictor of cardiovascular outcomes and the impact of ramipril: the HOPE randomized trial. Ann Intern Med 2001; 134:629–36.

19. Gerstein HC, Mann JF, Yi Q, Zinman B, Dinneen SF, Hoogwerf B, et al. Albuminuria and risk of cardiovascular events, death, and heart failure in diabetic and nondiabetic individuals. JAMA 2001; 286:421–6.

20. Hunsicker LG, Adler S, Caggiula A, England BK, Greene T, Kusek JW, et al. Predictors of the progression of renal disease in the modification of diet in renal disease study. Kidney Int 1997; 51:1908–19.

21. Woolhandler S, Pels RJ, Bor DH, Himmelstein DU, Lawrence RS. Dipstick urinalysis screening of asymptomatic adults for urinary tract disorders. I. Hematuria and proteinuria JAMA 1989; 262:1214–9.

22. Minetti EE, Cozzi MG, Granata S, Guidi E. Accuracy of the urinary albumin titrator stick 'Micral-Test' in kidney-disease patients. Nephrol Dial Transplant 1997;12:78–80.

23. Kost GJ, Vu HT, Inu M, DuPlantier R, Fleisher M, Kroll MH, Spinosa JC. Multicenter study of whole-blood creatinine, total carbon dioxide content, and chemistry profiling for laboratory and point-of-care testing in critical care in the United States. Crit Care Med 2000;28:2379–89.

24. Schaffar BP. Thick film biosensors for metabolites in undiluted whole blood and plasma samples. Anal Bioanal Chem 2002;372: 254–60.

25. Newman DJ, Pugia MJ, Lott JA, Wallace JF, Hiar AM. Urinary protein and albumin excretion corrected by creatinine and specific gravity. Clin Chim Acta 2000;294:139–55.

26. Ginsberg JM, Chang BS, Matarese RA, Garella S. Use of single voided urine samples to estimate quantitative proteinuria. New Engl J Med 1983;309:1543–6.

27. Ruggenenti P, Gaspari F, Perna A, Remuzzi G. Cross-sectional longitudinal study of spot morning urine protein:creatinine ratio, 24-h urine protein excretion rate, glomerular filtration rate, and end stage renal failure in chronic renal disease in patients without diabetes. BMJ 1998;316:504–9.

28. Claudi T, Cooper JG. Comparison of urinary albumin excretion rate in overnight urine and albumin creatinine ratio in spot urine in diabetic patients in general practice. Scan J Prim Health Care 2001;19:247–8.

29. Pugia MJ, Lott JA, Kajima J, Saambe T, Sasaki M, Kuromoto K, et al. Screening school children for albuminuria, proteinuria and occult blood with dipsticks. Clin Chem Lab Med 1999;37: 149–57.

30. Parsons M, Newman DJ, Pugia M, Newall RG, Price CP. Performance of a reagent strip device for quantitation of the urine albumin: creatinine ratio in a point of care setting. Clin Nephrol 1999;51:220–7.

31. Parsons MP, Newman DJ, Newall RG, Price CP. Validation of a point-of-care assay for the urinary albumin:creatinine ratio. Clin Chem 1999;45:414–7.

32. Harwell TS, Nelson RG, Little RR, McDowall JM, Helgerson SD, Gohdes D. Testing for microalbuminuria in 2002: barriers to implementing current guidelines. Am J Kidney Dis 2003;42: 392–4.

33. Hostetter TH. Detecting early chronic kidney disease: are clinical laboratories a problem? Am J Kidney Dis 2003;42:392–4.

34. Jafar TH, Stark PC, Schmid CH, Landa M, Maschio G, Marcantoni C, et al. Proteinuria as a modifiable risk factor for the progression of non-diabetic renal disease. Kidney Int 2001;60: 1131–40.

35. Guthrie RM, Lott JA. Screening for proteinuria in patients with hypertension or diabetes mellitus. J Fam Pract 1993;37:253–6.

36. Kissmeyer L, Kong C, Cohen J, Unwin RJ, Woolfson RG, Neild GH. Community nephrology: audit of screening for renal insufficiency in a high risk population. Nephrol Dial Transplant 1999; 14:2150–5.

37. Craig JC, Barratt A, Cumming R, Irwig L, Salkeld G. Feasibility study of the early detection and treatment of renal disease by mass screening. Intern Med J 2002;32:6–14.

38. Boulware LE, Jaar BG, Tarver-Carr ME, Brancati FL, Powe NR. Screening for proteinuria in US adults: a cost-effectiveness analysis. JAMA 2003;290:3101–14.

39. Garg AX, Kiberd BA, Clark WF, Haynes RB, Clase CM. Albuminuria and renal insufficiency prevalence guides population screening: results from the NHANES III. Kidney Int 2002;61: 2165–75.

40. Iseki K, Iseki C, Ikemiya Y, Fukiyama K. Risk of developing end-stage renal disease in a cohort of mass screening. Kidney Int 1996;49:800–5.

41. Iseki K, Ikemiya Y, Iseki C, Takishita S. Proteinuria and the risk of developing end-stage renal disease. Kidney Int 2003;63: 1468–74.

42. Ito K, Kawaguchi H, Hattori M. Screening for proteinuria and hematuria in school children—is it possible to reduce the incidence of chronic renal failure in children and adolescents? Acta Paediatr Jpn 1990;32:710–15.

43. Pugia MJ, Murakami M, Lott JA, Ohta Y, Kitagawa T, Yamauchi K, Suhara Y, Kasjima J. Screening for proteinuria in Japanese schoolchildren: a new approach. Clin Chem Lab Med 2000;389: 75–82.

44. Cho BS, Kim SD, Choi YM, Kang HH. Schoolurinalysis screening in Korea: prevalence of chronic renal disease. Pediatr Nephrol 2001;16:1126–8.

45. Lin CY, Sheng CC, Lin CC, Chen CH, Chou P. Mass urinary screening and follow-up for schoolchildren in Taiwan Province. Acta Paediatr Taiwan 2001;42:134–40.

46. Tomson CRV, Porter T. Asymptomatic microscopic hematuria or dipstick hematuria in adults: which investigations for which

patients? A review of the evidence. Br J Urol Int, 2002;90: 185–98.

47. Malmstrom PU. Time to abandon testing for microscopic haematuria in adults? BMJ 2003;326:813–5.

48. National Electronic Library for Health. http://www.nelh.nhs.uk/screening/adult_pps/bladder_cancer.html (accessed March 25, 2004).

49. McClellan WM, Hodgin E, Pastan S, McAdams L, Soucie M. A randomized evaluation of two health care quality improvement program (HCQIP) interventions to improve the adequacy of hemodialysis care of ESRD patients: feedback alone versus intensive intervention. J Am Soc Nephrol 2004;15:754–60.

50. Lambie SH, Taal MW, Fluck RJ, McIntyre CW. Analysis of factors associated with variability in haemodialysis adequacy. Nephrol Dial Transplant 2004;19:406–12.

51. McIntyre CW, Lambie SH, Taal MW, Fluck RJ. Assessment of haemodialysis adequacy by ionic dialysance: intra-patient variability of delivered treatment. Nephrol Dial Transplant 2003;18: 559–63.

52. Lindsay RM, Sternby J. Future directions in dialysis quantification. Semin Dial 2001;14:300–7.

53. Lambie SH, McIntyre CW. Developments in online monitoring of haemodialysis patients: towards global assessment of dialysis adequacy. Curr Opin Nephrol Hypertens 2003;12:633–8.

54. Garred LJ, Canaud B, Bosc JY, Tetta C. Urea rebound and delivered Kt/V determination with a continuous urea sensor. Nephrol Dial Transplant 1997;12:535–42.

55. Fernandez EA, Valtuille R, Willshaw P, Perazzo CA. Dialysate-side urea kinetics. Neural network predicts dialysis dose during dialysis. Med Biol Eng Comput 2003;41:392–6.

56. Olesberg JT, Arnold MA, Flanigan MJ. Online measurement of urea concentration in spent dialysate during hemodialysis. Clin Chem 2004;50:175–81.

57. Eddy CV, Arnold MA. Near-infrared spectroscopy for measuring urea in hemodialysis fluids. Clin Chem 2001;47:1279–86.

58. Fridolin I, Magnusson M, Lindberg LG. On-line monitoring of solutes in dialysate using absorption of ultraviolet radiation: technique description. Int J Artif Organs 2002;25:748–61.

59. Uhlin F, Fridolin I, Lindberg LG, Magnusson M. Estimation of delivered dialysis dose by on-line monitoring of the ultraviolet absorbance in the spent dialysate. Am J Kidney Dis 2003;41: 1026–36.

60. Arrigo G, Tetta C, Santoro A, Ghezzi P, Ronco C, Colasanti G, et al. Continuous urea monitoring in hemodialysis: a model approach to forecast dialytic performance. Results of a multi-center study. J Nephrol 2001;14:481–7.

61. Lindsay RM, Bene B, Goux N, Heidenheim AP, Landgren C, Sternby J. Relationship between effective ionic dialysance and in vivo urea clearance during hemodialysis. Am J Kidney Dis 2001; 38:565–74.

62. Katopodis KP, Hoenich NA. Accuracy and clinical utility of dialysis dose measurement using online ionic dialysance. Clin Nephrol 2002;57:215–20.

63. Kuhlmann U, Goldau R, Samadi N, Graf T, Gross M, Orlandini G, et al. Accuracy and safety of online clearance monitoring based on conductivity variation. Nephrol Dial Transplant 2001; 16:1053–58.

64. Hernandez-Herrera G, Martin-Malo A, Rodriguez M, Aljama P. Assessment of the length of each hemodialysis session by on-line dialysate urea monitoring. Nephron 2001;89:37–42.

65. Pobozy E, Radomska A, Koncki R, Glab S. Determination of dialysate creatinine by micellar electrokinetic chromatography. J Chromatogr B Analyt Technol Biomed Life Sci 2003;789: 417–24.

66. Farkas A, Vamos R, Bajor T, Mullner N, Lazar A, Hraba A. Utilization of lacrimal urea assay in the monitoring of hemodialysis: conditions, limitations and lacrimal arginase characterization. Exp Eye Res 2003;76:183–92.

67. Leypoldt JK, Lindsay RM. Hemodynamic monitoring during hemodialysis. Adv Ren Replace Ther 1999;6:233–42.

68. Sherman RA. Modifying the dialysis prescription to reduce intradialytic hypotension. Am J Kidney Dis 2001;38(Suppl 4): S18–25.

69. Santoro A, Mancini E, Basile C, Amoroso L, Di Guilio S, Usberti M, et al. Blood volume controlled hemodialysis in hypotension-prone patients: a randomized, multicenter controlled trial. Kidney Int 2002;62:1034–45.

70. Schroeder KL, Sallustio JE, Ross EA. Continuous haematocrit monitoring during intradialytic hypotension: precipitous decline in plasma refill rates. Nephrol Dial Transplant 2004;19:652–6.

71. Goldstein SL, Smith CM, Currier H. Noninvasive interventions to decrease hospitalization and associated costs for pediatric patients receiving hemodialysis. J Am Soc Nephrol 2003;14:2127–31.

72. Strippoli GF, Manno C, Schena FP, Craig JC. Haemoglobin and haematocrit targets for the anaemia of chronic renal disease. Cochrane Database Syst Rev 2003;(1):CD003967.

73. Collins AJ, Ma JZ, Ebben J. Impact of hematocrit on morbidity and mortality. Semin Nephrol 2000;20:345–9.

74. Collins AJ. Influence of target hemoglobin in dialysis patients on morbidity and mortality. Kidney Int 2002;80(Suppl):44–8.

75. Horl WH, Macdougall IC, Rossert J, Rutkowski B, Wauters JP, Valderrabano F. Predialysis survey on anemia management: patient referral. Am J Kidney Dis 2003;41:49–61.

76. Marooney M. Comparative analysis between centrifuged hematocrit and "point-of-care" hemoglobin: impact on erythropoietin dosing. ANNA J 1998;25:479–81.

77. Agarwal R, Heinz T. Bedside hemoglobinometry in hemodialysis patients: lessons from point-of-care testing. ASAIO J 2001;47:240–3.

78. Lacson E Jr., Ofsthun N, Lazarus JM. Effect of variability in anemia management on hemoglobin outcomes in ESRD. Am J Kidney Dis 2003;41:111–24.

79. Turco TF. Health care outcomes case study: anemia in end-stage renal disease. Am J Health Syst Pharm 1995;52(Suppl 4): S19–23.

80. Frankenfield DL, Johnson CA. Current management of anemia in adult hemodialysis patients with end-stage renal disease. Am J Health Syst Pharm 2002;59:429–35.

81. Balshaw-Greer A, Casey J. Encouraging self-administration of erythropoietin. EDTNA ERCA J 2003;29:96–9.

82. Chuang P, Parikh C, Reilly RF. A case review: anticoagulation in hemodialysis patients with heparin-induced thrombocytopenia. Am J Nephrol 2001;21:226–31.

83. Abramson S, Niles JL. Anticoagulation in continuous renal replacement therapy. Curr Opin Nephrol Hypertens 1999;8:701–7.

84. Holt AW, Bierer P, Glover P, Plummer JL, Bersten AD. Conventional coagulation and thromboelastograph parameters and longevity of continuous renal replacement circuits. Intensive Care Med 2002;28:1649–55.

85. Bommer J, Schwab M. Bedside testing with the new CoaguChek Pro activated clotting time assay in dialysis. Artif Organs 2002; 26:387–90.

86. Furuhashi M, Ura N, Hasegawa K, Yoshida H, Tsuchihashi K, Miura T, Shimamoto K. Sonoclot coagulation analysis: new bedside monitoring for determination of the appropriate heparin dose during haemodialysis. Nephrol Dial Transplant 2002;17: 1457–62.

87. Farmer CKT, Hobbs H, Mann S, Newall RG, Ndawula E, Mihr G, et al. Leucocyte esterase reagent strips for early detection of peritonitis in patients on peritoneal dialysis. Perit Dial Int 2000; 20:237–9.

88. Razek T, Olthoff K, Reilly PM. Issues in potential organ donor management. Surg Clin North Am 2000;80:1021–32.

89. Rosendale JD, Chabalewski FL, McBride MA, Garrity ER, Rosengard BR, Delmonico FL, et al. Increased transplanted organs from the use of a standardized donor management protocol. Am J Transplant 2002;2:761–8.

90. Baier KA, Markham LE, Flaigle SP, Nelson PW, Shield CF, Muruve NA, et al. Point-of-care testing in an organ procurement organization donor management setting. Clin Transplant 2003; 17(Suppl 9):48–51.

91. Viola RA, Abbott KC, Welch PG, McMillan RJ, Sheikh AM, Yuan CM. A multidisciplinary program for achieving lipid goals in chronic hemodialysis patients. BMC Nephrol 2002; 3:9–15.

92. National Kidney Foundation. K/DOQI clinical practice guidelines for bone metabolism and disease in chronic kidney disease. Am J Kidney Dis 2003;42(Suppl 3):S1–201.

Chapter **39**

Point-of-Care Testing in Oncology

Gilbert E. Wieringa

Point-of-care testing (POCT) in oncology provides opportunities to ensure a better quality of life and more effective resource utilization for a patient population that is rapidly increasing. In defining POCT, this chapter includes both geographic and time elements to highlight the opportunities for diagnostic tests to move closer to patients and better affect cancer outcomes. The limited literature on the subject belies the emerging potential of advances in phenotypic testing technology, which increasingly are being supplemented with rapid molecular diagnostic tests of alterations to DNA, the basis of all cancer.

SETTING THE SCENE

Worldwide Perspectives

The world burden of cancer is increasing, particularly in developing countries (1). From an estimated 10 million new cases in 1998, the incidence is set to double over the next two decades and the death rate will rise from 6 million to 10 million per annum. Until the mid 1990s, 50% of new cases came from developed countries. However, at that time, these countries represented only approximately one-quarter of the world's 5.6 billion population, highlighting cancer's preponderance as a disease of older people (65% of diagnoses are made in people over the age of 65 years) from more affluent societies. The likely shift in burden is perhaps reflected in worldwide population estimates that will see the currently defined developing world representing 85% of the predicted 7.8 billion population in 2025 (2).

Cancer Incidences in the Developed World

Cancer affects more than one in three people at some stage in their life. For the United Kingdom, the age-standardized incidence (i.e., the number of new cases per year) rose 1.6% for men and 6.3% for women every year between 1989 and 1999 (Figure 39-1). There are more than 200 recorded types of cancer, but four of these—breast (15%), lung (14%), colorectal (13%), and prostate (9%)—accounted for over half of all new cases in 2001 (3). For women, breast cancer was by far the most common (29% of all new cases) followed at some distance by colorectal cancer (12%). For the first time in 1999, prostate cancer in men superseded lung cancer as the most common type, 19% and 18%, respectively. Part of this reflects the decreasing lung cancer rate, but it may also be due to the rise in prostate cancer incidence reported above the age of 50

and increases in testing for prostate specific antigen (PSA). Across the European Community (EC), similar trends emerge but with some regional disparities (4).

In the United States, cancer incidence declined on average 1.1% between 1992 and 1998 (5). Similar to Europe, breast, lung, prostate, and colorectal cancer accounted for 56% of all new cases. Similar long-term trends are seen for lung cancer, i.e., a falling incidence, particularly in men, reflecting altered smoking patterns. For women, breast cancer incidence increased by 40% between 1973 and 1998 but mortality rates continue to decrease. For prostate cancer, the sharp rise in incidence in the 1980s perhaps reflected the earlier interest and the beginning of more PSA testing.

CHALLENGES TO DELIVERING CANCER STRATEGIES

As survival continues to improve due to advances in care (Figure 39-2), cancer will become a much longer term, chronic illness that imposes additional burdens on existing services. Evidence of the ongoing burden in the United Kingdom was the inability during 2002 to reduce the percentage of cancer patients waiting for longer than two months between referral and first treatment (6). For those already diagnosed, the challenges for many health systems are to ensure:

- More effective deployment of existing resources across and within different healthcare sectors (7). For example, advances in surgical and medical treatments allow a greater use of day-case and outpatient settings (Figure 39-3) but require a redeployment of resources to support such developments.
- New investment: The UK government, in part fueled by data from the EUROCARE-2 study showing relatively poor 5-year survival for several common cancers (8), identified an additional £1.26 billion in 2000 for its NHS Cancer Plan for faster, more convenient, higher-quality cancer care for patients at the center (9). Determining the balance of investment between additional staff, facilities, and technologies has been identified by others as the greater challenge to ensuring optimum clinical and financial outcomes in cancer care (6).

Preventive education programs can successfully influence incidence rates. These have been the central themes of strate-

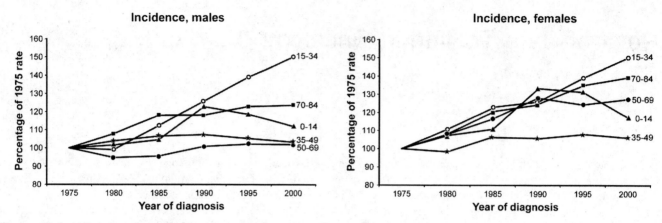

Figure 39-1   All malignant neoplasms except melanoma skin cancer incidence in England and Wales, 1975–2000. Modified by Cancer Research UK; reproduced with permission.

gies to reduce the incidence of lung cancer in the developed world. Awareness campaigns in Australia and New Zealand have highlighted excessive sunlight exposure as a risk factor for malignant melanoma, and these models are increasingly being adopted across Europe and in the United States (10).

Future challenges will also be to identify further cost-effective cancer screening programs that use state-of-the-art diagnostic tests and treatment. Controversy still surrounds the contribution of mammography-based programs in reducing breast cancer incidence, and a recent report of survival trends worldwide shows that individual national programs do not necessarily exploit best practice and policy (11). However such reports provide further baselines for refining and developing best practice.

Contribution of Diagnostics

Advances in laboratory medicine and diagnostic radiology technologies have provided much of the oncologist's means for achieving better outcomes in cancer care. Examples are positron emission tomography imaging, which now allows

sites for chemotherapy and/or surgery to be targeted with pinpoint accuracy, and modern linear accelerators, which allow radiation doses to be accurately delivered to cancerous tissue. In laboratory medicine, a greater understanding of malignancy has seen the emergence of new phenotypic and genotypic biomarkers that can aid in the following:

- Screening
- Diagnosis and staging
- Management
- Prognosis

Many of the technological advances allow such biomarkers to be taken closer to patients. However translating this benefit into altered clinical practice requires an understanding of the contribution of diagnostics that goes beyond technical performance (12). Although conventional outcome measures such as morbidity and mortality may often be inappropriate for diagnostics, there are numerous surrogate markers that allow near patient testing to present its contribution. These include:

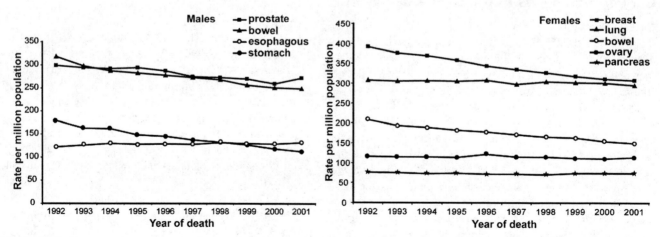

Figure 39-2   European age-standardized mortality rates for selected cancers, United Kingdom, 1992–2001. Not shown, male lung cancer rates fell from 840 per million in 1992 to 620 per million in 2001. Cancer Research UK; reproduced with permission.

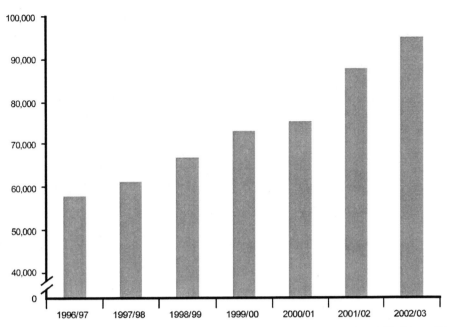

Figure 39-3 Day-case and outpatient treatment numbers from 1996–2003 at Christie Hospital NHS Trust, Western Europe's largest stand-alone cancer treatment center. Reproduced with permission.

- Faster and more informed clinical decisions
- Greater patient and clinician satisfaction
- Reduced length of hospital stay
- Reduced length of clinic stay
- Reduced referrals to hospitals and clinics
- Reduced cost of care

Such measures are more closely associated with, for example, clinical decisions to justify altered treatment protocols and organizational decisions in the deployment of new and existing resources. Rainey (13) has highlighted the opportunities for matching advances in POCT to clinical and financial need (outcomes) at a time when conventional laboratory testing can still be used as the control or gold standard. For cancer services, the most relevant of advances in laboratory testing should allow greater contributions to screening, diagnosis, and management. A consideration of these issues forms the focus of this chapter.

POINT-OF-CARE TESTING APPLICATIONS IN CANCER SCREENING

In the main, diagnostic tests are used as first-line tests to rule out the need for further investigations that may lead to a diagnosis. Their attraction is that they are relatively cheap compared with investigations such as biopsy, and continuing advances in technology allow aspects of the testing process to be offered nearer to patients. This section discusses those cancers for which POCT devices/opportunities are available. For laboratory medicine, the responsibility is to ensure that a favored test can meet its expected requirements.

Colorectal Cancer

There is little argument that screening for colorectal cancer (CRC) meets Wilson and Jungner's criteria of an appropriate condition, treatment option, and screening program organization (14). The presymptomatic phase of CRC, when screening would take place, may last many years, during which time many individuals will have resectable bowel wall–contained disease (Duke's A CRC stage) for which 5-year survival is 83%. However, 90% of those who currently present with CRC already have bowel wall penetration or spread of the disease to lymph nodes or elsewhere; up to 27% have metastatic spread at presentation (Duke's D) for which 5-year survival is 3%. Treatment costs of CRC in the United Kingdom exceed £250 million per annum, and the cost per year of life saved through screening is estimated at £6500, which compares well with many other established treatments such as renal transplantation.

The controversy is in the choice of screening test (14, 15). The gold standard is colonoscopy, which has the capacity to visualize the full length of the colon and detect many if not all lesions, particularly adenomatous polyps from which 70–90% of CRC appears to develop. Flexible sigmoidoscopy, which examines only the lower part of the bowel, is less effective and detects ≈66% CRC. Overall, endoscopic techniques could achieve a 70–80% cancer mortality reduction, but widespread introduction would require massive resource investment (staff, facilities, technology). The currently favored cost–benefit approach is a combination of fecal occult blood testing and sigmoidoscopy. Frazier et al. (16) calculate that of 22 potential screening strategies, addition of flexible sigmoidoscopy every 5 years to annual fecal occult blood testing in patients older than 50 years could produce an 80% reduction in CRC mortality. Winawer's approach, endorsed by many US healthcare organizations, is annual testing of two stool samples from each of three consecutive stools, with colonoscopy (or sigmoidoscopy) follow-up for any positive sample (17).

Many features of fecal occult blood testing make it suitable as a point-of-care test. The self-testing element is relatively easy to carry out, and samples are stable for prolonged periods. The analytical element is also relatively easy to carry out, requires no dedicated instrumentation, and is reported as a semiquantitative result. Taking such a diagnostic test closer to patients provides opportunities for greater engagement in the clinical process, part of which must be to inform of its many limitations (14, 15). A significant issue is poor sensitivity, i.e., false negatives (e.g., from nonbleeding tumors or poor sampling) that give false reassurance, leading to delayed/missed diagnosis and worse prognosis. The Haemoccult II method (Smith Kline Diagnostics, Munich, Germany) used in both the Nottingham (76,000 people in each of the screened and non-screened groups) and the Danish (31,000 in each group) randomized control trials has a reported sensitivity of 37.1% for detecting clinically proven CRC; mortality reduction in these trials was 15% and 18%, respectively. Sensitivity also varies across methods, as does their assay principle. False positives may occur due to dietary heme/peroxidases, non–colorectal-related bleeding, iron supplements, ascorbic acid, and rehydration of samples (to increase analytical sensitivity). The 4.2% false-positive rate reported by Rozen et al. (18) causes concern for the "worried well" and can lead to unnecessary (and expensive) follow-up. These issues highlight the laboratory contribution in providing informed communication and close participation in the delivery of the appropriate diagnostic test, the choice of which lies within the jurisdiction of individual trial organizers.

No trial has sought to use self-testing/interpretation kits available via Internet advertising and/or some pharmacies (19). These methods require a color interpretation of a test pad placed in the lavatory bowl after a bowel movement. Extensive performance data are not available, and concern has been expressed about their potential to misinform purchasers (20).

Given the reasonably well-understood limitations of fecal occult blood testing, the still-awaited cost–benefit analysis of endoscopy-based screening, and the potential for a future screening program based on a combination of these two tests, the UK government in 2003 recommended a second phase to its pilot study evaluating the feasibility of fecal occult blood testing. An important issue to emerge from the first pilot has been the low (60%) compliance rate that has perhaps highlighted the need for greater concordance (engagement and agreement) with patients to ensure their participation.

Prostate Cancer

Few cancers generate greater controversy than prostate cancer. It is perhaps a reflection of the weakness of the current evidence base for screening and the influence of public opinion that so many different policy recommendations have emerged.

In the United Kingdom, more centralized medical decision making has led to the introduction of a single prostate cancer risk-management program based on informed patient choice. In the United States, a more devolved medical culture, along with an engaged public and commercial lobbying, has ensured a variety of practices. Proponents of screening advocate that the rise and then fall in both incidence and mortality in the United States can be attributed to PSA testing and treatment changes (21). Opponents' concerns include the unnecessary detection of men who would die with, rather than from, the disease, the risks associated with carrying out prostate biopsy, the low number of individuals thought to benefit from radical treatment, and the costs of screening (22).

Digital rectal examination has little value as a screening test. Identifying at-risk individuals currently relies on serum PSA testing, but this also has its limitations. What represents an abnormal PSA is controversial. A 4-μg/L cutoff is widely used, seemingly on the basis of historical precedent rather than evidence (23). At this level, positive predictive values of 26% (sensitivity 44%, specificity 94%) can be achieved, but two-thirds of cancers can also be missed. In the European Randomised Study of Screening for Prostate Cancer, 36.5% of detectable cancers were found in the 87.5% of men with PSA <4 μg/L (24). This cutoff also ignores the effect of variability in results of different methods due to calibration differences (25). Use of the recently introduced First International Standard for PSA may rectify this situation. A single cutoff may also be inappropriate given the presumed physiological increase in PSA with age. However, defining age-specific reference ranges is made more challenging by the inability to confirm "normality" (identification of disease-free individuals) and the need to apply appropriate statistics to large data sets. Whether PSA and/or free PSA or complexed PSA or PSA velocity calculations are the most appropriate parameters also remains to be resolved (26).

Despite the number of societal and laboratory issues in prostate cancer screening, enthusiasm for the introduction of PSA home-testing kits has not been deterred, presumably reflecting public interest and demand. Given that issues of sensitivity, accuracy, and informed decision making are likely to be of relevance, literature reports vary in enthusiasm for their wider adoption. Reports of good agreement with laboratory-based methods across a wide range of values (27–29) have been tempered by closer evaluation of results around the 4-μg/L cutoff. Oberpenning et al. (30) reported that the agreement rate (concordance above and below 4 μg/L) between a laboratory-based assay and a semiquantitative immunochromatographic strip method in the range 0.1–11.3 μg/L was 53%, sensitivity 50%, and specificity 76%—barely superior to random chance. These authors also noted difficulties with test handling, results interpretation, the psychological distress for patients with false positives, and the risk of missed diagnoses due to false negatives. For the immediate future, it seems unlikely that these technologies can be recommended for rule-out testing, and any clinical application will more likely be in detection of unequivocally raised PSA values. Given the wider controversies surrounding prostate cancer screening programs and the already-recognized challenges to laboratory-based PSA testing, the contribution to the debate of POCT may not be realized at this time.

Cervical Cancer

Screening programs are widely exploited in the developed world and are aimed at detecting the largely asymptomatic, preinvasive phase of benign lesions that are amenable to treatment such as surgery and/or radiotherapy. Invasive cancer is associated with high mortality—only 27% 5-year survival for disease that has spread beyond the pelvis (stage 4), compared with 91% survival for those with stage 1 disease at diagnosis (31). The basis of screening is the cytological detection of dyskaryotic abnormalities in cells scraped from the cervix at the squamo-columnar junction. Specimens may be collected using the Papinacolaou (Pap) test, in which a spatula is used to collect cells that are spread and fixed on a microscope slide (the smear test) prior to being referred for laboratory interpretation. More recently, liquid-based cytology has been approved by the UK National Institute for Clinical Excellence (NICE) for sample processing (32). Specimens are collected by a brush-type device and transported to the laboratory in a preservative fluid. Liquid-based cytology is associated with fewer inadequately collected specimens (9.1% vs. 1.6%) and higher sensitivity and specificity.

Given the cost and anxiety caused by repeating inadequately collected specimens and the skill required to collect specimens from the appropriate site, screening programs demand trained healthcare professionals for their collection. Self-administered specimen collection devices have, however, been evaluated in a number of countries where the social stigma of participation in smear testing has affected screening program compliance. In Thailand, the Kato device has been reported as a successful alternative for women too shy to undergo pelvic examination or those who have limited time to visit health centers. An evaluation of this device showed a 78% agreement for detection of cellular changes (33). In Mexico, self-collecting vaginal sampling devices for the human papilloma virus (thought to be the essential causative agent in one or more stages of development of over 95% cases of cervical cancer) were much preferred by trial participants to Pap testing (34), but comparative sensitivity and specificity data have not been reported. Perhaps the most important contribution of such self-testing approaches is that they ensure a greater participation in screening programs, albeit with remaining concern about missed diagnoses.

Bladder Cancer

There are no formal screening programs, and protocols for the detection of new cases are dictated by local imperatives and stringencies. It is the sixth-commonest malignancy worldwide, the second most common cancer in men in France, and the fourth-commonest in the United Kingdom (4). The gold standard for diagnosis is cystoscopy and histology, which is an invasive, labor-intensive, and uncomfortable procedure for patients. At diagnosis, ≈75% of transitional cell carcinomas (TCCs, the commonest cell type in developed countries) are superficial, ≈20% are muscle-infiltrating (half of these will develop into metastatic disease), and ≈5% are already metastatic (35). Superficial cancers are amenable to conservative treatment (tumor removal with bladder retention), but clinical outcome varies considerably.

Diagnostic tests to identify superficial TCCs have included laboratory-based cytology of voided urine and hematuria detection by dipstick, but, given the poor evidence base, no hierarchical policies for their application have emerged. Although specific (>90%), cytology's poor sensitivity (48–62%) makes it inadequate as a rule-out screening test (36). It also requires trained personnel and has a poor record of interobservational variability. Self-testing may detect hematuria, but this is a common incidental finding with broad differential diagnoses (37).

Of interest is the advent of new urine markers with reported sensitivities greater than cytology, albeit in only a limited number of studies. Examples are the qualitative bladder tumor antigen BTA stat self-test (Polymedco, Cortlandt Manor, NY, USA; Figure 39-4) and the quantitative nuclear matrix

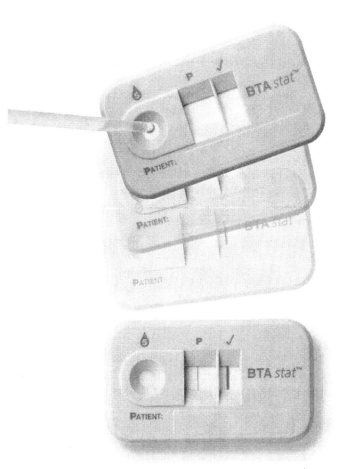

Figure 39-4 Polymedco's BTA-stat bladder cancer self-test. Registered trademark of Polymedco Inc., Cortland Manor, New York, USA; reproduced with permission.

protein NMP-22 test (Matritech, Cambridge, MA, USA) with respective sensitivities of 66–74% and 60–73% (38). Overall, such markers might potentially replace urine cytology, although none have the sensitivities that would normally be considered adequate for a screening program. Combined test approaches could increase predictive values and, in this regard, use of telomerase assays (with a sensitivity of ≈75%, but using a laboratory-based PCR assay) and cytology has been advocated (36). Further studies are required to assess the contribution of these and other emerging markers such as fibrin degradation products, cytokeratins, and NMPs such as BLCA4.

POINT-OF-CARE TESTING APPLICATIONS AS AIDS IN CANCER DIAGNOSIS

Histology remains the gold standard. However, the diagnostic process is increasingly being enhanced by rapid molecular diagnostic techniques able to identify the 25–30% of common cancers with a heritable component for which earlier detection of germ-line mutations allows prophylactic treatment and/or chemoprevention to be offered (39). These include breast cancer (the BRCA1/2 predisposition genes), bowel cancer (familial adenomatous polyposis and hereditary nonpolyposis colorectal cancer), prostate cancer, and testicular cancer. The *bcr-abl* gene rearrangement to produce the Philadelphia oncogene in chronic myeloid leukemia (CML) is the best-recognized example among hematological malignancies. Here a reciprocal exchange (translocation) occurs between chromosome 9's *abl* and chromosome 22's *bcr* that promotes overproduction of leukemic cells. Rarer family cancer syndromes (1% of all cancers) with high penetrance include multiple endocrine neoplasias, neurofibromatosis, and retinoblastoma. Such techniques allow more informed diagnoses, accurate staging, and prognostic assessment. Further, the information gathered is then potentially applicable to pharmacogenomic studies (see later section).

Concerns that commercial expediency in exploiting rapid technological advances in genetic testing might adversely affect patient protection have led the UK Human Genetics Commission to conclude that such tests should not be sold directly to the public (40). Their report highlights the role of regulatory and professional bodies in ensuring stricter controls, discouraging home testing and sampling, and engaging in consumer education.

POINT-OF-CARE TESTING APPLICATIONS IN CANCER MANAGEMENT

The potential of technological and methodological advances being implemented closer to patients has only recently begun to be reported. An emerging theme is the potential of diagnostics closer to patients to influence therapeutic decisions. The overriding theme of all applications is their effect on clinical and financial outcomes.

Parathyroid Hormone Measurements During Surgery

Unsuccessful parathyroidectomy, marked by persistently raised serum calcium postoperatively, occurs in 5–10% of patients and usually requires reoperation. The availability of real-time parathyroid hormone (PTH) measurements may allow preoperative tumor localization studies, recognition of suspicious nonparathyroid tissue, and confirmation of successful surgery (PTH has a half-life of ≈3.5 min). The assay (14 min analysis time from venepuncture) may be carried out during surgery and has been shown to improve the success rate of repeat surgery from 76% to 94% (41). In addition, it has enabled parathyroidectomy to become a day-case procedure with improved patient and clinician satisfaction and reduced costs (42).

C-reactive Protein and Full Blood Count Measurement at Hematological Oncology Clinics

Raised C-reactive protein (CRP) levels can provide an early indication of bacterial infection in patients with hematological malignancies, who frequently are immune-compromised and anemic (43). Whole blood CRP and full blood count testing at the point of care (ABX Micros-CRP, ABX Diagnostics, Shefford, Bedfordshire, UK; Figure 39-5) in outpatient settings has proven to be a valuable adjunct in reducing the number of samples referred to the central microbiology laboratory, improving patient throughput by 30%, hence providing scope for greater utilization planning, enhancing patient satisfaction, and encouraging greater ownership of results (44).

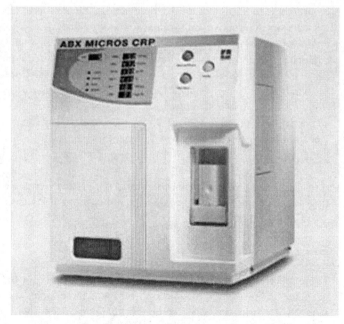

Figure 39-5 ABX Diagnostics' Micros-CRP whole blood analyzer. ABX Diagnostics, Shefford, Bedfordshire, UK; reproduced with permission.

Renal Function Tests to Aid Chemotherapy Dosing Decisions

The common action of all chemotherapeutics is to interfere with DNA replication. Frequency and size of dosing are dictated by the potential toxicity to normal tissue and the residual function of those tissues involved in drug metabolism and excretion (mainly the liver and kidney). Renal and electrolyte complications are not uncommon, as many agents are nephrotoxic. Factors governing dosing decisions include age, weight, surface area, and surrogate indices of renal function such as serum creatinine, which is sometimes used in conjunction with nomograms to calculate the glomerular filtration rate. Rapid access to measurements of whole blood urea, electrolytes, blood gases, and creatinine will enable faster management decisions, enhanced patient satisfaction, increased clinic capacity, and better organized chemotherapy preparation services.

Therapeutic Drug Monitoring

Most chemotherapeutic agents used in oncology exert their action across a sufficiently broad toxic/therapeutic window such that surrogate markers of adverse effects at the point of care such as serum creatinine are able to provide the necessary diagnostic support that contributes to better outcomes. For others direct monitoring is warranted, the results of which in turn influence the outcome of further therapeutic interventions. An example is the use of high-dose methotrexate to inhibit dihydrofolate reductase activity, in turn depleting reduced folate pools and hence DNA synthesis. Decisions to prescribe folinic acid rescue to replenish overdepleted pools are based on results of methotrexate assays, which act as the surrogate marker of reserve (45). Rapid diagnostics allow earlier interventions and also advice on toxic adverse effects such as renal impairment, gastrointestinal obstruction, pleural effusion, and ascites. Dosing of cyclosporin, a nephrotoxic immunosuppressant widely used during peripheral blood stem cell transplantation, is increasingly based on 2-h postdose single-point sampling to determine further interventions that ensure a favorable balance between toxic and therapeutic effects (46). The continued development of new agents challenges the laboratory to consider the potential contribution of POCT

Free Light-Chain Determinations in Multiple Myeloma

Sensitive (1.5-mg/L detection limit) latex-enhanced immuno-turbidimetric assays for κ and λ light chains with 13-min analysis times can now be offered nearer to patients as part of biochemical profile testing (47). The new assays could provide:

- *Earlier detection of treatment response.* Traditionally, response to chemotherapy is monitored through changes in the relevant intact serum immunoglobulin and/or urine Bence Jones protein by electrophoresis/densitometric scanning. The shorter half-life of light chains (4–6 h vs. 23, 6, and 5 days for IgG, IgA, and IgM, respectively) allows

opportunities for one set of serum assays to provide earlier information on the success of treatment for >99% of myeloma types.

- *Improved monitoring of Bence Jones myeloma.* Bence Jones protein in urine only becomes detectable when the renal reabsorptive threshold is exceeded and/or renal function is sufficiently compromised. As such, serum is the preferred medium for earlier detection of disease activity.

Initial evaluations suggest the assays are applicable on a variety of available analyzers. Such assays could have an impact on clinical outcomes (earlier decisions on treatment choices, prognostic assessment, and disease relapse detection), financial outcomes (earlier cessation of unsuccessful treatment), and organizational outcomes (resource implications of replacing electrophoresis-based quantification methods for Bence Jones protein and reduced number of clinic visits) (48, 49).

Serum Her-2/*neu* Measurements in Breast Cancer

The Her-2/*neu* receptor is expressed on the cell surface of tumors in $\approx$30% of women with breast cancer. Although associated with worse prognosis, tumor cells expressing Her-2/*neu* may be specifically targeted with Herceptin™ to inhibit further proliferation. When given in conjunction with standard chemotherapy such as taxanes, clear evidence emerges of significantly longer times to disease progression, a higher and prolonged rate of response, and improved overall survival (50). Such has been its success that UK's NICE recommended in 2002 that Herceptin should be made available to all Her-2–positive women with advanced breast cancer. Monitoring treatment is a potential application of serum Her-2/*neu* assays, which measure the extracellular domain of the receptor shed into the circulation (51). Some early observation studies warrant larger follow-ups. Esteva et al. (52) reported that serum Her-2/*neu* levels decreased significantly in 87% of women with metastatic breast cancer (MBC) who had responded clinically to Herceptin/docetaxel. Dnistrian et al. reported an 87.5% concordance between serum changes and the clinical course of disease in 54 MBC patients (53); Lüftner et al. (54) reported a 78.2% concordance.

The assays can be supplied as 20-min analyses on some immunoassay analyzers. With the increasing introduction of single-platform immunoassay and biochemistry analyzers, such diagnostics could be incorporated into stat analyses for influencing therapeutic decisions closer to the point of care. Earlier detection of those individuals not responding to Herceptin could enable clinicians to consider alternative, often less costly approaches. The cost of Herceptin was estimated in the United Kingdom at £20,000 per annum per patient in 2001. A readily accessible serum test could also provide earlier information for patients who might otherwise undergo radiological examination. Other applications of the assays, such as earlier detection of patients progressing to metastatic disease and in management of other cancers, require further investigation (55).

ADVANCES IN MOLECULAR DIAGNOSTICS

The increasing demand for, and supply of, rapid and accessible molecular diagnostics technologies provide new opportunities for translating the benefits of cancer research into clinical practice. Technologies such as Applied Biosystems' TaqMan (Foster City, CA, USA) and Roche's Light Cycler (Lewes, East Sussex, UK) allow point mutation detection in under 2 h, replacing separate, labor-intensive techniques for (a) DNA extraction from whole blood, (b) PCR for DNA amplification, and (c) electrophoretic techniques for identification of the PCR product. Single nucleotide polymorphisms (SNPs) are thought to account for >90% of genetic variation in the human chromosome. DNA sequencers and microchip array technologies, developed for example by Affymetrix (Santa Clara, CA, USA) and Incyte (Palo Alto, CA, USA), provide information on complex polymorphisms in <3 h. High-throughput arrays allow identification of clusters of differentially expressed genes that can act as biomarkers in their own right or from which phenotypic and/or genotypic biomarkers can be developed for analysis on single-platform analyzers. Such markers in turn can aid in discriminating cancer subtypes with different outcomes (see "Point-of-Care Testing Applications as Aids in Diagnosis," above) and potentially act as markers for a therapeutic target (pharmacogenomics applications, see below). A variety of samples may be used including blood, urine, buccal smears, and, increasingly, plasma. The contribution of newly emerging techniques such as surface-enhanced laser desorption ionization mass spectrometry (SELDI) awaits further evaluation (56).

For many cancers, a treatment plateau has been reached where different drug combinations often have little additional effect on survival. Significant advances are likely to come via pharmacogenomics using novel, targeted approaches (57). The determination of Her-2/*neu* status for Herceptin therapy is a recent example in clinical use and others are emerging. The use of the tyrosine kinase inhibitor Gleevec™ in CML, as a molecular target that recognizes the product of the *bcr-abl* gene rearrangement, is the most successful example of a designer drug that selectively attacks cancer cells (58). Rapid point mutation technologies can be used to identify such patients. Microarray technology has recently been successfully applied to subclassifying acute lymphoblastic leukemia responsiveness to chemotherapy and for prognostication (59). Such technology may also be applicable to bladder cancer staging, treatment selection, and monitoring of disease activity (60). Treatment outcomes to some platinum agents can be directly associated with SNPs in DNA excision repair genes (61). Although many such developments still sit on the interface between basic research and clinical practice, the ongoing translation process is likely to place new demands on diagnostic services

A further contribution of pharmacogenomics is in the detection of adverse drug reactions (ADRs) (57). For cancer therapy, ADRs are estimated to increase hospital running costs by 1.5% and drug costs by 15% (62), highlighting the need for faster diagnostic testing so as not to delay beneficial treatment. Examples of ADRs include severe or fatal toxicity to 5-fluorouracil due to dihydropyrimidine dehydrogenase (the drug's deactivating enzyme) gene polymorphisms; decreased survival during mercaptopurine treatment (used in childhood leukemias) due to polymorphisms in the thiopurine methyl transferase gene; increased chance of developing leukopenia and diarrhea during irinotecan therapy due to genotypic variation in hepatic UDP-glucoronosyltransferase (61)

CONCLUSIONS

Comparative evidence indicates the scope for greater efficiencies in individual healthcare systems (63) and the need to link health services research to clinical practice (64). Ham et al. (65), in comparing different delivery systems, have highlighted the strength of multidisciplinary approaches with evidence-based guidelines to determine the most appropriate level of clinical and diagnostic support needed to achieve more rapid and effective patient care. POCT provides opportunities for laboratory medicine to impact on healthcare outcomes by providing surrogate measures that can be readily integrated into cancer delivery strategies. Given the likely further advances in phenotypic and genotypic testing technologies, the opportunities to deliver diagnostics closer to patients are likely to increase and the examples cited here indicate only the beginning of the contribution of POCT to enhancing cancer care.

REFERENCES

1. World Health Report 1998. Life in the 21st century. a vision for all. Geneva, Switzerland: World Health Organization.
2. United Nations world population prospects: the 2002 revision population database. http://www.esa.un.org/unpp/p2k0data.asp (accessed January 2, 2004).
3. Cancer Research UK. Cancer incidence and mortality in England and Wales: trends and risk factors. http://cancerresearch.org.uk (accessed December 27, 2003).
4. Parkin DM, Bray FI, Devesa SS. Cancer burden in the year 2000: the global picture. Eur J Cancer 2001;37(Suppl 8):S4–66
5. Howe HL, Wingo PA, Thun MJ, Ries LA, Rosenberg HM, Fiegal E, et al. Annual report to the nation on the status of cancer, 1973–1998, featuring cancers with recent increasing trends. J Natl Cancer Inst 2001;93:824–42.
6. Sikora K, Bosanquet N. Cancer care in the United Kingdom: new solutions are needed. BMJ 2003;327:1044–6.
7. World Health Report 2003. Shaping the future. Geneva, Switzerland: World Health Organization.
8. Berrino F, Capocaccia R, Esteve J, Gatta G, Micheli A, Hakulinen T, et al. Survival of cancer patients in Europe. The EURO-CARE-2. Scientific Publication No. 151. Lyons: IARC, 1999
9. Department of Health. The NHS Cancer Plan. London: Department of Health, 2000.
10. Marks R. Campaigning for melanoma prevention: A model for a health education programme. J Eur Acad Dermatol Venereol 2004;18:44–7.

11. Coleman MP, Gatta G, Verdecchia A, Esteve J, Sant M, Storm H, et al. EUROCARE-3 summary: cancer survival in Europe at the end of the 20th century. Ann Oncol 2003;14(Suppl 5):V128–49

12. Price CP. Medical and economic outcomes of point of care testing. Clin Lab Med 2002;40:246–51.

13. Rainey PM. Outcomes assessment for point-of-care testing. Clin Chem 1998;44:1595–6.

14. Starkey BJ. Screening for colorectal cancer. Ann Clin Biochem 2002;39:351–65.

15. McArdle CS. Debate: faecal occult blood testing for colorectal cancer. Ann Oncol 2002;13:35–9.

16. Frazier LA, Colditz GA, Fuchs CS, Kuntz KM. Cost-effectiveness of screening for colorectal cancer in the general population. JAMA 2000;284:1954–61.

17. Winawer SJ, Fletcher RH, Miller L, Godlee F, Stolar MH, Mulrow CW, et al. Colorectal cancer screening with faecal occult blood testing and sigmoidoscopy. Gastroenterology 1997;112:594–642.

18. Rozen P, Knaai J, Samuel Z. Comparative screening with a sensitive guaiac and specific immunochemical occult blood test in an endoscopic study. Cancer 2000;89:46–52.

19. EZ DETECT™. www.craigmedical.com/occult_blood.htm (accessed December 23, 2003).

20. Howald K, Salkeld G. Home bowel cancer test and informed choice—is current information enough? Aust NZJ Public Health 2003;27:513–6.

21. Littrup PJ. Future benefits and cost-effectiveness of prostate carcinoma screening. Cancer 1997;80:1864–70.

22. Neal DE, Donovan JL. Prostate cancer: to screen or not to screen? Lancet Oncol 2000;1:17–24

23. Brawer MK, ed. Prostate specific antigen. New York: Marcel Dekker, 2001;1–327

24. Frankel S, Davey Smith G, Donovan J, Neal D. Screening for prostate cancer. Lancet 2003;361:1122–8.

25. Roddam AW, Price CP, Allen NE, Milford Ward A. Assessing the clinical impact of prostate specific antigen assay variability and non-equimolarity: a simulation study based on the population of the United Kingdom. Clin Chem 2004;50:102–6.

26. Price CP, Allard J, Davies G, Dawnay A, Duffy MJ, France M et al. Pre- and post-analytical factors that may influence use of serum prostate specific antigen and its isoforms in a screening programme for prostate cancer. Ann Clin Biochem 2001;38:188–216.

27. Berg W, Linder C, Escholz G, Link S, Schubert J. Possibility of improving the acceptance rate of early detection testing for prostate cancer with a one-step test for prostate specific antigen in whole blood. Urol Int 1999;63:102–6.

28. Dok An C, Yoshiki T, Lee G, Okada Y. Evaluation of a rapid prostate specific antigen assay: the One-Step PSA™ test. Cancer Lett 2001;162:135–9.

29. Jung K, Zachow J, Lein M, Brux B, Sinha P, Lenk S et al. Rapid detection of elevated prostate-specific antigen levels in blood: performance of various membrane strip tests compared. Urology 1999;53:155–60.

30. Oberpenning F, Hetzel S, Weining C, Brandt B, De Angelis G, Heinecke A, et al. Semi-quantitative immunochromatographic tests for prostate specific antigen in whole blood: tossing the coin to predict prostate cancer? Eur Urol 2003;43:478–84.

31. Cancer Research UK. CancerStats report. Cervical cancer. London: Cancer Research UK, 2003;1–8. Available at http://www.cancerresearchuk.org/aboutcancer/statistics/cancerstatsreport/ (accessed May 2004).

32. National Institute for Clinical Excellence. 2003/54 NICE guidance on liquid based cytology contributes to modernisation of cervical screening services for women. www.nice.org.uk.

33. Pengsaa P, Sriamporn S, Kritpetcharat O, Kamsa-Ard S, Suwanrunguang K, Noda S, Kakudo K. A comparison of cytology with pap smears taken by a gynecologist and with a self-sampling device. Asian Pac J Cancer Prev 2003;4:99–102.

34. Dzuba IG, Diaz EY, Allen B, Leonard YF, Ponce ECL, Shah KV, et al. The acceptability of self-collected samples for HPV testing vs. the Pap test as alternatives in cervical cancer screening. J Women's Health Gend Based Med 2003;11:265–75.

35. Landis SH, Murray T, Bolden S, Wingo PA. Cancer statistics 1999. CA Cancer J Clin 1999;49:8–31.

36. Glas AS, Roos A, Deutekom M, Zwinderman AH, Bossuyt PMM, Kurth KH. Tumor markers in the diagnosis of primary bladder cancer. A systematic review. J Urol 2003;169:1975–82.

37. Cohen RA, Brown RS. Microscopic Hematuria. N Engl J Med 2003;348:2330–8.

38. Lotan Y, Roehrborn CG. Cost-effectiveness of a modified care protocol substituting bladder tumor markers for cystoscopy for transitional cell carcinoma of the bladder: a decision analytical approach. J Urol 2002;167:75–9.

39. Cancer Research UK. CancerStats report. Genes and cancer. London: Cancer Research UK, 2002. http://cancerresearchuk.org (accessed May 2004).

40. Human Genetics Commission. Genes direct. Ensuring the effective oversight of genetic tests supplied directly to the public. London: Human Genetics Commission, 2003;1–78. Available at http://www.hgc.gov.uk/genesdirect/genesdirect_full.pdf (accessed May 2004).

41. Irvin GL, Molinari AS, Figueroa C, Carneiro DM. Improved success rate in reoperative parathyroidectomy with intraoperative PTH assay. Ann Surg 1999;229:874–8.

42. Chen H, Sokoll LJ, Udelsman R. Outpatient minimally invasive parathyroidectomy: a combination of sestamibi-SPECT localization, cervical block anesthesia, and intraoperative parathyroid hormone assay. Surgery 1999;126:1016–22.

43. Rintala E, Irjala K, Nikoskelainen J. Value of measurement of C-reactive protein in febrile patients with haematological malignancies. Eur J Clin Microbiol Infect Dis 1992;11:973–8.

44. British In Vitro Diagnostics Association. Cancer patients benefit from new management of diagnostic testing. Br In Vitro Diagn Assoc Spring Newsletter 2003;10:3. Available at http://www.bivda.co.uk/interest/index.cfm?ccs=152 (accessed May 2003).

45. Hallworth MJ, Capps NE. Therapeutic drug monitoring and clinical biochemistry. London: Association of Clinical Biochemists Venture Publications, 1993:70–3.

46. Andrews DJ, Cramb R. Cyclosporin: revisions in monitoring guidelines and review of current analytical methods. Ann Clin Biochem 2002;39:424–36.

47. Bradwell AR, Carr-Smith HD, Mead GP, Tang LX, Showell PJ, Drayson MT, et al. Highly sensitive, automated immunoassay for immunoglobulin free light chains in serum and urine. Clin Chem 2001;47:673–80.

48. Bradwell AR, Carr-Smith HD, Mead GP, Drayson MT. Serum free light chain immunoassays and their clinical application. Clin Appl Immunol Rev 2002;3:17–33.

49. Harland BE, Anderson JM, Overton J, Carr-Smith HD, Wieringa GE, Bradwell AR. The effect on laboratory organisation of introducing serum free light chain assays. Clin Chem 2004;50:A76.

50. Slamon DJ, Leyland-Jones B, Shak S, Fuchs S, Paton V, Bajamonde A, et al. Use of chemotherapy plus a monoclonal antibody against HER2 for metastatic breast cancer that over expresses HER2. N Engl J Med 2001;344:783–92.

51. Carney WP, Neumann R, Lipton A, Leitzel K, Ali S, Price CP. Potential clinical utility of serum HER-2/neu oncoprotein concentrations in patients with breast cancer. Clin Chem 2003;49: 1579–98.

52. Esteva FJ, Valero V, Booser D, Guerra LT, Murray JL, Pusztai L, et al. Phase II study of weekly docetaxel and trastuzumab for patients with HER-2 over-expressing metastatic breast cancer. J Clin Oncol 2002;20:1800–8.

53. Dnistrian AM, Schwartz MK, Schwartz DC, Ghani F, Kish L. Significance of serum HER-2/neu oncoprotein, CA 15-3 and CEA in the clinical evaluation of metastatic breast cancer. J Clin Ligand Assay 2003;25:215–20.

54. Lüftner D, Luke C, Possinger K. Serum Her-2/neu in the management of breast cancer patients. Clin Biochem 2003;36:233–40.

55. Molina R, Jo J, Zanon G, Filella X, Farrus B, Munoz M, et al. Utility of c-erbB-2 in tissue and serum in the early diagnosis of recurrence in breast cancer patients: comparison with carcinoembryonic antigen and CA15.3. Br J Cancer 1996;74:1126–31.

56. Diamandis EP. Proteomic patterns in biological fluids: do they represent the future for cancer diagnostics. Clin Chem 2003;49: 1272–8.

57. Marsh S, Mcleod HL. Cancer pharmacogenetics. Br J Cancer 2004;90:8–11.

58. Druker BJ. ST1571 (Gleevec) as a paradigm for cancer therapy. Trends Mol Med 2002;8:S14–8.

59. Yeoh EJ, Ross ME, Shurtleff SA, Williams WK, Patel D, Mahfouz R, et al. Classification, subtype discovery, and prediction of outcome in pediatric acute lymphoblastic leukaemia by gene expression profiling. Cancer Cell 2002;1:133–43.

60. Sánchez-Carbayo M. Use of high-throughput DNA microarrays to identify biomarkers for bladder cancer. Clin Chem 2003;49: 23–31.

61. Watters JW, Mcleod HL. Cancer pharmacogenomics: current and future applications. Biochem Biophys Acta 2003;1603: 99–111.

62. Wiffen P, Gill M, Edwards J, Moore A. Adverse drug reactions in hospital patients: a systematic review of the prospective and retrospective studies. Bandolier Extra at http://www.jr2.ox.ac.uk/bandolier/extra.html (accessed January 14, 2004).

63. Feachem RG, Sekhri NK, White KL. Getting more for their dollar: a comparison of the NHS with California's Kaiser Permanente. BMJ 2002;324:135–41.

64. Dash P, Gowman N, Traynor M. Increasing the impact of health services research. BMJ 2003;327:1339–41.

65. Ham C, York N, Sutch S, Shaw R. Hospital bed utilization in the NHS, Kaiser Permanente, and the US Medicare program: analysis of routine data. BMJ 2003;327:1257–60.

Chapter 40

Point-of-Care Testing in Hematology

Wouter W. van Solinge and Albert Huisman

The modern hematology laboratory can be divided into three different areas: hemocytometry [measuring the complete blood count CBC)], hemostasis and thrombosis, and blood transfusion (erythrocytes, plasma, and thrombocytes). These three areas differ markedly in their characteristics in respect to the need for a short turnaround time (TAT), accuracy, precision, automation, costs, 24-h availability, and other factors. Consequently, different aspects are important when considering the need of point-of-care testing (POCT) in these areas of hematology and laboratory medicine.

This chapter will focus on possible roles of POCT for those analytes measured in the hemocytometry and blood transfusion sections. In addition, some examples of special tests in hematology will be discussed. Aspects of POCT in hemostasis and thrombosis are dealt with in Chapters 41 and 42, respectively.

POCT can only be useful in those circumstances where the central laboratory cannot fulfill urgent clinical needs due to constraints in the organization's infrastructure, situations outside a hospital setting where no central laboratory is available, areas where results are urgently needed to improve patient outcome, or as a tool in direct patient management. The clinical need is based on the question of whether POCT speeds up decision making and results in better counseling, fewer visits to the hospital, better therapy, and in general affects patient outcome in a positive way. No matter how fast test results are generated, after reporting results to the clinic it must be kept in mind that treatment delays can still occur. The goal of laboratory testing is not achieved until the appropriate caregiver receives and reviews the results and takes any necessary clinical action. Several studies have raised concerns that responses to serious laboratory abnormalities may be inappropriate or delayed (1, 2).

In addition, POCT may improve work flow in the central laboratory because the number of stat samples will decrease, allowing for a more rational way of sample processing. Because the most common tests to be ordered outside routine hours are complete blood counts and clotting screens (3), introduction of hematology POCT may help to further reduce the number of staff needed in the central laboratory during evening or night shifts. We believe, however, that the value of POCT in hematology is rather limited, as discussed later.

HEMOCYTOMETRY ANALYTES: COMPLETE BLOOD COUNT

The CBC includes a variety of parameters as measured by modern hematology analyzers: these include hemoglobin (Hb), hematocrit (Hct), red blood cell (RBC; erythrocyte) count, erythrocyte indices [mean cell volume (MCV) of red cells, mean cell hemoglobin (MCH) content of red cells, and mean cell hemoglobin concentration (MCHC) of red cells], red cell distribution width (RDW), white blood cell (WBC; leucocyte) count, differential leucocyte count, platelet (thrombocyte) count, and mean platelet volume (MPV). The CBC is requested on a routine basis by physicians for a wide variety of diseases and indications. These include (among many others) the suspicion of anemia, changes in hemodilution/hemoconcentration, unexplained bleeding, infection, inflammation, leukemia (including myeloproliferative and lymphoproliferative disease), and bone marrow depression (induced by irradiation, cytotoxic drugs, immunosuppressive drugs, or antithyroid drugs). However, not all of these measured analytes are of clinical relevance in settings where POCT hematology testing may be required. Moreover, a recent survey indicated that many clinicians do not use all of the data provided in the routine CBC/differential investigation. Only Hb, Hct, platelet count, and WBC count were perceived as useful in daily clinical practice. Among primary care physicians, the MCV was also perceived as useful for the evaluation of anemia (4).

Laboratory requests for a CBC are among the most requested tests in daily practice. As the CBC in the central laboratory is performed by sophisticated automated hematology analyzers and preanalytical sample processing is not necessary, results generally can be reported within 15 min.

Several clinical settings are candidates for implementing POCT, as discussed throughout this book. Hematology POCT may be of use in the outpatient clinic, the intensive care and neonatal intensive care units (ICU/NICU), the emergency room (ER), the operating room (OR), the delivery ward, and the general practitioner or primary care physician's practice (rural environment) (Table 40-1).

HEMATOLOGY POCT IN THE OUTPATIENT CLINIC

In considering the effects of POCT in hematology, it is important to realize that the usefulness of POCT depends highly on the patient groups, where there is a clinical need and benefit may be demonstrated. Patients visiting the outpatient clinics generally already have a diagnosis and visit the clinicians for follow-up or to receive their next therapy. Alternatively, no diagnosis has been made and patients are referred to a consultant to be evaluated. In either case, it is likely that several laboratory tests will be requested, some of which cannot be undertaken using POCT. This may limit the rationale for POCT.

Fast hematology results are generally required at the outpatient clinic for hemato-oncology and oncology patients. These patients visit the clinic in order to receive their next treatment. The decision to start treatment is (among others) based on the WBC count, the WBC differential count, and the platelet count. Even modern state-of-the-art hematology analyzers may have serious difficulty in measuring CBCs and WBC differential count in patients with leukemia, undergoing chemotherapy, or being treated with hematopoietic growth factors. This is because these analyzers use algorithms based on a normal distribution of white cells and platelets. Invariably, these cells are either very low or absent, or severely abnormal in their characteristics in these patients and thus are difficult to measure accurately. No POCT devices currently on the market are capable of measuring these samples reliably. A word of caution is required here, since some companies market their equipment stating it is of value in hemato-oncology settings. No studies confirming these claims have been published to date.

Apart from these technical limitations, in our opinion, POCT testing is of no value in these patients, since invariably more laboratory tests will be requested when the patients comes to the outpatient clinic for follow-up and treatment.

Issues of fast TAT in these setting can be solved locally by use of, e.g., pneumatic tubing systems transporting samples to the central laboratory or, as in our hospital, by installing a dedicated state-of-the-art hematology analyzer on site (TAT < 15 min). This highly sophisticated analyzer may only be operated by trained laboratory technicians, since data generated by the machines in this clinical setting require professional review. This is effectively POCT using a benchtop analyzer for which the clinic staff can be trained or, alternatively, laboratory staff can attend the clinic at the relevant times.

Samples taken from other patient categories seen at the outpatient clinics may provide a fruitful opportunity for POCT, but again, there will in general be a need for a more elaborate test panel. The measurement of solely Hb or a WBC count will be rare, and even so, the result will not need to be available immediately. In addition, a patient's samples in other clinical diseases may have been taken a week in advance, making sure that the results are with the clinician when the patient visits. However, while this approach has been used for many years, e.g., in the diabetes clinic, it is now recognized that this may be inconvenient for the patient, and not in line with the patient-centered style of care which is now commonplace. In addition, when patients travel a distance to work, having to attend a phlebotomy service may involve taking time off work, which again is not popular.

HEMATOLOGY POCT IN THE INTENSIVE CARE AND NEONATAL INTENSIVE CARE UNITS

POCT in the ICU is widely implemented for blood gases and electrolyte measurements. In general, these POCT devices measure Hb as well as blood gases. Most currently available POCT devices produce accurate and reliable Hb and/or Hct results (5–7), provided that staff are appropriately trained in specimen handling as well as test performance. However, special care must be taken with neonatal specimens, as will be discussed later in this chapter. It has been shown that bedside measurement of Hb increases efficiency in patient care, decreases risk of blood-transmitted infection for staff, and decreases cost to the patient (8–12).

Table 40-1 POCT in Hematology

Clinical setting	Remarks
Outpatient clinic	No need for POCT hemocytometry. When short TAT is needed, optimization of logistics is required (e.g., pneumatic tubing system or a dedicated hemocytometer onsite).
Intensive care unit/neonatal intensive care unit	Hemoglobin is useful. WBC count, WBC differential count, and platelet count are not useful.
Emergency room/operating room	Hemoglobin is useful
	ER: WBC count, WBC differential count, and platelet count are not useful when adequate central laboratory facilities are available.
	OR: Point-of-care platelet function tests in cardiovascular surgery are currently under discussion.
Delivery room	Hemoglobin is useful.
General practitioner	Hemoglobin, if possible in combination with MCV, is useful.

Some patients may benefit when a fast test result for Hb is obtained. For instance, patients with active bleeding avoid delays when transfusion products are ordered from the laboratory. The clinical need for POCT WBC count is less clear. In most instances, a delay of 15 min in waiting for the result from the central laboratory is acceptable and will not influence direct medical intervention at the ICU. Again, in those patients where infection parameters are needed to assess further therapy, this decision will not be based on a WBC count alone; additional analytes will be requested as well.

The same reasoning applies to the clinical need for a platelet count at the bedside. When interpreting platelet counts at the ICU, invariably other analytes are needed in order to guide valid clinical decision making. In the case of the larger ICU, invariably there will be a hematology analyzer, or at least a rapid specimen transport arrangement.

When considering POCT in the NICU, again it is important to realize that even in the central clinical laboratory, samples from premature neonates may require special treatment before reliable blood counts can be generated. The erythrocytes are difficult to lyse and in addition, erythroblast and aberrant leucocytes are present in the circulation of these patients. These cells require modern hematology analyzers, as well as trained staff to interpret complex results.

A great advantage of POCT in the NICU, however, is the potential for reducing neonatal blood loss and, possibly, transfusion needs (13), because in general POCT devices use a smaller volume compared to standard laboratory equipment. This is of great clinical importance and improves the quality of care (14). However, it must be kept in mind that most hematology analyzers in the central laboratory can use volumes as little as 250 μL, although it may be the "dead volume" in the specimen collection tube that results in an unnecessarily large specimen volume being required.

The staff that perform the assays must adhere to the standard of practice to minimize errors in the measurements (15). Although this small-volume potential is very appealing, the results for Hb and Hct in this patient group are also less accurate (16). This seems to be dependent on the technology used. Photometric and centrifugation methods provide the closest approximation to the central laboratory hemocytometer. In contrast to conductivity methods (17), POCT devices based on the former technologies may produce more accurate results in this special patient group (18, 19).

In general, the need for hematology POCT in the IC/NICU is very limited. The only exception may be tests for coagulation.

HEMATOLOGY POCT IN THE EMERGENCY ROOM AND OPERATING ROOM

In the emergency room, POCT for Hb is useful when a patient is, or may be, bleeding. However, it must be kept in mind that immediately after an acute hemorrhage, the Hb levels are normal (20). Approximately 30 min after large blood loss, fluid shifts occur to correct the blood volume deficit for 12–36 h. As a result, there is a continuous decline in Hb levels (21). In trauma patients, there is in general a low prevalence of laboratory abnormalities. Considering the hematological laboratory parameters, only the Hb/Hct is sufficient for evaluation and management of the injured patient (22–24), and POCT is sufficient in the majority of cases (25). A study performed in trauma patients showed that Hb (among other POCT) measurements in patients with severe blunt trauma occasionally reduces morbidity and results in resource-conserving management changes (26).

The use of WBC count and WBC differential count in emergencies is limited. In general, results of these tests will not change therapy in an acute situation. However, the WBC count may be of use as a parameter of severity or as a predictive parameter in various types of injury (27–30). Reporting results within 1 h will most likely not change outcome. Because a central laboratory can generate a WBC count and in most cases a WBC differential count within 15 min after receiving the sample, POCT for WBC count and WBC differential count will not affect treatment. For example, antibiotics (infection) and antitumor therapy (leukemia) have an influence on the status of the patient on a larger time scale. In emergency room decision making, the WBC differential count is no more clinically significant than information obtained from the absolute WBC count alone (31, 32). Because of these observations, there is no need for POCT WBC count and WBC differential count in a hospital situation with a central laboratory facility, as is the case when an ER is operational. The situation may be different in situations were there are no laboratory facilities available; under these circumstances, a WBC count is sufficient.

The same reasoning for POCT in hematology support in the emergency room can be applied to the operating room: There is no requirement for POCT for leucocytes in the operating room.

Literature concerning the use of platelet count is scarce. Abnormalities in platelet count are rare. In common with WBC differential count, platelet count results will generally not change therapy or patient management on an acute basis. During extensive cardiac surgery, for instance, POCT evaluation of platelets (among others) can enable physicians to rapidly assess bleeding abnormalities. This facilitates optimal administration of pharmacological and transfusion-based therapy, identifies patients with surgical bleeding, and reduces the unnecessary use of blood products (33). Therefore, POCT for platelet count is not considered essential if adequate central laboratory facilities are available.

Interestingly, several POCT devices to rapidly determine platelet function have been developed (34–38). Especially during cardiovascular surgery, it is claimed that POCT to assess platelet function has added value in rapidly assessing bleeding abnormalities and thereby facilitating optimal intervention (33, 39–41). However, this is not confirmed in several other studies (42–47). In the light of the limited scope of these tests (only during cardiovascular surgery), their disputable efficacy, and complicated sample handling, it is not advisable to broadly introduce these specific tests into the clinic setting. However, since the central laboratory has no real alternative for rapid platelet function analysis, these tests are of interest. The laboratory should always be involved in evaluating these devices, the training of operators, and quality control.

HEMATOLOGY POCT IN THE DELIVERY UNIT

During delivery of the baby, rapid assessment of the Hb concentration can be mandatory. Usually, POCT is already undertaken in the delivery unit for blood gases and glucose. In general, only the measurement of Hb in the mother will be useful, since measurement of Hb using POCT devices in the neonate is prone to error (see under NICU). In addition, if anemia in the newborn is suspected, usually more laboratory tests will be needed, not all of which can be done by POCT.

HEMATOLOGY POCT FOR THE GENERAL PRACTITIONER

Because the incidence of anemia in the general population is high, the determination of Hb /Hct in the general practitioner's office may be useful. By ruling out anemia by means of POCT, unnecessary follow-up diagnostic procedures can be avoided. A recent study indicated that Hb alone is a valuable primary screening test, and a CBC is required only when anemia is present or when the patient's history and clinical signs indicate the need for further investigation. With this procedure, it is unlikely that any serious error in diagnosis will be made or the diagnosis of a clinically significant condition will be missed (48).

A large portion of laboratory tests requested by general practitioners involve a CBC. From a patient's point of view it would be convenient if the laboratory tests could be performed on site so that adequate therapy and clinical decision making in primary care can be established instantaneously. In practice, however, prescription of antibiotic therapy by the general practitioner is based solely on clinical evaluation and rarely on laboratory evaluation of the patient. If other diseases are suspected, e.g., leukemia, more tests will be requested and the patient will be referred to the hospital.

If POCT for Hb were done by the general practitioner, the MCV would be a useful parameter (4). Unfortunately, no such devices to measure this parameter are on the market to date.

TRANSFUSION

During or after a large hemorrhage, a decision must be made concerning transfusion therapy. Younger patients with a nor-

mal cardiovascular system tolerate an Hb decrease without hypoxic organ damage. However, transfusions with packed cells may be more urgently needed, for example, in elderly patients with cardiovascular disease. When a transfusion is needed, a specimen should be taken for ABO and Rhesus D typing and for antibody screening, cross match, and, if necessary, antibody typing. These elaborate tests may take a considerable amount of time. In situations compelling immediate action, transfusion may be necessary before laboratory results have become available. In these situations, there may be a limited clinical need for POCT at first sight. Several pretransfusion bedside compatibility tests are available. However, many publications indicate that the use of these tests is an unsafe procedure, and this should therefore be discouraged (49–51). Therefore, in our opinion, since transfusion laboratory procedures and techniques are complex and prone to errors, they require skilled and highly trained staff. Mistakes may be fatal to the patient, thus there is no place for these kinds of tests in a point-of-care setting. For situations requiring urgent transfusion with no time to wait for laboratory results, laboratory specialists and clinicians should establish guidelines for optimal patient treatment.

CONCLUSIONS

Since hematology laboratory tests are prone to erroneous results in certain patient groups (neonates, hemato-oncology patients, etc.), even when using state-of-the-art hemocytometers in the central laboratory, an important element of the hematology service is the interpretative function, including the impact of preanalytical factors. However, as has been described, there are several clinical settings in which a full hematological panel is extremely valuable, and in these situations there is often a bench-top analyzer installed, effectively creating an onsite, or stat, laboratory. At present, POCT in hematology is of limited value when considering handheld devices and can only be useful in a few clinical settings. Thus, when measuring hemoglobin concentrations, rapid results obtained using POCT will be of clinical value and improve patient outcome. This situation may change with the advent of miniature analyzers, described elsewhere in this book, enabling a full profile of tests, together with intelligent software to interrogate the data produced and report against well-validated diagnostic algorithms. This is being seen in other clinical settings, but in transfusion medicine there is no place for POCT.

REFERENCES

1. Kuperman GJ, Boyle D, Jha A, Rittenberg E, Ma'Luf N, Tanasijevic MJ, et al. How promptly are inpatients treated for critical laboratory results? J Am Med Inform Assoc 1998;5:112–9.
2. Lundberg GD. Critical (panic) value notification: an established laboratory practice policy (parameter). JAMA 1990;263:709.

3. Shirley J, Wing S. Workload, organisation, and cost of haematology laboratory out of hours services. J Clin Pathol 2001;54: 647–9.

4. Sandhaus LM, Meyer P. How useful are CBC and reticulocyte reports to clinicians? Am J Clin Pathol 2002;118:787–93.

5. Despotis GJ, Alsoufiev A, Hogue CW, Jr., Zoys TN, Goodnough LT, Santoro SA, et al. Evaluation of complete blood count results from a new, on-site hemocytometer compared with a laboratory-based hemocytometer. Crit Care Med 1996;24:1163–7.

6. Despotis GJ, Saleem R, Bigham M, Barnes P. Clinical evaluation of a new, point-of-care hemocytometer. Crit Care Med 2000;28: 1185–90.

7. Briggs C, Kunka S, Pennaneach C, Forbes L, Machin SJ. Performance evaluation of a new compact hematology analyzer, the Sysmex pocH-100i. Lab Hematol 2003;9:225–33.

8. Gehring H, Hornberger C, Dibbelt L, Rothsigkeit A, Gerlach K, Schumacher J, et al. Accuracy of point-of-care-testing (POCT) for determining hemoglobin concentrations. Acta Anaesthesiol Scand 2002;46:980–6.

9. Ray JG, Post JR, Hamielec C. Use of a rapid arterial blood gas analyzer to estimate blood hemoglobin concentration among critically ill adults. Crit Care 2002;6:72–5.

10. Agarwal R, Heinz T. Bedside hemoglobinometry in hemodialysis patients: lessons from point-of-care testing. ASAIO J 2001;47: 240–3.

11. Lardi AM, Hirst C, Mortimer AJ, McCollum CN. Evaluation of the HemoCue for measuring intra-operative haemoglobin concentrations: a comparison with the Coulter Max-M. Anaesthesia 1998;53:349–52.

12. Marooney M. Comparative analysis between centrifuged hematocrit and "point-of-care" hemoglobin: impact on erythropoietin dosing. ANNA J 1998;25:479–81.

13. Widness JA, Kulhavy JC, Johnson KJ, Cress GA, Kromer IJ, Acarregui MJ, et al. Clinical performance of an in-line point-of-care monitor in neonates. Pediatrics 2000;106:497–504.

14. Alex CP, Manto JC, Garland JS. Clinical utility of a bedside blood analyzer for measuring blood chemistry values in neonates. J Perinatol 1998;18:45–8.

15. Krenzischek DA, Tanseco FV. Comparative study of bedside and laboratory measurements of hemoglobin. Am J Crit Care 1996; 5:427–32.

16. Papadea C, Foster J, Grant S, Ballard SA, Cate JC, Southgate WM, et al. Evaluation of the i-STAT Portable Clinical Analyzer for point-of-care blood testing in the intensive care units of a university children's hospital. Ann Clin Lab Sci 2002;32:231–43.

17. McNulty SE, Torjman M, Grodecki W, Marr A, Schieren H. A comparison of four bedside methods of hemoglobin assessment during cardiac surgery. Anesth Analg 1995;81:1197–202.

18. Rechner IJ, Twigg A, Davies AF, Imong S. Evaluation of the HemoCue compared with the Coulter STKS for measurement of neonatal haemoglobin. Arch Dis Child Fetal Neonatal Ed 2002; 86:F188–9.

19. Gong AK. Near-patient measurements of methemoglobin, oxygen saturation, and total hemoglobin: evaluation of a new instrument for adult and neonatal intensive care. Crit Care Med 1995;23: 193–201.

20. Foltin GL, Cooper A. Abdominal trauma. In: Barkin RM, ed. Pediatric emergency medicine: concepts and clinical practise. St. Louis: Mosby, 1997:335–54.

21. Thomas L. Hematology. In: Thomas L, ed. Clinical laboratory diagnostics. Frankfurt am Main: TH-Books, 1998:463–547.

22. Bryant MS, Tepas JJ, III, Talbert JL, Mollitt DL. Impact of emergency room laboratory studies on the ultimate triage and disposition of the injured child. Am Surg 1988;54:209–11.

23. Jacobs IA, Kelly K, Valenziano C, Chevinsky AH, Pawar J, Jones C. Cost savings associated with changes in routine laboratory tests ordered for victims of trauma. Am Surg 2000;66:579–84.

24. Rothrock SG, Green SM, Morgan R. Abdominal trauma in infants and children: prompt identification and early management of serious and life-threatening injuries. Part I: Injury patterns and initial assessment. Pediatr Emerg Care 2000;16:106–15.

25. Frankel HL, Rozycki GS, Ochsner MG, McCabe JE, Harviel JD, Jeng JC, et al. Minimizing admission laboratory testing in trauma patients: use of a microanalyzer. J Trauma 1994;37:728–36.

26. Asimos AW, Gibbs MA, Marx JA, Jacobs DG, Erwin RJ, Norton HJ, et al. Value of point-of-care blood testing in emergent trauma management. J Trauma 2000;48:1101–8.

27. Rovlias A, Kotsou S. The blood leukocyte count and its prognostic significance in severe head injury. Surg Neurol 2001;55: 190–6.

28. Rainer TH, Lam PK, Wong EM, Cocks RA. Derivation of a prediction rule for post-traumatic acute lung injury. Resuscitation 1999;42:187–96.

29. Shah S, Miller PR, Meredith JW, Chang MC. Elevated admission white blood cell count in pregnant trauma patients: an indicator of ongoing placental abruption. Am Surg 2002;68:644–7.

30. Despotis GJ, Levine V, Goodnough LT. Relationship between leukocyte count and patient risk for excessive blood loss after cardiac surgery. Crit Care Med 1997;25:1338–46.

31. Badgett RG, Hansen CJ, Rogers CS. Clinical usage of the leukocyte count in emergency room decision making. J Gen Intern Med 1990;5:198–202.

32. Wenz B, Gennis P, Canova C, Burns ER. The clinical utility of the leukocyte differential in emergency medicine. Am J Clin Pathol 1986;86:298–303.

33. Despotis GJ, Skubas NJ, Goodnough LT. Optimal management of bleeding and transfusion in patients undergoing cardiac surgery. Semin Thorac Cardiovasc Surg 1999;11:84–104.

34. Peters AJ, Borries M, Gradaus F, Jax TW, Schoebel FC, Strauer BE. In vitro bleeding test with PFA-100-aspects of controlling individual acetylsalicylic acid induced platelet inhibition in patients with cardiovascular disease. J Thromb Thrombolysis 2001; 12:263–72.

35. Coiffic A, Cazes E, Janvier G, Forestier F, Lanza F, Nurden A, Nurden P. Inhibition of platelet aggregation by abciximab but not by aspirin can be detected by a new point-of-care test, the hemostatus. Thromb Res 1999;95:83–91.

36. Wheeler GL, Braden GA, Steinhubl SR, Kereiakes DJ, Kottke-Marchant K, Michelson AD, et al. The Ultegra rapid platelet-function assay: comparison to standard platelet function assays in patients undergoing percutaneous coronary intervention with abciximab therapy. Am Heart J 2002;143:602–11.

37. Carville DG, Schleckser PA, Guyer KE, Corsello M, Walsh MM. Whole blood platelet function assay on the ICHOR point-of-care hematology analyzer. J Extra Corpor Technol 1998;30:171–7.

38. Smith JW, Steinhubl SR, Lincoff AM, Coleman JC, Lee TT, Hillman RS, et al. Rapid platelet-function assay: an automated and quantitative cartridge-based method. Circulation 1999;99: 620–5.

39. Avidan MS, Alcock EL, Da Fonseca J, Ponte J, Desai JB, Despotis GJ, et al. Comparison of structured use of routine laboratory tests or near-patient assessment with clinical judgement in the management of bleeding after cardiac surgery. Br J Anaesth 2004;92:178–86.

40. Despotis GJ, Levine V, Saleem R, Spitznagel E, Joist JH. Use of point-of-care test in identification of patients who can benefit from desmopressin during cardiac surgery: a randomised controlled trial. Lancet 1999;354:106–10.

41. Despotis GJ, Joist JH, Goodnough LT. Monitoring of hemostasis in cardiac surgical patients: impact of point-of-care testing on blood loss and transfusion outcomes. Clin Chem 1997;43:1684–96.

42. Saleh N, Hansson LO, Kohut M, Nilsson T, Tornvall P. Platelet function and myocardial injury during percutaneous coronary intervention. J Thromb Thrombolysis 2002;13:69–73.

43. Fattorutto M, Pradier O, Schmartz D, Ickx B, Barvais L. Does the platelet function analyser (PFA-100) predict blood loss after cardiopulmonary bypass? Br J Anaesth 2003;90:692–3.

44. Cammerer U, Dietrich W, Rampf T, Braun SL, Richter JA. The predictive value of modified computerized thromboelastography and platelet function analysis for postoperative blood loss in routine cardiac surgery. Anesth Analg 2003;96:51–7.

45. Forestier F, Coiffic A, Mouton C, Ekouevi D, Chene G, Janvier G. Platelet function point-of-care tests in post-bypass cardiac surgery: are they relevant? Br J Anaesth 2002;89:715–21.

46. Serebruany VL, Alford AB, Meister AF, Fuzaylov SY, Gattis WA, Gurbel PA, et al. Clinical utility of the platelet function analyzer (PFA-100) for the assessment of the platelet status in patients with congestive heart failure (EPCOT trial). Thromb Res 2001;101:427–33.

47. Isgro F, Rehn E, Kiessling AH, Kretz KU, Kilian W, Saggau W. Platelet function test HemoSTATUS 2: tool or toy for an optimized management of hemostasis? Perfusion 2002;17:27–31.

48. Lewis SM, Osei-Bimpong A. Haemoglobinometry in general practice. Clin Lab Haematol 2003;25:343–6.

49. Ingrand P, Surer-Pierres N, Houssay D, Salmi LR. Reliability of the pretransfusion bedside compatibility test: association with transfusion practice and training. Transfusion 1998;38:1030–6.

50. Dujardin PP, Salmi LR, Ingrand P. Errors in interpreting the pretransfusion bedside compatibility test: an experimental study. Vox Sang 2000;78:37–43.

51. Migeot V, Ingrand I, Salmi LR, Ingrand P. Reliability of bedside ABO testing before transfusion. Transfusion 2002;42:1348–55.

Chapter 41

Point-of-Care Testing for Self-Monitoring of Oral Anticoagulation Therapy

Christopher P. Price and Andrew St John

Point-of-care testing (POCT) to assess anticoagulation status is now well established for a range of assays in hematology and hemostasis practice, including the operating room (Chapter 25) and the emergency room (Chapter 24), as well as in the primary care setting (Chapter 28). The latter development reflects the change in the approach to chronic disease management being seen in many healthcare systems throughout the world, and the demands of patients for a more user-friendly service. Thus, whereas in the past most patients on Coumadin (warfarin) therapy would have had to attend an outpatient clinic in a secondary care setting, today they may be able to visit their primary care center or even perform the tests themselves in their own homes or workplaces. In the secondary care setting, the "anticoagulation clinic" would usually be set up close to the hematology laboratory so that the patient's blood specimens could be taken, the analysis performed, and any dosage change made within a short time frame. However, this approach was still inconvenient for the patient, as it often required travel as well as time off work. In addition, many ambulance or hospital care journeys are devoted to transporting old or more infirm patients to the anticoagulation clinic.

DEVELOPMENTS IN TECHNOLOGY

The development of POCT has been a result of the advances in instrumentation, and of equal importance, advances in disposable reagent systems, particularly in relation to standardization of assay systems. A number of devices are now available for the POCT of prothrombin time (PT) that assess the integrity of the extrinsic and common pathways of coagulation, and some of these have been described in Chapter 3. The most common causes of abnormal PT are aberrations in oral anticoagulation therapy, vitamin K deficiency, liver dysfunction, and disseminated intravascular coagulation. A recent summary of the systems available for measurement of PT indicates the range of systems available for monitoring oral anticoagulation therapy, all of which use 10 to 65 μL of whole blood obtained from a fingerstick sample (1).

One of the main issues that has concerned laboratory personnel regarding the POCT systems for PT has been the variation in the quality and sensitivity of reagents. The result is that there can be a high inter–reagent lot variability in the PT results for any given patient's specimen. The sensitivity is represented by the international sensitivity index, with a low

level indicating a sensitive reagent. The international normalized ratio (INR), which is calculated from the PT reading and the international sensitivity index, can be used to nullify the effect of differences in reagent sensitivities. This was not so much of an issue when PT measurements were made in the laboratory, as it was possible to choose reagents with a required sensitivity, together with the use of a thromboplastin reference preparation for calibration. The European Concerted Action on Anticoagulation Group investigated the number of lyophilized plasma samples required for reliable international sensitivity index calibration in two POCT PT measuring systems—the CoaguChek Mini (Roche Diagnostics, Mannheim, Germany) and the TAS PT-NC (Pharmanetics, Morrisville, NC, USA). They found that the former required 30 Coumadin samples and 10 normal samples, whereas the latter required 20 Coumadin® or artificially depleted samples together with 7 normal samples to make it possible to obtain a reliable measure of the international sensitivity index (2). These estimates were significantly lower than the 80 samples recommended by the World Health Organization. The same group had checked the agreement in the INR values of the two systems and had found that correcting for the international sensitivity index reduced the variability between the two systems from 21.0% to 3.5% (3). The authors still believed that there was variability between the systems, which highlighted the need to maintain external quality assurance. The group went on to test a total of 60 lyophilized artificially depleted and 60 lyophilized Coumadin plasmas at 10 centers on the same systems, using subsets of three and five samples for quality assurance purposes (4). Although there was considerable variability in the INR values using the common set of 55 plasmas, it was shown that the lyophilized depleted samples could be used to provide useful quality assurance. Clearly there is a need for careful calibration of such systems as well as good quality assurance (5).

A number of studies have been published evaluating the use of devices for the assessment of INR. In a prospective multicenter study, Cosmi et al. (6) showed the CoaguChek to have a mean bias of −0.0675, +0.018, and +0.039 at INRs in the regions of <2.0, 2.0 to 3.0, and >3.0, respectively, with an overall coefficient of variation across the centers of 6.5%. Furthermore, they reported variations in performance among centers. In a prospective trial involving three laboratories and nine primary care centers, Hobbs et al. (7) compared more than 400 test results using POCT and the same laboratory procedure. Although the correlation between the results was good, it was estimated that 53% of the results obtained by POCT would have led to a different management decision, depending on the site and method of testing, with the method bias varying from 0.28 to 1.5. The authors stressed the importance of close liaison between the laboratory and the POCT site, especially with regard to training and quality assurance. The Oral Anticoagulation Monitoring Study Group recruited 386 patients to a multicenter study of POCT for PT (8). They found that the identification of the patient's therapeutic status based on INR was equivalent for POCT and the local hospital laboratory service, with 77% of the POCT results falling within 0.4 INR of the reference method. Overall, 93% of the results differed by <0.7 INR. In addition, the patients reported greater satisfaction with the POCT system. Shiach et al. (9) found a similar experience in a crossover study in which patients were managed on POCT and laboratory systems. The proportion of patients within the target range was 60.9% using POCT and 59.3% using a laboratory coagulometer for management. Patient questionnaires showed greater satisfaction with the community-based POCT monitoring program.

TRAINING AND QUALITY ASSURANCE

In a multicenter study, Cosmi et al. (10), using a portable PT monitor, evaluated the patient's capability to self-adjust oral anticoagulant dosage. A total of 78 patients were studied and were given three instruction sessions using a Coagucheck. They undertook the analysis at home and telephoned in their suggested dosage changes on the basis of the PT results obtained. They were then prescribed a change in dose that the health professional deemed appropriate. The authors found that the dosage changes suggested were within ±6% of the mean weekly dose in 80% and 82% of the suggestions for Coumadin and acenocoumarol, respectively. Similar findings were reported by Hasenkam et al. (11) and Morsdorf et al. (12). The latter group recruited 50 patients into a structured training program and tested their performance against a laboratory procedure. They found good agreement between the two testing modalities in most of the patients, although the POCT INRs were significantly lower compared with the venous samples tested by the laboratory. They found that the older patients took longer to master the technical details of the system. Sawicki described a structured teaching and self-management program for patients receiving oral anticoagulation therapy (13). The results of the randomized single-blind multicenter trial involving 179 patients showed that the deviation from the mean of the INR target range was significantly lower in the intervention group (trained) at 3 months (squared INR deviation 0.59 vs. 0.95, $P < 0.001$) and at 6 months (0.65 vs. 0.83, $P = 0.03$), compared with the control group. The intervention group also had INRs within the target range more often, with less frequent suboptimal INRs, compared with the control group (32% vs. 50% at 3 months and 34% vs. 48% at 6 months). The treatment satisfaction scores were also significantly higher in the intervention group.

Tripodi et al. (14) investigated the feasibility of a quality assurance program for PT POCT devices used by patients for self-testing. The patients were asked to analyze three recalcified plasma samples used as quality assurance samples together with analyzing their own blood, and also supply a sample to the laboratory for analysis. The results obtained by the patients for the quality assurance pilot study material were all within 20% of the laboratory consensus values. Furthermore, there were no significant differences between the results obtained by the patients on their own samples and those produced by the laboratory; all were within 20% of the laboratory value. The authors considered the program suitable for use by patients involved in self-monitoring, with an overall benefit for the patient. Murray et al. (15) undertook a similar study with 23 patients and 75 healthcare professionals contributing to an external quality assurance program. The study took place over 26 weeks, and the patients were trained in program participation. There was no significant difference between the median results on National External Quality Assessment Service samples obtained by the patients and those obtained by professionals, and three patients were outside of the consensus value for the INR (>15%) on more than one occasion. The coefficient of variation across the patient samples varied from 5.4% to 22.3%. The authors suggested that more research was required to determine the effect of the level of performance shown in the program and the clinical outcome.

Some of the factors that should be taken into account in delivering a reliable PT monitoring service are identified in Table 41-1.

USE OF TREATMENT ALGORITHMS AND DECISION SUPPORT TOOLS

A number of "test-and-treat" algorithms have been described, typically linked with some form of computerized dosage protocol. Fitzmaurice et al. (16) evaluated a computerized decision support tool in primary care in one health center practice, while in a second practice patients were randomly assigned to receive either computerized decision support or conventional care us-

Table 41-1 Important Issues Associated with Reliable Performance in the Self-Monitoring of INR

Training and certification of operator
Establishment of robust international sensitivity index for reagents and system used
Review of international sensitivity index for new reagent batches
Use of appropriate plasma samples for checking international sensitivity index
Regular maintenance of PT measuring equipment
Use of appropriate patient sample
Regular use of quality control
Participation in external quality assurance program
Regular audit (review) of clinical data
Regular contact with local laboratory professional

ing the local laboratory. There was a significant improvement in INR control (from 23% to 86%, $P < 0.001$) at the center using decision support. At the center where patients were randomly assigned to be managed with decision support, logistic regression showed a significant improvement ($P < 0.001$) compared with the patients managed by conventional care. There was also a notable extension of recall time in the decision support patients, with no difference in adverse events. In a larger randomized controlled trial involving more health centers (nine intervention and three control), Fitzmaurice et al. (17) showed an increase in time spent in the INR range for the intervention group ($P = 0.08$). The authors concluded that the approach was generally applicable to primary healthcare centers operating in developed healthcare systems. In a further paper, Fitzmaurice et al. (18) investigated whether their approach could work outside trial conditions. The study was undertaken as a form of retrospective audit over an 18-month period. Interestingly there was no difference in the time spent in range between the health center and hospital-based care (69% and 64%, respectively) but the proportion of tests in range was greater for the health center (61% vs. 57% for hospital-based care). Follow-up time did not differ between the groups. The authors concluded that this was a safe form of patient management.

Poller et al. (19) performed a randomized study of computerized support in five European centers involving 285 patients. Combining the data from all of the centers, the computerized support resulted in greater achievement of the target INR ($P = 0.004$), and the mean time within range was greater ($63.3 \pm 28.0\%$ vs. $53.2 \pm 27.7\%$, respectively) compared with the conventional treatment group. Manotti et al. (20) undertook a multicenter randomized controlled trial of computer-aided management involving 1251 patients, of whom 335 had been treated for only 3 months. Patients were randomly assigned to receive either computerized support or dosing based on the usual physician support. The investigators found faster stabilization of therapy ($P < 0.01$) in the computerized support group, and this group spent more time within the therapeutic range ($P < 0.001$). As seen in earlier studies, the improvement was attributable mainly to decreased time at a subtherapeutic level of oral anticoagulant. There was also a significant reduction in the number of appointments required ($P < 0.001$). Kovacs et al. (21) assessed a warfarin initiation nomogram in 105 consecutive referrals to outpatients. In their study, 83% of the patients reached the treatment goal in 5 days, and 98% reached the goal in 8 days. Furthermore, there were no reported incidents of bleeding, and the INR rose above 4.5 in only six cases. The authors concluded that the program was worthy of further study.

HEALTH OUTCOME STUDIES

It is clear from the studies already described that a number of outcome measures have been used in assessing POCT in the monitoring of oral anticoagulation therapy. Fitzmaurice et al. (22) performed a systematic review of the outcome measures

reported in relation to the therapeutic effectiveness of oral anticoagulants. The main outcome measures were the mean INR value, the time spent in the range, the proportion of patients in the range, and the mean Coumadin dose. Fifteen papers met the quality criteria, but fewer than 50% of these papers reported any one of these criteria. Six papers reported one outcome, six reported two outcomes, two reported three, and one paper reported four outcomes. Clearly, the objectives of the study will determine the outcome measures chosen, but the authors observed that more than one outcome measure is generally required for the results to be useable in practice. Some of the outcome measures that have been used to assess the utility of PT monitoring in monitoring oral anticoagulation therapy are indicated in Table 41-2.

Watzke et al. (23) undertook a prospective controlled trial of weekly self-monitoring and self-dosing, compared with the conventional approach to anticoagulation management. They studied only patients with stable anticoagulation status, including 49 patients using self-monitoring and dosing, compared with 53 patients on conventional management. Different target ranges were used for patients following heart valve replacement (INR = 2.5–4.5) than for patients with atrial fibrillation (INR = 2.0–3.0). The patients on weekly self-testing and self-dosing had more INR values within the therapeutic range than patients on standard management (86.2% vs. 80.1% at INR = 2.5–4.5; 82.2 vs. 68.9 at INR = 2.0–3.0). The mean INR achieved was almost identical to the target INR in the patients on self-management but was significantly ($P < 0.005$) below the target INR in the high-intensity anticoagulation group on standard management. The investigators concluded that weekly self-monitoring and self-dosing was a better approach to anticoagulation management than that using an anticoagulation clinic. Piso et al. (24) from the same group analyzed the quality of anticoagulation over a period of 3 years when patients were first managed using a clinic approach, then using self-management, and then returned to the clinic approach. The mean proportion of INR values within the therapeutic target range was higher in the self-management phase (0.69 ± 0.11) compared to the first clinic (0.40 ± 0.20) and

Table 41-2 Some Outcome Measures to Assess the Utility of Anticoagulant Self-Monitoring with Decision Support Systems Compared with Clinic-Based Management

Mean, median, and range of INR values
Point prevalence
Proportion of INR values in preferred therapeutic range
Proportion of time spent in preferred therapeutic range
Deviation of INR from mean of therapeutic range
Mean Coumadin (warfarin) dose
Dose changes per month
Number of visits to the clinic or specialist
Time between visits to the clinic or specialist
Bleeding events
Thromboembolic events

second clinic (0.56 ± 0.18; $P < 0.05$) phases. Time in the therapeutic target range was also higher in the self-management phase (0.70 ± 0.10) compared to first clinic (0.43 ± 0.25) and second clinic (0.60 ± 0.17; $P < 0.05$) phases. Furthermore, the mean square deviation from target value was lower in the self-management phase (0.39 ± 0.17) compared to the first clinic (0.81 ± 0.44) and second clinic (0.64 ± 0.39, $P = 0.05$) phases. The study showed that self-management was superior to clinic-based management, using a number of outcome measures. The authors also noted that the performance deteriorated after the self-management was stopped but not to such a poor level as the initial clinical phase.

Cromheecke et al. (25) also performed a randomized crossover study comparing self-management with management in a specialist anticoagulation clinic. They studied 50 patients on long-term oral anticoagulation therapy for 3-month periods on either self-management or specialist anticoagulation clinic management, returning back to the other option after the second 3-month period. The investigators found that patients were within the target treatment for 55% and 49% of the time in the self-management and clinic management phases, respectively ($P = 0.06$). The proportion of patients who spent the most time in the therapeutic range was larger during the self-management phase, and the odds ratio for better control of coagulation (defined as time within the therapeutic range) during self-management compared with clinic management was 4.6 (95% CI = 2.1–10.2). In addition, patient satisfaction was greater in the self-management phases of the study.

Fitzmaurice et al. (26) conducted a randomized controlled trial of self-management compared with primary care management over a period of 6 months. The 49 patients were given two training sessions and allowed to undertake self-management after successful completion of training as well as participation in internal and external quality assurance. There was no difference in the INR control, as judged by the proportion of time spent in control (74% vs. 77% for self-management and clinic management, respectively). There were no serious adverse events in the intervention group, compared with one in the control group, but the costs were greater in the clinic management group [£425 ($680) vs. £90 ($144) at 2002 prices].

Gadisseur et al. (27) compared self-management with management provided by a specialist clinic, using a randomized design and involving two clinics. They recruited 341 patients receiving long-term anticoagulant therapy and used a complex randomization design. There was a moderate improvement in the INR in the self-managed group, and the quality of the INR was dependent on the type of Coumadin used, with phenprocoumon outperforming acenocoumarol. In a subsequent paper, the same authors also showed increased patient satisfaction with self-management, using a number of indices (28). Rosendaal (29), from the same group, came to the same conclusions in another small study. Siebenhofer et al. (30) performed a systematic review of studies of self-management of oral anticoagulation therapy and found nine relevant randomized controlled trials, but only four met the inclusion

criteria. In a comparison of the four studies, there was no difference in oral anticoagulation control between self-management and management by a specialized anticoagulation clinic. In comparison with routine care by general practitioners, self-management was found to be better. Data from two studies showed that self-management could clearly improve treatment-related quality of life. Furthermore, patient self-management can improve the quality of oral anticoagulation as an indirect parameter of a reduced risk for thromboembolic and bleeding complications. The authors concluded that self-management oral anticoagulation treatment is safe and improves treatment-related quality of life. However, the authors did note that there were no valid long-term studies that demonstrated reduction of bleeding and thromboembolic events, the major risks associated with anticoagulation therapy.

Several studies have focused on patients receiving heart valve replacements. Sidhu and O'Kane (31) undertook a 2-year prospective randomized trial of self-managed anticoagulation therapy in 100 patients following valve replacement. The self-managed group demonstrated better control as judged by the number of test results in the target range (67.6% vs. 58.0%) and time in the range (76.5% vs. 63.8%), compared with the conventionally managed group. There was no difference in morbidity or mortality between the two groups. Kortke et al. (32) studied self-management in a group of patients with mechanical heart valve replacements. A randomization scheme was used to assign patients to self-management or to the control group, with management by a family practitioner. There was a higher incidence of INR values within range in the self-managed group compared with the control group (80% vs. 62%), and the incidence of complications (hemorrhage and thromboembolic events) was also reduced ($P < 0.05$). Christensen et al. (33), in another small study, followed 24 patients with mechanical heart valve replacements for a total of 4 years. They found that the self-managed patients were within the target INR range for a mean of 78% (range 36.1–93.9%) of the time, compared with 61.0% (range 37.4–2.9%) for the control group. They concluded it was a feasible and safe approach to anticoagulation management. In a later study, Koertke et al. (34) reported data on 1818 patients who had received mechanical heart valve replacements. They performed a randomized controlled trial, assigning patients to specific treatment target INRs depending on the valve replaced. The investigators concluded that the early initiation of INR self-management after mechanical heart valve replacement enables patients to stay within a lower and smaller INR target range. In addition, the reduced anticoagulation level that could be achieved resulted in fewer grade III bleeding complications without increasing thromboembolic event rates.

CONCLUSIONS

This brief review illustrates many of the important features of the successful use of POCT. It has been stressed how important standardization of methodology is to the delivery of reliable results for therapy management. This is particularly the case with PT measurement as the reagents vary in their sensitivity. It is also important to maintain good links with the laboratory, which can provide valuable backup, helpful advice, and expertise, as well as contributing to quality control, quality assurance, and training of operators. This may prove to be a valuable extended role for clinical scientists in the future, bringing them into closer contact with the patient.

A number of studies, including randomized controlled trials, have shown that POCT in the form of patient self-management, both testing and making dosage adjustments, can lead to improved clinical outcomes. Several of the studies are small in terms of patient numbers, but the ability to deliver the service in this way has been clearly demonstrated. Studies with larger numbers of patients, possibly through the use of clinical auditing, are now needed to determine whether there are any significant adverse events associated with this modality of treatment. In this respect, the need for continuing patient education and its effect on maintaining clinical outcomes is worthy of further study. Douketis (35) summarized the advantages of anticoagulation self-monitoring as contributing to patient convenience with regard to visits to anticoagulation clinics and for laboratory monitoring, as well as fewer INR values outside of the therapeutic range. In addition, and equally important, there is the potential for a reduction in bleeding and thromboembolic events. If there is a downside to this approach to chronic disease management, it is that it may be limited to those patients who have the cognitive and physical capabilities to perform the tests—and there will undoubtedly be ways in the future of combating these potential drawbacks, such as through the use of simpler devices and decision support software.

Finally, there is the possibility that self-monitoring will not be required, or will at least be less common, with the future introduction of new anticoagulants such as ximelagatran that are currently undergoing clinical trials (36)

REFERENCES

1. Van Cott EM. Coagulation point-of-care testing. Clin Lab Med 2001;21:337–50.
2. Poller L, Keown M, Chauhan N, van den Besselaar AM, Tripodi A, Jespersen J, Shiach C. European concerted action on anticoagulation. Minimum numbers of lyophilized plasma samples for ISI calibration of CoaguChek and TAS point-of-care whole blood prothrombin time monitors. Am J Clin Pathol 2003;119:232–40.
3. Poller L, Keown M, Chauhan N, Van Den Besselaar AM, Tripodi A, Shiach C, Jespersen J, ECCA Steering Group Members. European Concerted Action on Anticoagulation. Correction of displayed international normalized ratio on two point-of-care test whole-blood prothrombin time monitors (CoaguChek Mini and TAS PT-NC) by independent international sensitivity index calibration. Br J Haematol 2003;122:944–9.
4. Poller L, Keown M, Chauhan N, van den Besselaar AM, Tripodi A, Shiach C, Jespersen J. European concerted action on anticoagulation. Quality assessment of the CoaguChek Mini and TAS PT-NC point-of-care whole-blood prothrombin time monitors. Clin Chem 2004;50:537–44.
5. Poller L. International normalized ratios (INR): the first 20 years. J Thromb Haemost 2004;2:849–60.
6. Cosmi B, Palareti G, Moia M, Carpenedo M, Pengo V, Biasiolo A, et al. Accuracy of a portable prothrombin time monitor (Coagucheck) in patients on chronic oral anticoagulant therapy: a prospective multicenter study. Thromb Res 2000;100:279–86.
7. Hobbs FD, Fitzmaurice DA, Murray ET, Holder R, Rose PE, Roper R. Is the international normalised ratio (INR) reliable? A trial of comparative measurements in hospital laboratory and primary care settings. J Clin Pathol 1999;52:494–7.
8. Oral Anticoagulation Monitoring Study Group. Point-of-care prothrombin time measurement for professional and patient self-testing use. A multicenter clinical experience. Oral Anticoagulation Monitoring Study Group. Am J Clin Pathol 2001;115:288–96.
9. Shiach CR, Campbell B, Poller L, Keown M, Chauhan N. Reliability of point-of-care prothrombin time testing in a community clinic: a randomized crossover comparison with hospital laboratory testing. Br J Haematol 2002;119:370–5.
10. Cosmi B, Palareti G, Carpanedo M, Pengo V, Biasiolo A, Rampazzo P et al. Assessment of patient capability to self-adjust oral anticoagulant dose: a multicenter study on home use of portable prothrombin time monitor (COAGUCHECK). Haematologica 2000;85:826–31.
11. Hasenkam JM, Knudsen L, Kimose HH, Gronnesby H, Attermann J, Andersen NT, Pilegaard HK. Practicability of patient self-testing of oral anticoagulant therapy by the international normalized ratio (INR) using a portable whole blood monitor. A pilot investigation. Thromb Res 1997;85:77–82.
12. Morsdorf S, Erdlenbruch W, Taborski U, Schenk JF, Erdlenbruch K, Novotny-Reichert G, et al. Training of patients for self-management of oral anticoagulant therapy: standards, patient suitability, and clinical aspects. Semin Thromb Hemost 1999;25:109–15.
13. Sawicki PT. A structured teaching and self-management program for patients receiving oral anticoagulation: a randomized controlled trial. Working Group for the Study of Patient Self-Management of Oral Anticoagulation. JAMA 1999;281:145–50.
14. Tripodi A, Bressi C, Carpenedo M, Chantarangkul V, Clerici M, Mannucci PM. Quality assurance program for whole blood prothrombin time-international normalized ratio point-of-care monitors used for patient self-testing to control oral anticoagulation. Thromb Res 2004;113:35–40.
15. Murray ET, Kitchen DP, Kitchen S, Jennings I, Woods TA, Preston FE, Fitzmaurice DA. Patient self-management of oral anticoagulation and external quality assessment procedures. Br J Haematol 2003;122:825–8.
16. Fitzmaurice DA, Hobbs FD, Murray ET, Bradley CP, Holder R. Evaluation of computerized decision support for oral anticoagulation management based in primary care. Br J Gen Pract 1996;46:533–5.
17. Fitzmaurice DA, Hobbs FD, Murray ET, Holder RL, Allan TF, Rose PE. Oral anticoagulation management in primary care with the use of computerized decision support and near-patient testing: a randomized, controlled trial. Arch Intern Med 2000;160:2343–8.
18. Fitzmaurice DA, Murray ET, Gee KM, Allan TF. Does the Birmingham model of oral anticoagulation management in primary care work outside trial conditions? Br J Gen Pract 2001;51:828–9.
19. Poller L, Shiach CR, MacCallum PK, Johansen AM, Munster AM, Magalhaes A, Jespersen J. Multicentre randomised study of

computerised anticoagulant dosage. European Concerted Action on Anticoagulation. Lancet 1998;352:1505–9.

20. Manotti C, Moia M, Palareti G, Pengo V, Ria L, Dettori AG. Effect of computer-aided management on the quality of treatment in anticoagulated patients: a prospective, randomized, multicenter trial of APROAT (Automated Program for Oral Anticoagulant Treatment). Haematologica 2001;86:1060– 70.

21. Kovacs MJ, Anderson DA, Wells PS. Prospective assessment of a nomogram for the initiation of oral anticoagulation therapy for outpatient treatment of venous thromboembolism. Pathophysiol Haemost Thromb 2002;32:131–3.

22. Fitzmaurice DA, Kesteven P, Gee KM, Murray ET, McManus R. A systematic review of outcome measures reported for the therapeutic effectiveness of oral anticoagulation. J Clin Pathol 2003; 56:48–51.

23. Watzke HH, Forberg E, Svolba G, Jimenez-Boj E, Krinninger B. A prospective controlled trial comparing weekly self-testing and self-dosing with the standard management of patients on stable oral anticoagulation. Thromb Haemost 2000;83:661–5.

24. Piso B, Jimenz-Boj E, Krinninger B, Watzke HH. The quality of oral anticoagulation before, during and after a period of patient self-management. Thromb Res 2002;106:101–4.

25. Cromheecke ME, Levi M, Colly LP, de Mol BJ, Prins MH, Hutten BA et al. Oral anticoagulation self-management and management by a specialist anticoagulation clinic: a randomised cross-over comparison. Lancet 2000;356:97–102.

26. Fitzmaurice DA, Murray ET, Gee KM, Allan TF, Hobbs FD. A randomised controlled trial of patient self management of oral anticoagulation treatment compared with primary care management. J Clin Pathol 2002;55:845–9.

27. Gadisseur AP, Breukink-Engbers WG, van der Meer FJ, van den Besselaar AM, Sturk A, Rosendaal FR. Comparison of the quality of oral anticoagulant therapy through patient self-management and management by specialized anticoagulation clinics in the Netherlands: a randomized clinical trial. Arch Intern Med 2003; 163:2639–46.

28. Gadisseur AP, Kaptein AA, Breukink-Engbers WG, van der Meer FJ, Rosendaal FR. Patient self-management of oral anticoagulant care vs. management by specialized anticoagulation clinics: positive effects on quality of life. J Thromb Haemost 2004;2:584–91.

29. Rosendaal FR. Patient self-management of oral anticoagulation care vs. management by specialized anticoagulation clinics: positive effects on quality of life. J Throm Haemost 2004;2:584–91.

30. Siebenhofer A, Berghold A, Sawicki PT. Systematic review of studies of self-management of oral anticoagulation. Thromb Haemost 2004;91:225–32.

31. Sidhu P, O'Kane HO. Self-managed anticoagulation: results from a two-year prospective randomized trial with heart valve patients. Ann Thorac Surg 2001;72:1523–7.

32. Koertke H, Minami K, Boethig D, Breymann T, Seifert D, Wagner O et al. INR self-management permits lower anticoagulation levels after mechanical heart valve replacement. Circulation 2003;108(Suppl 1):1175–8.

33. Christensen TD, Attermann J, Pilegaard HK, Andersen NT, Maegaard M, Hasenkam JM. Self-management of oral anticoagulant therapy for mechanical heart valve patients. Scand Cardiovasc J 2001;35:107–13.

34. Koertke H, Koerfer R. International normalized ratio self-management after mechanical heart valve replacement: is an early start advantageous? Ann Thorac Surg 2001;72:44–8.

35. Douketis JD. Patient self-monitoring of oral anticoagulant therapy: potential benefits and implications for clinical practice. Am J Cardiovasc Drugs 2001;1:245–51.

36. Salam AM, Al Mousa EN. The therapeutic potential of ximelagatran to become the anticoagulant of choice in medicine: a review of recently completed clinical trials. Expert Opin Pharmacother 2004;5:1423–30.

Chapter **42**

Point-of-Care Testing and Venous Thromboembolic Disease

James C. Boyd

The term *venous thromboembolic disease* (VTE) is applied to clinical conditions in which blood clots (thrombi) form, often in the deep veins of the thigh or calf, and, subsequently, may dislodge and flow centrally through the inferior vena cava and right side of the heart to lodge in the pulmonary arterial circulation as pulmonary emboli. Pulmonary embolism (PE) is a serious clinical event that occurs in 1 to 2 persons per 1000 annually in the United States (1, 2). The mortality rate for untreated PE has been reported to be as high as 26% and an additional 26%, of patients develop nonfatal recurrent emboli (3). When treated using anticoagulants, mortality rates are reduced to 8% at 3 months (4), and the recurrence rate for thromboembolic events is cut to 6% over 3 months (5). Because anticoagulation is associated with a 7% annual incidence rate of major bleeding complications (6), it is important to avoid the risks of unnecessary anticoagulant therapy. Thus, diagnostic modalities are needed that can rapidly confirm or exclude PE in patients who are suspected to have the disorder.

The clinical signs and symptoms of PE are not specific for the diagnosis. Chest pain and shortness of breath occur in ~70% of patients; cough, tachycardia, and sweating in ~40%; hemoptysis and syncope in ~10% (7). Thus, diagnosing PE on clinical grounds alone is difficult (7–9). A high clinical suspicion predicts PE correctly in only 68% of cases (10).

Only about one-third of patients presenting with suspected pulmonary embolism are diagnosed to actually have the disease (10). This low rate of confirmed PE can lead to presumptive anticoagulation, hospital admission, and testing of many patients without pulmonary embolism. Thus, recently investigated diagnostic approaches have focused on how to identify patients most likely not to have pulmonary embolism and, who, therefore, do not require anticoagulant therapy (11).

TESTS EMPLOYED IN THE DIAGNOSIS OF VTE

Pulmonary angiography and contrast venography remain the gold-standard tests for the diagnosis of PE and deep vein thrombosis (DVT), respectively. However, these tests are expensive, invasive, and associated with small but significant risks of complications (12). For these reasons they are no longer widely used as the first tests to be applied in the diagnosis of venous thromboembolic disease. Noninvasive alternatives are available, including lower-limb compression ultrasound for suspected DVT and ventilation-perfusion (VQ) scanning for suspected PE. However, the latter tests are rarely able to rule in or rule out the diagnosis of VTE by themselves. Compression ultrasound studies are negative initially in more than three-fourths of patients with suspected DVT (13), making their application very expensive. They must be repeated one or more times because about 2% to 6% of DVT becomes apparent within 1 week of initial presentation. In addition, 70% of patients with suspected PE have a nondiagnostic VQ scan (10) and require further imaging with ultrasonography or pulmonary angiography for definitive diagnosis.

In light of the shortcomings of imaging and ultrasonography studies, a noninvasive test has been sought for VTE that is simple and reliable. Measurements of plasma D-dimer have shown clinical promise in the diagnosis of intravascular fibrinolysis and recently have emerged the front-runners as adjunctive measures to exclude suspected VTE. The remainder of this chapter will review D-dimer testing in relation to VTE.

D-DIMER

During the blood clotting process, fibrinogen is converted to fibrin by the activation of thrombin. Fibrin monomers elaborated in this process polymerize into a soluble gel of noncrosslinked fibrin (14) (Figure 42-1). The blood coagulation Factor XIII, activated by thrombin, converts the noncrosslinked fibrin to crosslinked fibrin, which forms an insoluble fibrin clot. Lysis of the formed clot occurs through the action of plasmin. Plasmin is a fibrinolytic enzyme that cleaves both fibrinogen and fibrin to form degradation products. Because D-dimer is formed only by the degradation of crosslinked fibrin, it is a specific marker of the endogenous fibrin removal process. Approximately 2% to 3% of plasma fibrinogen is degraded daily to fibrin (15). Thus, small amounts of D-dimer can be measured in the plasma of healthy individuals. D-dimer fragments appear to be cleared primarily by the reticuloendothelial system of the liver, but they are also excreted in the urine (16)

Conditions in which fibrin is formed and then degraded by plasmin are associated with increased concentrations of D-dimer. D-dimer concentrations in VTE rise in proportion to the extent of thrombosis and usually normalize within 2–3 weeks following treatment of a thrombotic event (17). However,

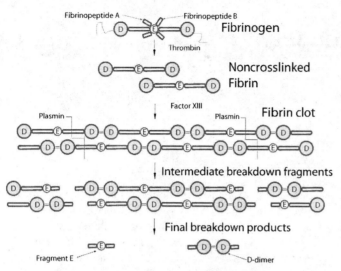

Figure 42-1 Schematic representation of the formation and degradation of fibrin. Fibrinogen is characterized by three globular domains and two D domains separated by a central E domain, all linked by α-helical coils. Fibrinogen is converted by the action of thrombin to noncrosslinked fibrin monomer with the liberation of fibrinopeptides A and B. Factor XIIIa crosslinks D domains of fibrin monomers with a covalent bond, and the fibrin protofibrils organize in an offset fashion into a fibrin clot. The action of plasmin breaks the fibrin clot into a set of intermediate forms that are further degraded to the final fibrinolytic products, fragment E and D-dimer. Adapted from (14).

D-dimer may also be elevated in other conditions (Table 42-1), making the diagnosis of VTE difficult in patients who also have one or more of these conditions present (15, 18). The study of Schrecengost et al. (19) demonstrated that D-dimer measurements did not have appreciable diagnostic value for VTE in hospital inpatients (who often have conditions listed in Table 42-1). Additional factors associated with decreases in the diagnostic utility of D-dimer measurements in hospital inpatients are increasing length of hospital stay and elevations in C-reactive protein concentration (20).

Assays for D-Dimer

D-dimer assays utilize monoclonal antibodies specific for various epitopes of the D-dimer antigen. When used as a screening test for VTE, a D-dimer assay should be highly sensitive with a high negative predictive value. In addition, the assay method should be quantitative, rapid, and easy to perform. Methods for measurement of D-dimer can be divided into several groups (Table 42-2): (*i*) classical microplate ELISA assays, (*ii*) first- and second-generation latex agglutination assays, (*iii*) red-blood-cell agglutination assays, (*iv*) membrane ELISA assays, (*v*) rapid ELFA assays, (*vi*) immunochromatographic assays, and (*vii*) dendrimer-enhanced radial partition immunoassays. Microplate ELISA has been the gold standard for the measurement of D-dimer concentrations and has high sensitivity (93–100%). However, microplate ELISA tests are not routinely used because they are labor intensive and time-consuming to perform (2–3 h). Other test formats have proven to provide

more rapid analysis (5–35 min) with equivalent sensitivity to the microplate ELISA.

Given the differences in monoclonal antibodies utilized across the various D-dimer assays, it is not surprising that results vary between assays. Some assays are reported, for example, in ng/mL fibrinogen equivalent units (FEUs), and others are reported in D-dimer units (1 FEU = ~0.5 D-dimer unit). Standardization of assays will require the development of international standards and careful evaluation of their commutability between assays. Until assay standardization has been accomplished, different assays will utilize different thresholds for the exclusion of VTE. Derivation of assay thresholds for each assay has typically been accomplished by retrospective data analysis aiming to set the sensitivity of the assay to a high value (say, >90%) while maintaining as much assay specificity as possible.

Point-of-Care Assays for D-Dimer

Red blood cell agglutination assays can be performed at the bedside on whole blood, but they have shown more variability in clinical studies than other assay formats, perhaps due to variability from one person to another in visually reading the assays (21).

Recently developed immunochromatographic assays also may be used at the bedside. These assays are based upon the binding of gold-labeled monoclonal antibodies to D-dimer in the patient sample. In the Agen assay (Agen Biomedical, Brisbane, Australia), the D-dimer/antibody complexes migrate through the filter membrane in an aqueous phase until they are captured and concentrated in a zone where a second D-dimer monoclonal antibody has been bound. Concentration of complexes at this zone causes the appearance of a visible line on the membrane. Uncaptured gold/antibody conjugate continues to flow to the end of the membrane, where it is bound by antimurine antibody at the procedural control zone. Formation of a visible line at the procedural control zone gives an indi-

Table 42-1 Conditions Other Than Venous Thromboembolism Associated with Elevated D-Dimer Concentrations

Malignancy
Disseminated intravascular coagulation
Severe infection
Heart failure
Renal failure
Acute coronary syndrome
Acute nonlacunar stroke
Liver disease
Sickle cell crisis
Connective tissue disease
Pregnancy
Postoperative state
Trauma
Recent bleeding
Advanced age

Table 42-2   D-Dimer Assay Characteristics

Assay format	Examples[a]	Sensitivity	Specificity	Comments
Microplate ELISA	Asserachrom, Dimertest GOLD EIA	High	Moderate	Regarded as the gold standard; performed in batch analysis; slow to perform
First-generation latex agglutination	Dimertest, Minutex	Moderate	Moderate	Rapid; insufficiently sensitive to be clinically useful
Second-generation latex agglutination	AutoDimertest, BC D-dimer, IL Test, Liatest, LPIA, Tinaquant	High	Moderate	Rapid; comparable sensitivity to microplate ELISA
Red blood cell agglutination	SimpliRED	Moderate to High	Moderate	Rapid; can be used with whole blood
Membrane ELISA	NycoCard	High	Moderate	Rapid; comparable sensitivity to microplate ELISA
ELFA	Automated Rapid ELFA Assay VIDAS	High	Moderate	Rapid; comparable sensitivity to microplate ELISA
Immunochromatographic	Simplify D-Dimer, Cardiac D-dimer	Insufficient data	Insufficient data	Rapid; preliminary results indicate comparable sensitivity to microplate ELISA; can be used with whole blood
Dendrimer-enhanced radial partition immunoassay	Stratus CS D-dimer	Insufficient data	Insufficient data	Rapid; preliminary results indicate comparable sensitivity to ELFA; can be used with whole blood

[a] Manufacturers: Dimertest GOLD EIA, Dimertest, AutoDimertest, SimpliRED, Simplify D-dimer (Agen Biomedical, Brisbane, Australia); NycoCard (Axis Shield, Dundee, Scotland); IL Test (Beckman Coulter, Fullerton, CA, USA); Automated Rapid ELFA Assay VIDAS (bioMerieux, Marcy-'Etoile, France); BC D-dimer, Stratus CS D-dimer (Dade Behring, Deerfield, IL, USA), Asserachrom, Liatest (Diagnostica Stago, Parsippany, NJ, USA), Minutex (DiaPharma Group, West Chester, OH, USA); LPIA (Mitsubishi Kasei, Tokyo, Japan), Tinaquant, Cardiac D-dimer (Roche Diagnostics, Indianapolis, IN, USA). Adapted from (15).

cation that the device is working properly. The Cardiac D-Dimer Test (Roche Diagnostics, Mannheim, Germany) also incorporates gold-labeled antibodies but uses biotin-labeled second antibodies to bind the gold/antibody conjugate to the streptavidin signal line. A reflectance measurement of the accumulated complex is made on the cardiac reader instrument and this reflectance is then converted into concentration via a lot-specific calibration curve (22).

Another recent D-dimer assay that can be used at the bedside uses the radial partition immunoassay format (Dade Behring, Inc., Deerfield, IL, USA). In this assay procedure, dendrimer-linked monoclonal antibody to D-dimer is bound to the central portion of a square piece of glass fiber paper furnished with the test pack. The sample is then added to the paper and D-dimer is bound to the dendrimer-linked antibody. After a short incubation time, a conjugate reagent containing enzyme-labeled monoclonal antibody directed against a second distinct antigenic site on D-dimer is pipetted onto the reaction zone of the paper. During a second incubation period, an enzyme-labeled antibody reacts with the bound analyte of interest to form an antibody-antigen–labeled antibody sandwich. The unbound, labeled antibody is eluted from the reaction zone by applying a wash solution that includes a fluorescent substrate for the enzyme. The reaction rate is measured by monitoring front-surface fluorescence and comparing the rate

of the fluorescent signal produced by the bound enzyme fraction with the stored calibration curve to determine the concentration of analyte in the sample. Because centrifugal separation of blood cells from plasma is required for the performance of other assay formats, these are less suitable for performance at the bedside.

D-Dimer in the Diagnostic Evaluation of VTE

Most clinical studies have focused on the evaluation of patients with suspected pulmonary embolism because PE can pose an immediate life-threatening risk. The initial focus in this chapter will be on the diagnostic evaluation of PE, with the diagnosis of DVT covered second.

As pointed out earlier, information derived from taking the clinical history and performing a physical examination often proves inaccurate in diagnosing or excluding pulmonary embolism (23, 24), and various radiological and ultrasonographic tests proposed for the diagnosis also have their limitations. Most recent approaches to the diagnosis of PE have combined a clinical assessment of risk with one or more diagnostic tests (25). Using one of several empirical or standardized approaches, patients are placed into three risk groups (low, intermediate, or high risk for PE) based on clinical information.

Combining a 10% or lower risk of PE in the low-risk group with a negative result for a highly sensitive diagnostic test can reduce the net risk of PE in a person with this combination to 2% or less. [For a detailed discussion on how to compute the post-test probability of PE, given a pre-test probability and test sensitivity and specificity, see Boyd and Deeks (26).] Thus, the negative test result can be used in a rule-out strategy for PE. This has been the most common approach taken in applying the D-dimer assay in the diagnosis of PE.

Clinical Studies of the Accuracy and Economic Benefits of D-Dimer in the Diagnosis of PE

As with all laboratory tests, evaluation of D-dimer as a diagnostic test for PE has been hampered by limited numbers of high-quality clinical studies (27, 28).

Only one clinical study has considered the diagnostic value of D-dimer as a stand-alone test in pulmonary embolism (29). In this study, radiological studies and treatment were withheld in 159 (36%) of 444 outpatients with negative VIDAS® d-d assay (bioMérieux, Durham, NC, USA) results and suspected PE. In the overall group of patients with negative D-dimer results, no cases of VTE were noted during 3 months of follow-up. Although this study suggests that a negative result for the stand-alone VIDAS assay may be a safe means to exclude PE, further studies are warranted in different populations to confirm these results,

Two recent systematic reviews have evaluated ELISA-based and turbidimetric latex-based assays for the diagnosis of PE (30, 31). The systematic review of ELISA-based assays found only 11 studies out of 52 met the study inclusion criteria (30). Meta-analysis of the subgroup of nine studies that used traditional ELISA D-dimer methods using a random-effects model gave a pooled estimate of sensitivity of 0.94 [95% confidence interval (CI), 0.88–0.97] and a pooled estimate of specificity of 0.45 (95% CI, 0.36–0.55). Boyd and Deeks (26), in a reanalysis of the combined data for the 11 studies, found an overall sensitivity of 0.96 (95% CI, 0.91–1.00) and an overall specificity of 0.44 (0.35–0.54). Forest plots in Figure 42-2 show a consistent pattern in sensitivities from study to study but a diverse spectrum of specificities. The overall high estimate of average sensitivity for the D-dimer test and its relative consistency from study to study suggest that a negative test result can be used with a fair amount of confidence in ruling out PE. Brown et al. (30) concluded that the ELISA D-dimer test was highly sensitive but nonspecific for the detection of PE in a clinical setting, and could be used to help clinicians rule out PE in cases of low to moderate pre-test probabilities of disease.

In a systematic review of turbidimetric latex methods, Brown et al. (31) found only 9 of 264 studies met the inclusion criteria. Meta-analysis using a random-effects model gave an overall sensitivity of 0.93 (95% CI, 0.89–0.96) and an overall specificity of 0.51 (95% CI, 0.42–0.59). The authors concluded that given a negative likelihood ratio for turbidimetric tests in the range of 0.1–0.15, the turbidimetric test could be used to reduce the post-test probability of PE to <1% when used in a patient population with a pre-test probability of <10%.

CLINICAL STUDIES ON THE DIAGNOSTIC EVALUATION OF DVT

Various studies have combined information from a negative D-dimer test with normal ultrasound (29, 32, 33), with low clinical probability assessment (34–36), moderate clinical probability assessment (37), or low to moderate clinical probability assessment (38, 39) as effective tools in ruling out DVT. When low to moderate clinical probability assessment was combined with D-dimer measurement, the occurrence of VTE over 3 months of follow-up in patients in whom DVT was

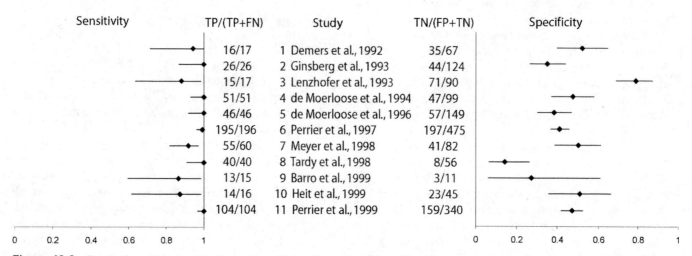

Figure 42-2 Forest plots of the sensitivities and specificities from 11 studies of D-dimer as reviewed by Brown et al. (30). The estimated mean values for each study are shown by the diamonds, and the 95% confidence intervals by the whiskers on either side of the diamonds. Reproduced with permission from (26).

ruled out by this approach ranged from 0% (35, 37) to 0.9% (36). Following this same approach for ruling out DVT, 11% (37) to 69% (36) of patients were spared from having ultrasound studies.

Of these studies, only the study by Wells et al. (36) was a randomized controlled trial (RCT). These investigators evaluated D-dimer testing in 1096 patients with suspected DVT and used either the SimpliRED red blood cell agglutination test (Agen Biomedical, Brisbane, Australia) or the IL Test latex agglutination test for D-dimer testing (Instrumentation Laboratory, Lexington, MA, USA). All patients were evaluated using a clinical model for predicting the pre-test probability of DVT. Then, patients were randomly assigned to undergo ultrasound imaging alone (control group) or to undergo D-dimer testing (D-dimer group), followed by ultrasound imaging, unless the D-dimer test was negative and the patient was considered to have a low clinical probability of deep-vein thrombosis, in which case ultrasound imaging was not performed. The overall prevalence rate of DVT or PE was 15.7%. In those patients for whom VTE had been ruled out by the initial diagnostic strategy, there were two confirmed VTE events in the 218 patients in the low-probability, negative D-dimer group (0.9%, 95% CI, 0.01–3.3%) during 3 months of follow-up. Of the patients in the low probability, negative D-dimer group, 69% did not require ultrasound imaging. This study represents the first RCT that has been carried out to evaluate D-dimer testing to rule out deep-vein thrombosis, and it provides strong evidence that negative D-dimer testing combined with a low pre-test probability of VTE is effective for ruling out VTE and can significantly reduce the need for imaging studies. Taken together, the results of Wells et al. (36) and the other studies listed earlier suggest that D-dimer combined with clinical probability assessments in a rule-out approach can achieve modest to major cost savings in the evaluation of DVT.

Cost-Effectiveness of D-Dimer Testing

In contrast with studies suggesting that D-dimer testing can reduce the need for imaging studies, Goldstein et al. (40) found that use of D-dimer testing may actually result in an increased number of imaging studies. One important drawback of the latter study is that it was performed in a hospital inpatient population. As previously outlined, D-dimer testing appears to have limited diagnostic value in hospital inpatients, giving many more falsely positive results in this patient group (19). In addition, an editorial accompanying the study of Goldstein et al. points out that fewer than 50% of patients in the cohort were followed up, diagnostic criteria for PE were not clearly defined, and the diagnostic workup was not standardized (41). The editorial writer also points out that the absolute number of patients found to have PE was almost twice as high in the patient group (where D-dimer testing was used) as it was in the control group, suggesting that diagnostic resources may have been underutilized in the control group rather than overutilized in the group where D-dimer testing was used. Clearly, such contradictory results between studies suggest a need for further investigations that clearly delineate the economic benefits of

D-dimer testing. Nevertheless, based on the quality of studies, the cost savings of D-dimer testing appear to be better supported by the RCT conducted by Wells et al. (36) and the systematic reviews conducted by Brown et al. (30, 31).

Anticoagulation and D-Dimer Testing

Anticoagulation therapy is known to lower D-dimer concentrations, and the use of D-dimer testing in the anticoagulated population is controversial. In patients with chronic atrial fibrillation, mean plasma D-dimer concentrations in untreated patients or patients on low-dose coumadin with aspirin are higher than those of control individuals and decrease to concentrations similar to those of the controls when patients are put on standard coumadin therapy (42, 43). Couturaud et al. (44) determined from a literature review that the mean concentration of D-dimer decreases by 25% when patients are started on anticoagulant therapy. These investigators estimated that a mean decrease of 25% in D-dimer concentrations would reduce the sensitivity of D-dimer testing from 96% to 89% within 24 h after starting heparin therapy. Although such a drop in test sensitivity could have a negative impact on the potential value of D-dimer testing in anticoagulated patients, the findings of Schrecengost et al. (19) suggest that the impact is minimal. The latter investigators found D-dimer to be elevated in 32 of 45 patients on anticoagulation treatment. The higher D-dimer results expected if these patients were not anticoagulated would not have changed their classifications. Of 13 patients with negative D-dimer results, two had evidence of VTE. Exclusion of these two patients from their overall study results only slightly changed assay sensitivity and negative predictive value.

OVERALL STRATEGY FOR THE DIAGNOSTIC EVALUATION OF VTE

Because the sensitivity of D-dimer tests is not 100%, in order to obtain sufficiently low post-test probabilities when ruling out VTE, use of D-dimer tests must be combined with other approaches that ensure the pre-test probability of VTE is relatively low. Various combinations of approaches have been proposed as reviewed by Fedullo and Tapson (26). In some cases, clinical assessment of the probability of VTE has been combined with CT angiographic studies, ventilation-perfusion scanning, or ultrasonography. However, there is a developing consensus that measurement of D-dimer, when combined with a preclinical assessment of the probability of disease using either an empirical approach or a clinical model for predicting the pre-test probability, can be used successfully in the diagnosis of PE and DVT (25, 36, 45, 46). If the clinical risk is judged to be low (less than 10%), then a negative D-dimer test can be used to effectively exclude the diagnosis of VTE and a protocol similar to that illustrated in Figure 42-3 can be followed.

When the D-dimer test is positive, further testing is necessary, including ventilation-perfusion scanning, CT scanning, ultrasonography, venography, or pulmonary angiography. Var-

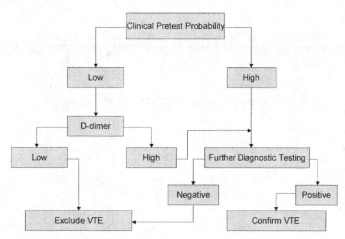

Figure 42-3 Diagnostic strategy for venous thromboembolic disease.

ious coexisting conditions listed in Table 42-1, hospitalization for longer than 3 days, and elevations in CRP are all factors that tend to increase the number of nondiagnostic positive D-dimer results. Because the prevalences of these factors vary depending on what population of patients is being examined, the potential cost savings of D-dimer testing will also vary. Due to these considerations, the D-dimer testing strategy will likely be most cost-effective in ruling out VTE when it is performed in outpatients in whom there is a relatively low clinical suspicion for VTE.

As indicated above, several D-dimer assays are available for use at the point of care. Clinical application of these point-of-care tests appears warranted as long as their sensitivities and specificities are demonstrated to be comparable to microplate ELISA methods.

REFERENCES

1. Anderson FA Jr., Wheeler HB, Goldberg RJ, Hosmer DW, Patwardhan NA, Jovanovic B, et al. A population-based perspective of the hospital incidence and case-fatality rates of deep vein thrombosis and pulmonary embolism. The Worcester DVT Study. Arch Intern Med 1991;151:933–8.

2. Silverstein MD, Heit JA, Mohr DN, Petterson TM, O'Fallon WM, Melton LJ III. Trends in the incidence of deep vein thrombosis and pulmonary embolism: a 25-year population-based study. Arch Intern Med 1998;158:585–93.

3. Barritt DW, Jordan SC. Anticoagulant drugs in the treatment of pulmonary embolism: a controlled trial. Lancet 1960;1:1309–12.

4. Goldhaber SZ, Visani L, De Rosa M. Acute pulmonary embolism: clinical outcomes in the International Cooperative Pulmonary Embolism Registry (ICOPER). Lancet 1999;353:1386–9.

5. Douketis JD, Foster GA, Crowther MA, Prins MH, Ginsberg JS. Clinical risk factors and timing of recurrent venous thromboembolism during the initial 3 months of anticoagulant therapy. Arch Intern Med 2000;160:3431–6.

6. Linkins LA, Choi PT, Douketis JD. Clinical impact of bleeding in patients taking oral anticoagulant therapy for venous thromboembolism: a meta-analysis. Ann Intern Med 2003;139:893–900.

7. Manganelli D, Palla A, Donnamaria V, Giuntini C. Clinical features of pulmonary embolism. Doubts and certainties. Chest 1995;107(Suppl):25S 32S.

8. Goldhaber SZ, Visani L, De Rosa M. Acute pulmonary embolism: clinical outcomes in the International Cooperative Pulmonary Embolism Registry (ICOPER). Lancet 1999;353:1386–9.

9. Carman TL, Deitcher SR. Advances in diagnosing and excluding pulmonary embolism: spiral CT and D-dimer measurement. Cleveland Clinic J Med 2002;69:721–9.

10. The PIOPED Investigators. Value of the ventilation/perfusion scan in acute pulmonary embolism. Results of the prospective investigation of pulmonary embolism diagnosis (PIOPED). JAMA 1990;263:2753–9.

11. Kruip MJ, Leclercq MG, van der Heul C, Prins MH, Buller HR. Diagnostic strategies for excluding pulmonary embolism in clinical outcome studies: a systematic review. Ann Intern Med 2003; 138:941–51.

12. American Thoracic Society. The diagnostic approach to acute venous thromboembolism: clinical practice guideline. Am J Respir Crit Care Med 1999;160:1043–66.

13. Cogo A, Lensing AW, Koopman MM, Piovella F, Siragusa S, Wells PS, et al. Compression ultrasonography for diagnostic management of patients with clinically suspected deep vein thrombosis: prospective cohort study. Brit Med J 1998;316: 17–20.

14. Bockenstedt P. D-dimer in venous thromboembolism. N Engl J Med 2003;349:1203–4.

15. Kelly J, Rudd A, Lewis RR, Hunt BJ. Plasma D-dimers in the diagnosis of venous thromboembolism. Arch Intern Med 2002; 162:747–56.

16. Pasqua JJ, Pizzo SV. The clearance of human fibrinogen fragments X and Y in mice: a process mediated by the fragment D receptor. Thromb Haemost 1983;49:78–80.

17. The DVTENOX Study Group. Markers of haemostatic system activation in acute deep venous thrombosis evolution during the first days of heparin treatment. Thromb Haemostasis 1993;70: 909–14.

18. Frost SD, Brotman DJ, Michota FA. Rational use of D-dimer measurement to exclude acute venous thromboembolic disease. Mayo Clin Proc 2003;78:1385–91.

19. Schrecengost JE, LeGallo RD, Boyd JC, Moons KG, Gonias SL, Rose CE Jr, et al. Comparison of diagnostic accuracies in outpatients and hospitalized patients of D-dimer testing for the evaluation of suspected pulmonary embolism. Clin Chem 2003;49: 1483–90.

20. Brotman DJ, Segal JB, Jani JT, Petty BG, Kickler TS. Limitations of D-dimer testing in unselected inpatients with suspected venous thromboembolism. Am J Med 2003;114:276–82.

21. De Monye W, Huisman MV, Pattynama PM. Observer dependency of the SimpliRed D-dimer assay in 81 consecutive patients with suspected pulmonary embolism. Thromb Res 1999;96: 293–8.

22. Bucek RA, Quehenberger P, Feliks I, Handler S, Reiter M, Minar E. Results of a new rapid D-dimer assay (cardiac D-dimer) in the diagnosis of deep vein thrombosis. Thromb Res 2001;103:17–23.

23. Goldhaber SZ. Pulmonary embolism. N Engl J Med 1998;339: 93–104.

24. Moser KM, Fedullo PF, LittleJohn JK, Crawford R. Frequent asymptomatic pulmonary embolism in patients with deep vein thrombosis. J Amer Med Assoc 1994;271:223–5.

25. Fedullo PF, Tapson VF. The evaluation of suspected pulmonary embolism. N Engl J Med 2003;349:1247–56.

26. Boyd JC, Deeks JJ. Analysis and presentation of data. In: Price CP, Christenson RH. Evidence-based laboratory medicine: from principles to outcomes. Washington, DC: AACC Press, 2003:115–36.

27. Reid MC, Lachs MS, Feinstein AR. Use of methodological standards in diagnostic test research. Getting better but still not good. J Am Med Assoc 1995;274:645–51.

28. Lijmer JG, Mol BW, Heisterkamp S, Bosel GJ, Prins MH, van der Meulen JH, et al. Empirical evidence of design-related bias in studies of diagnostic tests. JAMA 1999;282:1061–6.

29. Perrier A, Desmarais S, Miron M, de Moerloose P, Lepage R, Slosman D, et al. Non-invasive diagnosis of venous thromboembolism in outpatients. Lancet 1999;353:190–5.

30. Brown MD, Rowe BH, Reeves MJ, Bermingham JM, Goldhaber SZ. The accuracy of the enzyme-linked immunosorbent assay D-dimer test in the diagnosis of pulmonary embolism: a metaanalysis. Ann Emerg Med 2002;40:133–44.

31. Brown MD, Lau J, Nelson RD, Kline JA. Turbidimetric D-dimer test in the diagnosis of pulmonary embolism: a meta-analysis. Clin Chem 2003;49:1846–53.

32. Kraaijenhagen RA, Piovella F, Bernardi E, Verlato F, Beckers EA, Koopman MM, et al. Simplification of the diagnostic management of suspected deep vein thrombosis. Arch Intern Med 2002;162:907–11.

33. Bernardi E, Prandoni P, Lensing AW, Agnelli G, Guazzaloca G, Scannapieco G, et al. D-dimer testing as an adjunct to ultrasonography in patients with clinically suspected deep vein thrombosis: prospective cohort study. The Multicentre Italian D-dimer Ultrasound Study Investigators Group. BMJ 1998;317:1037–40.

34. Kearon C, Ginsberg JS, Douketis J, Crowther M, Brill-Edwards P, Weitz JI, Hirsh J. Management of suspected deep venous thrombosis in outpatients by using clinical assessment and D-dimer testing. Ann Intern Med 2001;135:108–11.

35. Janes S, Ashford N. Use of a simplified clinical scoring system and D-dimer testing can reduce the requirement for radiology in the exclusion of deep vein thrombosis by over 20%. Br J Haematol 2001;112:1079–82.

36. Wells PS, Anderson DR, Rodger M, Forgie M Kearon C, Dreyer J, et al. Evaluation of D-dimer in the diagnosis of suspected deep-vein thrombosis. N Engl J Med 2003;349:1227–35.

37. Aguilar C, Martinez A, Martinez A, Del Rio C, Vazquez M, Rodriguez FJ. Diagnostic value of D-dimer in patients with a moderate pretest probability of deep venous thrombosis. Br J Haematol 2002;118:275–7.

38. Schutgens RE, Ackermark P, Haas FJ, Nieuwenhuis HK, Peltenburg HG, Pijlman AH, et al. Combination of a normal D-dimer concentration and a non-high pretest clinical probability score is a safe strategy to exclude deep venous thrombosis. Circulation 2003;107:593–7.

39. Bates SM, Kearon C, Crowther M, Linkins L, O'Donnell M, Douketis J, et al. A diagnostic strategy involving a quantitative latex D-dimer assay reliably excludes deep venous thrombosis. Ann Intern Med 2003;138:787–94.

40. Goldstein NM, Kollef MH, Ward S, Gage BF. The impact of the introduction of a rapid D-dimer assay on the diagnostic evaluation of suspected pulmonary embolism. Arch Intern Med 2001;161:567–71.

41. Perrier A, de Moerloose P, Bounameaux H. Introduction of D-dimer assay: does it increase resource utilization or correct identification of pulmonary embolism? Arch Intern Med 2001;161:2049–50.

42. Lip GYH, Lip PL, Zarifis J, Watson RDS, Bareford D, Lowe GD, et al. Fibrin D-dimer and B-thromboglobulin as markers of thrombogenesis and platelet activation in atrial fibrillation. Circulation 1996;94:425–31.

43. Li-Saw-Hee FL, Blann AD, Lip GY. Effects of fixed low-dose warfarin, aspirin-warfarin combination therapy, and dose-adjusted warfarin on thrombogenesis in chronic atrial fibrillation. Stroke 2000;31:828–33.

44. Couturaud F, Kearon C, Bates SM, Ginsberg JS. Decrease in sensitivity of D-dimer for acute venous thromboembolism after starting anticoagulant therapy. Blood Coagul Fibrinolysis 2002;13:241–6.

45. Kelly J, Hunt BJ. A clinical probability assessment and D-dimer measurement should be the initial step in the investigation of suspected venous thromboembolism. Chest 2003;124:1116–9.

46. Kline JA, Wells. Methodology for a rapid protocol to rule out pulmonary embolism in the emergency department. Ann Emerg Med 2003;42:266–75.

Chapter 43

Clinical Drug Testing at the Point of Care

Ian D. Watson

CLINICAL AND DIAGNOSTIC QUESTIONS

Point-of-care testing (POCT) is based on the premise that the immediacy of a result enhances the doctor–patient interaction. It provides a valuable addition to the clinical armamentarium when compared to obtaining the same result from a laboratory based at a distance, physically or temporally, from the clinical examination.

The issues surrounding POCT have been the subject of recent reports (1, 2). The issues of proven clinical effectiveness, cost-effectiveness, and medicolegal implications are now being vigorously addressed. A recent report by the National Academy of Clinical Biochemistry found that, although high-quality evidence for the economic benefits of POCT is still very limited, there are clearly clinical situations in which clinical and economic benefits can accrue from its adoption (3). The majority of available studies on POCT for toxicological substances still concentrate on the analytical performance of devices. Given the poor results for some products, this is a valid first step.

However, the organizational and economic effects of POCT on drugs and alcohol services using appropriate devices have the potential to have a positive effect on clinical relationships and service economics.

Testing for substance abuse has been the most popular area of usage. POCT devices are widely used in preemployment and employment screening, as well as in prisons and other controlled environments. The potential for clinical applications is also widespread. However, there have been fewer examples of their application in clinical toxicology and therapeutic drug monitoring—certainly from the standpoint of the peer-reviewed literature.

It is generally true that POCT devices are analytically sophisticated yet easy to use. In drug POCT a typical format in use today is solid-phase immunoassay with a visible endpoint in a disposable cartridge, commonly referred to as a "stick test." Surprisingly, few devices can provide positive subject identification or a printed record of the result, or can be downloaded into a patient information system.

Drugs of Abuse

Drugs-of-abuse (DOA) testing encompasses the substances commonly misused recreationally, i.e., heroin, cocaine, amphetamines, cannabis, and benzodiazepines. The emphasis in societal-based DOA testing is to ensure substance abusers comply with regulatory and/or employer requirements to be drug free with the imposition of penalties for failure to comply, such as loss of employment or imprisonment. There is a very different focus for clinical applications.

Patients abusing substances may present to the health system either as acute admissions through the emergency room (ER) or as drug-dependent users enrolled in a substance abuse program. Where history and symptomatology are insufficient in acute presentations, DOA screening enables assistance with diagnosis and patient disposition, particularly if there is a high prevalence in the population served, e.g., if malignant hyperpyrexia produced by methylenedioxymethamphetamine (MDMA) is suspected, or if administration of an antagonist may be appropriate, e.g., for opiates. Chronic DOA users may prefer particular types of drugs. Programs for opiate addiction may be delivered in a number of ways, for example, in drop-in clinics, outpatient clinics, or through a community physician. Harm minimization programs encourage a nonchaotic lifestyle and self-control of the types, and amounts, of substances used, often through a methadone maintenance program. Testing is required to confirm compliance with drug-team/client agreed-on goals and also to ensure that compliance with the methadone program is being adhered to, thus reinforcing a decreased reliance on other opiates. The ability to detect 2-ethylidene-1,5-dimethyl-3,3-diphenylpyrrolidine (EDDP), a metabolite of methadone, has circumvented the common ploy of spiking urine with methadone linctus to ensure a positive result, thereby ensuring further methadone prescription. An assay for this substance is currently available as an automated cloned enzyme donor immunoassay (CEDIA), but the introduction as a POCT device is being explored. The immediacy that this technology will give would greatly enhance the benefits of testing. With the advent of buprenorphine programs one can expect development of POCT devices to detect it or its more abundant metabolite, norbuprenorphine.

Inevitably clients attempt to beat the system, and reference to underground publications and the Internet will reveal information on how their authors believe one can beat the "urine police." The client's goal may be to stop using methadone, but it might also be to stockpile supplies of methadone by not taking it or to appear to continue on a program but also misuse substances at the same time. The motivations are complex and vary between individuals; examples from experience in our own unit include concern over social services intervention in child-safety situations or obtaining methadone supplies for onward illegal sale; the former raises medicolegal issues similar to those found in workplace testing.

Referrals through community physicians may relate to behavioral changes in young people (4). The initial presentation may be attributable to mental illness (5), and dual diagnosis is not uncommon.

The aesthetics of observed urine collection for both donor and observer are not pleasant, and alternative matrices have been sought: hair, sweat, and saliva; of these only the last is readily adaptable to POCT (6). The recognized POCT benefits of immediacy are linked to an acceptable observable collection medium. Further, it is claimed that detection of the parent compound, such as cocaine or a unique metabolite (e.g., 6-monoacetylmorphine, from heroin), enables less equivocal interpretation of detected substances. However the concentrations to be detected are much lower than in urine. There is, as yet, no true consensus over issues such as passive exposure or detection windows. There is also the issue of analytical sensitivity required for confirmation of a positive screening result.

The ultimate goal for many substance misusers is abstinence. For many users, particularly of opiates, this may require a period as an in-patient in a drug-free area; it is vital to the success of such units that the patients remain drug free and frequent mandatory testing is conducted.

Clinical Toxicology

The most common causes of poisoning include carbon monoxide, ethanol, analgesics, antidepressants, and hypnotics (7). Poisoning is a common ER presentation and the discrimination of drugs as primary or contributory factors to the presentation may help management. In the majority of cases, analyses are confined to a very few compounds (Table 43-1). Quantitative information on these analytes has definitive prognostic or management value. Thus acetaminophen concentration determines whether the use of the antidote, N-acetylcysteine, is required (8). A recent POCT device enables ER physicians to safely rule out acetaminophen and salicylate ingestion (Henry JA, www.euromed.ltd.uk); however, to date, there is no peer-reviewed publication validating this claim. Because of the pharmacokinetic and predictive factors in treating acetaminophen poisoning such devices are not advised for quantitation to determine the need for intervention, i.e., rule-in.

Carboxyhemoglobin values may assist in determining the need for referral for hyperbaric oxygen.

Ethanol is a significant contributory factor to many cases of poisoning, but also to injuries resulting from accidents and fights. In some circumstances, such as head injury, it is difficult to discriminate clinical causes for symptoms from the contribution of ethanol to the clinical presentation without measuring the ethanol level. Breath ethanol measurement using handheld devices is one way of determining the contribution of alcohol to a patient's condition; saliva testing also appears to be a promising alternative (9).

Qualitative drug-class detection (e.g., for benzodiazepines or tricyclic antidepressants), although possible, rarely affects patient management (10).

Table 43-1 Clinical Toxicology: Drugs for Which Qualitative or Quantitative Analysis Is Clinically Useful

Qualitative: urine
  Benzodiazepines
  Barbiturates
  Tricyclic antidepressants
  Drugs of abuse
    Opiates
    Amphetamines
    Cocaine
    Methadone
    Cannabis
    Phencyclidine
Quantitative: serum
  Benzodiazepines
  Tricyclic antidepressants
Quantitative: serum—24-h availability necessary
  Carbon monoxide (as carboxyhaemaglobin)
  Digoxin
  Ethylene glycol
  Iron
  Lithium
  Methanol
  Methemoglobin
  Acetaminophen (paracetamol)
  Phenobarbitone
  Phenytoin
  Salicylate
  Theophylline

Therapeutic Drug Monitoring

Therapeutic drug monitoring (TDM) is based on a relationship between desired effects, or avoidance of undesirable effects, and a target concentration (11). Such a relationship has been established for relatively few drugs (Table 43-2). There is evidence to suggest that monitoring of these drugs is of real clinical value (12). Compliance is advanced as another reason for TDM although there are considerable difficulties in interpretation; however, knowledge that treatment failure is related to noncompliance helps clinical management by enabling the reasons for this to be examined. Clinical drug trials are an area in which compliance is vital to ensure an effective comparison between therapies.

THE APPROPRIATENESS OF POCT FOR DRUGS

The immediacy of POCT lends itself to many of the clinical situations described above. Thus the ability to confirm or exclude ethanol or DOA as part of an ER patient's problem, checking the veracity of a DOA clinic user, proving an in-patient area is drug free, that a patient's medication is at an effective target concentration, or that an overdose of acetaminophen has occurred and requires treatment can all be seen as beneficial to both patient and healthcare professional alike.

Table 43-2 Drugs for Which Therapeutic Drug Monitoring Is Widely Accepted and Practiced

Anticonvulsants
  Phenytoin
  Carbamazepine
  Phenobarbital
  Lamotrigine
Immunosuppressants
  Cyclosporin A
  Tacrolimus
  Sirolimus
Antibiotics
  Gentamicin
  Vancomycin
Antiretrovirals
Others
  Digoxin
  Theophylline
  Lithium

POCT devices for drugs rarely have instrumental measurement. In the case of DOA, positivity is determined as a color change that occurs above the Substance Abuse and Mental Health Services Administration (SAMHSA) limits. Different cutoff limits are operative in Europe, notably for morphine, which makes global application of DOA POCT devices problematic. The result from a urine sample is, however, qualitative and, even if positive, it gives no information on timing, frequency, or size of dose. The development of saliva (oral fluid) as a testing matrix and the detection of far lower concentrations requires instrumental measurement (Figure 43-1). This lends itself to printed output and therefore a permanent record. Currently the preceding three factors cannot be implied from salivary data either.

POCT for DOAs in urine gives a window of detection of no more than 2 to 3 days for most DOAs (cannabis, 2 to 3 weeks). The compound to be detected may be a metabolite that may enable detection for a longer period of time and confer some specificity on the analysis. Methadone detection is used to confirm compliance with therapy and here detection of its metabolite, EDDP, is definitive. The analysis is currently available only in the laboratory, but it may soon be available as a POCT.

POCT in this and other DOA testing is effectively screening, and confirmation of positive results *must* be performed, even for clinical samples, if any substantive action (e.g., discharge or withdrawal of methadone) is contemplated. Interpretation requires an awareness of pharmacokinetics and pharmacogenetics and a clear, equitable policy based on this knowledge (13).

In establishing client veracity in a DOA clinic, the reviewer may find qualitative information adequate to enable a challenge: "Your test for opiates is positive." If the client agrees, clinical management can then proceed immediately. However, if the client disagrees, the POCT screen has to be confirmed using a laboratory method based on different analytical principles (i.e., noncorrelated), such as chromatography. This will reinforce the validity of the POCT screen in this situation to the client, who is more likely to agree the next time illicit substance use is detected by POCT. Good client–reviewer relationships are important (14). By a similar process, detection of the methadone metabolite EDDP in urine may be taken as confirmation of compliance. This enables appropriate dispensing of methadone at the time of the consultation.

As noted in the previous section, ethanol breath meters or saliva strips in an ER can rapidly provide evidence of the degree of intoxication, or rule it out as a contributory factor in the clinical presentation. Carboxyhemoglobin measured using a blood gas analyzer is commonly available in an ER to detect carbon monoxide poisoning.

Acetaminophen (paracetamol) POCT provides a cautionary tale. The authors of one report found poor correlation with the laboratory method and advised against its use (15). Subsequent correspondence suggested that the device significantly overestimated acetaminophen concentrations when compared to a reference high-performance liquid chromatographic method, whereas the routine laboratory method was satisfactory. In addition, other ER users of this POCT system found that, even with good performance, reinforced with an algorithm card for users, "in economic terms, and in accelerating care pathways to referral, it [the device] should not replace the standard, cheaper, laboratory method. . ." (16). However, a different perspective in which exclusion of the presence of acetaminophen in the ER allows effective patient disposition through rule-out using a POCT device has been claimed to be effective. It may be used in advance of the requirement for 4 hours to have elapsed as is required for quantitative measurement and use of the risk curve. Salicylates may be similarly

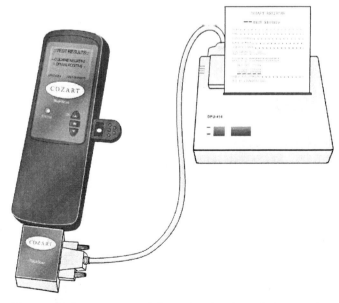

Figure 43-1 Cozart oral fluid device for drug-of-abuse testing, connected to a printer. Cozart Bioscience Ltd, Abingdon, UK.

ruled out using a POCT approach. A broad-spectrum device to detect overdose might appear appropriate, but to provide the appropriate breadth it would be prohibitively expensive— whether this might be accounted for by a reduced stay in the ER would require a good evidence base.

The limited range of drugs suitable for TDM would appear to make the use of POCT in clinics and community care attractive. However, the need for consistent acceptable quantitation by analytically inexperienced staff, yet at an acceptable cost, has meant that the two devices developed for this area, the Seralyzer (Ames, now Bayer Diagnostics, Elkhart, IN, USA) and Acculevel (Syva, now Dade Behring, Deerfield, IL, USA), have been discontinued.

ORGANIZATION AND MANAGEMENT OF POCT FOR DRUGS

Policy

The need for adequate, traceable recording of the result is a constantly recurring theme for POCT and applies equally to the use of POCT for drugs. Where blood gas analyzers are used to measure carboxyhemoglobin, the values and controls can be incorporated in the laboratory information system, if interfaced. However, a major concern is the frequent disconnection of data obtained from POCT devices from the laboratory or patient record. The information obtained usually requires the use of high-reagent-cost POCT, which if not recorded, is a loss of patient relevant data but may also be considered a waste of resources.

Introduction of any POCT device must be undertaken in cooperation with the laboratory serving that clinical area to ensure comparability of results between POCT and the laboratory. This cooperation ensures that the clinical needs and skills of the physician are matched by the clinical skills and needs of the laboratory to ensure a good quality system is chosen. Involvement of the laboratory staff with training and quality assurance ensures an ongoing dialogue reinforcing support to the users of the POCT systems (17). This is particularly relevant for POCT for drugs because the potential for false-positives and -negatives results from the variation in cross-reactivity between different antibodies. The liabilities associated with device-specific performance characteristics, and the significance of POCT results, means that there is a need for clear organization-wide policies on the introduction and use of POCT. In some countries use of in vitro diagnostic devices is governed by national guidelines (18).

Nonadherence to the requirements of the POCT policy should be considered as serious a problem as nonadherence to any other clinical policy. This is a quality management, a clinical risk, and ultimately a disciplinary issue, and therefore the responsible executive must be aware of, and support, such policies in full.

Drugs of Abuse

In workplace testing there is a need to ensure the integrity of the specimen. This entails use of chain-of-custody procedures.

For clinical situations such procedures are rarely used; however, the knowledge available to clinic users means that great care is required in the preanalytical phase. Urine must be collected under indirect observation, i.e., watching in a mirror, to avoid the many adulteration options practiced (19), or indeed substitutions with "clean" urine (20). Some individuals drink large volumes of water to lower concentrations of drugs below the positive threshold; creatinine measurement or post-collection concentration has been advocated as a way to circumvent the problem (21).

For POCT to be applied to clinical DOA testing it is therefore necessary to perform a number of preanalytical checks including pH, specific gravity, foaming, aroma, and appearance, to detect attempts to circumvent testing by adulterating the specimen and thereby disrupting the analytical system. Proof that a result, particularly a positive result, has come from a particular individual requires careful logging of patients' results in a systematic, auditable fashion, ensuring that the quality assurance procedures used are also documented.

The limitations of urine testing for DOAs are well known. Testing for DOAs in saliva is aesthetically more pleasing and therefore more acceptable to donor and observer. However, the window of detection is different from that for urine: drugs may be detected sooner, but not for as long as in urine. Saliva is a poor medium for detecting cannabis use. The preanalytical variables affecting saliva DOA testing are not as well characterized as for urine, nor are the opportunities for manipulation and avoidance of detection. No doubt the drug users will come up with many attempts; it remains to be seen which work.

POCT devices may be analytically inadequate, or subject to significant interindividual variation in reading (22). Adequate initial and continuing training is essential. Some devices include positive and negative controls; these are usually proof that the reaction works and not confirmation that a particular drug can be detected. It is highly advisable, although rarely practiced, that users of POCT for DOAs should participate in an external quality assurance (EQA) scheme (23). EQA participation directly in an EQA scheme, or through a central laboratory in a laboratory network configuration, are options that need to be explored to ensure that POCT is not only rapid but is also of good quality.

A clear policy for handling positive POCT results must be delineated and the required procedure for confirmatory analyses should be followed. In workplace testing there can be significant financial liability for acting on an erroneous POCT result. However, incorrect results obtained in a clinical setting may also result in significant financial penalties. Therefore good organization and management of all the aspects of the POCT program are essential.

Toxicology

DOA POCT devices are used in ERs to identify causes of symptoms. In this situation it is the pharmacological effect that is important, and confirmation of a positive screen is rarely required. Exclusion of acetaminophen and salicylate poisoning with POCT devices provides an opportunity to triage suspected analgesic overdoses more effectively.

OUTCOMES AND BENEFITS FROM POCT FOR DRUGS

There is much claimed as to the outcomes and benefits of POCT in a clinical DOA testing setting. Thus the ability POCT gives to challenge veracity and reinforce the client–physician relationship is highly valuable provided those performing the tests are aware of the limitations. If there is client denial the sample must be referred for confirmation *before* definitive challenge. The delay in returning negative or predictable results from a central laboratory means any reinforcement is retrospective. To date, there is no evidence as to whether POCT or central laboratory testing yields the greater benefit in terms of outcome. Whichever is used, analysis is superior to relying on user self-report (24).

POCT ensures effective outcomes for substance abusers presenting for admission to hospital; the use of DOA POCT in the ER to detect cocaine or heroin use immediately directs medical intervention. Where opiate misusers have access to a methadone maintenance program it is important to confirm prior exposure to methadone to ensure continuity of use. However, users can claim methadone use without previous or recent use; this is dangerous and potentially fatal. A facility prescribing methadone without evidence of use would therefore be negligent and liable to a lawsuit. Use of a POCT device for methadone, or preferably EDDP, ensures identification of the correct categorization of the patient.

Support of an anticonvulsant clinic using laboratory personnel with a simple laboratory analyzer has been shown to be cost effective (25), offering the opportunity for the clinician to review the patient in light of the drug concentration, history, and examination and to make any dosage adjustments immediately. As with other forms of clinic-based POCT, this minimizes patient attendances, provides a more meaningful letter to the community physician, and maximizes patient throughput per physician. A short outcomes study did show a significant reduction in the time to achieve optimal phenytoin levels in a group of newly diagnosed epileptic individuals compared with using a laboratory service. In addition, there was a reduction in the number of clinical visits and drug dosage changes (26). The disadvantage is that although there is an additional cost to the institution for the POCT device, this cannot be recovered from the laboratory; for the latter it is a minor revenue saving. Furthermore it is challenging to recover the saving from the clinical area in which POCT has been introduced, as a result of the reduction in clinic visits, although it might be claimed that such an approach could help to reduce waiting lists. There is no evidence offered to suggest a patient's long-term outcome is better, as it has not been studied; however, it is likely that there will be improved patient satisfaction—and possibly improved long-term compliance. These papers illustrated the use of POCT for anticonvulsants in a clinic setting operated by lab-

oratory personnel. Where there are focused groups of a reasonable number of patients, such an approach may offer organizational advantages, ensure quality results, and draw laboratory personnel out to be part of the clinical team. The Acculevel device offered the opportunity of TDM for infrequent use, but the lack of successors to this device suggest this was not a commercially attractive option.

An interesting study reported by Cope et al. (27) looked at the use of POCT for nicotine in a program intended to reduce cigarette smoking during pregnancy. A cross-sectional randomized controlled trial was set up involving 856 pregnant women. Patients were tested for smoking using a urine nicotine concentration testing device that gave both visual and numerical results. Only smokers were subsequently enrolled in the study. The intervention group participants were given the test results and received smoking reduction counseling, while the control group participants were not given the results and received conventional counseling. A target date to quit smoking was agreed to (usually within 14 days), and the protocol was repeated on subsequent clinic visits. The urine nicotine results also showed a strong correlation with self-reported cigarette consumption. Self-reported cigarette consumption—the outcome measure employed in the study—fell significantly in the intervention group, with 16.2% giving up smoking and 33.3% reducing their consumption, compared with only 8% and 23%, respectively, in the control group ($P < 0.001$).

WHERE IS POCT FOR DRUG TESTING NOW?

Prior to the Vietnam war, analyses for drugs were performed in central laboratories using chromatography or wet chemistry methods. A few simple color tests for use on urine had been developed in the 1950s allowing POCT for salicylate, phenothiazines, and neuroleptics. Immunoassays relied on radioisotopes and were the domain of specialized laboratories with slow turnaround times. At this time there was little significant illegal substance abuse in the population of the Western world; overdoses were usually caused by salicylates and barbiturates. Laborious quantitative methods existed for the latter while a simpler colorimetric assay existed for the former. TDM had only just been identified as relevant for anticonvulsant dosing (28).

Testing of the US military in Vietnam for substance abuse required a reliable, rapid-throughput methodology. This need was met with the development of the enzyme multiplied immunoassay technique (EMIT), which was applied to, and helped develop, TDM. Extra-laboratory testing needs were met with a briefcase-sized package that enabled suitably trained individuals to perform testing near to the subject. As programs were developed to deal with the increasing incidence of substance abuse, this technology lent itself to clinic use.

Laboratory and POCT DOA assays utilized the cutoff limits recommended by the National Institute of Drug Abuse (NIDA). Consequently, clinical management philosophies of dealing with positive results were, and still are, influenced by the demands of forensic workplace testing. These guidelines have been adopted worldwide. The reason in part is that the initial laboratory assays for DOAs in urine were sold by US companies, but also because NIDA, now SAMHSA, conducted unique research into DOA pharmacokinetics and pharmacodynamics, which enabled the identification of cutoff concentrations that maximized the efficiency of the tests. These guidelines are the subject of occasional review; workplace cutoffs have also been developed in Europe and a divergence is developing. SAMHSA has recently considered the cutoff values appropriate for oral fluid (saliva) testing; this is complicated by the fact that POCT compatible testing utilizes saliva, while oral fluid is a hypertonically induced transudate for central laboratory analysis. However, typically the term "oral fluid" is used.

The clinical philosophy in dealing with substance misuse has recognized that there are different groups of users: cocaine users, amphetamine users, or opiate users who abuse heroin intravenously or by smoking. Some use quantities of codeine linctus orally or dihydrocodeine; the last two are legally available and offer a defense in the case of a positive screen. The harm-minimization needs of the different users may be addressed in different ways.

The use of chromatography allows separation of opiates that cross-react in immunoassay systems and in particular indicates codeine–morphine ratios, which can be used to distinguish whether heroin or codeine was more likely to have been used. A definitive heroin metabolite, 6-monoacetylmorphine, is preferred in workplace testing although it has a short half-life; this view is reflected in clinical DOA testing.

The structural side chain of amphetamines is variously substituted to produce different congeners; unfortunately the epitope is similar to other compounds and cross-reactions with ephedrine, ranitidine, and other compounds are well known to laboratory personnel. In programs where *d*-amphetamine is prescribed to amphetamine users, immunoassays such as used in POCT cannot distinguish between this and the street supply, which is racemic.

A further difficulty with class-specific antibodies is the need for up to 25-fold differences in concentration to trigger a positive result (e.g., antidepressant or benzodiazepine POCT immunoassays). This was a particular issue when immunoassays designed for the North American market were applied in Europe, where different compounds within the class were misused; consequently, analytical performance was often poor (29). However, these issues are being addressed. The antibodies used in central laboratory methods are also used in POCT, which enables comparability of accuracy and sensitivity between field and laboratory methods.

Users of POCT devices frequently lack knowledge of the limitations of analytical systems including the POCT assay and make inappropriate care decisions (4, 19, 21, 30). This situation is exacerbated by an ever-increasing range of POCT sticks and cartridges for the common DOA tests being produced.

Comparisons of POCT DOA devices with laboratory immunoassay procedures indicate that some are unacceptable for use (22, 31, 32), and even those that are said to be acceptable will perform differently from each other and from labora-

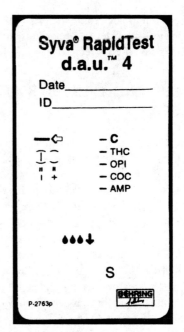

Figure 43-2 Drug-of-abuse multitest cartridge: C, control; THC, tetrahydrocannibinol carboxylic acid; OPI, opiates; COC, cocaine; AMP, amphetamines. Dade Behring, Deerfield, IL, USA.

tory immunoassay methods (30, 33, 34). Although some claim good comparison, (35) even these devices have operational problems (36).

Most POCT devices for DOAs use immunochromatography with migration of the compound of interest to a point where it can react with the antibody. These may be for a single analyte or have a selection of drugs on the same slide. The Syva Rapid Test (Figure 43-2) has various drug combinations, allowing a degree of customization to clinical needs; other devices, e.g., Triage, have fixed combinations. Visualization of positives may occur either as a developing color zone, or as a zone that disappears; i.e., negatives give a line. Clearly there is the potential for confusion, although both types of systems are available. This reinforces the need for a coherent policy on the introduction and use of POCT in the clinical or workplace environment.

As indicated earlier, DOA users have various motivations for cheating the system. To address this problem, Roche has developed the OnTrak TesTCup (Figure 43-3) to circumvent tampering by clients and to ensure sample integrity. Any positives identified on the integral immunochromatographic strip can be sealed and sent for subsequent confirmation (37, 38).

Although the use of such sophisticated devices may be justified in workplace testing, such rigor is unlikely to be thought economically justifiable in routine clinical testing. However, there are clinical and social services situations in which it might be beneficial to all concerned, e.g., high-security mental institutions, child place-of-safety cases, and forensic psychiatric outpatient cases.

Because of the operator dependence of POCT for DOAs and the varied cross-reactivity and nondetection of substances

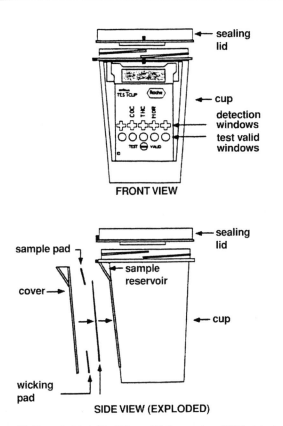

Figure 43-3   OnTrak TesTCup: COC, cocaine; THC, tetrahydro-cannibinol carboxylic acid; MOR, morphine. Reproduced with permission from (37).

not included in the POCT analytical profile, good clinical practice will require confirmation of positives and more extensive investigation for drugs not screened for, e.g., lysergic acid diethylamide (LSD), khat, and buprenorphine [for reviews see Braithwaite et al. (39) and Simpson et al. (40)].

The limitation to urine screening for DOA is the short window of positivity, with the exception of cannabis; many drug dependency units consider cannabis use to be ubiquitous and not relevant. Blood poses a far greater infection risk than urine and requires detection of far lower concentrations of drugs, with consequently greater demands on analytical systems. The last criticism can also be applied to saliva, sweat, and hair. Although these are noninvasive, saliva testing initially for ethanol is becoming important in clinical use through a POCT DOA device originally developed for police use. Hair provides a longitudinal record of substance use; at the very least this covers the last 7 days even if the head is shaved, but it does not lend itself to POCT, although it is more sensitive than urine testing (41). Sweat testing using patches has been shown to correlate with urine testing in outpatients (42). Its use may become more widely applied. There is a need for different antibodies in these matrices from those used in urine tests, because in the former the drug accumulates in greater quantities as the parent compound than as its metabolites, as occurs in urine.

What are the prospects? DOA testing, driven by workplace and police testing, will continue apace, and the systems will be

utilized in clinical settings. The main difficulty is that testing has to be done for appropriate clinical reasons; i.e., one must know the question before getting the answer! Clinical practice in drug-dependence clinics dispensing methadone in support of opiate addicts was undermined by the ease with which the clients of these services perfected the ability to add just sufficient linctus to their urine samples to obtain a positive urine methadone reading, thus ensuring a continuing supply, some or all of which could be resold. The advent of a POCT device to detect EDDP will greatly help clinics. The new alternative therapies to methadone being introduced, such as buprenorphine (43), in widespread use in some countries (e.g., France), demand the utility of POCT systems to demonstrate compliance. In clinical toxicology the continuing popularity of acetaminophen as an overdose agent and the proven success and safety of N-acetylcysteine has led to the development of a POCT device. Will similar devices be developed for other over-the-counter drugs (e.g., ibuprofen)? A broad spectrum of poisons encountered less frequently yet of clinical significance would be worth detecting and would require a broad-spectrum device. However, there is little evidence that such information changes management (7).

Classic TDM drugs are becoming used less frequently, although still in large numbers, and may not be an attractive area for commercial development. Immunosuppressant drug monitoring is widely practiced, particularly for cyclosporine, and use of sirolimus and tacrolimus is increasing as concentrations are critical to managing organ rejection and nephrotoxicity; if a sufficiently precise POCT device could be developed, this would be attractive. Antiretrovirals for use in HIV-positive patients may require monitoring; as many of these patients may not readily access healthcare, there might be a role for POCT.

Alternatives to immunoassay and color reaction–based POCT devices may be developed using field-effect transistor technology, but they may still show the same inherent specificity and narrow-spectrum problem of other devices. However, microchip technology has already given us handheld gas chromatographs and microcapillary electrophoresis, so that the separation power of these techniques could be harnessed to a wide variety of tasks and would transform POCT for drugs.

Pharmacogenomics is seen as a potentially economic way of determining metabolic clearance rates and susceptibility to drugs, thus enabling dosing regimens to be prospectively informed. It is not inconceivable that POCT genotyping could be used for detecting drugs if phenotypically significant differences are present (e.g., CYP2D6).

One area common to all and greatly neglected is the issue of quality. It is to be hoped that POCT for DOAs and other drugs will be the subject of self-regulated or legally required quality systems incorporating meaningful quality control. Experience of laboratory drug testing through EQA schemes has shown just how poor performance can be. It is likely the same or worse pertains in the arena of POCT. Involvement in an independent, relevant, and effective EQA system is essential if the credibility of POCT results seek comparability with central laboratory testing.

HEALTH ECONOMIC ANALYSIS OF POCT FOR DRUGS

Evidence-based medicine standards have been considered for TDM, toxicology, and DOA, and there is evidence that appropriate use can have beneficial clinical, economic, and disciplinary impacts; these are balanced by the disadvantages arising from uncritical, misinformed use. Formal health economic analysis has not been performed; the best evidence base is the NACB publication on evidence-based POCT (http://www.nacb.org/lmpg/poct_lmpg.draft.stm). Much of the POCT practiced is in relation to testing of substance misusers. The necessity for comprehensive toxicology screens was disproved by clinical practice many years ago; thus if the basis of the measurements as currently performed is not proven it is unlikely that use of POCT in these situations will be any better. There are benefits of POCT use versus laboratory analysis in all the situations addressed in this chapter; proof, although available, still requires more robust demonstration.

REFERENCES

1. Seamonds B. Medical, economic and regulatory factors affecting point-of-care testing. Clin Chim Acta 1996;249:1–19.
2. Blick KE. The essential role of information management in point of care/critical care testing. Clin Chim Acta 2001;307:159–68.
3. National Academy Clinical Biochemistry. Laboratory management practice guidelines. Evidence based practice for POCT. To report in summer 2004. http://www.nacb.org.lmpg/poct_lmpg.draft.stm (accessed June 2004).
4. Schwarz RH. Urine testing in the detection of drugs of abuse. Arch Intern Med 1988;148:2407–12.
5. Boutros N, Bonnett K, Mak T. Drug abuse: a significant variable in schizophrenia research. Biol Psychiatry 1996;39:1053–4.
6. Jehanli A, Brannan S, Moore L, Spiehler VR. Blind trials of an onsite saliva drug test for marijuana and opiates. J Forens Sci 2001;46:1214–20.
7. Watson ID. Laboratory support of the poisoned patient. Ther Drug Monit 1998;20:490–97.
8. Watson ID, Proudfoot AT. Poisoning and laboratory medicine. London: ACB Venture, 2002;107.
9. Bendtsen P, Hultberg J, Carlsson M, Jones AW. Monitoring ethanol exposure in a clinical setting by analysis of blood, breath, saliva, and urine. Alcohol Clin Exp Res 1999;23:1446–51.
10. Watson ID, Proudfoot AT. In: Sherwood RA, ed. Poisoning and laboratory medicine. London: ACB Venture, 2002:57, 133.
11. Watson ID, Potter J, Yatscoff R, Fraser, A et al. Definition of therapeutic drug monitoring. Ther Drug Monit 1997;19:25.
12. Watson ID. A case for therapeutic drug monitoring. In: Sunshine I, ed. Recent development in therapeutic drug monitoring and clinical toxicology. New York: Marcel Dekker, 1992:3–8.
13. Hedenmalm K, Sundgren M, Granberg K, Spigeset O, Dahlqvist R. Urinary excretion of codeine, ethylmorphine and their metabolites: relation to the CYP206 activity. Ther Drug Monit 1997;19:643–9.
14. Woody GE, McLellan AT, Luborsky L, O'Brien CP. Psychotherapy and counselling for methadone-maintained opiate addicts: results of research studies. NIDA Res Monogr 1990;104: 9–23.
15. Egleston CV, Browning C, Hamdi I, Campbell-Hewson G, Robinson SM. Comparison of two assays for measuring plasma concentrations of paracetamol. Br Med J 1997;315: 991–2.
16. Jones AL, Jarvie, DR, Simpson D, Prescott LF. Comparison of assays for measuring plasma paracetamol. Possibility of calibration error needs evaluation. Br Med J 1998;316:475.
17. Fitzpatrick R, Hassan T, Ward V, Bodiwala G. Training and education in use of assays are important. Br Med J 1998;316: 475–6.
18. Medical Devices Agency. Management and use of IVD point of care test devices. UK Department of Health, March 2002.
19. Kapur BM. Drug-testing methods and clinical interpretations of test results. Bull Narc 1993;45:115–54.
20. Council on Scientific Affairs. Scientific issues in drug testing. JAMA 1987;257:3110–4.
21. Luceri F, Godi F, Messeri G. Reducing false-negative tests in urinary drugs of abuse screening. J. Anal Toxicol 1997;21: 244–5.
22. Ros JJW, Pelders MG, Egberts ACG. Performance of drugs of abuse slide tests with particular emphasis on concentrations near the cut-off: comparison with FPIA-ADx and confirmation of results with GC-MS. J Anal Toxicol 1998;22:40–4.
23. Watson ID. Screening for drugs of abuse: how confident can you be in the results? Assoc. Clin Biochem News Sheet 1993; 36:10–4.
24. Ehrman RN, Robbins SJ, Cornish, JW. Comparing self-reported cocaine use with repeated urine tests in outpatient cocaine abusers. Exp Clin Psychopharmacol 1997;5:150–6.
25. Elliot K, Watson ID, Tsintis P, Gray J, Stewart MJ, Kadr H, Lawson DH. The impact of near patient testing on the organisation and costs of an anticonvulsant clinic. Ther Drug Monit 1990;120:434–7.
26. Patsalos PN, Sander JW, Oxley J. Immediate anticonvulsive drug monitoring in management of epilepsy. Lancet 1987;2:39.
27. Cope GF, Nayyar P, Holder R. Feedback from point-of-care test for nicotine intake to reduce smoking during pregnancy. Ann Clin Biochem 2003;40:674–9.
28. Barr WH. The pharmacokinetic basis for using blood anti-epileptic levels in monitoring and optimizing therapy. In: Pippenger CE, Penry JK, Kutt H, eds. Anti-epileptic drugs: quantitative analysis and interpretation. New York: Raven Press, 1978:237–51.
29. Hansen HJ, Caudill SP, Boone J. Crisis in drug testing. JAMA 1985:2382–7.
30. Fisher J. Immunoassay drug screen results: easy to get, hard to interpret. Clin Toxicol 1998;36:115–6.
31. Kintz P, Godelar B, Cirimele V. Evaluation of the Rapidrug cannabis non-instrumental immunoassay. J Anal Toxicol 1997; 21:243–6.
32. Jenkins AJ, Darwin WD, Huestis MA, Cone EJ, Mitchell JM. Validity testing of the accupPINCH THC test. J Anal Toxicol 1995;19:5–12.
33. Schwartz RH, Bogema S, Thorne MM. Evaluation of the EZ-SCREEN enzyme immunoassay test for detection of cocaine and marijuana metabolites in urine specimens. Pediatr Emerg Care 1990;6:147–9.

34. Wu AH, Wong SS, Johnson KG, Callies J, Shu DX, Dunn WE, Wong SH. Evaluation of the Triage system for emergency drugs of abuse testing in urine. J Anal Toxicol 1993;17:241–5.

35. De la Torre R, Domingo-Salvany A, Badia R, Gonzalez G, McFarlane D, San L, Torrens M. Clinical evaluation of the Triage analytical device for drugs of abuse testing. Clin Chem 1996;42:1433–8.

36. Poklis A, O'Neal C. Potential for false-positive results by the TRIAGE panel of drugs of abuse immunoassay. J Anal Toxicol 1996;20:209–10.

37. Towt J, Tsai SC, Hernandez MR, Klimov AD, Kravec CV, Rouse SL, et al. ONTRAK TESTCUP: a novel, on-site, multi-analyte screen for the detection of abused drugs. J Anal Tox 1995;19: 504–10.

38. Crouch DJ, Cheever ML, Andrenyak DM, Kuntz DJ, Loughmiller DL. A comparison of ONTRAK TESTCUP, Abuscreen ONLINE and GC/MS urinalysis test results. J Forens Sci 1998;43:35–40.

39. Braithwaite RA, Jarvie DR, Minty PSB, Simpson D, Widdop B. Screening for drugs of abuse. I: Opiates, amphetamines and cocaine. Ann Clin Biochem 1995;32:123–53.

40. Simpson D, Braithwaite RA, Jarvie DR, Stewart MJ, Walker S, Watson ID, Widdop B. Screening for drugs of abuse (II); cannabinoids, lysergic acid diethylamide, buprenorphine, methadone, barbiturates, benzodiazepines and other drugs. Ann Clin Biochem 1997;34:460–510.

41. Kintz P. Drug testing in addicts: a comparison between urine, sweat and hair. Ther Drug Monit 1996;18:450–5.

42. Taylor JR, Watson ID, Tames FJ, Lowe D. Detection of drug use in a methadone maintenance clinic: sweat patches versus urine testing. Addiction 1998;93:847–53.

43. Johnson RE, Fudala PJ. Development of buprenorphine for the treatment of opioid dependence. In: Blaine JD, ed. Buprenorphine: an alternative treatment for opioid dependence. NIDA Res Monogr 1992;121: 120–41.

Chapter 44

Point-of-Care Testing in Histopathology

Krsty P. Nale, Maria R. Calaminici, and Joanne E. Martin

Point-of-care testing (POCT) in histopathology does exist; it focuses not on the clinician taking a sample and sending it to the laboratory, but on the operator, often the pathologist, taking the sample and making a diagnosis. For the purposes of this chapter we exclude frozen sections, as they still involve the pathologist receiving the sample from the clinical team, even if the pathologist's laboratory is next to the operating room. This exclusion is not purely logical, as many classify frozen sections as point-of-care procedures, but it is pragmatic, and there are more interesting areas to cover.

POCT in histopathology (anatomical pathology) as discussed in this chapter encompasses primarily smear, scrape, and fine-needle aspiration (FNA) cytology (wet mounts). Many of these procedures may be classified as provider-performed microscopy procedures such as wet mounts, including preparations of vaginal, cervical, or skin specimens, as well as potassium hydroxide preparations for fungi (see, e.g., www.cms.hhs.gov/clia/ppmplst.asp). It has taken some time for many of these procedures to be accepted, and pioneers such as Stewart from New York did much to change practice, and to validate the techniques involved. Their widespread use is continuing with introduction in a range of areas, transforming the patient pathway and speeding care. A wealth of data about FNA is available in a variety of formats via the World Wide Web [see, e.g., University of Iowa Health Care (1)] and also in the medical literature.

FNA AND CLINICAL INVESTIGATION

In many settings fine-needle aspirate cytology remains the first choice for the initial investigation and diagnosis of both superficial and deep lesions (2–5). It is also a means of confirming a clinical suspicion of local recurrence or metastasis of known cancer without the need to subject patients to further surgical intervention. It is a tool not only in the primary and preoperative diagnosis of tumors but also in the diagnosis of nonneoplastic conditions, in monitoring graft rejection, and in diagnostic evaluation during intraoperative settings.

Superficial FNA is applicable to the superficial palpable lesions in skin, soft tissue, salivary glands, thyroid, breast, and lymph nodes. Using needle biopsy guided by ultrasound or by computed tomography, it is relatively easy to diagnose deep-located lesions (3–6). Intraoperative FNA cytology is a complement to frozen section where there is a need for definitive diagnosis in order to proceed with surgery.

Benefits and Limitations

FNA is relatively painless, inexpensive, and, in experienced hands, can approach histopathology in providing a conclusive diagnosis. With the immediate reading of preparations, the speed of diagnosis cannot be paralleled by conventional histopathological methods other than frozen section. The very low risk of complications is an additional advantage, allowing FNA to be performed in the outpatient department, where the majority of patients can be treated conservatively or referred to the hospital if found to have a serious disease, thus reducing the rate of surgery for benign disease. In a hospital setting, FNA can be used in debilitated patients as a preoperative or pretreatment investigation in planning surgery, radiotherapy, and chemotherapy (7).

In some fields, cytological morphological criteria for the diagnosis of malignancy remain to be defined, especially in difficult diagnostic areas such as soft tissue tumors and some cystic lesions (8), and in such cases, in the interest of the patient, it would be reasonable to send the patient to a center with specialized expertise. For FNA to be successful it is vital that an adequate specimen is taken and prepared according to strict guidelines. During the interpretation of FNA samples it must not be forgotten that diagnosis is the final piece of the puzzle, to be correlated with and validated against clinical and other investigations. Information obtained from FNA must play a decisive part in any final decision making at clinico-pathological meetings with a multidisciplinary team composed of surgeons, radiologists, and oncologists as well as others involved in patient care.

Serious consequences such as major hemorrhage, septicemia, bile peritonitis, acute pancreatitis, pneumothorax, and needle-track seeding occur very rarely. The incidence of needle-track seeding is increased if needles larger than 21 gauge are used, if the neoplastic growth is on the surface of the parenchymatous organ, and if multiple passes are attempted.

Some histopathologists still express skepticism about the level of diagnostic accuracy of FNA. Furthermore, specialized areas such as lymphoma subtyping and soft tissue and bone tumor diagnosis are best managed by tissue biopsy. Still more should be done to standardize reports and promote better communication between the pathologist and clinicians, who may sometimes not be aware of the morphological limitations of the technique.

FNA TECHNIQUE

The aim of FNA is to obtain maximum material from the lesion with minimum trauma to the patient. The pathologist must be given all the relevant clinical and radiological data beforehand to assess the feasibility of access. The clinical history should include the patient's age and gender, the anatomical localization, clinical findings, and previous therapy. For breast cytodiagnosis, pregnancy, lactation, and mammography findings are important data.

Disposable 25- to 21-gauge needles are used for palpable superficial lesions. When using cutting-core needles to obtain a core of tissue for paraffin embedding and sectioning, the risk of tumor implantation along the needle track, hemorrhage, and discomfort for the patient have to be taken into account. A 27-gauge needle is recommended for children; a 5- to 20-mL disposable plastic syringe producing a good negative pressure is convenient for routine aspiration technique. Different brands of syringe holders that allow precision in placing the needle are available. To obtain material for cell suspension or cell block, sterile containers containing physiological saline to rinse needles and syringes should be at hand. To smear the aspirate, two cleaned, dried slides and a coverslip for more even spread are required (see Figure 44-1). A 70% to 90% ethanol or spray fixative is used in routine wet fixation of smears. A microscope and Diff-Quick stain, or the equivalent, are used to assess the adequacy of the smear, and to make a preliminary diagnosis they should be available in the same room or in a separate suite near the patient. Preinjection swabs, sterile dressings, sterile scalpel blades, latex gloves, and face masks should also be on hand. All of these can be kept in a small toolbox that can conveniently be carried to clinics, wards (units), and radiology departments.

Before starting, the procedure should be explained to the patient, and the patient's consent and cooperation must be sought and documented. For superficial biopsies, preinjection swabs for simple skin disinfection are adequate. Local anesthesia (2% lignocaine) is very rarely necessary in superficial biopsies. A spray anesthetic is convenient for mucosa-covered surfaces, and an anesthetic ointment is useful in biopsies performed on children.

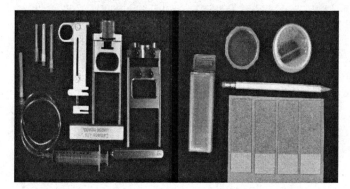

Figure 44-1   The equipment used for fine-needle aspiration.

Procedure

Superficial palpable lumps are immobilized between the thumb and the first two fingers. FNA is performed by passing a fine needle (27 to 23 gauge) alone without suction, or more often attached to the syringe and syringe holder, into the target tissue. Once positioned within the target tissue, the needle is moved within the lesion in a fan-shaped fashion and at the same time the plunger is pulled to apply negative pressure. The negative pressure in the syringe increases the yield.

Before exiting the lesion, negative pressure is released. Blood in the syringe is not desirable, and suction should stop if blood appears in the hub of the needle. After exiting the lesion, the needle is detached from the syringe, and air is drawn into the syringe. Finally, the needle is attached to the syringe, and the contents (aspirate) of the needle are blown onto a glass slide.

In sclerotic or necrotic lesions where cell yield is poor, aspiration should be repeated, aiming at the margins of the lesion.

Capillary Sampling.   For fine-needle sampling without aspiration, the needle is moved to and fro within the target lesion, varying the angle to cover a larger area. In this case capillary pressure in the fine needle keeps the cells inside the lumen. This technique is preferable for most neck lumps, especially from the thyroid gland, where aspiration inevitably yields to hemodilution. It is also routinely used for sampling all superficial lesions except for cystic lesions, soft tissue tumors, and some fibrous breast lesions.

As the needle is withdrawn, pressure is applied over the site to prevent bruising. To avoid this complication, it is important to stress that a good FNA technique is paramount; i.e., use a thin needle (25 to 23 gauge), and release negative pressure on the syringe and the needle before exiting the lesion.

Aspiration of a thyroid nodule might very rarely lead to accidental puncture of the trachea, which is harmless to the patient, except for causing a slight cough.

The diagnostic accuracy of FNA varies among different centers but on average reaches 95%, for example, in thyroid and salivary gland aspirates. Diagnostic accuracy is even higher when combined with clinical and radiological assessments, for example, FNA cytology of breast carcinoma combined with clinical assessment and mammography (the triple approach).

Skin Scraping.   Fungal lesions of the skin can be identified by incubating a scraping of the affected skin or hairs detached from the lesion in 10% KOH. Diagnostic cells from viral lesions are obtained from the base of a vesicle (Tzanck test).

Diagnostic material obtained from a direct scrape is preferred for ulcerated lesions, while subcutaneous nodules and soft tissue masses may be sampled by FNA. A permanent preparation is made by either the Papanicolau or Romanowsky method.

Sample Errors

If the needle passes the lesion tangentially, an adjacent tissue reaction will be sampled, and the lesion will be misdiagnosed as an inflammatory process. Some tumors are centrally necrotic or cystic, and the sample of such focus may not yield diagnostic cells. In such cases, aspiration is repeated, aiming at the margins of the lesion, which are representative. A benign tumor or cyst can overlie a small malignant tumor, producing false-negative results. Therefore, it is important to repeat the biopsy of any remaining palpable lesion after the apparently complete aspiration of a cyst.

Processing the Sample and Staining

Material obtained from the needle used for FNA is expelled onto a slide using air in the syringe, avoiding splashing. Sometimes the crucial part of the aspirate is in the hub of the needle and cannot be expelled. Such a sample must be retrieved using another needle. There are two kinds of aspirates, one referred to as "dry," consisting of numerous cells suspended in a small amount of tissue fluid, and another referred to as "wet," composed of a small number of cells suspended in fluid or blood.

A dry aspirate is best smeared with the flat side of a microscopic slide, avoiding the ridge of the glass and applying a light pressure to achieve a thin, even spread without blood clots. Applying too hard a pressure produces smearing (mechanical) artifacts.

A wet aspirate is smeared by moving the smearing slide from one end of the specimen slide at a blunt angle. In this way the cells follow the movement of the smearing slide. Concentrated cells are then smeared with the slide kept flat. The smearing technique must be done quickly to avoid coagulation and to enable adequate cell fixation and staining. If a small fragment of tissue is seen on the smearing slide, it can be picked up and either put on another slide and smeared, or added to a drop of blood to form a clot and then processed as a cell block. Thin fluid samples should be processed by centrifugation, which gives better results than filtration.

For lymph node aspirates, it is recommended to have a cell suspension in addition to direct smears. For cell suspension, an aspirate is mixed with Hank's balanced salt solution and 10% fetal calf serum. A smear is then prepared by centrifugation at low speed. The undiluted specimen shows clumping of cells with many smudged nuclei; therefore, dilution is required to obtain the dispersion of cells necessary for the adequate interpretation of lymphoid cells. Thick, bloody smears with clotting and unevenly spread smears are inadequate for interpretation.

In FNA cytology two methods of fixation and staining are routinely used, both having advantages and disadvantages. One method uses air drying followed by staining with May–Grunwald–Giemsa stain, Wright's stain, or Diff-Quick, and the other method uses 95% ethanol fixation followed by staining with Papanicolaou (Pap) or hematoxylin and eosin (H&E). With air drying, cells flatten on the glass slide and appear larger than cells fixed in ethanol; this cytological feature is useful in cytodiagnosis, but requires preparation by experienced technicians. Smearing artifacts, however, can also occur with wet fixation if the smearing has not been done properly.

In Giemsa-stained smears, the nuclear chromatin pattern is well demonstrated. Because tissue properties stained by the Giemsa and Pap methods look different when compared, the use of one stain cannot be favored over the other. The two methods of staining should ideally complement each other when the pathological process is interpreted under the microscope. To check the adequacy of a specimen obtained in the operating room or in a one-stop clinic, rapid-type stains (such as Diff-Quik) can be used.

Finally, it should not be forgotten that in the interest of the patient, the cytopathologist must be as much clinician as microscopist. New technologies (e.g., serial analysis of gene expression in small samples and proton magnetic resonance techniques) will make diagnostic work in specialized areas easier, and the interface with molecular pathology and genetics will become less distinct as biosensors and array technology move from the development stage into everyday use.

CLINICAL APPLICATIONS

A wide range of applications currently exist for POCT in histopathology and cytology. Some general and some specific examples are described and discussed in the following sections.

Central Nervous System

The main source of cytological specimens for the diagnosis of diseases involving the central nervous system is cerebrospinal fluid, which is obtained via a lumbar puncture or by aspirating ventricles via burr holes. In addition, crushed preparation of specimens can be obtained intraoperatively as an open biopsy during craniotomy or as an aspiration biopsy via stereotactic computed tomography (CT)-guided biopsy. Disease processes affecting meninges and subarachnoid spaces can be evaluated by sampling cerebrospinal fluid. However, aspiration biopsy with immediate study of the resultant sample is primarily used for the diagnosis of intracranial tumors.

FNA of the Salivary Gland

FNAs are a common source of diagnosis in the head and neck area because a wide range of primary and metastatic neoplasms first present in this area. In the salivary gland, FNA is a well-established and reliable technique (9). FNA is taken to obtain a preoperative diagnosis in order to distinguish benign disease (e.g., sialosis) and thus avoid the need for surgery (important in the elderly and in patients who are poor surgical risks) or confirm malignancy and thus the need for surgery (see Figure 44-2). In those undergoing surgery, preoperative FNA can enable the surgeon to plan wide surgical excision if the tumor is high grade. In this case, intraoperative confirmation of tumor type by frozen section is advised even though specific

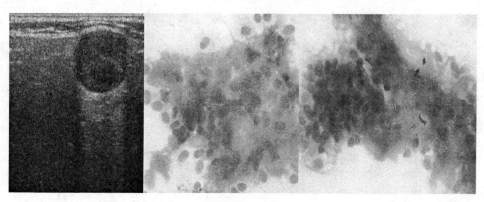

Figure 44-2   A pleomorphic adenoma of the parotid gland seen on ultrasound and on fine-needle aspirate preparation.

diagnosis will not alter the clinical management of the patient. Assessment of the completeness of excision after surgery is still performed using the conventional resection specimen. In the case of local recurrence, nodal metastasis of known cancer elsewhere, or high-grade malignancy, FNA will confirm the need for palliative treatment, and thus the need for further surgery is avoided.

When performing FNA on immunocompromised patients, caution should be exercised to avoid needle-stick injury. When sampling cystic lesions that can be nonneoplastic or neoplastic, the cyst wall should be reaspirated if possible to obtain the representative cells. This is important because, for example, a cystic tumor may be misdiagnosed as a retention cyst if the solid component is not sampled. In addition, the majority of cystic lesions are multicystic. Cytological morphology can closely mimic that of neoplastic tissue if the aspirated sample comes from a previously irradiated patient. Inflamed branchial cysts and necrosis of well-differentiated squamous cell carcinoma pose a special problem in differential diagnosis and are a common cause of misdiagnosis in this area. A more frequent problem is distinction between intraparotid lymphadenopathy (normally lymph nodes can be found within the parotid gland tissue owing to late encapsulation in fetal life) and inflammatory disease of the salivary gland. If a metastatic deposit is sampled from an intraparotid lymph node, distinction has to be made from a primary carcinoma. A clinical history of a primary tumor elsewhere can help when one is faced with a completely replaced carcinomatous lymph node. Rarely, ectopic salivary gland tissue anywhere in the neck may undergo malignant transformation. Tumors of other tissue can occur in proximity to the gland and mimic primary tumor of the gland; for example, basal cell carcinoma of the skin can closely mimic adenoid cystic carcinoma. The heterogeneous structure of tumors is yet another limit to the diagnostic accuracy. Attempts to classify tumors along the lines of histological classification are often impossible, owing to different histological appearances within individual tumors and because selective sampling can lead to misinterpretation. A type-specific diagnosis should be made only when there are unequivocal morphological criteria.

FNAs and biopsies are easy to perform, and the technique is the same as for other palpable superficial lesions mentioned earlier. Hematoma is the only rare complication that may occur. Facial nerve damage and implantation along the fine-needle track have not been reported. A more common serious complication for the unwary is torrential hemorrhage when biopsy of a carotid body tumor or paraganglioma is attempted in the belief that the lump is a neoplastic lymph node. Control of this bleeding by artery forceps then can result in occlusion of the carotid artery, with hemiplegia and death in 30% of patients. In this case, arteriography is useful to show splaying of the carotid bifurcation and the characteristic blush outlining abnormal blood vessels.

FNA of the Thyroid Gland

The technique developed in Scandinavia 30 years ago is simple and quick to perform in outpatient departments and is easily repeated. There are no absolute contraindications in a cooperative, well-informed, and consenting patient. The main role of FNA of the thyroid is in reducing the number of surgeries for benign disease, such as in diagnosis of diffuse nontoxic goiter or solitary thyroid nodule. It is also used to confirm diagnosis of malignancy (5). One example is shown in Figure 44-3.

Examination of the thyroid should be done with the patient in the upright position and FNA in the supine position with a pillow under the shoulders to extend the cervical spine and optimize exposure of the gland. The patient is asked to swallow to establish movement of the thyroid, along with other neck structures. Palpation is performed with the examiner standing behind the patient. A nodule in the posterior part of a lobe is made accessible by pushing the larynx toward the same side. Palpation of the lesion with the needle tip is important. The first needle pass occurs easily if the lesion is cystic, but it can be difficult to pierce it if the wall is fibrotic. A syringe in a pistol grip is attached to evacuate fluid when the wall of the cystic lesion is passed.

Ultrasound imaging reduces the risk of false-negative findings and also enables sampling of small nodules and enlarged parathyroid glands. In Hashimoto's thyroiditis and scle-

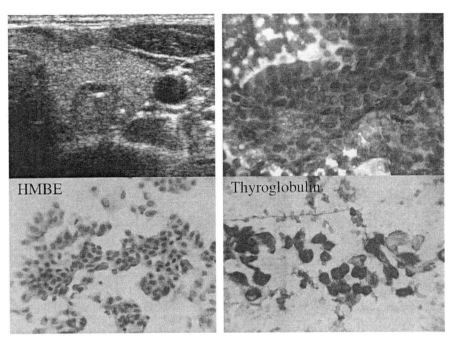

Figure 44-3 Thyroid papillary carcinoma seen on ultrasound, on conventional staining, and with human bone marrow endothelial (HMBE) and thyroglobulin immunostains.

rosing malignancies, more time may be needed to obtain material. Follicular neoplasms should be suspected if hemorrhage occurs easily in a solitary lesion. Consistency of the colloid should be observed during smear preparation.

The needle is held between the thumb and the index finger of the dominant hand. The nodule is immobilized with the index and middle fingers of the other hand. The needle is then moved back and forth several times within the nodule with a gentle stabbing motion. After the needle is withdrawn, an air-filled syringe with its plunger retracted is immediately attached to the needle, and the needle contents are expelled onto clean glass slides. Smears are prepared from the ejected material.

It is recommended that at least two punctures be performed for each nodule, and alcohol-fixed and air-dried smears are prepared from aspirated material. It has been reported that an increased number of passes may reduce the number of false-negative diagnoses. For alcohol fixation (as mentioned earlier), the smears must be placed promptly in 95% alcohol before air-drying occurs. ThinPrep processors are now widely used in many laboratories, allowing monolayer preparation. A disadvantage of this method is that the colloid (important for diagnosis) may not be preserved.

Indications for FNA Biopsy of the Thyroid Gland. Investigation of the thyroid nodule should involve a team approach, including a pathologist with proper training and a clinician with good technique. Using a nonsuction technique, taking into account the size of the nodule, and adopting standardized terminology for reporting are also essential for success.

An FNA report must be considered, bearing in mind the patient's clinical history. In clinical practice, an FNA biopsy can be used for diagnosis or triage. It should be remembered that follicular adenoma, well-differentiated carcinoma, and some hypercellular goiters are indistinguishable on an FNA biopsy. This distinction depends on the demonstration of capsular or vascular invasion, which requires histological sampling of the surgical excision.

FNA biopsy is used to distinguish a malignant thyroid nodule that would require surgical excision from a goitrous nodule, for example, which is managed medically, thus reducing the cost of patient care. In diffuse nontoxic goiter, FNA is a reliable means for distinction between colloid goiter and autoimmune thyroiditis. FNA biopsy is indicated not only for a solitary nodule but also for a nodule in a multinodular goiter that has grown steadily, become dominant, or changed in consistency. It is also indicated for a dominant localized change in autoimmune diseases and for diffuse, rapidly growing thyroid enlargement to rule out lymphoma or anaplastic carcinoma. However, the majority of nodules in which cytology is not definitely benign eventually will be excised for histological diagnosis. In this situation a frozen section or paraffin blocks may be helpful, especially when there is cytological ambiguity, before proceeding to the total thyroidectomy (e.g., thyroid adenoma with bizarre cells).

Different forms of thyroiditis can be confirmed if necessary, and at the same time material for microbiology can be obtained. Cytological diagnosis allows preoperative irradiation and palliative therapy, and can be used for identification of metastatic tumors in the thyroid. Other diagnostic methods such as antibody measurements, thyroid scanning, hormone levels, and ultrasound are used together with FNA to reach a reliable diagnosis.

A high rate of false-negative findings is reported in the literature if one diagnostic modality is used. For example, if antibody estimation is used as the sole investigation method, cases will be more frequently missed. On the other hand, antibodies have been found to be positive in a patient without thyroiditis.

Complications. FNA of the thyroid is a minimally invasive procedure; therefore, complications are extremely rare, although possible. The risk of hematoma formation should be borne in mind in those with large goiters or malignant tumors in the neck. In such cases the patient must not be discharged, because hematoma can lead to tracheal compression, necessitating emergency ligation of the superficial thyroid artery.

Bleeding caused by needling occurs only rarely and is self-limited if firm pressure is applied for 5 min to the aspiration site. Clotting status should be checked in all patients who are anticoagulated. Accidental puncture of the trachea may lead to transient coughing, and small amounts of blood can be coughed up. Other complications reported in the literature are transient laryngeal nerve palsy, hemorrhagic necrosis of adenomas (which may stimulate invasion), and infection. Surgeons who often worry about needle-track seeding and consequent tumor recurrence following FNA should be reassured that needle-track implantation is extraordinarily rare (only two cases have been reported). It is advisable to carry out scans if indicated before FNA, because needling may cause conversion of a "hot" nodule to a "cold" nodule on a scan.

Diagnostic accuracy varies among centers but reaches 96% in some larger series. About 10% of cancers are not diagnosed by FNA, and 40% of cystic neoplasms may be missed by FNA. The greatest diagnostic difficulty is with cystic papillary carcinoma. Follow-up of the patient is therefore recommended where there is negative cytology and with a tumor size of 4 cm or larger (taking into account the age and gender of the patient and other clinical criteria of malignancy), and a new FNA should be performed in 6 months. If the nodule persists or grows, surgery should be considered. Therefore, nodule size is an important consideration in selecting surgical or nonsurgical treatment.

The reason for advocating the removal of all follicular neoplasms is that it is rarely possible to distinguish between a follicular adenoma and carcinoma cytologically (as already mentioned, distinction usually depends on histological evidence of capsular or vascular invasion). In these circumstances, hard irregular swelling with fixation and recurrent laryngeal nerve paralysis are criteria to assist in the selection of a patient for surgery. Deep cervical lymphadenopathy along the internal jugular vein (this may be present in some patients with Hashimoto's thyroiditis), along with clinically suspicious swelling, are suggestive of papillary carcinoma. The incidence of thyroid carcinoma in women is about three times that in men, but a discrete swelling in a man is more likely to be malignant. The risk of carcinoma is also increased in patients at either end of the age range, in patients with a history of head and neck irradiation, and in patients with a family history of endocrine neoplasia syndrome (type 2A and 2B).

If a cyst is found during nonsuction FNA, suction with a larger needle is recommended to evacuate as much fluid as feasible. The residual solid area is then sampled with a 25- or 27-gauge needle without suction.

False-negative diagnoses can occur in low- or intermediate-grade lymphoma in the background lymphoma. Some studies suggest the paramount importance of experience in any great improvement in accuracy (each aspirator must perform at least 1 to 5 aspiration procedures per month).

A standardized terminology for reporting has been proposed that should be universally understood, which can be related to the probability of cancer and therefore can guide management of the patient. Ambiguous terms with no reference to the specific histological type should be avoided in FNA reports.

FNA of the Lymph Node

Advantages and Disadvantages. An FNA biopsy of a palpable peripheral node offers an immediate, preliminary diagnosis in the majority of cases with little trauma and cost, whereas surgical excision requires anesthesia, may leave a scar, and is considerably more expensive and time consuming. The primary purpose of an FNA biopsy is to decide whether surgical excision for histological examination is indicated. The age of the patient, presence of known infection, and the previous medical history must be considered when patients with enlarged lymph nodes are clinically managed. Lymph nodes can react to a variety of nonspecific stimuli by expansion of the follicle centers and/or interfollicular areas with resultant enlargement of lymph nodes. This is particularly true of children, who can present with massive local lymphadenopathy after mild infection. Elderly patients, in contrast, react to infection with only slight lymph node enlargement; therefore, lymphadenopathy in these patients indicates immediate needle biopsy because of suspected malignancy. Patients with reactive lymph node enlargement or metastasis from a known malignancy can be spared lymph node excision. The cytological examination in lymph node pathology has three major indicators: primary diagnosis (whether the lymphadenopathy is due to reactive hyperplasia, metastatic malignancy, or malignant lymphoma), staging of disease, and follow-up. In patients with lymphadenopathy of unknown cause, FNA is the first line of investigation. If the cytological diagnosis is malignant lymphoma or suspicious of lymphoma, this is followed by surgical excision of the node. Lymph nodes clinically suspicious of metastatic disease are one of the most common indications for FNA biopsy in routine practice. In patients with known histologically proven malignancy in whom enlarged nodes appear, FNA is indicated to confirm diagnosis. In patients without previous evidence of primary tumor, metastatic deposits can be confirmed, and the nature and the site of the primary tumor can also be detected. It is advisable to repeat an FNA biopsy after 2 to 3 weeks in cases with lymphadenopathy that cannot be diagnosed confidently. Conclusive diagnosis is achieved in the majority of patients with metastatic tumors and in cases of reactive lymphadenopathy.

Diagnostic sensitivity is significantly lower for lymphoma than for metastatic malignancy (10, 11). From a clinical standpoint, for an FNA to be of practical value the diagnosis of lymphoma must also include the subtype according to the current classification. Interpretation of immune straining is more difficult in cytological preparations than in sections. Samples obtained by FNA can be subjected to the supplementary techniques such as DNA analysis, optometry, and gene rearrangement studies (12). Commercially produced monoclonal antibodies to various antigens that are specific to cell lines assist in the identification of the source of tumor metastases to lymph nodes and in the distinction between malignant lymphoma, melanoma, and undifferentiated carcinoma.

The role of cytology in the diagnosis of lymphoma is to confirm a clinical suspicion of (Hodgkin's and non-Hodgkin's) or to exclude it (13). A negative cytological diagnosis must be supported by clinical findings. The lymph node can be sent to the laboratory fresh (not fixed) and a full immunological study can be undertaken, in cases in which a diagnosis of lymphoma is known beforehand. Imprints of such nodes can be used for cytonuclear details. Biopsies at different sites can be carried out for the staging of disease. This is particularly useful in the elderly where there is a need to avoid laparotomy only to obtain tissue for histological examination. Therefore, FNA together with radiological and clinical examinations can play an important role in therapeutic management of patients with advanced intraabdominal or mediastinal lymphoma without involvement of superficial lymph nodes. Virtually any lesion in any organ can be reached with a fine needle. With radiological guidance, long needles can reach deep sites of the body. Small, hard, and mobile masses (particularly in the lung) can be biopsied using a corkscrew-like needle (the shape of the needle tip also affects diagnostic yield). Deep lymph nodes are easily accessible to FNA when visualized by radiological imaging. Fibrosis in the node makes it difficult to obtain sufficient material for diagnosis. This often happens with reactive inguinal nodes and nodular sclerosing Hodgkin's disease.

FNA yields viable cells, and special studies can be performed with living material (e.g., cytochemistry and tissue culture). Immunophenotyping is also important, because follicular lymphoma, for example, can be mistaken for reactive follicular hyperplasia. Failure to obtain a representative sample is responsible for the majority of false-negative diagnoses. Most false-positive diagnoses are cases of reactive follicular hyperplasia that were reported as suspicious of lymphoma. Therefore, it is advisable to repeat the FNA if the lymphadenopathy does not show regression within several weeks. Because diagnosis and classification of lymphoma are dependent on the evaluation of fine nuclear and cytoplasm details of various cell types in the smear, cytological preparations of high quality must be prepared. Diagnostic sensitivity of metastatic disease in lymph nodes reported in the literature varies with different hospitals, but it is generally >95%. Both reactive nodes and nodes involved in metastatic malignancy or lymphoma are highly cellular and moderately vascular. Adequate material is therefore easily obtained with a 25- or 23-gauge needle without aspiration (except in the presence of fibrosis). An abundance of blood in the sample distorts the cells. If the cell concentration is low, the cells can be concentrated by centrifugation at 700 rpm for 3 to 5 min. Air-dried cytosine preparations can be stored at room temperature for up to 1 week. Aspirated cells can also be immunologically characterized by flow cytometry.

In addition to the diagnosis of infections (e.g., fungal, viral, protozoal), inflammations (e.g., granulomas in sarcoidosis), or infiltrations (e.g., amyloidosis), the practical importance of exclusion or confirmation of malignant lymphoma and other malignancies by FNA plays a vital initial step in HIV patients (14). In these patients lymph nodes can be also sampled when an opportunistic infection is suspected, but safety precautions (regarding technical problems) and confidentiality must be taken into account. Finally, FNA of lymph nodes can be useful in the evaluation of masses in pediatric practice and can be used as a method of postmortem examination. The aspirate from a thyroglossal cyst can be cytologically similar to that of a branchial cyst. Here, differential diagnosis can be based on the anatomical site of the lesion; lymph node metastasis of carcinoma undergoing necrosis is important in differential diagnosis and efforts should be made to reveal malignant squamoid cells. Smears obtained from an inflamed branchial cyst can contain atypical cells. The gross appearance of the aspirate from a branchial cyst (pus-like) may mimic suppurative lymphadenitis.

Problems are encountered if the patient had previous radiotherapy, because it is difficult to locate a small recurrence in an area of edema and fibrosis and it is very difficult to obtain a representative sample. Even when a sample is sufficient, differentiation between radiation-induced cellular abnormality and tumor recurrence is difficult. A small metastatic deposit in a reactive lymph node can be missed by the needle (15).

A major disadvantage of an FNA biopsy when compared with tissue is that architecture is lost, because the cells are pulled out from their surroundings. This can be overcome by paying attention to the degree of cohesion among cells. For example, lymphomas show a completely dissociated cellular pattern, benign epithelial tumors show a strong intercellular cohesion (less cellular aspirates composed of sheets of cells), and carcinomas are characterized by decreased intercellular cohesion (richly cellular aspirates). As a general rule, diagnosis should not be reached with a minimal number of abnormal cells, and interpretation should be an integral part of clinical judgment. Serious complications are generally more often reported with deep-target biopsies.

Contraindications. Contraindications are relative rather than absolute, and there are no well-established contraindications for FNA biopsy of superficial palpable lymph nodes.

Complications. Postaspiration hematoma, necrosis, and infection are very rare. Tumor implantation along the needle track has not been reported in the literature, unlike with other FNA sites [e.g., Ohlsson et al. (16), Nyland et al. (17), and Shinohara et al. (18)]. Occasionally, the patient will feel lightheaded during or after the procedure (vasovagal reaction) and may even faint. If the patient has brain metastases, the cytopathologist may witness the patient having seizures. Inadvertent penetration of the carotid artery or other major blood vessels is not a significant concern, but a death has been reported following aspiration of a carotid body tumor that resulted in carotid thrombosis (the moral of the story is to have appropriate investigations and to be certain to listen for a bruit).

REFERENCES

1. University of Iowa Health Care. www.uihealthcare.com/news/currents/vol3issue2/04fineneedleaspiration.html (accessed May 2004).
2. Brugge WR, Lewandrowski K, Lee-Lewandrowski E, Centeno BA, Szydlo T, Regan S, et al. Diagnosis of pancreatic cystic neoplasms: a report of the cooperative pancreatic cyst study. Gastroenterology 2004;126:1330–6.
3. Kuo FY, Chen WJ, Lu SN, Wang JH, Eng HL. Fine needle aspiration cytodiagnosis of liver tumors. Acta Cytol 2004;48:142–8.
4. Liu F, Gnepp DR, Pisharodi LR. Fine needle aspiration of parathyroid lesions. Acta Cytol 2004;48:133–6.
5. Hurtado-Lopez LM, Arellano-Montano S, Torres-Acosta EM, Zaldivar-Ramirez FR, Duarte-Torres RM, Alonso-De-Ruiz P, et al. Combined use of fine-needle aspiration biopsy, MIBI scans and frozen section biopsy offers the best diagnostic accuracy in the assessment of the hypofunctioning solitary thyroid nodule. Eur J Nucl Med Mol Imaging 2004; May 6 (Epub ahead of print).
6. Yoder M, Zimmerman RL, Bibbo M. Two-color immunostaining of liver fine needle aspiration biopsies with CD34 and carcino-embryonic antigen. Potential utilization in the diagnosis of primary hepatocellular carcinoma vs. metastatic tumor Anal Quant Cytol Histol 2004;26:61–4.
7. Vazquez-Sequeiros E, Wiersema MJ. EUS FNA staging of esophageal cancer. Gastroenterology 2004;126:1499–500.
8. Agarwal B, Abu-Hamda E, Molke KL, Correa AM, Ho L. Endoscopic ultrasound-guided fine needle aspiration and multidetector spiral CT in the diagnosis of pancreatic cancer. Am J Gastroenterol 2004;99:844–50.
9. Zbaren P, Nuyens M, Loosli H, Stauffer E. Diagnostic accuracy of fine-needle aspiration cytology and frozen section in primary parotid carcinoma. Cancer 2004;100:1876–83.
10. Stelow EB, Lai R, Bardales RH, Mallery S, Linzie BM, Crary G, Stanley MW. Endoscopic ultrasound-guided fine-needle aspiration of lymph nodes: the Hennepin County Medical Center experience. Diagn Cytopathol 2004;30:301–6.
11. Schafernak KT, Kluskens LF, Ariga R, Reddy VB, Gattuso P. Fine-needle aspiration of superficial and deeply seated lymph nodes on patients with and without a history of malignancy: review of 439 cases. Diagn Cytopathol 2003;29:315–9.
12. Borovecki A, Kardum-Skelin I, Sustercic D, Hitrec V, Lasan R, Jaksic B. Chromosomal abnormalities and DNA image cytometry of haematological neoplasms in fine needle aspirates of lymph nodes. Cytopathology 2003;14:320–6.
13. Crapanzano JP, Lin O. Cytologic findings of marginal zone lymphoma. Cancer 2003;99:301–9.
14. Nayak S, Mani R, Kavatkar AN, Puranik SC, Holla VV. Fine-needle aspiration cytology in lymphadenopathy of HIV-positive patients. Diagn Cytopathol 2003;29:146–8.
15. Gupta RK, Naran S, Lallu S, Fauck R. The diagnostic value of fine needle aspiration cytology (FNAC) in the assessment of palpable supraclavicular lymph nodes: a study of 218 cases. Cytopathology 2003;14:201–7.
16. Ohlsson B, Nilsson J, Stenram U, Akerman M, Tranberg KG. Percutaneous fine-needle aspiration cytology in the diagnosis and management of liver tumours. Br J Surg 2002;89:757–62.
17. Nyland TG, Wallack ST, Wisner ER. Needle-tract implantation following us-guided fine-needle aspiration biopsy of transitional cell carcinoma of the bladder, urethra, and prostate. Vet Radiol Ultrasound 2002;43:50–3.
18. Shinohara S, Yamamoto E, Tanabe M, Maetani T, Kim T. Implantation metastasis of head and neck cancer after fine needle aspiration biopsy. Auris Nasus Larynx 2001;28:377–80.

Chapter 45

Point-of-Care Testing: A Patient's Perspective

Helen Spriggs

I am 30 years of age, and I was diagnosed with diabetes at the age of 13. I left school at the age of 18 and moved from North Lincolnshire to London to study for a BSc Social Sciences degree at South Bank University. After graduation, I went to work for Diabetes UK, the largest diabetes charity registered in the United Kingdom, as its Youth Services Project Leader. In 2000, I joined a diagnostics company as a sales executive for diabetes products. I lead what I consider to be a very active life, have lots of leisure interests, and really throw myself into the London social scene. I would probably consider myself a determined person and one of my passions is running. I have run a total of seven marathons, and my best time is 3 h, 45 min; I have run in both the London and New York marathons. You can see that I also enjoy travel.

LEARNING ABOUT DIABETES

Some people might think that being diagnosed as a diabetic at the age of 13 was unlucky, and I certainly felt that way for quite a long time. You might also think it to be particularly bad timing. The last thing that a teenage girl wants to be bothered with is injections, diet restrictions, clinic appointments, and tests. I certainly found the whole experience very difficult to deal with—the responsibility, a personal responsibility, of having to manage a chronic condition day and night, every day, every week—forever. At an early stage I was made aware that diabetes was a serious condition, and I was constantly reminded that complications of the disease was the fourth leading cause of death. At this stage in my life, boys and boy bands were more at the top of my agenda.

My first reaction to learning that I had diabetes was "Why me? Couldn't someone, anyone else, have it instead?" You might think this to be an embarrassing or selfish reaction, but remember I was 13 years of age with a very active social life and about to discover the world. In the last 7 years I have met many kids who have had very similar reactions—and frankly they have found it very difficult to come to terms with the fact that their life has changed. Overnight, there was a huge amount of information to take in, a whole new lifestyle to learn. It was an enormous burden to put on the shoulders of a 13-year-old

This chapter was written by a young woman with diabetes mellitus. It is a reflection on her life as a diabetic and her experience with point-of-care testing.

child. It was very obvious that this was a permanent change, I didn't receive any get-well cards; it wasn't going to get better no matter how hard I wished for someone to put a sticking plaster on my pancreas and tell me that everything was going to be okay. The only upside was the amount of attention I was getting from family, school friends, and showing off all this very scientific medical equipment that I was charged to use. Friends would say in amazement, "Wow, you can take blood and then test it for sugar! Do mine! Do mine!" My parents were incredibly supportive, but it is now clear to me that they had as much of a problem coming to terms with the situation as I did. However, they would never outwardly show this to me.

Soon all of the novelty and celebrity status wore off—both for me and my friends. By the time I was 16 years old diabetes had become a definite bore. I was fed up with the pressure of responsibility, having to think of "it" constantly, sticking to a strict regimen that was imposed on me like a school timetable. I wasn't able to choose what I wanted to do, my daily routine—my life was all mapped out for me, unlike school, where you have some understanding of what you are taking the lessons for, what you are working towards. You also realize you can influence your examination results. Living with diabetes is not like that. There are always questions: Why was I eating at a certain time? What would happen if I ate 5 minutes later? Why did I have to inject that amount of insulin in the morning and a different amount at night? Why the hell did I have to test my blood? These are a lot of questions to be answered at a time when I wanted to reject the knowledge that my life had changed irrevocably. I also had to understand the feelings and concerns of my parents and friends, as well as take in the fact that there was a group of health professionals that was trying to help me: What did my diabetes specialist nurse get from looking at a diary page of numbers?

DIABETES, THE DIFFICULT YEARS

Diabetes didn't make sense to me. I began to feel helpless, and I rapidly lost interest. I found the whole process of learning to live with my disease very difficult. I felt great pain—no, not from the injections—from having to prick my finger with something that I regarded as tantamount to a skewer for meat. Then I would have to wait for 3 minutes to get a glucose result, unlike the 15 seconds of today—a result that I was told was "only as accurate as the technique employed by the person doing the test." What does that mean? For someone who didn't have a second hand on their watch and got confused with certain colors, my result didn't make a lot of sense. In addition, and to top it all, the method chosen to test my blood was determined by what someone else thought was best for me. Someone—the diabetes specialists, the clinical biochemist in the local laboratory, the general practitioner on the local PCT purchasing committee, or even a procurement officer—had decided what blood glucose system I should use. On the one hand, there was a great deal of care taken to try to make me understand what it meant to have diabetes, to teach me how to manage my disease. However, when I look back on those early years, no thought whatsoever was given to what I wanted, no apparent thought into how testing was going to affect my life or what would be the best equipment for me to use.

I should point out that there were many others in the same position as me, people whom I met in later life, although I did not get a chance to meet them in those early days. You have to remember I was in a rejection phase. Life was a nightmare in those early years, and so testing just didn't get done. As I reflect on it now, I think it was US President Richard Nixon who said, "There are lies, damn lies, and statistics." For "statistics," read "my blood glucose test diary;" I was expected to keep a diary of all of my test results, and I was testing myself four times a day. I made up the results, on the way to the clinic, equipped with an assortment of colored pens and a smudge of blood and a coffee cup stain in all the right places. If I obtained a high result, even if it was a real result, I did not record it as such but rather added it to the other fictitious results dotted all over the page. At this point it never occurred to me to think that a high reading was a sign of weakness and a low one of virtue. I went for weeks, maybe even months at my worst, without testing my blood. I seemed to adopt this strange sort of logic, which said that if I stopped taking insulin I would become ill quickly and so would know something was wrong. This is clearly a very short-term view, but with blood testing there is not the same motivating influence as there is with insulin. Indeed, at one time I felt so confident about not testing that I would even boast that I would be able to guess my reading without testing. My doctor and my nurse, on the rare occasions that I would actually make it to my appointment, reinforced this; they lectured me on how I should do this and that and if I didn't then I would be in trouble later in life. Can you imagine what that said to me as a teenager who knew everything and felt capable of ruling the world? My reaction was to go ahead and raise hell now and worry about complications later. At the time, life was fun.

I was partly in the disowning phase. I felt far removed from diabetes. I thought that testing was for other people's benefit—it helped them to have a diary full of numbers. I did not see them as being of any benefit to me; they were not made to feel anything to me. I therefore cast aside, with relative ease, all of these burdens that I was living with. I was having a good time; life couldn't have been better. I was at university, away from the people who cared about my diabetes and in with a crowd that didn't even know that I had diabetes. Therefore, like many fellow students, I went for it, but because I felt I had more to prove, I went for it even more than the rest. It was a matter of pride to drink the most and stay out partying more often and later than anyone else. I do not think my experience in the early years is particularly unique and have since met many people of all ages living with diabetes who tell of similar experiences, some better, some worse. We are all different, and diabetes manifests itself in different people in different ways. However, I am convinced that there are some things common to most people, and one is that we all have some degree of difficulty in coming to terms with the recognition that we have an illness, especially when we have it for life. In addition, our parents, friends, neighbors, and peers are all individuals, and there is no "one case fits all" in dealing with a person who has diabetes.

This couldn't go on forever and—thankfully—this phase in my life was relatively short lived. I moved into the realization that I needed to be more compliant with my readings. I cannot pinpoint what changed, but I happened to change when at the diabetes clinic I attended, I met a diabetes specialist nurse who understood. She understood what it was like for a young person to live with diabetes. Furthermore, I would go so far as to say that not only did she understand, but also she understood what it was like for me to live with diabetes at this moment in my life.

She took an interest in me—the individual—not the statistic, not the label on my file stamped "Diabetic." I never heard her say what I thought was part of the patter for diabetes: "How many hypos [hypoglycemic readings] have you had in the last month? How many tests have you been doing each day? Why do you have a high reading? Have you lost any weight?"

My response to all of these questions used to be no. With every question asked, I would feel worse and worse about how I was living with *my* diabetes. It was almost like I'd borrowed something from them, something that they regarded as precious, and on my handing it back to them there were a million and one questions fired at me that made me feel inadequate and incapable of caring for the thing I had borrowed. I had violated something that did not belong to me. The new specialist nurse helped me to take ownership of my diabetes—that thing I had previously borrowed was my diabetes. I had originally been made to feel that I wasn't the one in control of my diabetes, that diabetes belonged to the health service and not me; I hadn't been given the tools to think any differently. However, I had now met someone who did things differently and suggested it be all about give and take. It was obviously incredibly important that I, as the patient, was ready to accept change. You might say that I was growing up at the time.

I look upon this as the adoption phase. This was a new world of diabetes, and where my life has been for the last 8 years. The change has taught me to put value into *me* being in control. Blood glucose testing does mean something; trying to get a reading between 4 and 8 mmol/L (72 and 144 mg/dL) does mean something to me. In the past it was easier than picking the winning lottery numbers. I was taught what I should have been taught way back, back to the basics—step by step. I learned what insulin did in my body, how it did it, when it did it, and why. I learned about different foods and what they did. Then it started to come together, and I was given the space to allow this to come together. I began to see that what I ate and what I injected, directly affected my blood glucose levels—I had *control* over my blood glucose levels. I was encouraged to take control. At this time I also began to understand the meaning of the HbA1c results and how they provided another tool for me to manage my disease. It's just like a set of bathroom scales, really!

TODAY . . . IN CONTROL

I am now in the control phase. I lead a full professional and social life. Life is good! In terms of my diabetes I test myself on average about six times a day. I keep a regular diary of my glucose results using a memory meter and an additional software program allowing me to download my results onto my computer for analysis—for my benefit. I visit my primary care physician about once every 3 months and my diabetes specialist every 6 months. I have my HbA1c tested annually in secondary care and using point-of-care testing equipment (the Bayer DCA 2000+). My own primary care physician and his team perform the HbA1c within minutes right there at his desk every few months. Originally, I used to get my HbA1c result in the mail about 2 weeks after my visit to the specialist, but now it is done at the time of my visit and I get the result while I am discussing all of the other aspects of my life.

As stated earlier, I have run seven marathons between 1997 and 2001. I will describe a little of this experience because I think it is a superb demonstration of being in control and one I am incredibly proud of. I ran my first marathon in London in 1997 to mark the 10th year since my diagnosis of diabetes, and it was the greatest learning experience of my life. I was the one who set the agenda. This was me saying how I wanted to live my life with diabetes. I set the goals for the team. I use the word *team* as it was understood at the outset—that this was a team effort involving my specialists and me. Through this challenge I defined what blood glucose control meant to me and what I understood of it. Frankly, I think it was as much a learning experience for them as it was for me, but more than ever before—*me*, the patient, and the health care specialists. We discovered what blood glucose testing was all about in this more extreme environment. I think the answer lay in the diabetes team focusing on the behavior that required me to achieve my goal of running the marathon—and doing it without causing my diabetes to become an issue. Thus, success was measured by my ability to eat, exercise, adjust insulin, and test in a way that was going to achieve my goal. I became empowered; I made the connection that I could control my behavior. As a result, I could make sense of my blood glucose results and the end point was the payoff. I could see that I had influenced those results and that I could use them for my benefit. Through this understanding I found that I stuck to achieving my goals.

I don't think I am that different from the majority of runners in marathons today—perhaps a little more motivated. It involved a lot of trials and along the way I learned through my mistakes. The 1999 London Marathon didn't go too well for me. I suffered a real roller-coaster ride of high and low glucose readings throughout the race. At one point I thought my glucose would never rise above 2 mmol/L (36 mg/dL). It was the closest I had come to giving up but I was determined to not let diabetes win. It was as if there were two people running those marathons—Helen Spriggs and Diabetes; we were neck and neck and on that particular day Diabetes was winning for the majority of the race! As you have probably gathered, I wasn't going to give in to Diabetes that easily, so I ate and drank everything and anything in my reach in order to raise my glucose levels and complete the 26.2 miles. I, Helen Spriggs, crossed the finish line on the Mall before Diabetes! However, instead of feeling I had done wrong, I spent time looking at why it all fell apart. Did I eat sufficiently before the race? What about the night before? Was I more stressed than usual because a BBC TV documentary crew was shadowing my every move? Did I put more effort into the race earlier on? In the past I would never have known to ask these questions. Being able to ask them felt incredibly powerful. I now know why the specialists enjoy asking those questions of me so much—they become the patient, it is their diabetes in my hands—they have the power. I took it back. It was never easy, and it took time for me to stick with it long enough to reap the rewards of my management.

What Does Blood Glucose Testing Mean to Me?

There is a simple answer to this question. Blood glucose testing has given me the answers to achieve all that I wanted in life. It has put me in control to achieve what I want and, more important, it all makes sense. On a practical day-to-day level, blood glucose testing helps me to see that I am on track. If I am doing anything more unusual, as when running a marathon, testing gives me a tool to use in conjunction with my insulin and diet. It is therefore a tool and a support to enable me to lead my life the way I want to lead it. In many ways it is not any different from everyone being encouraged to take control of their life, health, or well-being. In the United Sates, everyone is encouraged to know their cholesterol number.

What Does HbA1c Testing Mean to Me?

Obviously the HbA1c gives a broader picture of my glycemic control and so it becomes more of a backup because I have really come to grips with my glucose testing. I think it also gives my specialists the equivalent of an external quality assurance snapshot. When I was younger and in my rejection and disowning phases, I think that the HbA1c results were particularly helpful to my specialists as they indicated the level of my noncompliance with what they were asking me to do. I certainly know that being presented with my HbA1c results was a way of making me think—and indeed helped me understand what was going on in my body. Today it is more of a support, and I always feel better when I see my result and know that it is within the range that my specialist team and I are aiming for. I feel confident that what action I have taken is paying off, and it gives me the basis to set new goals for my diabetes management.

What Does My Specialist Team Mean to Me?

I think you have the picture of the transition that has occurred in my relationship with my diabetes specialist team. They have become a great asset for me, helping me through some difficult times and also getting involved to help when I have wanted to stretch things a little. My husband, family, and friends have also been part of this team. The glucose and HbA1c testing has been a help and a support for all of us. It is also obvious that being able to test at the point of care is crucial to this relationship.

CONCLUSIONS

Obviously, I have gotten to know a large number of people with diabetes, and many share my experiences to varying degrees—others have even run marathons. However, we are all different, and I am convinced that we each have individual needs. I am also convinced, however, that personal ownership of one's body is vital for everyone, whether you have diabetes or not. We all look for some tools to indicate that our health is what we would want it to be. Blood glucose and HbA1c testing are just two of the important tools, especially when they can be done by me or my diabetes specialist, when I am present.

Part **Five**

Conclusions

Chapter 46

Point-of-Care Testing: The Future

Christopher P. Price, Andrew St John, and Jocelyn M. Hicks

In the first edition of this book we pointed out that the main objective of point-of-care testing (POCT) was to deliver results more quickly and to reduce the time between request and decision. The stated justification was that this would lead to improved outcomes for the patient, the healthcare provider, and the purchaser. As is the case with the majority of innovations seen in healthcare, the transition from an idea through a technology, device, or intervention to a product with a demonstrated efficacy and then to routine application is a very lengthy procedure. Typical cycle times are anything from 10 to 15 years, and this is no different for POCT systems. Thus, although POCT devices for many analytes have been around for several years, the routine application appears to be limited, at least from the perspective of the peer-reviewed literature. In addition, the adoption of POCT varies throughout the world, which may reflect the differing approaches to healthcare funding and delivery. However, it is now clear that major change is underway in healthcare, both toward a greater focus on patient demands and also to the ways in which healthcare is delivered (1, 2).

CHANGING DEMANDS FROM THE PATIENT

The patient is becoming a more demanding customer of healthcare services, and this reflects a dissatisfaction with the way that existing healthcare is delivered in many countries, as well as increasing access to healthcare- and disease-related information. Thus, there is no doubt that placing the patient at the top of the agenda is now an explicit objective in healthcare (3) and represents a similar force for change to that of concerns about the increasing expenditure on healthcare. While the increasing age of the population will demand more resources for healthcare, this can only be sustained by more efficient use of those resources. As a consequence of these pressures, there are targets set by governments in relation to many aspects of healthcare provision (4).

It is also clear that a long-term objective is to place greater emphasis on good health and well-being (5), as there are considerable concerns about the effect on health of aspects of the modern lifestyle. The rising incidence of obesity and the reduction in the amount of exercise taken are prime examples. The effect of increasing airline travel and general population migration are also seen as having major implications for healthcare. This is a major sociological challenge, and one in

which it is not clear what role laboratory medicine might play. However, the concept of well-being is one that has to be taken up by all those involved in healthcare, as are the issues around changing behavior if the wellness agenda is to be pursued. It is also part of the ethos of individual empowerment.

CHANGES TO THE DELIVERY OF HEALTHCARE

All developed countries are facing similar pressures to change the way healthcare is delivered (Table 46-1), and this includes changes to laboratory medicine. It is acknowledged that the rising cost of healthcare is a major factor (6), but changes in clinical practice and a greater emphasis on outcomes are also high on the agenda (7).

While this might involve the hospital providing a better patient experience and reducing the risk of hospital-acquired infections, it is also about processes outside of tertiary care, such as more effective care in the community and in the home.

Hospital Process Reengineering

From an organizational standpoint, hospitals are clearly looking to reduce length of stay (8). The profile of the length of stay in a teaching hospital in the United Kingdom is shown in Figure 46-1. It has been argued that both reducing the number of people requiring admission (very short stay—*period A*) and the average length of medium stay (*period B*) could have a significant effect on total costs. The data were used as the core of the argument for the fundamental redesign of the hospital buildings (it was a very old hospital), as well as for methods of working. It was argued that there was less likelihood of radically changing the longer lengths of stay, with exception of those elderly patients whose need for long-term nursing (but not hospital) care prevented them from being transferred home. Length of stay varies across the world, but the average values have fallen in many countries over the past decade (6, 9). Efforts to address these issues are seen in the evolution of triage protocols in the emergency room and admissions unit, which are aimed at identifying those who do not require admission, along with a more efficient approach for those that do require admission (10).

The adoption of a more patient-centered approach to care is also seen as having an effect on the hospital process, as well as being more desirable for the patient (3). The essence of this strategy from an organizational standpoint is having the service

Table 46-1   Key Trends in Healthcare

An aging population, an increasing incidence of:
  Diabetes
  Cancer
  Cardiovascular disease
  Osteoporosis
  Dementia
Changes in social behavior
  Diet
  Exercise
  Sexual activity
  Drug abuse
  Population mobility
New technology
  Human genome
  Drugs
  Diagnostic tests
  Organ replacement
  Tissue regeneration
Increasing costs of healthcare
  Equipment, devices, therapies
  Labor
  Buildings and infrastructure
Increasing patient expectations
  Knowledge
  Quality
  Accountability
  Convenience

come to the patient, rather than the reverse. This places the patient at the center of activities and requires a total reorganization of the siting and approaches to the delivery of service. Thus, in an ideal situation, the diagnostic services are located close to the point of entry of the patient into the hospital. If one then adds in the other times at which the diagnostic services interact with the patient, you have a locational framework, as set out in Figure 46-2. The diagnostic services must be readily available for intensive and emergency care, nonelective care, and surgery. Depending on the geographical location of the laboratory and the specific process of care at the level of the clinician–patient interaction, either the laboratory must be close by, or POCT becomes the only option to fulfill the clinical need.

One of the changes in healthcare provision that has evolved from this philosophy is the increasing use of day-case surgery, and in certain situations diagnostic support at the point of care is critical to that success, e.g., parathyroidectomy (11). There is an increasing demand for testing as part of the triage protocols in the emergency room, e.g., in the case of patients with chest pain (12). The third case where change is occurring is in the devolution of chronic disease management, e.g., diabetes (13), Coumadin® (warfarin) management (14), and hyperlipidemia management (15).

Primary Care Reengineering

The changes in the basic approaches to healthcare extend far beyond the boundaries of the hospital, which for many years

was seen as the main healthcare provider. The primary care sector is now seen as the first point of entry into the healthcare system and one where more care can be provided at less cost than admission to the hospital (16) Its importance and the possible utilization of POCT is reflected in the recent decision of the Australian government to conduct a randomized controlled trial of POCT for certain analytes in 60 general practices across Australia (17). Included within this broad definition of primary care is the use of telephone support services such as NHS Direct in the United Kingdom (18) and Health Direct in Australia (19), where people are encouraged to use this point of contact for minor ailments and advice on nonurgent issues. Primary care is also the bridgehead for more care in the home, which can include posthospital discharge or chronic disease management, as well as a point of introduction into the long-term goal of health education and encouraging individuals to take greater responsibility for their health and well-being (20). This concept includes the involvement of other organizations in healthcare delivery, such as the community pharmacy (21).

Laboratory Services Reengineering

In parallel with the changes being seen in frontline healthcare provision, changes are also occurring in the way laboratory services are provided. The style, progress, and extent of change vary from country to country across the world, but there are several common themes. Clinical demand and technological innovation have both led to the proliferation of laboratories, in part reflecting the development of hospitals. However, more recent centralization and consolidation of hospital facilities have been accompanied by similar changes in laboratory services (22–24). Thus, in the United States and Australia we already have large reference or service laboratories handling workloads in excess of 10,000 specimens shipped in from all over the country by air. Such laboratories are then complemented, in terms of more local and faster delivery, by smaller satellite laboratories, physician office laboratories, and POCT. In the United Kingdom the original thoughts on modernizing pathology centered on the creation of core laboratories and laboratory networks, although the thinking has resolved toward networks more recently—which might include large automated laboratories (25). This reflects similar changes in countries such as Germany, the Netherlands, Australia, and the United States.

There does seem to be some contradiction between the way in which clinical care provision is envisioned for the future and the way in which laboratory diagnostic services may be provided (Figure 46-3). Thus, on the one hand we are seeing a considerable commitment to managing patients in the community and closer to home—which in itself may be more beneficial, as well as more acceptable to the patient—while on the other hand we are seeing a consolidation of laboratory services. If diagnostic test results are to be helpful to patient care and enable decisions to be made, then they must be available at the time of the consultation. The alternative is that the patient and/or the clinician is inconvenienced. The alternative has to be a huge commitment to logistics support so that

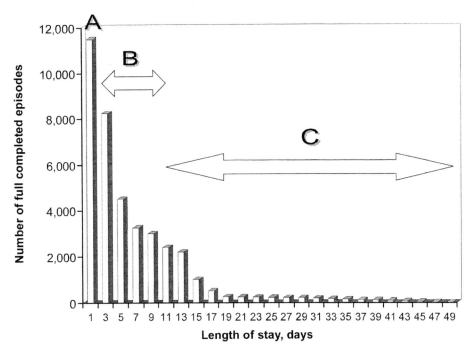

Figure 46-1 Profile of the lengths of stay at the Royal London Hospital in 1998 according to the full completed episodes, which equates to discharge rates.

the samples and test results can be transported extremely quickly. The alternative could be a major proliferation of POCT to satisfy the need for the rapid triage of patients and the commitment to patient-centered care.

QUALITY NEEDS

The issue of quality has risen on the healthcare agenda, and there are several reasons for this development. One is the greater focus on reducing medical errors, referred to in several chapters of this book. Another is the increased desire and needs of patients, as indicated previously. These higher expectations from healthcare delivery have led to a philosophy of greater patient choice (26). The advent of the Internet and access to

information has also changed the way in which many patients interact with their physicians (27).

The rise in patient expectations is also complemented by the rise of evidence-based practice and the production of clinical practice guidelines (28). This enables patients to see the level of evidence supporting a particular diagnostic tool or therapy and request its adoption in their case. One of the best examples of this is the growth of testing for prostate-specific antigen in screening for prostate cancer. The guidelines also have the effect of increasing compliance with best practice among healthcare providers, as well as increasing the confidence of patients in the care they are receiving. Quality can also be built into both regulatory and reimbursement programs, the format of which may depend on the country and the type of healthcare system. Thus, in the United States the Federal Drug

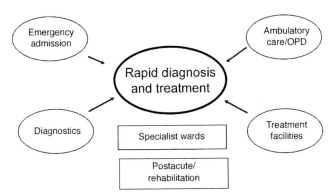

Figure 46-2 The conceptual design for a hospital that is patient centered and that seeks to make the stay in hospital as efficient as possible.

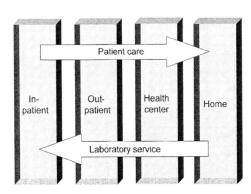

Figure 46-3 Illustrating the apparent paradoxical trends in clinical care and the delivery of laboratory services.

Administration requires evidence of efficacy before it will register a test or a device (29). Reimbursement is heavily dependent on this acknowledgement of efficacy through product registration. Agencies such as the Agency for Health Research and Quality provide reviews of evidence to inform healthcare provider organizations in the United States (30).

At a different level, the new contract for primary care physicians in the United Kingdom includes a section on reimbursement for undertaking certain tasks in relation to chronic disease management, e.g., regular HbA1c measurement in diabetics (31).

IMPLICATIONS FOR POINT-OF-CARE TESTING

All of the changes outlined above have the potential to affect the utilization of POCT. The commitment to improving the efficiency and effectiveness of all aspects of healthcare delivery is firmly based on more rapid and accurate decision making. The emphasis on efficiency of process means that a faster turnaround time will be required for many investigations. It is clear that the era when rapid testing was only required for medical emergencies has now passed. Speed of response is now a prerequisite for many facets of healthcare provision, including emergency care, improving the clinician-patient interaction, and helping the patient individually (Table 46-2).

Reference has already been made on several occasions in this book to the potential outcomes that can be gained from POCT. The easiest outcomes to identify are those associated with the reduction in the time to make a clinical management decision, and particularly reduction in the length of stay. This can then translate into a reduction in use of beds by a reduction in the number of admissions to a particular unit (e.g., coronary care unit) (12). Although this might appear to be a straightforward argument, the challenges in carrying through the observation to a change in resource allocation and possible change in bed availability should not be underestimated. There are other possible operational benefits that may also accrue from POCT that are not necessarily as challenging in terms of change of practice or resource utilization, e.g., decreasing delays in specimen transport, decreasing delays in obtaining results, and reducing the need for other diagnostics modalities.

The transition of care away from the centralized hospital facility is, of itself, a powerful driver for the use of POCT, since in many situations testing must accompany the devolved care process. This devolution of care will include both early diagnostic triage for new patients presenting to primary care and secondary care, as well as management of chronic disease. POCT in the latter is not so much concerned with the speed of the service but rather with having the result available at the time of the consultation. It has been suggested that this can be achieved by having the patient attend a phlebotomy clinic a few days before their consultation, but this may be inconvenient for the patient and also risks nonattendance. The extension of the convenience argument may also be used for the use of the community pharmacy as a venue for testing, the visit

Table 46-2   Reasons for Providing Results Quickly

The Justification for POCT

Clinical
  Faster stabilization of life-threatening crises
  Immediate risk stratification
  Fewer intraoperative complications
  Fewer postoperative complications
  Closer therapeutic management
  Greater patient compliance
Operational
  Optimized patient triage
  Optimized intensive care stay
  Reduced unnecessary length of stay
  Optimized clinical appointments
  Optimized usage of pharmaceuticals
  Optimized use of clinical specialist's time
  Reduced transport costs
  Fewer errors (e.g., lost samples)
Economic
  Reduced testing required
  Reduced drug utilization
  Reduced staff requirement
  Fewer clinical visits
  Faster hospital turnaround
  Fewer complications
  Fewer working days lost
  Improved life expectancy

being integrated into other routine aspects of life—at a time chosen by the patient rather than the healthcare provider.

ADVANCES IN POCT TECHNOLOGY

In the early days of POCT there were major concerns about the quality of the results from testing outside of the laboratory. This was in part due to the complexity of the testing process that was being conducted by operators with a limited background in using analytical equipment. The earlier chapters describe a whole raft of innovations that have been incorporated into newer types of POCT testing devices with the purpose of making the systems more robust and their operation less complex. Thus, devices are now more stable, both in terms of storage and also routine use, do not require special preparation, and are simpler to use. In some cases only a single step is required.

As well as becoming fit for use by nonlaboratory personnel, POCT devices are now being made smaller and less invasive for the patients. The advent of miniaturization and nanotechnology for diagnostics makes the idea of a mobile testing unit possible and thus makes any location suitable for testing. In certain instances nanotechnology is likely to result in the ability to implant the testing device, possibly linked to a feedback loop for therapy. Miniaturization will also enable a larger repertoire of tests to be encapsulated within the same device.

One of the observations that can be made from studies using POCT is that invariably a clinical decision is delayed because one of the diagnostic tests was only provided from the central laboratory (32). Thus, the full gain from POCT will only really be achieved when all of the required tests can be provided at the point of care. It is now possible to utilize all of the main analytical techniques within a POCT device, and the main challenge is now to identify those panels of tests that are required at the point of care in different clinical settings. An example is the "wish list" identified in Chapter 24 for the emergency department.

An important achievement since the first edition of this book has been the development of an interfacing standard for all POCT devices that will enable them to be easily linked directly to the laboratory or hospital information system so that results are entered into the patient record. There are likely to be other substantial organizational and management benefits to come from better connectivity that will address many of the quality concerns about POCT, such as lack of patient identification. Concurrent developments in information technology may soon make it feasible to transmit a patient result to the requesting clinician's PDA or mobile telephone so that he or she can take action immediately.

THE IMPORTANCE AND CHALLENGE OF DETERMINING OUTCOMES

There are several analogies from other walks of life that suggest that the arguments between the use of centralized laboratory testing and POCT may always be controversial. Examples would include the rise of the supermarket compared with the local grocery store, the use of mass transport systems versus the use of the private car, and even the development of large hospital complexes serving widely distributed areas of population. The underlying arguments will always revolve around the economy of scale using this approach, whether it is simply in the cost of care or the availability of a greater critical mass of expertise in a larger employment unit. The counterarguments are based on the wider benefits that can be seen from a more distributed style of care.

This was often the picture in the early days of POCT, with claims for the high cost of testing in addition to the poor quality of results. There were few papers that addressed the outcomes of POCT—other than the high cost of consumables. This preoccupation with cost meant that few of the early papers addressed the reasons for which POCT was being used (33, 34). The increasing focus on the cost and quality of care has changed that view. In an era of evidence-based practice, questions are now being asked concerning the benefit to the patient (34).

This is not a challenge for POCT alone but is something facing the whole of diagnostic medicine (28). There have been several reviews on the use of diagnostic tests that have shown that there is a very limited amount of literature available relating diagnostics to outcomes (28, 33–5). It is also obvious that this is not an easy subject to address in formal studies. The difficulties include identifying the clinical question through to the robust study design, and ensuring compliance with the study protocol so that the appropriate outcome measures are collected (28).

HEALTH ECONOMICS AND IMPLEMENTATION

It has been clearly shown in several of the chapters in this book that POCT can improve clinical outcomes for patients, with a concomitant reduction in the healthcare resources required for individual patient care. In many instances where economic analysis of a particular disease diagnostic and management protocol has been undertaken, the costs of the diagnostic tests do not appear, and in others the costs apportioned do not reflect the true cost. Certainly there is very little discussion of the value of the test. This is in part because no study has been undertaken that compares care with and without the contribution made by the diagnostic test. In fairness, this also reflects the way in which diagnostic testing is resourced in routine clinical practice, namely as an independent budget from the clinical team. Consequently, any change in testing that raises the potential resource requirement, albeit saving money in another part of the organization's budget, is likely to be problematic. There are numerous examples where an operational benefit has been demonstrated and where the potential reduction in the cost of care can be first modeled and then implemented, e.g., the transition to day-case surgery for parathyroidectomy (11, 36, 37).

It is only by implementing the whole change in the model of care that the full benefit of POCT is likely to be realized (38). However, this is also likely to prove the most challenging aspect of introducing POCT. Several authors have pointed out that it is only when there is wholesale process change that the real benefits will begin to be seen. This is a challenge beyond POCT and applies equally to the whole of laboratory medicine, namely the need to develop a more outcomes-oriented approach not just to demonstrating efficacy and effectiveness but also to reimbursement (39).

CONCLUSIONS

It is clear that the technology for POCT is now reaching the level of reliability and performance such that the testing devices can take their place alongside the other tools used by the healthcare professional in the care of patients. Furthermore, guidelines and managerial tools are now available with which to ensure that practice can be assured if followed properly, as is the case with any other facet of care. In addition, there are now a number of studies that illustrate the crucial role that POCT can play in patient care and identify the benefits that can accrue from its application. The style of care and the way in which it is delivered will be the main determinants of how extensively POCT is employed. This should be founded on evidence-based guidelines and the improved outcomes that are demonstrated. The key challenges to delivering this style of patient-focused care are devices that offer a complete panel of tests and devices with simple operating routines that match other devices used in day-to-day life. Furthermore, there must be a reimbursement strategy that takes a more holistic view of the patient care pathway and those elements that are crucial to achieving the best quality of care and outcomes.

REFERENCES

1. Committee on Leading Health Indicators for Healthy People 2010. Leading health indicators for healthy people 2010: second interim report. Washington, DC: Institute of Medicine, 1999.
2. Wanless D. Securing our future health: taking a long term view. 2002. http://www.hm-treasury.gov.uk/Consultations_and_Legislation/wanless/consult_wanless_final.cfm (accessed April 30, 2004).
3. Lewin SA, Skea ZC, Entwistle V, Zwarenstein M, Dick J. Interventions for providers to promote a patient-centered approach in clinical consultations. Cochrane Database Syst Rev 2001;(4): CD003267.
4. Yoong KKY, Heyman T. Targets can seriously damage your health. BMJ 2003;327:680.
5. Kemper HC, Stasse-Wolthuis M, Bosman W. The prevention and treatment of overweight and obesity: summary of the advisory report by the Health Council of the Netherlands. Neth J Med 2004;62:10–7.
6. Dixon A, Mossialos F, eds. Health care systems in eight countries: trends and challenges. London: European Observatory on Health Care Systems, 2002.
7. Rowan K, Harrison D, Brady A, Black N. Hospitals' star ratings and clinical outcomes: ecological study. BMJ 2004; 328:924–5.
8. Discher CL, Klein D, Pierce L, Levine AB, Levine TB. Heart failure disease management: impact on hospital care, length of stay, and reimbursement. Congest Heart Fail 2003;9:77–83.
9. Clarke A, Rosen R. Length of stay: how short should hospital care be? Eur J Public Health 2001;11:166–70.
10. Cannon CP, Hand MH, Bahr R, Boden WE, Christenson R, Gibler WB, et al. Critical pathways for management of patients with acute coronary syndromes: an assessment by the National Heart Attack Alert Program. Am Heart J 2002;143:777–89.
11. Chen H, Sokoll LJ, Udelsman R. Outpatient minimally invasive parathyroidectomy: A combination of sestamibi-SPECT localization, cervical block anesthesia, and intraoperative parathyroid hormone assay. Surgery 1999;126:1016–22.
12. Ng SM, Krishnaswamy P, Morissey R, Clopton P, Fitzgerald R, Maisel AS. Ninety-minute accelerated critical pathway for chest pain evaluation. Am J Cardiol 2001;88:611–7.
13. Griffin S. Diabetes care in general practice: meta-analysis of randomised control trials. BMJ 1998;317:390–6.
14. Fitzmaurice DA, Hobbs FD, Murray ET, Holder RL, Allan TF, Rose PE. Oral anticoagulation management in primary care with the use of computerized decision support and near-patient testing. Arch Intern Med 2000;160:2343–8.
15. Mason CM. Managing the spectrum of dyslipidemia in primary care. J Vasc Nurs 2003;21:81–9.
16. Showstack J, Anderson Rothman A, Hasmiller SB, eds. The future of primary care. San Francisco, CA: Jossey Bass, 2004.
17. Australian Government Department of Health and Ageing. Point of care testing trial general information and updates. http://www.health.gov.au/pathology/poctt/info.htm (accessed May 2, 2004).
18. NHS Direct Online. The NHS Direct self-help guide. Available at http://www.nhsdirect.nhs.uk/SelfHelp/index.asp (accessed April 30, 2004).
19. Turner VF, Bentley PJ, Hodgson SA, Collard PJ, Drimatis R, Rabune C, et al. Telephone triage in Western Australia. Med J Aust 2002;176:100–3.
20. Whitlock EP, Polen MR, Green CA, Orleans T, Klein J, U.S. Preventive Services Task Force. Behavioral counseling interventions in primary care to reduce risky/harmful alcohol use by adults: a summary of the evidence for the U.S. Preventive Services Task Force. Ann Intern Med 2004;140:557–68.
21. Anderson C, Blenkinsop A, Armstrong M. The contribution of community pharmacy to improving the public's health. London: Pharmacy HealthLink and the Royal Pharmaceutical Society of Great Britain, 2003.
22. Kricka LJ, Parsons D, Coolen RB. Healthcare in the United States and the practice of laboratory medicine. Clin Chim Acta 1997; 267:5–32.
23. Price CP, Barnes IC. Laboratory medicine in the United Kingdom: 1948–1998 and beyond. Clin Chim Acta 2000; 290: 5–36
24. Fagg KL, Gordon P, Reib B, McGann JT, Higa TE, Kinniburgh DW, et al. Laboratory restructuring in metropolitan Edmonton: a model for laboratory reorganization in Canada. Clin Chim Acta 1999;290:73–91.
25. DH Pathology Modernisation Team. Modernising pathology services. www.dh.gov.uk/assetRoot/04/07/31/12/04073112.pdf (accessed April 30, 2004).
26. The Employment and Social Affairs Directorate General of the European Commission. The future of health care and care for the elderly: guaranteeing accessibility, quality and financial viability. Information section, 200 Rue de la Loi, B-1049 Brussels, 2001.
27. Kiley R, Graham E. The patient's internet handbook. London: Royal Society of Medicine, 2002;1–302.
28. Price CP, Christenson RH, eds. Evidence-based laboratory medicine: from principles to outcomes. Washington: AACC Press, 2003;1–279.
29. US Food and Drug Administration Center for Devices and Radiological Health. Overview of regulations. Available at http://www.fda.gov/cdrh/devadvice/overview.html (accessed April 30, 2004).
30. Agency for Healthcare Research and Quality. Outcomes research fact sheet. What is outcomes research? Available at http://www.ahrq.gov/clinic/outfact.htm (accessed April 30, 2004).
31. British Medical Association. Quality and outcomes framework guidance. Investing in general practice. The new General Medical Services contract. Annex A: Quality indicators—summary of points. Available at http://www.bma.org/uk/ap.nsf/Content/NewGMScontract/$file/gpcont.pdf (accessed April 30, 2004).
32. Murray RP, Leroux M, Sabga E, Palatnick W, Ludwig L. Effect of point of care testing on length of stay in an adult emergency department. J Emerg Med 1999;17:811–4.

33. Hobbs FD, Delaney BC, Fitzmaurice DA, Wilson S, Hyde CJ, Thorpe GH, et al. A review of near patient testing in primary care. Health Technol Assess 1997;1:1–230.

34. Price CP. Point-of-care testing. BMJ 2001;322:1285–8.

35. Price CP. Point of care testing: potential for tracking disease management outcomes. Dis Manage Health Outcomes 2002;10:749–61.

36. Howell MR, Quinn TC, Brathwaite W, Gaydos CA. Screening women for *Chlamydia trachomatis* in family planning clinics: the cost-effectiveness of DNA amplification assays. Sex Transm Dis 1998;25:108–17.

37. Zarich S, Bradley K, Seymour J, Ghali W, Traboulsi A, Mayall ID, et al. Impact of troponin T determinations of hospital resource utilization and costs in the evaluation of patients with suspected myocardial ischemia. Am J Cardiol 2001;88:732–6.

38. Nichols JH, Kickler TS, Dyer KL, Humbertson SK, Cooper PC, Maughan WL, et al. Clinical outcomes of point-of-care testing in the interventional radiology and invasive cardiology setting. Clin Chem 2000;46:543–50.

39. Lundberg GD. The need for an outcomes research agenda for clinical laboratory testing. JAMA 1998;280:565–6.

Index